Food and Food Additive Intolerance in Childhood

TJ DAVID MB ChB PhD MD FRCP DCH
Professor of Child Health,
University of Manchester;
Honorary Consultant Paediatrician,
Booth Hall Children's Hospital,
Charlestown Road,
Blackley,
Manchester M9 2AA

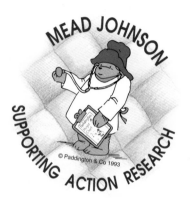

© Paddington & Co 1993

OXFORD

Blackwell Scientific Publications

LONDON EDINBURGH BOSTON

MELBOURNE PARIS BERLIN VIENNA

© 1993 by
Blackwell Scientific Publications
Editorial Offices:
Osney Mead, Oxford OX2 0EL
25 John Street, London WC1N 2BL
23 Ainslie Place, Edinburgh EH3 6AJ
238 Main Street, Cambridge
   Massachusetts 02142, USA
54 University Street, Carlton
   Victoria 3053, Australia

Other Editorial Offices:
Librairie Arnette SA
2, rue Casimir-Delavigne
75006 Paris
France

Blackwell Wissenschafts-Verlag
Meinekestrasse 4
D-1000 Berlin 15
Germany

Blackwell MZV
Feldgasse 13
A-1238 Wien
Austria

First published 1993

Set by Excel Typesetters Company
Hong Kong
Printed and bound in Great Britain
by The Bath Press, Bath and London

DISTRIBUTORS

Marston Book Services Ltd
PO Box 87
Oxford OX2 0DT
(*Orders*: Tel: 0865 791155
        Fax: 0865 791927
        Telex: 837515)

USA
Blackwell Scientific Publications, Inc.
238 Main Street
Cambridge, MA 02142
(*Orders*: Tel: 800 759-6102
        617 876-7000)

Canada
Times Mirror Professional Publishing, Ltd
130 Flaska Drive
Markham, Ontario L6G 1B8
(*Orders*: Tel: 800 268-4178
        416 470-6739)

Australia
Blackwell Scientific Publications Pty Ltd
54 University Street
Carlton, Victoria 3053
(*Orders*: Tel: 03 347-5552)

A catalogue record for this title
is available from the British Library

ISBN 0–632–03487–4

Contents

Preface

Aim of the book   This book attempts to delineate food and food additive intolerance, and establish its importance in the context of paediatric symptoms and disorders. The author has sifted through the mountain of published information about food intolerance, and picked out the few most reliable studies, where these existed. Information from these reports was, if necessary, supplemented by the author's experience, bearing in mind that experience has been defined as the ability to go on making the same mistakes with increasing confidence. It is hoped that the result is a practically orientated book, with sufficient factual information to enable the reader to make some sense of a generally confusing area, and also to allow the reader to make a personal assessment of the strength of evidence on any major issue.

Controversial subject   The subject of food intolerance is highly contentious, and one aim of this book is to replace *ex-cathedra* statements which abound by information about actual experimental data. Regrettably, sound data is all too often not available, and one may have to settle, at least for the time being, for anecdotal and therefore unreliable information. Worse still, there are problem areas where even anecdotal reports cannot be found, and another aim of this book has been to highlight some interesting areas of uncertainty.

Fact or opinion?   The reader needs to be able to distinguish between statements for which there is published evidence, and the author's personal recommendations or opinions. Where published evidence is available, it is cited. Anecdotal or uncontrolled studies are not referred to unless there is a lack of anything better. Where a statement or opinion is unreferenced, for example 'It is uncommon for coughing or wheezing to be the sole manifestation of cow's milk protein intolerance', or 'most children with egg intolerance can tolerate cooked chicken', then it must be taken as meaning in the personal experience or opinion of the author.

The context   The book is also an attempt to set food intolerance into its context. It seeks to examine the relative importance of food intolerance in specific disorders such as, eczema, migraine or the nephrotic syndrome. This results in an unexpectedly long section on urticaria, where unravelling the cause and putting food intolerance into perspective requires some description of the myriad of other causes and triggers. The chapter on salicylates is also disproportionately longer than would be justified purely by its relevance to food intolerance, again because a discussion of the importance (if any) of naturally occurring salicylates is difficult without an examination of intolerance to aspirin and other non-steroidal anti-inflammatory agents.

Practical approach

Some doctors have hoped that the current popular vogue for food intolerance, if ignored studiously enough, would go away. Others are inclined to see reactions to food around every corner. But all doctors dealing with children are confronted by parents who are concerned about possible food or additive intolerance. There is a real need for a book about the practical management of children with genuine or suspected adverse reactions to food, and it is hoped that this book will fill this gap.

Mechanisms usually not examined

Given the poor quality of published data, attempting to delineate the clinical features of food intolerance has been a more than adequate challenge, and an important first step. Reliable information about the underlying mechanisms is much harder to obtain. Our understanding of why some children are unable to tolerate certain foods, or of how they often grow out of this intolerance, is very poor. We do not know why peanuts and fish are more capable of inducing violent reactions than lamb or potato. The molecular acrobatics that make one antigen an allergen and another antigen a non-allergen are not known. Simplistic but unproven explanations abound. For example, all too often the presence of circulating IgE antibodies is assumed, without any proof, to indicate that an adverse reaction is IgE-mediated. Given the shaky nature of the clinical data on food intolerance, the regurgitation of speculation about mechanisms was not felt to be helpful in this practically orientated book, although a detailed review of this area would be most useful.

Paediatric orientation

Whenever possible, reference has been made to studies in childhood, in preference to observations in adults. Nevertheless, the book does quite often refer to adult studies, either because of their importance or because of a dearth of sound paediatric data.

How is this book constructed?

The layout is similar to that in Mygind's textbook *Essential Allergy*, which is a landmark of clarity of presentation. One difference in the present book is the addition of detailed referencing, an essential feature in view of the contentious nature of the subject. To facilitate reading, the book consists of short chapters (78 mini-chapters), each with a summary and a list of key references (if there are any). The remaining references are given at the end of each of the 18 sections. The names of authors are cited in the text, rather than using the Vancouver system of numerical referencing. This risks interrupting the flow of reading, but is intended to help those who already have some familiarity with the literature. Single authorship has enabled repetition to be minimized, but there are some topics where repetition was necessary to minimize inconvenience to the reader. Thus, for example, the relationship between various disorders and additive intolerance is discussed both in sections on specific disorders and sections on specific food additives.

Why intolerance and not allergy?

Strictly speaking, the term *allergy* applies only to adverse reactions caused by an immunological response. As the mechanism of many adverse reactions to food is poorly understood, and as proof of an immunological mechanism is often lacking, the term *food intolerance* is preferred here because it makes no assumptions about the mechanism.

Apology to North American readers

Apologies are offered to North American readers, who will be familiar with a different terminology, in which *food sensitivity* is the term which embraces all adverse reactions to foods, and which is subdivided into food hypersensitivity or allergy (immunologically mediated) and food intolerance (non-immunologically mediated).

Other terminology intolerance to or of?

In this book, the word intolerance is followed by the preposition *to*. A few reviewers of sections of the manuscript were uncomfortable with this and preferred *intolerant of*. To them and any like-minded readers I apologize. When consulted, the editors of the *Lancet* and the *British Medical Journal* did not express a strong preference for either usage. Sidney Greenbaum, Quain Professor of English Language and Literature at University College London, and co-editor of the third edition of *The Complete Plain Words*, ruled in favour of the preposition *to* in the context of this book, and commented that *of* is used when the word has the more general sense, as in, for example, intolerance of other people's opinions.

empirical

To those who use the word *empirical* in its medical sense to mean 'based on the results of observation and experiment only', I apologize. In this book, empirical is used in its more general sense to mean 'guided by experience'. Both definitions are cited by the *Shorter Oxford Dictionary*, as is a third, 'to practice medicine without scientific knowledge', or *quackery*, which I fear comes alarmingly close to my own usage of the word.

Omissions or errors

Please write to me at the address below if you feel that there are any important omissions or errors. Any comments or suggestions would be welcome, whether relating to simple omissions or substantive disagreements.

Grateful thanks All that one needs to write a book, according to Christie, is 'a measure of self-discipline, a few sheets of paper and a long-suffering wife'. However, this particular book would not have been written had it not been for the initial suggestion and continued encouragement of Vicky Reeders and John Harrison at Blackwell Scientific Publications, and for the real support and enthusiasm of my parents, wife and sons. I am also especially grateful to my father and my wife for their translation of numerous papers. I am indebted to numerous colleagues who have read and commented upon various sections, namely Dr Michael Addison, Dr Michael Beck, Miss Franscine Brown, Professor Robert Boyd, Dr Michael Clarke, Dr Jon Couriel, Mr Peter Davenport, Dr Jim Devlin, Professor Anne Ferguson, Dr Jonathan Green, Dr Mansel Haeney, Dr Lennox Holt, Dr Meriel Jenney, Dr Cameron Kennedy, Mr John Lendrum, Dr Jim Littlewood, Mr John Lockwood, Professor Maurice Longson, Dr David Mabin, Dr Michael Marsh, Dr Victor Miller, Dr David Pearson, Dr Barbara Phillips, Dr Helen Roper, Dr Claire Smith, Mr John Stanton, Mrs Adele Sykes, Professor John Walker-Smith, Dr Ian Ward, Dr Robert Warin, Mr John Wells, and Mr Andrew Zarod. One of the pleasures in writing has been to have their help. Particular thanks must go to Professor Robert Boyd for his help, support, encouragement and meticulous but kindly criticism, but especially for his incessant enquiries as to the evidence for a particular statement, and to Mrs Valerie Smith for her help in running a computerized database of some 10 000 references on food intolerance. Many of these references were obtained with the help of the libraries at Booth Hall Children's Hospital, the University of Manchester, the British Medical Association, and the Royal Society of Medicine. I gratefully thank them all, but especially Mrs Valerie Hicklin and Mrs Marcia Dooley, past and present librarians at the Post-Graduate Centre at Booth Hall Children's Hospital.

TJ David
University Department of Child Health
Booth Hall Children's Hospital
Blackley
Manchester M9 2AA, UK

Part 1 Definitions, Mechanisms, Prevalence and Unsolved Problems

1 Definitions
The term 'food allergy' is best avoided

Allergy
An allergic response is a reproducible adverse reaction to a substance mediated by an immunological response, irrespective of the precise mechanism. The substance provoking the reaction may have been ingested, injected, inhaled or merely have come into contact with the skin or mucous membranes.

Food allergy
Food allergy is a form of adverse reaction to food in which there is evidence that the reaction is caused by an immunological response to a food.

Misuse of 'allergy'
The word allergy is robbed of any useful meaning if it is applied indiscriminately to any adverse reaction, regardless of the mechanism. Since evidence of a specific immunological response is often not sought, the term allergy is best reserved for those relatively rare occasions where the immunological nature of the response is clear.

Food intolerance
Food intolerance is a reproducible adverse reaction to a specific food or food ingredient, and it is not psychologically based. Food intolerance occurs even when the subject cannot identify the type of food which has been given.

dosage
This definition does not take into account dosage. Large quantities of certain foods may result in disease in certain individuals, although such disorders are not always included in the category of food intolerance. Thus an increased consumption of purine-rich foods is one factor which contributes to hyperuricaemia and gout (Simmonds 1990), a disorder which is not usually regarded as a form of food intolerance. Certain fruits such as pears, and other foods such as honey, contain fructose, which is relatively poorly absorbed, and increased intake may result in loose stools (see chapter 31), a situation that might reasonably be regarded as a form of food intolerance. Clearly any food in vast excess will cause a reproducible adverse reaction (e.g. raised intracranial pressure due to vitamin A intoxication in two 3-month-old infants who were fed 120 g chicken liver daily for 4 months; see Mahoney *et al.* 1980). Such events are not generally covered by the term food intolerance.

Food sensitivity
In this book, the term food sensitivity is taken to mean exactly the same as food intolerance. However, in North America the terminology is different. There, food sensitivity is the term used to cover all

1

adverse reactions to food, which are then subdivided into food hypersensitivity (i.e. immunologically mediated) and food intolerance, which implies a non-immunologically mediated event (Sampson 1988).

Food aversion   Food aversion comprises food avoidance, where the subject avoids a food for psychological reasons such as distaste or a desire to lose weight, and psychological intolerance. The latter is an unpleasant bodily reaction caused by emotions associated with the food rather than the food itself. Psychological intolerance will normally be observable under open conditions, but will not occur when the food is given in an unrecognizable form. Psychological intolerance may be reproduced by suggesting (falsely) that the food has been administered.

necessary avoidance   It is helpful to distinguish between necessary food avoidance, for example the avoidance of cow's milk by someone with lactose intolerance, and unnecessary food avoidance as described above.

Anaphylaxis   In this book, and in the clinical situation, the term anaphylaxis or anaphylactic shock is taken to mean a severe reaction of rapid onset, with circulatory collapse. In the past the term anaphylaxis was used to describe any IgE-mediated allergic reaction, however mild, but such usage fails to distinguish between, for example, trivial urticaria, and a life-threatening event.

Antigen   An antigen is a substance which is capable of provoking an immune response. Antigens are usually proteins but are sometimes polysaccharides.

Antibody   An antibody is an immunoglobulin which is capable of combining specifically with certain antigens.

Allergen   An allergen is a substance which provokes a harmful (allergic) immune response.

Immunological tolerance   Immunological tolerance is a process which results in the immunological system becoming specifically unreactive to an antigen which is capable in other circumstances of provoking antibody production or cell-mediated immunity. The immunological system nevertheless reacts to unrelated antigens given simultaneously and via the same route.

Atopy   Atopy is generally taken to mean the ability to produce a weal and flare response to skin-prick testing with a common antigen such as house-dust mite or grass pollen.

Atopic disease The atopic diseases are asthma (but not all adult cases), atopic eczema, allergic rhinitis, allergic conjunctivitis and some cases of urticaria.

Double-blind challenge A double-blind challenge is an objective test performed to exclude a psychological explanation for a supposed allergy or intolerance. The test comprises exposing the subject to a challenge substance, which is either the item under investigation or an indistinguishable, inactive (placebo) substance. Neither the subject nor the observer knows the identity of the administered material at the time of the challenge or during the subsequent period of observation.

Open challenge Where the subject and the observer know the identity of the administered material at the time of the challenge, the procedure is said to be an open challenge.

Usage in this book The term food allergy is avoided throughout this book, because proof of an immunological basis for an adverse reaction to food is rare. An immunological basis is often assumed, on the basis of the presence of IgE antibodies, the speed of the reaction, or the nature of the reaction, e.g. urticaria or anaphylactic shock. However, none of these constitute proof of an immunological cause of the reaction. One aim of this book is to try and sift out the hard evidence from the mass of anecdotal information, and it is essential for this purpose to avoid unproven assumptions. The term food intolerance, which makes no immunological assumptions, is the preferred one in this book.

Key references 1.1 Royal College of Physicians *et al.* (1984) Food intolerance and food aversion. A Joint Report of the Royal College of Physicians and the British Nutrition Foundation. *J Roy Col Phys Lond* **18**:83–134. *A key report which attempts to define food intolerance, to assess its frequency, and to consider the biological and psychological mechanisms.*

1.2 PEARSON DJ (1987) Problems with terminology and with study design in food sensitivity. In Dobbing J (ed) *Food Intolerance: Current Research and Paediatric Practice*, pp. 1–23, Baillière Tindall, London. *A review of the problems associated with the latest British terminology (described in the reference above) and current North American terminology, which are unfortunately quite different. There seems to be no prospect for general international agreement about terminology. The chapter is particularly useful for its comments about the design and statistical analysis of double-blind studies of food intolerance.*

Summary 1 Food intolerance is a reproducible adverse reaction to a specific food and it is not psychologically based. Food intolerance occurs even when the subject cannot identify the type of food which has been given. The term allergy implies the presence of a definite immunological mechanism. Food aversion comprises food avoidance (for example, distaste for a food) and psychological intolerance, an unpleasant reaction caused by emotions associated with food rather than by food itself. Anaphylaxis is a rapid-onset, severe, life-threatening allergic reaction. A double-blind challenge is an objective test to verify a specific allergy or intolerance. Atopic diseases comprise asthma, atopic eczema, allergic rhinitis, allergic conjunctivitis, and urticaria.

2 Mechanisms of food intolerance
Uncertain in most cases

Poor understanding   As will become clear, it is often difficult to find proof that a specific food intolerance actually exists. It is hardly surprising that in this situation our understanding of the mechanisms is poor, and in many cases of food intolerance the precise mechanism is obscure. A book on the more practical and clinical aspects of food intolerance is not the place for a detailed examination of speculative immunological, pharmacological and other mechanisms. Where possible, the reader is referred in the text and in the key references to useful reviews.

Immunological tolerance   Humans of all ages are frequently exposed to antigens, whether by ingestion, inhalation or skin contact. Our ignorance of the cause of inappropriate immunological responses (allergy) is matched by a poor understanding of the mechanisms involved in the development of immunological tolerance to ingested antigens in man (for reviews see Strober *et al.* 1981; Strobel 1986; Strobel 1989). Unfortunately most textbooks of allergy studiously avoid the counterpart of allergy; tolerance.

Sensitization   Possible factors which contribute to immunological sensitization leading to food intolerance include:
1 genetic predisposition;
2 immaturity of the immune system or gastrointestinal mucosal barrier, either in term or pre-term infants (see Rieger & Rothberg 1975; Eastham *et al.* 1978; Udall *et al.* 1981; Roberton *et al.* 1982; Stern 1989; Lucas *et al.* 1990), but the reverse may be true – pre-term birth may protect against severe atopic disease (see David & Ewing 1988);
3 dosage of antigen, e.g. high dosage leading to development of

tolerance, and low dosage leading to sensitization (Firer *et al.* 1981; Lindfors & Enocksson 1988);

4 certain antigens especially likely to lead to sensitization (e.g. egg);

5 triggering event, e.g. viral infection (Barnetson *et al.* 1981);

6 alteration in gut permeability (Dupont *et al.* 1989), possibly permitting abnormal antigen access.

Principal mechanisms   The principal mechanisms resulting in food intolerance are:

1 food allergy;

2 enzyme defect;

3 pharmacological;

4 irritant;

5 effect of drug;

6 toxic.

food allergy   The mechanism is immunological (by definition), and examples of possible effectors of the immunological response are food-specific antibodies, the production of immune complexes, and mucosal T-cell mediated reactions. It is often unclear whether immunological abnormalities are the cause of the adverse reaction, the result of the reaction, or simply epiphenomena.

enzyme defects   Inborn errors of metabolism may affect the digestion and absorption of carbohydrate, fat or protein. In some the disorder is primarily gastrointestinal, causing defects in digestion or absorption (for example, lactase deficiency – see chapter 6 and Flatz 1989). In others the defect is systemic (for example, fructosaemia – see Gitzelmann *et al.* 1989).

pharmacological   In the context of food intolerance, the best known example of a pharmacological agent found in food is caffeine. Other examples are vasoactive amines such as tyramine, serotonin, tryptamine, phenylethylamine and histamine, found in many foods such as tuna, pickled herring, sardines, anchovy fillets, bananas, cheese, yeast extracts (such as Marmite), chocolate, wine, spinach, tomato and sausages – see Table 2.1 (Undenfriend *et al.* 1959; Taylor *et al.* 1978; Moneret-Vautrin 1983; Malone & Metcalfe 1986). Another example which has been studied recently is the inhibition of the enzyme 11β-hydroxysteroid dehydrogenase by liquorice, which can result in sodium and water retention, hypertension, hypokalaemia, and suppression of the renin-aldosterone system (Edwards 1991; Farese *et al.* 1991).

irritant   Certain foods have a direct irritant effect on the mucous membranes of the mouth or gut, such as the irritant effect of coffee or curry

Table 2.1 Histamine levels in sausages[1]

	Histamine level (mg/100 g)	
	Mean	Range
Cooked sausages[2]		
Bologna	0.55	0.19–0.84
Cooked salami	0.83	0.47–5.86
Kosher salami	0.50	0.33–0.97
Semi-dry sausages[2]		
Thuringer cervelat	2.35	1.03–3.63
Thuringer	1.19	0.31–2.56
Dry sausages[2]		
Italian dry salami	2.14–24.5[3]	0.42–36.4[3]
Pepperoni	1.03–38.1[3]	0.72–55.0[3]
Chorizo	2.29	0.60–8.08

[1] Source: Taylor *et al.* (1978).
[2] The sausages were obtained from retail markets in the San Francisco Bay area.
[3] Depending upon the brand tested.
Semi-dry sausages are fermented for varying periods. During this sausage ripening process the histamine concentration increases, depending upon the length of the ripening process. It is estimated that 70 mg to 1000 mg of histamine ingested in a single meal is necessary for the onset of toxicity, depending on individual sensitivity. Thus 130 g of the pepperoni sample that contained 55.0 mg histamine per 100 g would be necessary to cause symptoms in the most sensitive individuals.

(Bjarnason *et al.* 1988). In certain cases, food intolerance only occurs in the presence of a co-existing medical disorder. For example, the ingestion of coffee, orange juice or a spicy drink provokes oeso-phageal pain in some patients with reflux oesophagitis; the effect is unrelated to temperature, acidity or effect on the lower oesophageal sphincter (Price *et al.* 1978).

effect of drug   Examples of drug-induced food intolerance are potentiation of the pressor effects of tyramine-containing foods (e.g. cheese) by mono-amine oxidase inhibitors (Horwitz *et al.* 1964), and flushing and nausea which occur when patients receiving disulfiram ingest alcohol.

toxic   Many foods contain naturally occurring toxins, for example solani-dine in potatoes (Liener 1980), cyanide in tapioca (Hall 1987), myco-toxins in mushrooms and cereal grains (Ciegler 1975), protease inhibitors in soya (Friedman 1986), haemagglutinating lectins in in-adequately cooked red kidney beans (Noah *et al.* 1980) and photo-toxic furocoumarins in angelica, parsley, dill and celeriac (Knudson

Table 2.2 Examples of toxic constituents of plant foodstuffs and their role in plant physiology[1]

Toxic constituent	Type of food containing toxic constituent	Physiological role of toxic constituent	Role in plant defence: mechanism of toxic constituent
Protease inhibitors	Legumes, cereals, potatoes, pineapple	?Prevents degradation of storage protein during seed maturation	Part of defence against invading microbes following mechanical damage to leaves
Haemagglutinins	Legumes, cereals, potatoes	(a) Attach glycoprotein enzymes (b) Role in embryonic development/differentiation (c) Role in sugar transport or store (d) ?Involved in root nodule nitrogen-fixing bacteria symbiosis	(a) Counteract soil bacteria (b) Antifungal (c) Protect against seed predators
Glucosinolates	Radish, horseradish, turnip, cabbage, rape seed	?Disease & insect resistance role	
Cyanogens	Almonds, cassava, corn, peas, butter beans, bamboo shoots		
Saponins	Alfalfa, French beans, soya beans		

[1] Source: Leiner (1980).

& Kroon 1988), which in sufficient quantities can give rise to a wide variety of toxic reactions (Tables 2.2 & 2.3). Although there is clearly some overlap between toxic reactions and pharmacological reactions, toxic reactions are not generally included under the category of food intolerance.

Food storage   Chemical changes in food during storage can produce substances which cause food intolerance. An example is intolerance to ripe or stored tomatoes in subjects who can safely eat green tomatoes, where ripening of the fruit produces a new active glycoprotein (Bleumink *et al.* 1967). Some adverse reactions resulting from food storage come into the category of toxic reactions, such as the rise in levels of histamine and tyramine in certain foods during storage as a result of bacterial decarboxylation. An example of this is the production of histamine in badly stored mackerel and other fish, scombroid fish poisoning (Taylor 1986). Contamination of food by antigens such as storage mites or microbial spores may give rise to adverse effects, particularly asthma and eczema. Contamination of food by micro-organisms may result in adverse effects. For example, celery, parsnip and parsley may become infected with the fungus *Sclerotinia sclerotiorum* ('pink rot'), resulting in the production of

Table 2.3 Some examples of foodborne toxins or toxin-producing organisms, excluding plant foodstuffs

Pathogen or toxin	Principal symptoms	Common food source	Reference
Bacillus cereus	(a) Diarrhoea	Proteinaceous food vegetables, sauces, puddings	Lund (1990)
	(b) Vomiting	Fried rice	Lund (1990)
Bacillus subtilis	Vomiting, diarrhoea, flushing, sweating	Meat & pastry, meat/seafood with rice	Lund (1990)
Bacillus licheniformis	Diarrhoea	Cooked meat and vegetables	Lund (1990)
Clostridium botulinum	Neuroparalytic disease (botulism)	Meat, fish, vegetables hazelnut conserve	Lund (1990)
Clostridium perfringens	Diarrhoea, abdominal pain	Meat, poultry	Lund (1990)
Salmonella enteridis	Diarrhoea, abdominal pain, fever, vomiting	Poultry, eggs	Coyle *et al.* (1988) Baird-Parker (1990)
Staphylococcus aureus	Vomiting, abdominal pain, diarrhoea	Numerous, but especially cooked high-protein foods	Tranter (1990)
Verotoxin-producing *Escherichia coli*	Haemorrhagic colitis	Ground beef	Sekla *et al.* (1990)
Listeria monocytogenes	Listeriosis	Unpasteurised cheese, undercooked meat	Linnan *et al.* (1988) Schwartz *et al.* (1988)
Dioxins and dibenzofurans	Adverse effects uncertain when consumed in quantities found in food	Fish	Svensson *et al.* (1991)
Cantharidin	Sensitivity to urethra and genitalia; priapism	Frogs which have Meloidae (blister beetles)	Eisner *et al.* (1990)
Methyl mercury	Brain damage	Fish, bread	Clarkson (1990)
Toxic alkaloid (saxitoxin) in dinoflagellates and plankton	Diverse neurological disorders (paralytic shellfish poisoning)	Clams, oysters, scallops and mussels	Morgan & Fenwick (1990) Mills & Passmore (1988)
Brevetoxins	Paraesthesia, abdominal pain, diarrhoea, transient blindness, paralysis, death (neurotoxic shellfish poisoning)	Clams, oysters, scallops and mussels	Scoging (1991)
Ciguatera toxin	Diverse gastrointestinal and neurological disorders	Fish (especially reef predators)	Morgan & Fenwick (1990) Ruff (1989) Hashimoto *et al.* (1969)
Tetrodotoxin	Diverse gastrointestinal and neurological disorders	Puffer fish, certain newts	Scoging (1991) Mills & Passmore (1988)
Domoic acid	Vomiting, diarrhoea, hyperexcitation, seizures, memory loss (amnesic shellfish poisoning)	Mussels	Scoging (1991) Teitelbaum *et al.* (1990) Perl *et al.* (1990)

continued on p. 9

Table 2.3 *Continued*

Pathogen or toxin	Principal symptoms	Common food source	Reference
Okadaic acid, dinophysis toxins, yessotoxin, pectenotoxins	Diarrhoea, vomiting, abdominal pain (diarrhoetic shellfish poisoning)	Mussels, scallops	Scoging (1991)
Scombrotoxin (usually histamine)	Headache, palpitations, gastrointestinal disturbance	Mackerel, tuna and related species	Morrow *et al.* (1991) Morgan & Fenwick (1990) Taylor *et al.* (1989) Gilbert *et al.* (1980) Arnold & Brown (1978)
Tetramine (red whelk poisoning)	Diplopia, dizziness, leg pains	Whelks	Black *et al.* (1991) Reid *et al.* (1988)
Grayanotoxins (in honey from areas of Turkey where Rhododendrons are grown)	Hypotension, bradycardia, vomiting, sweating	Honey	Yavuz *et al.* (1991)
Unknown (? in algae) (turtle flesh poisoning)	Cardiorespiratory failure, death	Turtles	Chandrasiri *et al.* (1988)

the photosensitizing chemicals psoralen, 5-methoxypsoralen and 8-methoxypsoralen (Ashwood-Smith *et al.* 1985).

What makes a food antigenic?

Where an adverse reaction to a food has an immunological basis, the question arises as to what makes a food antigen antigenic? The little information we have about the importance of molecular size and three-dimensional structure of proteins in relation to antigens in cow's milk, fish, egg, legumes, cereals and tomatoes are reviewed elsewhere (Bleumink 1970; Stanworth 1973; King 1980; Metcalfe 1985; Taylor *et al.* 1987a, b; Aas 1989).

Heat treatment

Heat treatment clearly affects certain (but not all) foods, rendering them less likely to provoke adverse reactions in a subject who is intolerant. Occasionally the reverse occurs, as in the celebrated case of Professor Heinz Küstner, who was allergic to cooked and not raw fish (Prausnitz & Kustner 1921). The effect of heat is discussed elsewhere in this book; in relation to cow's milk protein in chapter 16, egg in chapters 22 and 23 and soya in chapter 20. Heat appears to render a large number of fruits and vegetables less likely to provoke adverse reactions in subjects who are intolerant. For example, it is a personal observation that most children with intolerance to fresh pineapple can tolerate tinned pineapples. It has been suggested that heating inactivates or destroys the potent allergens in sesame seeds (Kägi & Wüthrich 1991). In some situations it appears that heat can accelerate a process of denaturation which can in time occur on its own. Tuft and Blumstein (1942) reported patients who reacted to fresh melon, pear, peach, pineapple, grape and banana. In each case, stewed or tinned fruit caused no reaction. Studies of fresh extracts of these fruits showed that, when stored in a refrigerator, the extracts lost their ability to provoke a positive skin test after approximately 3 days.

Key references 2.1 CHALLACOMBE SJ & TOMASI TB (1987) Oral tolerance. In Brostoff J & Challacombe SJ (eds) *Food Allergy and Intolerance*, pp. 255–268, Baillière Tindall, London. *Review of current knowledge, based mainly on animal studies rather than human data.*

2.2 HOLT PG & MCMENAMIN C (1989) Defence against allergic sensitization in the healthy lung: the role of inhalation tolerance. *Clin Exper Allergy* **19**:255–262. This is a review of experimental studies in animals. These studies indicate that initial encounters with non-pathogenic antigens such as pollens do not trigger immune responses, but instead activate antigen-specific suppressor T cells which protect against subsequent sensitization by inducing a state of immunological tolerance to the inhaled antigen. *The authors suggest that inhalation and oral tolerance mechanisms are relatively slow to develop postnatally in man, providing a possible basis for sensitization in infancy.*

2.3 METCALFE DD, SAMPSON HA & SIMON RA (eds) (1991) *Food Allergy: Adverse Reactions to Foods and Food Additives*, Blackwell, Boston. *Multi-author book, with sections of relevance to this chapter which review the roles of mucosal immunity, mast cells, basophils, IgE, antigen absorption and the pharmacological properties of foods.*

2.4 AAS K (1989) Biochemical characteristics of food allergens. In Harms HK & Wahn U (eds) *Food Allergy in Infancy and Childhood*, pp. 1–12, Springer, Berlin. *Review of current knowledge about what makes a food allergenic.*

2.5 TAYLOR SL (1986) Histamine food poisoning: toxicology and clinical aspects. *CRC Crit Rev Toxicol* **17**:91–128. *Detailed review of chemical intoxication resulting from the ingestion of food that contains unusually high levels of histamine. The term scombroid fish poisoning is eschewed, since nonscombroid fish and cheese have also been implicated.*

2.6 GILBERT RJ, HOBBS G, MURRAY CK, CRUICKSHANK JG & YOUNG SEJ (1980) Scombrotoxic fish poisoning: features of the first 50 incidents to be reported in Britain (1976–9). *Br Med J* **281**:71–72. Scombrotoxic poisoning results from eating fish of the families Scomberesocidae and Scombridae which include tuna, bonito and mackerel, the flesh of which has become toxic as a result of incorrect storage. Details are given of 196 cases. The fish consumed was smoked mackerel in 90% of cases. The major symptoms were diarrhoea, hot flushing, sweating, bright-red rash, nausea, headache and abdominal pain. Freshly caught fish, or fish stored at 0°C, contains low concentrations of histamine (up to 3–4 mg/100 g). However, at room temperature high concentrations of histamine are rapidly reached and the fish becomes toxic, even though the flavour may still be acceptable to the consumer.

2.7   RICE SL, EITENMILLER RR & KOEHLER PE (1976) Biologically active amines in food: a review *J Milk Food Technol* **39**:353–358. The authors describe the mechanisms of formation and catabolism of biologically active amines normally present in food, tyramine, histamine, and phenethylamine. These amines do not represent any hazard to individuals unless large quantities are ingested or natural mechanisms for their catabolism are inhibited or genetically deficient.

2.8   PRICE SF, SMITHSON KW & CASTELL DO (1978) Food sensitivity in reflux esophagitis. *Gastroenterol* **75**:240–243. Sixty-six adults with possible oesophageal pain were studied. Those in whom acid infusion provoked symptoms were significantly more likely also to be sensitive to infusions of coffee, orange juice or a spicy drink (Tabasco Bloody Mary mix), even when these solutions were adjusted to a pH of 7. The mechanism of pain associated with ingestion of these foods is unrelated to temperature, acidity, or effect on the lower oesophageal sphincter.

2.9   LEINER IE (ed) (1980) *Toxic Constituents of Plant Foodstuffs*, 2nd edn, Academic Press, New York. *A major review of naturally occurring toxic substances present in plant materials.*

2.10   SOCKETT PN (1991) Food poisoning outbreaks associated with manufactured foods in England and Wales: 1980–1989. *Communicable Disease Report* **1**:105–109. In the 10-year period, 294 reported outbreaks of food poisoning were associated with eating precooked sliced meats, meat products and other manufactured foods in England and Wales. *Salmonella* was the most commonly reported agent, causing 45% of outbreaks. The number of outbreaks associated with manufactured foods accounted for less than 5% of food poisoning outbreaks. *Useful review of food sources of food poisoning.*

2.11   SCOGING AC (1991) Illness associated with seafood. *Communicable Disease Report* **1**:117–122. *Most useful review of infectious diseases and toxic syndromes as a result of eating seafood.*

2.12   NOAH ND, BENDER AE, REAIDI BG & GILBERT RJ (1980) Food poisoning from raw red kidney beans. *Br Med J* **281**:236–237. *Report of investigation into seven outbreaks of food poisoning due to consumption of raw or inadequately cooked red kidney beans. The clinical features were nausea and vomiting followed by diarrhoea, with onset 1 to 3 hours after ingestion.*

Summary 2   In many cases of food intolerance the precise mechanism is obscure. The principal mechanisms which cause food intolerance are food allergy (i.e. immunologically mediated reactions), enzyme defects, pharmacological effects, irritant effects, the effect of drugs, and toxic effects. Heat treatment makes a number of foods less likely to provoke an adverse reaction in a subject who is intolerant.

3 History, prevalence and natural history
Need for scepticism, prevalence uncertain, prognosis usually good

History The concept that certain foods can produce adverse reactions in susceptible individuals has a long history. Hippocrates (460–370 BC) reported that cow's milk could cause gastric upset and urticaria. Later, Galen (131–210 BC) described a case of intolerance to goat's milk (Bahna & Heiner 1980). It was Lucretius (96–55 BC) who said 'What is food to one man may be fierce poison to others'.

early reports Early reports of food intolerance in the medical literature were anecdotal, but even at the beginning of this century there were some noteworthy attempts to study individual cases (Schloss 1912).

Controversy In the 1920s and 1930s a fashion developed of blaming food intolerance for a large number of hitherto unexplained disorders. The uncritical and overenthusiastic nature of the claims, plus the anecdotal evidence upon which they were based, generally discredited the whole subject. Indeed, the field of food intolerance at that time has been described as 'a model of obstruction to the advancement of learning' (May 1982). Since then the whole area has provoked much controversy. The introduction of double-blind provocation tests has placed studies on a more scientific footing, but they are impractical in routine management. The lack of objective and reproducible diagnostic laboratory tests which could eliminate bias has ensured that controversy about food intolerance continues.

Need for scepticism It is common for parents to believe that foods are responsible for a variety of childhood symptoms. It is a paediatric maxim that parents are usually right, but on the subject of food intolerance this is not always so. Parents beliefs can often be shown to be wrong, and parents find it difficult to be objective about their childrens' symptoms. Double-blind provocation tests in children with histories of reactions to food confirm this story in only one-third of all cases (May & Bock 1978). In the case of purely behavioural symptoms the proportion that could be reproduced under blind conditions was zero (David 1987). The same is true of adults' beliefs about their own symptoms (Bentley *et al.* 1983; Young *et al.* 1987). If unnecessary dietary restrictions are to be avoided, the doctor has to be sceptical, and may need to seek objective confirmation of food intolerance.

12

Prevalence   The most common foods leading to reports of intolerance in childhood are cow's milk, eggs, nuts and fruit. However, the true prevalence of food intolerance is unknown, and it is a subject which has attracted little systematic study.

difficult to study   The major difficulties in establishing the prevalence of food intolerance are the individual variation in tolerance of feelings and symptoms, the unreliability of unconfirmed parental observations, and the lack of definition of what constitutes a reaction to food. All eating causes reactions, for example satiety, the urge to defaecate, a feeling of warmth and weight gain. In the context of this book we are dealing with unwanted reactions, but families vary in their tolerance of events. For some, flatus is unacceptable, but to others it is the normal effect of eating baked beans.

general observations   The prevalence is said to be higher in infants than in adults, and it appears to be higher in atopic children than in non-atopic children.

specific studies   The parents of 866 children from Finland were asked to provide a detailed history of food intolerance, and for certain foods the diagnosis was further investigated by elimination and open challenge at home. Food intolerance was reported in 19% by the age of 1 year, 22% by 2 years, 27% by 3 years, and 8% by 6 years (Kajosaari 1982). In a prospective study of 480 children in the USA up to their third birthday, 16% were reported to have had reactions to fruit or fruit juice and 28% to other food (Bock 1987). However open challenge confirmed reactions in only 12% of the former and 8% of the latter.

cow's milk protein intolerance   Estimates of the prevalence of cow's milk protein intolerance are reported to range from 0.3% to 7.5% of subjects (Bahna & Heiner 1980), but if all reactions, however trivial, are included, the prevalence may be higher. However, the majority of these reactions are never proved to be due to food intolerance. They are frequently presumed to have such a basis by both parents and doctors because no other reason is found, and the symptoms improve when cow's milk is removed from the diet.

Natural history   The natural history of food intolerance has been little studied. It is well known that a high proportion of children with food intolerance in the first year of life lose their intolerance in time. The proportion of children to which this happens varies with the food and probably with type of symptoms which are produced. Thus it is common for intolerance to cow's milk or egg to spontaneously disappear with time, whereas nut or fish intolerance is more likely to persist, peanut intolerance usually being life-long (Bock & Atkins 1989).

intolerance is temporary in most cases

The best data on the natural history of food intolerance come from the North American study referred to above (Bock 1987). The most striking finding was the brief duration during which reactions could be reproduced. It was found that the offending food or fruit was back in the diet after only 9 months in half the cases, and virtually all the offending foods were back in the diet by the third birthday. A further study of nine children with very severe adverse reactions to food showed that despite the severity, three were later able to tolerate normal amounts of the offending food and a further four became able to tolerate small amounts (Bock 1985). Whilst it is clear that the majority of children with food intolerance spontaneously improve, it remains to be established to what extent this depends on the age of onset, the nature of the symptoms, the food itself and other factors.

Key references 3.1   SCHLOSS OM (1912) A case of allergy to common foods. *Am J Dis Child* **3**:341– 362. *This describes severe urticarial reactions to egg, almonds and oatmeal in a boy. The report is remarkable for the enormous efforts which were made to identify the mechanisms involved.*

3.2   MAY CD & BOCK SA (1978) A modern clinical approach to food hypersensitivity. *Allergy* **33**:166–188. A detailed review of the mechanisms, manifestations, diagnosis and treatment of food intolerance, written by the two people who have done most to provide objective evidence of food intolerance and a rational basis for management. In the paper, the authors include data on double-blind food challenges in 81 children reported by their parents to have adverse reactions to food. In only 27 (33%) could symptoms be provoked by double-blind challenge. *Not only were the parents histories shown to be unreliable, but the physicians' opinions were no more accurate than the parents.*

3.3   DAVID TJ (1987) Reactions to dietary tartrazine. *Arch Dis Child* **62**:119–122. Double-blind challenges with tartrazine and benzoic acid were performed in 24 children whose parents gave a definite history of a purely behavioural immediate adverse reaction to one of these substances. In no patient was any change in behaviour noted either by the parents or the nursing staff after the administration of active substances or placebo (the placebo response was conditioned out by repeated administration of vehicle). Twenty-two patients returned to a normal diet without problems, but the parents of two children insisted on continuing to restrict the diet. *Objective verification is required to prevent overdiagnosis of harmful behavioural effects of food additives.*

3.4   KAJOSAARI M (1982) Food allergy in Finnish children aged 1 to 6 years. *Acta Paediat Scand* **71**:815–819. *The prevalence of food intolerance in 866 Finnish children was reported to be 19% at 1 year, 27% at 3 years, and 8% at 6 years. Open food challenges were only done for three foods, but they demonstrated a marked discrepancy between the parents' reports and actual symptoms provoked by challenge.*

Summary 3   Food intolerance has been known from ancient times. Over-enthusiastic and uncritical claims, accompanied by a serious lack of reproducible diagnostic tests, soon discredited the whole subject. The introduction of double-blind provocation tests has placed the subject on a more scientific footing. Double-blind provocation studies also demonstrate that parents' beliefs about food intolerance in their child are only correct in about one-third of all cases, and far less in the case of suspected food additive intolerance. If unnecessary dietary restriction is to be avoided, the doctor has to be sceptical and may need to seek objective confirmation of food intolerance. Food intolerance affects up to 10% of children by the age of 12 months, but in over a half the intolerance lasts less than 9 months, and most can tolerate the offending food by the age of 3 years. The prevalence in older children is far less, although precise figures are unavailable.

4   Interesting areas of uncertainty
Important gaps in our knowledge about food intolerance

Personal selection

This chapter outlines a few interesting areas of uncertainty. The selection is a personal one, and is not intended to be comprehensive. There are many other unanswered questions, as will be evident throughout this book.

Natural history

There is very poor data on the natural history of food intolerance. We know that a large proportion of children grow out of their food intolerance, but that life long intolerance can occur, particularly in the case of peanut intolerance. Are the chances of growing out of food intolerance related to:

1 the nature of the symptoms, for example, is one more or less likely to grow out of food intolerance if the main symptoms are gastrointestinal, respiratory, etc;

2 does the age of onset affect the chances of growing out of food intolerance;

3 to what extent does the nature of the food antigen affect the chances of growing out of food intolerance, for example, why do children usually grow out of egg but not peanut intolerance;

4 does repeated exposure to small quantities of the food increase, decrease, or have no effect upon the chances of growing out of food intolerance?

Tolerance resulting from repeated exposure

The regular administration of salicylates to patients with salicylate intolerance quickly leads to a state of tolerance to salicylate (see chapter 38). The mechanism is thought to be pharmacological rather than immunological. Could a similar phenomenon apply to some children with food intolerance? The answer is not known, but is germane to the issue of whether foods or food additives need to be avoided before challenge tests are performed. The observation that adverse reactions are occasionally greatly enhanced after a period of strict avoidance (David 1989) suggests that frequent administration of a trigger food may at least affect the response if not actually lead to tolerance. A possible mechanism could be that repeated release of inflammatory mediators could prevent their accumulation. Strict avoidance would then allow such accumulation, which would in turn result in a much more severe reaction upon re-exposure.

Cross-reactions

The degree of cross-reactions between different foods, whether of the same family or not, is very poorly documented. Double-blind challenge studies have demonstrated that cross-reactivity is less common than previously believed (see chapter 71), but this information is of little use. A child is found to have severe reactions to peanut: should he or she avoid other nuts? At present we are poorly equipped to give a scientifically based answer to the question. Erring on the side of safety is likely to entail needless avoidance of foods which can be eaten safely, whilst a more robust approach may risk a serious and possibly life-threatening reaction.

Dose of food and speed of adverse reaction

The precise relationship between the quantity of milk (or any other food for that matter) taken and the speed of onset of symptoms in those with intolerance is poorly documented. Further information on this subject might help one to understand the different mechanisms which operate in food intolerance. For example, it is highly likely that the process requiring only micrograms of food to produce a response differs from that which requires large quantities. The topic is of interest in relation to the growing out of food intolerance, for it appears that some patients at least do so by developing increasing tolerance. Indeed some patients have apparently been successfully treated by oral hyposensitization – for example, the administration of gradually increasing volumes of cow's milk (Brodribb 1944; Bahna & Heiner 1980), although this approach has never been objectively investigated.

Additive effect of multiple foods – does it exist?

The line taken in this book is that, at any particular time, a child either is, or is not, intolerant to an individual food. It is acknowledged that for a reaction to occur to that food, other conditions might have to be met. For example, a reaction might only occur if food ingestion occurs just before vigorous exercise – see food-dependent exercise-provoked anaphylaxis, discussed in chapter 58. Another less well-documented example would be the failure to react to a known food trigger if the associated disease (e.g. urticaria or atopic eczema) is inactive. If one accepts the received wisdom of an all-or-none effect, then cases which are inconsistent with this tend to be discounted, e.g. as being due to a mistaken parental belief. For example, how should one evaluate a parental report that ingestion of cow's milk provokes eczema on some occasions but not others? Can one assume that the parents' belief of cow's milk protein intolerance is incorrect? Is it possible, for example, for intolerance to a food to be confined to occasions when the pollen count is high or when the child consumes certain other foods? At present there are no objective studies which address the complex issue of the possible additive effect of orally ingested and possibly inhaled antigens. As far as examples of severe immediate reactions to single foods, it is difficult to interpret personal experience. The author has seen children with marked intolerance to single foods in whom the severity of adverse reactions clearly varies from time to time. The reasons for this variability are not known. Does it depend on the presence of other trigger foods? In this context, the documentation of the additive effect of antigens in patch testing (see chapter 42) is important. Similar studies are needed in the context of food and food additive intolerance.

The relationship between reactions in the skin and intolerance to ingested food

It is clear that not all patients who exhibit positive skin-prick tests to a food are intolerant to the same food when it is ingested. This phenomenon and the practical problem of false positive skin-prick test results are discussed particularly in chapter 41. The reasons for the different behaviour of the skin and the gastrointestinal tract when they are exposed to the same food are poorly understood. The same uncertainty applies to allergic contact urticaria. The fact that a food causes allergic contact urticaria does not necessarily imply that it cannot be eaten safely by the same patient (see chapter 59).

Is oil safe?

It is unclear whether or not oil can be given safely to subjects who are intolerant to the food item from which the oil was derived, such as soya or peanut.

statistical problems

It is difficult to prove a negative. Studies in which small numbers of subjects (see below) intolerant to a food protein are challenged with the oil derived from the same food without developing adverse effects are not very reassuring in practice. This particularly applies when the price of inappropriate reassurance is a potentially fatal reaction. The statistical problems in assessing safety are addressed in Table 30.1, but in short, to be 99.9% sure that peanut oil is safe in 99.9% of those with peanut intolerance, one would need to test 6905 individuals with peanut intolerance.

soya oil   Very limited data (only seven patients were studied) on soya oil originally suggested that a number of people who are intolerant to soya can tolerate soya oil (Bush *et al.* 1985 and see chapter 21). However, several studies have identified small quantities of soya protein in soya oil (Tattrie & Yaguchi 1973; Porras *et al.* 1985). This implies that soya oil must be avoided in those with soya intolerance, especially those who are sensitive to very small quantities of protein.

peanut oil   Peanut oil does not usually contain detectable protein (Tattrie & Yaguchi 1973), and is therefore said to be a highly unlikely source of danger to subjects with peanut intolerance (Taylor *et al.* 1981). A study of 10 adults with peanut intolerance failed to demonstrate any adverse reactions to ingestion of peanut oil (Taylor *et al.* 1981). However, there is one report of a local painful and erythematous reaction, accompanied by urticaria, following injection of adrenaline in peanut oil in an adult with asthma and peanut intolerance (Chafee 1941). Furthermore, there is a recent report of two infants who developed generalized skin rashes 15 min after ingestion of 1 ml of peanut oil (Moneret-Vautrin *et al.* 1991). On data currently available, it is evident that peanut oil cannot be safely given to those with peanut intolerance. Moneret-Vautrin *et al.* (1991) reported that the vegetable lipids of 11 out of 45 infant milk formulae included peanut oil, but whether this oil is responsible for sensitization to peanut or intolerance to milk formulae is unknown.

corn oil   There is one report of a subject with intolerance to corn who was able to tolerate corn oil (Loveless 1950), but there has been no systematic study of corn oil in subjects intolerant to corn.

cottonseed oil   A study of two adults with intolerance to cottonseed indicated that cottonseed oil could be tolerated (Bernton *et al.* 1949).

sesame oil   There are no data on the effects of sesame oil in subjects who are intolerant to sesame, but sesame oil has been shown to contain sesamolin, sesamin and sesamol, all of which may act as contact allergens causing contact dermatitis (Hayakawa *et al.* 1987).

cashew nuts   For the sake of completeness, one should mention a very different situation found with cashew nuts, where the oil from the shell of the nut is more likely to cause an adverse reaction than the nut itself. Cashew nuts are covered by a double-layered shell, and between these two layers is an oil which causes dermatitis after skin contact or ingestion, whereas the nut itself does not unless it becomes contaminated with the oil during processing (Marks *et al.* 1984).

Food consumed by cows

It is recognized that small amounts of foods consumed by a nursing mother may pass into her breast milk, leading to an adverse reaction if the infant is intolerant to the food. The question arises as to whether the diet of cows may have any influence on adverse reactions in human infants who receive cows' milk (see The diet of cattle, chapter 7).

Are small doses of gluten safe?

So-called 'gluten-free' bread may, surprisingly, contain small quantities of gluten (see chapter 26). It has been assumed by most workers that such small quantities of gliadin are safe, but a threshold dose has not been established. There is no evidence to confirm or refute the possibility that small quantities of gluten may be harmful if given long term.

Are oats safe in coeliac disease?

In the short term, oats have been given to small numbers of adults with coeliac disease without harm, but the long term safety of oats in coeliac disease is unknown. Finding the crucial amino acid sequence or sequences in the storage proteins of cereals might help to clarify this issue.

Long-term effect of diets in atopic eczema

Do elimination diets have any effect on the long-term outcome in atopic eczema, or is any benefit solely a short-term one? Is a child more likely (or less likely) to grow out of eczema if treated with a diet? There is no good data to address this question. The answer could be an important determinant in helping to decide whether or not to employ a diet.

Dose of fructose for breath hydrogen testing

Fructose malabsorption (see chapter 31) can be confirmed by a sharp rise in the breath hydrogen excretion after an oral fructose load. However, we lack age or weight related population-derived data for the ability to absorb different quantities of fructose, an ability which is in turn known to be affected by the quantity of glucose taken at the same time (glucose facilitates fructose absorption). Thus the test is at present poorly standardized.

Summary 4

Interesting areas of uncertainty include the natural history of food intolerance; the question of whether repeated exposure to a food trigger can lead to the development of tolerance; the degree to which cross-reactions occur to different foods, the relationship between the dose of food required to provoke a reaction and the speed of that reaction; the additive effect of food and other food or non-food triggers; the relationship between reactions in the skin and clinical intolerance to a food; the question of whether oil can be given safely to those who are intolerant to the food from which the oil was derived; the question of whether the diet of cows has any effect on the antigenicity of cows' milk; the question of whether oats or small doses of gluten are safe in coeliac disease; the question of whether dietary treatment has any effect on the natural history of atopic eczema; and the uncertainty about the correct dose of fructose to be used when testing for food intolerance.

References to Chapters 1–4

AAAS K (1989) Biochemical characteristics of food allergens. In Harms HK & Wahn U (eds) *Food Allergy in Infancy and Childhood*, pp. 1–12, Springer, Berlin.

ARNOLD SH & BROWN WD (1978) Histamine (?) toxicity from fish products. *Adv Food Res* **24**:113–154.

ASHWOOD-SMITH MJ, CESKA O & CHAUDHARY SK (1985) Mechanism of photosensitivity reactions to diseased celery. *Br Med J* **290**:1249.

BAHNA SL & HEINER DC (1980) *Allergies to Milk*, Grune & Stratton, New York.

BAIRD-PARKER AC (1990) Foodborne salmonellosis. *Lancet* **2**:1231–1235.

BARNETSON RStC, HARDIE RA & MERRETT TG (1988) Late-onset atopic eczema and multiple food allergies after infectious mononucleosis. *Br Med J* **283**:1086.

BENTLEY SJ, PEARSON DJ & RIX KJB (1983) Food hypersensitivity in irritable bowel syndrome. *Lancet* **2**:295–297.

BERNTON HS, COULSON EJ & STEVENS H (1949) On allergy to cottonseed oil. *J Am Med Ass* **140**:869–871.

BJARNASON I, LEVI S, SMETHURST P, MENZIES IS & LEVI AJ (1988) Vindaloo and you. *Br Med J* **297**:1929–1631.

BLACK NMI, O'BRIEN SJ & BLAIN P (1991) Red spells danger for whelk eaters. *Communicable Disease Report* **1**:125.

BLEUMINK E (1970) Food allergy. The chemical nature of the substances eliciting symptoms. *World Rev Nutr Diet* **12**:505–570.

BLEUMINK E, BERRENS L & YOUNG E (1967) Studies on the atopic allergen in ripe tomato fruits. II. Further chemical characterization of the purified allergen. *Int Arch Allergy* **31**:25–37.

BOCK SA (1985) Natural history of severe reactions to foods in young children. *J Pediat* **107**:676–680.

BOCK SA (1987) Prospective appraisal of complaints of adverse reactions to foods in children during the first 3 years of life. *Pediatrics* **79**:683–688.

BOCK SA & ATKINS FM (1989) The natural history of peanut allergy. *J Allergy Clin Immunol* **83**:900–904.

BRODRIBB HS (1944) Allergic vomiting in an infant. *Arch Dis Child* **19**:140–142.

BUSH RK, TAYLOR SL, NORDLEE JA & BUSSE WW (1985) Soybean oil is not allergenic to soybean-sensitive individuals. *J Allergy Clin Immunol* **76**:242–245.

CHAFEE FH (1941) Sensitivity to peanut oil with the report of a case. *Ann Intern Med* **15**:1116–1117.

CHANDRASIRI N, ARIYANANDA PL & FERNANDO SSD (1988) Autopsy findings in turtle flesh poisoning. *Med Sci Law* **28**:142–144.

CIEGLER A (1975) Mycotoxins: occurrence, chemistry, biological activity. *Lloydia* **38**:21–35.

CLARKSON TW (1990) Mercury – an element of mystery. *New Engl J Med* **323**: 1137–1139.

COYLE EF, PALMER SR, RIBEIRO CD *et al.* (1988) *Salmonella enteritidis* phage type 4 infection: association with hens' eggs. *Lancet* **2**:1295–1297.

DAVID TJ (1987) Reactions to dietary tartrazine. *Arch Dis Child* **62**:119–122.

DAVID TJ (1989) Hazards of challenge tests in atopic dermatitis. *Allergy* **9** (suppl.):101–107.

DAVID TJ & EWING CI (1988) Atopic eczema and preterm birth. *Arch Dis Child* **63**:435–436.

DUPONT C, BARAU E, MOLKHOU P, RAYNAUD F, BARBET JP & DEHENNIN L (1989) Food-induced alterations of intestinal permeability in children with cow's milk-sensitive enteropathy and atopic dermatitis. *J Pediat Gastroenterol Nutr* **8**:459–465.

EASTHAM EJ, LICHAUCO T, GRADY MI & WALKER WA (1978) Antigenicity of infant formulas: role of immature intestine on protein permeability. *J Pediat* **93**:561–564.

EDWARDS CRW (1991) Lessons from licorice. *New Engl J Med* **325**:1242–1243.

EISNER T, CONNER J, CARREL JE *et al.* (1990) Systemic retention of ingested cantharidin by frogs. *Chemoecology* **1**:57–62.

FARESE RV, BIGLIERI EG, SHACKLETON CHL, IRONY I & GOMEZ-FONTES R (1991) Licorice-induced hypermineralocorticoidism. *New Engl J Med* **325**: 1223–1227.

FINE AJ (1987) Hypersensitivity reaction to kiwi fruit (Chinese gooseberry, *Actinidia chinensis*). *J Allergy Clin Immunol* **68**:235–237.

FIRER MA, HOSKING CS & HILL DJ (1981) Effect of antigen load on development of milk antibodies in infants allergic to milk. *Br Med J* **283**:693–696.

FLATZ G (1989) The genetic polymorphism of intestinal lactase activity in adult humans. In Scriver CR, Beaudet AL, Sly WS & Valle D (eds) *The Metabolic Basis of Inherited Disease*, 6th edn, pp. 2999–3006, McGraw Hill, New York.

FRIEDMAN M (ed) (1986) *Nutritional and Toxicological Significance of Enzyme Inhibitors in Foods*, Plenum Press, New York.

GILBERT RJ, HOBBS G, MURRAY CK, CRUICKSHANK JG & YOUNG SEJ (1980) Scombrotoxic fish poisoning: features of the first 50 incidents to be reported in Britain (1976–9). *Br Med J* **281**:71–72.

GITZELMANN R, STEINMANN B & VAN DEN BERGHE G (1989) Disorders of fructose metabolism. In Scriver CR, Beaudet AL, Sly WS & Valle D (eds) *The Metabolic Basis of Inherited Disease*, 6th edn, pp. 399–424, McGraw Hill, New York.

HALL MJ (1987) The dangers of cassava (tapioca) consumption. *Bristol Med-Chi J* **102**:37–39, 50.

HASHIMOTO Y, KONOSU S, YASUMOTO T & KAMIYA H (1969) Ciguatera in the Ryukyu and Amami Islands. *Bull Jap Soc Sci Fish* **35**:316–326.

HAYAKAWA R, MATSUNAGA K, SUZUKI M *et al.* (1987) Is sesamol present in sesame oil? *Contact Derm* **17**:133–135.

HORWITZ D, LOVENBERG W, ENGELMAN K & SJOERDSMA A (1964) Monoamine oxidase inhibitors, tyramine, and cheese. *J Am Med Ass* **188**:1108–1110.

KAJOSAARI M (1982) Food allergy in Finnish children aged 1 to 6 years. *Acta*

Paediat Scand **71**:815–819.

KING TP (1980) Chemical and biological properties of some atopic allergens. *Adv Immunol* **23**:77–105.

KNUDSON EA & KROON S (1988) In vitro and in vivo phototoxicity of furocoumarin-containing plants. *Clin Exper Dermatol* **13**:92–96.

LEINER IE (ed) (1980) *Toxic Constituents of Plant Foodstuffs*, 2nd edn, Academic Press, New York.

LINDFORS A & ENOCKSSON E (1988) Development of atopic disease after early administration of cow milk formula. *Allergy* **43**:11–16.

LINNAN MJ, MASCOLA L, LOU XD *et al.* (1988) Epidemic listeriosis associated with Mexican-style cheese. *New Engl J Med* **319**:823–828.

LOVELESS MH (1950) Allergy for corn and its derivatives: experiments with a masked ingestion test for its diagnosis. *J Allergy* **21**:500–511.

LUCAS A, BROOKE OG, MORLEY R, COLE TJ & BAMFORD MF (1990) Early diet of preterm infants and development of allergic or atopic disease: randomised prospective study. *Br Med J* **300**:837–840.

LUND BM (1990) Foodborne disease due to *Bacillus* and *Clostridium* species. *Lancet* **336**:982–987.

MAHONEY CP, MARGOLIS MT, KNAUSS TA & LABBE RF (1980) Chronic vitamin A intoxication in infants fed chicken liver. *Pediatrics* **65**:893–986.

MALONE MH & METCALFE DD (1986) Histamine in foods: its possible role in non-allergic adverse reactions to ingestants. *New Engl Reg Allergy Proc* **7**:241–245.

MARKS JG, DEMELFI T, MCCARTHY MA *et al.* (1984) Dermatitis from cashew nuts. *J Am Acad Dermatol* **10**:627–631.

MAY CD (1982) Food allergy: lessons from the past. *J Allergy Clin Immunol* **69**:255–259.

MAY CD & BOCK SA (1978) A modern clinical approach to food hypersensitivity. *Allergy* **33**:166–188.

METCALFE DD (1985) Food allergens. *Clin Rev Allergy* **3**:331–349.

MILLS AR & PASSMORE R (1988) Pelagic paralysis. *Lancet* **1**:161–164.

MONERET-VAUTRIN DA (1983) False food allergies: non-specific reactions to foodstuffs. In Lessof MH (ed) *Clinical Reactions to Food*, pp. 135–153, John Wiley & Sons, New York.

MONERET-VAUTRIN DA, HATAHET R, KANNY G & AIT-DJAFER Z (1991) Allergenic peanut oil in milk formulas. *Lancet* **338**:1149.

MORGAN MRA & FENWICK GR (1990) Natural foodborne toxicants. *Lancet* **336**:1492–1495.

MORROW JD, MARGOLIES GR, ROWLAND J & ROBERTS LJ (1991) Evidence that histamine is the causative toxin of scombroid-fish poisoning. *New Engl J Med* **324**:716–720.

NOAH ND, BENDER AE, REAIDI BG & GILBERT RJ (1980) Food poisoning from raw red kidney beans. *Br Med J* **281**:236–237.

PERL TM, BÉDARD L, KOSATSKY T, HOCKIN JC, TODD ECD & REMIS RS (1990) An outbreak of toxic encephalopathy caused by eating mussels contaminated with domoic acid. *New Engl J Med* **322**:1775–1780.

PORRAS O, CARLSSON B, FÄLLSTRÖM SP & HANSON LÅ (1985) Detection of soy protein in soy lecithin, margarine and, occasionally, soy oil. *Int Arch Allergy Appl Immunol* **78**:30–32.

PRAUSNITZ C & KÜSTNER H (1921) Studien über die Ueberempfindlichkeit. *Centralbl Bakt Parasitol* **86**:160–169.

REID TMS, GOULD IM, MACKIE IM, RITCHIE AH & HOBBS G (1988) Food poisoning due to the consumption of red whelks (*Neptunea antiqua*). *Epi-*

demiol Infect **101**:419–423.

RIEGER CHL & ROTHBERG RM (1975) Development of the capacity to produce specific antibody to an ingested food antigen in the premature infant. *J Pediat* **87**:515–518.

ROBERTON DM, PAGANELLI R, DINWIDDIE R & LEVINSKY RJ (1982) Milk antigen absorption in the preterm and term neonate. *Arch Dis Child* **57**:369–372.

RUFF TA (1989) Ciguatera in the Pacific: a link with military activities. *Lancet* **1**:201–204.

SAMPSON HA (1988) Food sensitivity in children. In Lichtenstein LM & Fauci AS (eds) *Current Therapy in Allergy, Immunology and Rheumatology-3*, pp. 52–56, Decker, Toronto.

SCHLOSS OM (1912) A case of allergy to common foods. *Am J Dis Child* **3**:341–362.

SCHWARTZ B, CIESIELSKI CA, BROOME CV *et al.* (1988) Association of sporadic listeriosis with consumption of uncooked hot dogs and undercooked chicken. *Lancet* **2**:779–782.

SCOGING AC (1991) Illness associated with seafood. *Communicable Disease Report* **1**:117–122.

SEKLA L, MILLEY D, STACKIW W, SISLER J, DREW J & SARGENT D (1990) Verotoxin-producing *Escherichia coli* in ground beef – Manitoba. *Canada Diseases Weekly Report* **16–22**:103–105.

STANWORTH DR (1973) *Immediate Hypersensitivity. The Molecular Basis of the Allergic Response*, North Holland Publishing Company, Amsterdam.

STERN M (1989) Mucosal passage and handling of food-protein antigens. In Harms HK & Wahn U (eds) *Food Allergy in Infancy and Childhood*, pp. 13–23, Springer, Berlin.

STROBEL S (1986) Allergenicity of feeds and gastrointestinal immunoregulation in man and experimental animals. *Hum Nutr Appl Nutr* **40A** (suppl. 1):45–54.

STROBEL S (1989) Immune responses of the young to foods: developmental aspects of food allergy. In Harms HK & Wahn U (eds) *Food Allergy in Infancy and Childhood*, pp. 25–38, Springer, Berlin.

STROBER W, RICHMAN LK & ELSON CO (1981) The regulation of gastrointestinal immune responses. *Immunol Today* **2**:156–162.

SVENSSON BG, NILSSON A, HANSSON M, RAPPE C, ÅKESSON B & SKERFVING S (1991) Exposure to dioxins and dibenzofurans through the consumption of fish. *New Engl J Med* **324**:8–12.

TATTRIE NH & YAGUCHI M (1973) Protein content of various processed edible oils. *J Inst Can Sci Technol Aliment* **6**:289–290.

TAYLOR SL (1986) Histamine food poisoning: toxicology and clinical aspects. *CRC Crit Rev Toxicol* **17**:91–128.

TAYLOR SL, BUSSE WW, SACHS MI, PARKER JL & YUNGINGER JW (1981) Peanut oil is not allergenic to peanut-sensitive individuals. *J Allergy Clin Immunol* **68**:372–375.

TAYLOR SL, LEATHERWOOD M & LIEBER ER (1978) A survey of histamine levels in sausages. *J Food Protection* **41**:634–637.

TAYLOR SL, LEMANSKE RF, BUSH RK & BUSSE WW (1987a) Food allergens: structure and immunologic properties. *Ann Allergy* **59**:93–99.

TAYLOR SL, LEMANSKE RF, BUSH RK & BUSSE WW (1987b) Chemistry of food allergens. In Chandra RK (ed) *Food Allergy*, Nutrition Research Foundation, pp. 21–44, St. John's, Newfoundland.

TAYLOR SL, STRATTON JE & NORDLEE JA (1989) Histamine poisoning (scombroid fish poisoning): an allergy-like intoxication. *Clin Toxicol* **27**:225–240.

TEITELBAUM JS, ZATORRE RJ, CARPENTER S et al. (1990) Neurologic sequelae of domoic acid intoxication due to the ingestion of contaminated mussels. *New Engl J Med* **322**:1781–1787.

TRANTER HS (1990) Foodborne staphylococcal illness. *Lancet* **336**:1044–1046.

TUFT L & BLUMSTEIN GI (1942) Studies in food allergy. II. Sensitisation to fresh fruits: clinical and experimental observations. *J Allergy* **13**:574–582.

UDALL JN, PANG K, FRITZE L, KLEINMAN R & WALKER WA (1981) Development of gastrointestinal mucosal barrier. I. The effect of age on intestinal permeability to macromolecules. *Pediat Res* **15**:241–244.

UDENFRIEND S, LOVENBERG W & SJOERDSMA A (1959) Physiologically active amines in common fruits and vegetables. *Arch Biochem Biophys* **85**:487–490.

YAVUZ H, ÖZEL A, AKKUS I & ERKUL I (1991) Honey poisoning in Turkey. *Lancet* **337**:789–790.

YOUNG E, PATEL S, STONEHAM M, RONA R & WILKINSON JD (1987) The prevalence of reaction to food additives in a survey population. *J Roy Coll Phys* **21**:241–247.

Part 2 Cow's Milk Intolerance

5 Composition of cow's milk
Constituents of milk and milk formulae

Cow's milk Cow's milk is a complex mixture of water, carbohydrates, proteins, lipids, enzymes, vitamins, pigments and minerals (Lee 1983; Swaisgood 1985; Kitchen 1985; Cremin & Power 1985). This chapter is confined to milk components relevant to food intolerance; the many other constituents of cow's milk are not discussed here. It is worth pointing out that the composition of cow's milk is affected by a large number of factors such as the breed of the animal, the type of feed being given, the stage of lactation, the time of day the milk is drawn, and the season of the year (Egan *et al.* 1987).

Carbohydrate In cow's milk (and goat's milk or human milk) the principal carbohydrate present is lactose. Other carbohydrates are glucose and galactose, various oligosaccharides, and in addition several carbohydrate-protein combinations (Lee 1983).

modified cow's milk In practice, many infants receive modified cow's milk formulae or other commercial forms of cow's milk (such as sweetened condensed milk). Other infants may receive cow's milk substitute infant feeds (such as soya or casein hydrolysate-based formulae). Many infant formulae, whether based on cow's milk, soya or casein hydrolysate, may contain other forms of added carbohydrate, such as sucrose, malto-dextrin, amylose, glucose, corn starch and tapioca starch. The range of carbohydrates to be found in cow's milk and cow's milk formulae gives rise to a variety of different possible forms of carbohydrate intolerance (see chapter 6).

Fat The fat content is made up mainly of triglycerides, which comprise 95% of the total milk lipids. In addition there are small amounts of diglycerides, monoglycerides, keto acid glycerides and phospholipids (Lee 1983; Swaisgood 1985).

intolerance to fat Intolerance to the fat components of cow's milk but not to other fats does not appear to be a clinically recognized problem. Some artificial cow's milk formulae also contain added fat in the form of vegetable oil, soya lecithin, butter fat, beef fat, corn oil, coconut oil or medium chain triglyceride. In theory, intolerance to these added fats could occur (e.g. if oil is contaminated by small quantities of protein), but if this happens at all it must be very rare. Intolerance to fat does occur in patients with lipase deficiency, cystic fibrosis or Shwachman's syndrome, but these patients are unable to digest all fats, not just the fat in milk.

Table 5.1 Concentrations of the major proteins in cow's milk[1]

Protein	Concentration (g/l)
Caseins	24–28
α-caseins	15–19
α_1-caseins	12–15
α_2-caseins	3–4
β-caseins	9–11
κ-caseins	3–4
γ-caseins	1–2
Whey proteins	5–7
β-lactoglobulins	2–4
α-lactalbumin	1–1.5
Proteose – peptones	0.6–1.8
Serum albumin	0.1–0.4
Immunoglobulins	0.6–1.0

[1] Source: Swaisgood (1985).

Table 5.2 Some current uses of whey in manufactured food[1]

1 Bread: the improvement in baking properties of bread by the addition of whey is attributed to its lactic acid and riboflavine content
2 Sausages
3 Vinegar
4 Coffee whitener
5 Frozen desserts, e.g. sherbet, soft serve ice cream
6 Beverages

Name	Country of origin
Rivella	Switzerland
Whey champagne	Poland
Bodrost	Russia
Boychu	Russia

[1] Source: Smith (1976).

Protein   About 80% of cow's milk protein is casein (Swaisgood 1985). Bovine casein is not a single protein, and it can be separated into five main components (Table 5.1). All the caseins exist with calcium phosphate in a highly hydrated spherical complex known as a micelle.

whey   Whey is the fluid portion of milk which is obtained after coagulation and removal of most of the casein during the manufacture of cheese or casein. Whey is used in a variety of foodstuffs (Table 5.2). β-lactoglobulin and α-lactalbumin are the major whey proteins. Cow's milk also contains small quantities of immunoglobulins and serum albumin (see Table 5.1).

Vitamins, minerals   Animal milks contain vitamins and minerals. In theory, added vitamins of yeast origin in artificial milk formulae (by contamination with protein impurities) could give rise to intolerance in yeast intolerant subjects, but this remote possibility has not been documented.

Key references 5.1   ROSE D, BRUNNER JR, KALAN EB *et al.* (1970) Nomenclature of the proteins of cow's milk: third revision. *J Dairy Sci* **53**:1–17. *A detailed description of the structure and nomenclature of the various proteins present in cow's milk.*

5.2   SMITH G (1976) Whey protein. *Wld Rev Nutr Diet* **24**:88–116. *A major review of the composition, nutritional value and commercial uses of whey protein.*

Summary 5   Although the principal carbohydrate in animal milk is lactose, milk formulae which are commonly given to infants may contain a range of other carbohydrates, which can result in a number of different forms of carbohydrate intolerance. The major proteins in cow's milk are casein, β-lactoglobulin, α-lactalbumin, serum albumin and immunoglobulin.

6 Carbohydrate intolerance
Monosaccharide, disaccharide and starch intolerance

Types of sugar   The simplest carbohydrates are the monosaccharides. These have between three and eight carbon atoms. Most carbohydrates in food, for example glucose, fructose, galactose, mannose, have six carbon atoms, and are therefore called hexoses. Arabinose, xylose and ribose have only five carbon atoms and are thus pentoses (Coultate 1984).

Disaccharides   One monosaccharide may be combined with another to produce a disaccharide, such as sucrose, lactose, maltose and isomaltose.

Trisaccharides   A trisaccharide consists of three monosaccharide units joined together, for example raffinose and maltotriose.

Polysaccharides   When two to 10 monosaccharide units are joined together they form the class of oligosaccharides (oligo meaning few). When more than 10 monosaccharide units are joined together they produce a polysaccharide (poly meaning many). Starch is the principal polysaccharide found in food. Some polysaccharides contain only one type of monosaccharide, and these are termed homopolysaccharides or homoglycans. The 'an' ending denotes a polysaccharide, and glycose is the general name for any monosaccharide. Examples of homoglycans are starch and cellulose, but they do not have the proper 'an' ending because they were named before this nomenclature was instituted. Both starch and cellulose are polymers of glucose (Whistler & Daniel 1985).

Starch structure   Starch consists of two types of glucose polymer, amylose which is essentially linear, and amylopectin which is highly branched, usually in a proportion of one part of amylose to three parts of amylopectin.

Reducing sugars   When a solution of a reducing sugar is heated with an equal volume of mixed Fehling's solution in boiling water the cupric salt is reduced to red cuprous oxide. The reaction is given by the monosaccharides (e.g. glucose, fructose, galactose, mannose, arabinose), and by disaccharides with a free reducing group (e.g. lactose and maltose but not sucrose). When testing urine for reducing sugars it must be remembered that several drugs (e.g. a number of antibiotics such as the cephalosporins and nalidixic acid) will also give a positive reaction.

Source of sugars   Monosaccharides occur naturally in food in only small amounts; and they are usually present almost entirely as units in polysaccharides rather than as free sugars.

disaccharides   Common disaccharides in food are sucrose (cane or beet sugar), maltose (from corn syrup), and lactose (milk sugar).

Monosaccharide absorption   Glucose and galactose are actively transported by an energy- and sodium-dependent pump mechanism (Gray 1983). Fructose has its own transport mechanism, a form of facilitated diffusion, which is not as efficient as the glucose pump (Gray 1983). Intolerance to fructose is dealt with in chapter 31. Mannose and ribose are absorbed by free diffusion.

other carbohydrates   All other carbohydrates, that is disaccharides, other oligosaccharides and polysaccharides, require hydrolysis before quantitatively important absorption can occur.

Disaccharide absorption   Under normal conditions, the intestine is almost impermeable to disaccharides, but trace amounts may be absorbed without hydrolysis (Gray 1983). The amount absorbed may increase in patients with intestinal damage (for example coeliac disease, or in those with a high intraluminal concentration of disaccharide as may happen in disaccharidase deficiency (for example lactase deficiency – see Gray 1983). There is little, if any, metabolism of absorbed disaccharides, which are excreted in the urine. However, the presence of disaccharides in the urine is a non-specific finding and this is therefore not a useful clinical test (Gray 1983).

Disaccharide hydrolysis

Disaccharides and other oligosaccharides are hydrolysed to monosaccharides by the enzymes lactase, sucrase, isomaltase and maltase, all of which are located in the brush border membrane of the small intestine.

Starch hydrolysis

Hydrolysis of starch is achieved by the action of salivary amylase and pancreatic amylase. This results in the production of oligosaccharides maltose, glucose and a highly branched complex known as limit dextrin.

Causes of loose stools

Non-hydrolysed oligosaccharides and polysaccharides pass unabsorbed from the small intestine to the large intestine where they provide bulk (fibre). Loose stools can then be the result of a combination of the following mechanisms.

1 The osmotic action of non-hydrolysed disaccharides, oligosaccharides and polysaccharides (especially the former) in the lumen of the large intestine which induces a net fluid secretion into the gut lumen (Gray 1983).

2 Rapid intestinal transit which in turn may cause secondary malabsorption of fat (Gray 1983).

3 Non-hydrolysed oligosaccharides and polysaccharides provide fibrous bulk and increase the volume of the stool (Whistler & Daniel 1985).

4 The action of bacteria on disaccharides and oligosaccharides in the large intestine, to produce metabolites such as acetic, lactic butyric and propionic acids (Whistler & Daniel 1985), which if present in sufficient quantities may cause loose stools.

5 Bacterial action may also produce gases such as carbon dioxide or hydrogen, which results in flatulence. This tends to occur with particular oligosaccharides, such as raffinose and stachyose present in beans (Whistler & Daniel 1985).

Causes of carbohydrate intolerance

There are basically four steps in carbohydrate absorption (see above) and utilization, and faults can occur at each step.

1 *Pancreatic amylase deficiency*: hydrolysis of polysaccharides (for example starch) to produce oligosaccharides.

2 *Disaccharidase deficiency*: hydrolysis of oligosaccharides to produce monosaccharides.

3 *Monosaccharide malabsorption*: transport or diffusion of monosaccharides from the gut lumen into the bloodstream.
4 *Utilization* of the monosaccharide, once it has entered the bloodstream:

   (a) *galactosaemia* (reviewed elsewhere; see Segal 1989);

   (b) *hereditary fructose intolerance* (reviewed elsewhere; see Gitzelman *et al.* 1989).

excessive ingestion   A further theoretical cause of carbohydrate intolerance is excessive ingestion, overloading one of the pathways described above, but in otherwise normal children this does not seem to occur, with the possible exception of fructose (see chapter 31).

Symptoms   The main symptoms of carbohydrate intolerance are watery loose stools, abdominal distension, vomiting and poor weight gain. The acid character of the stools is said to be the cause of the excoriation of the peri-anal skin and buttocks (Carre *et al.* 1984).

Breast-fed neonates are different   The stools of normal newborn infants, particularly those who are breast-fed, often contain reducing substances. In one series, reducing substances in amounts greater than 0.5% were found in the stools of 14 out of 22 (64%) breast-fed newborns and two out of 11 (11%) formula-fed newborns (Whyte *et al.* 1978). Thin-layer chromatography of faecal extracts demonstrated two oligosaccharides, one of which was present in 85% of samples, and which was identified as containing fucose, glucose and galactose. This oligosaccharide was also identified in breast milk. All but two stools had a pH between 5.0 and 6.0. A previous study had shown that newborn infants commonly had acid stools with 0.5% to 0.75% reducing substances (Counahan & Walker-Smith 1976). The practical implication is that finding reducing substances up to 0.75% in the stools of newborn infants is normal, and at this age only concentrations of 1% or more are supportive of a diagnosis of carbohydrate intolerance (see below). There is a report of an otherwise normal, breast-fed newborn infant who was admitted to hospital because she was passing profuse watery loose stools five times a day (Barfoot *et al.* 1988). An oligosaccharide which contained fucose was found in her stools, and her symptoms disappeared when breast-feeding was stopped. Some observers felt that these symptoms were physiological, and that stopping breast-feeding had not been necessary (Baumer 1988), but it was pointed out that the symptoms were sufficient to cause hospitalization, and that once improvement had occurred the mother had been unwilling to resume breast-feeding (McEnery & Seakins 1988).

Monosaccharide intolerance
diagnosis

Thin-layer chromatography of faecal extracts will enable identification to be made of the sugar present, and therefore reveal the probable cause of the carbohydrate intolerance. The diagnosis of monosaccharide intolerance is made by the detection of excess amounts (0.5% or more; except in neonates – see above) of reducing substances in the watery stools, while the child is having a feed known to contain only a single monosaccharide, such as an electrolyte solution containing glucose (Walker-Smith 1988). Removal of this monosaccharide from the diet should relieve the loose stools, but if there are other mechanisms contributing to the diarrhoea (e.g. bacterial overgrowth) then resolution may not occur.

congenital glucose-galactose malabsorption

Congenital glucose-galactose malabsorption is inherited as an autosomal recessive trait, and is very rare. The absorptive defect is confined to glucose and galactose, and fructose is absorbed normally. Severe symptoms may lead to severe dehydration with neurological complications or even death in infancy, but milder cases may only be diagnosed in adulthood. Management consists of elimination of glucose and galactose from the diet, using fructose as a substitute. A special fructose-containing cow's milk formula (Galactomin 19, Cow & Gate – not nutritionally complete) may be used in infancy. Alternatively, a modular feed may be constructed (for example based on comminuted chicken), using fructose as the source of carbohydrate (Walker-Smith 1988).

secondary monosaccharide intolerance

Temporary monosaccharide intolerance is common after gastroenteritis. For example, in one series 16 out of 200 (8%) of children who were admitted to hospital with gastroenteritis developed this intolerance (Trounce & Walker-Smith 1985). It is usually mild and short-lived and can almost be regarded as part of the natural history of the disease (Walker-Smith 1988). The mechanism is thought to be temporary impairment of the active transport mechanism for glucose absorption. Temporary monosaccharide intolerance can also occur in newborn infants following gastrointestinal surgery (Walker-Smith 1988).

management

In mild cases, temporary avoidance of oral carbohydrate suffices. In severe cases, intravenous fluids may be required. A period of carbohydrate avoidance is followed by gradual re-introduction of glucose and fructose. In severe and protracted cases, intravenous feeding may be necessary (Walker-Smith 1988).

Disaccharide intolerance
secondary lactase deficiency

Lactase deficiency (more commonly called lactose intolerance) is by far the most common form of carbohydrate intolerance in childhood. It often occurs secondary to a number of disorders (Table 6.1

Table 6.1 Causes of secondary lactose intolerance[1]

Viral gastroenteritis
Neonatal gastrointestinal surgery
Extensive small intestinal resection
Cow's milk protein intolerance
Coeliac disease
Giardiasis
Protein-calorie malnutrition
Immunodeficiency syndromes

[1] Source: Walker-Smith (1988).

and Walker-Smith 1988). The most common of these is viral gastro-enteritis, in which the lactose intolerance is temporary.

incidence

In a study of post-gastroenteritis lactose intolerance in London in 1973, 38 out of 348 (10.9%) children admitted to hospital with gastro-enteritis were diagnosed as having lactose intolerance (Gribbin *et al.* 1976). In a similar further study from the same unit in 1985, 15 out of 200 (7.5%) children were diagnosed as having lactose intolerance (Trounce & Walker-Smith 1985). A further 16 children (8%) had monosaccharide intolerance. These data accord with the general impression that the incidence of lactose intolerance has fallen, possibly because of the diminishing severity of gastroenteritis which in turn may be partly due to more appropriate management (Manuel & Walker-Smith 1980). It has been suggested that some infants formerly diagnosed as lactose intolerant may in fact have had cow's milk protein intolerance, which may also be a sequel to gastroenteritis (Trounce & Walker-Smith 1985). The suggestion is that misdiagnosis may have resulted in a falsely high incidence of lactose intolerance, and that cow's milk protein intolerance as a sequel to gastroenteritis may be diminishing in frequency because of the introduction of more modern and less sensitizing modified cow's milk formulae (Trounce & Walker-Smith 1985).

clinical relevance?

The patients in the above series were highly selected, both because they were admitted to hospital and also because the figures come from a unit with a special interest in paediatric gastroenterology and are therefore likely to include unusual or atypical cases. Furthermore, these were prospective studies where sugar intolerance was being specially sought, and it is questionable whether making the diagnosis had any influence on the management. In all cases where re-introduction of milk was followed by a recurrence of loose stools, the action was simply to return to giving a glucose electrolyte mixture, and then to try milk again when the loose stools had settled. Lactose intolerance persisted long enough for milk re-introduction to fail three times in only one out of 200 children (Trounce & Walker-Smith 1985).

diagnosis

If gastroenteritis is treated with withdrawal of milk and substitution of a glucose electrolyte mixture, then lactose intolerance should be suspected if loose stools recur within 3 days of re-introduction of a lactose-containing milk (Trounce & Walker-Smith 1985). If milk is not withdrawn at all, for example in a breast-fed infant, then persistent loose stools should raise the suspicion of lactose intolerance. The diagnosis can be made by testing the watery portion of the stool with Clinitest tablets, while the child is on a lactose-containing feed and finding 0.5% or more (1% or more in neonates) of reducing substances (Kerry & Anderson 1964; Trounce & Walker-Smith 1985). If reducing substances are found while the child is only receiving a glucose electrolyte mixture, this indicates monosaccharide intolerance.

management

In cases of post-gastroenteritis lactose intolerance, simple withdrawal of milk containing feed for 24 hours followed by re-introduction of milk should suffice in most cases, although it may be necessary to repeat the procedure once or twice. Where lactose intolerance persists, then a lactose-free diet will be required. Avoidance of lactose will fail if the lactose intolerance is secondary to cow's milk protein intolerance, which may be a sequel to gastroenteritis, and in such infants loose stools will only abate when cow's milk protein is also withdrawn from the diet. Treatment of other cases of lactose intolerance is with a lactose-free diet, pending treatment of the underlying cause if this is possible.

late-onset lactase deficiency

A degree of deficiency of lactase is common in adults, particularly non-Caucasians (Flatz 1989). The management is reduction or elimination of dietary lactose, but this is only necessary if the symptoms are a nuisance.

congenital alactasia

Congenital alactasia is inherited as an autosomal recessive, and is very rare (Levin *et al*. 1970). Incomplete forms (i.e. hypolactasia) can occur. From the first few days of life the stools are loose, and the condition is permanent. Treatment is with a lactose-free diet.

glucose-polymer intolerance

Temporary intolerance to glucose polymer, which is included in certain artificial milk formulae, has been described. The intolerance can be demonstrated by stool chromatography (Walker-Smith 1988).

sucrase-isomaltase deficiency

Sucrase-isomaltase deficiency is inherited as an autosomal recessive, and is rare except in Greenland Eskimos, up to 10% of whom may be affected (Gudmand-Hoyer 1985). Symptoms only appear when food containing sucrose is introduced into the child's diet, usually when solids are introduced. The severity of the symptoms depends on the quantity of sucrose in the diet. Treatment is by restriction of sucrose. In theory this needs to be lifelong, but in practice patients often tolerate small quantities of sucrose without undue symptoms. In theory starch restriction is also required, but in practice exclusion of starch is usually not required because there is sufficient maltase to ensure hydrolysis and normal absorption of maltose and maltotriose derived from dietary starch (Walker-Smith 1988).

Lactose contamination   Lactose itself is not antigenic, but commercial lactose may contain small amounts of cow's milk protein as well as other antigens distinct from known milk proteins. In one study, commercial reagent grade lactose was found to contain β-lactoglobulin and α-lactalbumin as well as four other unidentified antigens (Spies 1971), and it is known that pharmaceutical grade lactose also contains traces of protein. These protein impurities are often 'built-in' to the crystal lattice structure during crystallization, and indeed may form the nucleus for the initial crystallization of lactose (Lactochem 1988). Thus it is theoretically possible that lactose, either added to a cow's milk substitute or used as an excipient in a tablet or capsule, could cause intolerance in subjects with cow's milk protein intolerance, although this has never been documented.

Key references 6.1   GRAY GM (1983) Intestinal disaccharidase deficiencies and glucose-galactose malabsorption: In Stanbury JB, Wyngaarden JB, Fredrickson DS, Goldstein JL & Brown MS (eds) *The Metabolic Basis of Inherited Disease*, 5th edn, pp. 1729–1742, McGraw Hill, New York. *Very clearly written comprehensive review.*

6.2   LEE PC, NORD KS & LEBENTHAL E (1981) Digestibility of starches in infants. In Lebenthal E (ed) *Textbook of Gastroenterology and Nutrition in Infancy*, pp. 423–433, Raven Press, New York. *Useful review of the physiology of starch digestion in infancy.*

6.3   TROUNCE JQ & WALKER-SMITH JA (1985) Sugar intolerance complicating acute gastroenteritis. *Arch Dis Child* **60**:986–990. Sugar intolerance, defined as loose watery stools containing 0.5 % or more reducing substances, occurred in 31 of 200 children admitted to hospital with acute gastroenteritis. In 28 this was transient and settled rapidly, but in the remaining three there was a more serious and persistent problem. A common trigger was rotavirus infection.

6.4   SERRANO J & ZETTERSTROM R (1987) Disaccharidase activities and intestinal absorption in infants with congenital intestinal obstruction. *J Pediat Gastroenterol Nutr* **6**:238–243. Biopsies were taken from the gut above the site of obstruction at the time of surgery in 12 infants with congenital duodenal or jejunal obstruction. Activities of maltase, isomaltase, sucrase, trehalase and lactase were all very low, especially the latter two. One month after surgery the absorption of glucose was markedly impaired in those with gut atresia, but not those with incomplete obstruction.

6.5   HARMS H-K, BERTELE-HARMS R-M & BRUER-KLEIS D (1987) Enzyme-substitution therapy with the yeast *Saccharomyces cerevisiae* in congenital sucrase-isomaltase deficiency. *New Engl J Med* **316**:1306–1309. The oral administration of 0.3 g of lyophilized yeast cells in water, given after loading with 2 g of sucrose per kilogram of body weight, reduced intestinal hydrogen production by 70% and abolished or greatly reduced clinical symptoms in eight children with sucrase-isomaltase deficiency. *In vitro*, fresh yeast had appreciable sucrase activity, a low isomaltase and maltase activity, and virtually no lactase activity. This study was prompted by the discovery of an 11-year old girl with sucrase-isomaltase deficiency who was unable to maintain a low sucrose diet, and who found that the addition of fresh baker's yeast to a diet containing sucrose led to the disappearance of diarrhoea and abdominal pain. *It appears that patients with sucrase-isomaltase deficiency can ameliorate the effects of sucrose consumption by the ingestion of a small amount of viable yeast cells, preferably on a full stomach.*

6.6   BARILLAS C & SOLOMONS NW (1987) Effective reduction of lactose maldigestion in preschool children by direct addition of beta-galactosidases to milk at bedtime. *Pediatrics* **79**:766–772. The addition to milk of microbial β-galactosidase *in vitro* can produce a lactose-free milk, with the inconvenience that it has a sweeter flavour and requires a 24-hour incubation period at 4°C. *This study demonstrated that the direct addition of β-galactosidase to milk is just as effective as in vitro hydrolysis at digesting lactose in both normal children and those with lactase deficiency.*

Summary 6   Intolerance to monosaccharides or disaccharides, can, rarely, be a primary autosomal recessive disorder, or more commonly a secondary phenomenon, usually following viral gastroenteritis. The features are loose watery stools, abdominal distension, vomiting and poor weight gain. The diagnosis rests upon the demonstration of abnormal carbohydrate in the stools, and the response to exclusion of the particular carbohydrate from the diet.

7   Antigens in cow's milk
Nature, cross-reactivity and sensitization

Milk proteins   Cow's milk contains at least 25 separate proteins which can induce specific antibody production in man (Hanson & Mansoon 1961; Bahna & Heiner 1980). Some of these proteins are specific to cow's milk, but others are also found in bovine serum. The serum proteins tend to be heat labile, whereas milk-specific proteins are more heat stable (Bahna & Heiner 1980). The most common antigens in cow's milk are β-lactoglobulin, casein, α-lactalbumin, bovine serum albumin and bovine gamma globulin (Bahna & Heiner 1980).

Digestion

In theory, digestion may result in the production of additional antigens. For example, in one series of 10 patients with cow's milk protein intolerance, only four had antibodies to β-lactoglobulin, but all 10 had antibodies to enzymatic digests of β-lactoglobulin (Haddad *et al.* 1979).

Cross-reactivity — goats' milk
observations in guinea-pigs

In the guinea-pig model (see chapter 16), after orally sensitizing with cow's milk, a challenge with goat's milk resulted in anaphylactic shock in 70% of the animals. Orally sensitizing with goat's milk and challenging with cow's or goat's milk gave comparable results: 80% of the animals reacted with anaphylactic shock (McLaughlan *et al.* 1981).

observations in human

Objective information is unavailable about the number of cow's milk protein intolerant children who are also intolerant to goat's milk. However in 1939, Hill reported that 25 of 44 eczematous infants with positive skin-prick tests to cow's milk whey proteins also exhibited identical positive skin tests to the whey protein fraction of goat's milk (Hill 1939). These findings were supported by those of Gjesing *et al.* (1986), who showed that anti-cow's milk protein IgE antibody produced by cow's milk allergic children reacted with goat's milk proteins. Juntunen and Ali-Yrkkö (1983) performed provocation tests in 28 children with cow's milk protein intolerance, and found that 22 were also intolerant to goat's milk. The marked antigenic similarity between cow's and goat's milk proteins (Saperstein 1960; Crawford *et al.* 1961; Uusi-Rauva *et al.* 1970) suggests that goat's milk is unlikely to be tolerated in most children with genuine cow's milk protein intolerance.

Cross-reactivity — sheep's milk

An even greater antigenic similarity appears to exist between bovine and sheep β-lactoglobulins (Bahna & Heiner 1980).

Cross-reactivity — human milk

Cow's milk proteins and human milk proteins apparently do not cross-react (Bahna & Heiner 1980).

Cross-reactivity — cow's hair

Cross-reactivity between cow's milk proteins and cow's hair has been shown, and in one study inhalation of a cow's hair extract caused marked bronchospasm in seven out of 10 children with cow's milk protein intolerance (Osvath *et al.* 1972).

Heat treatment

Heat treatment reduces the immunological activity of some milk proteins, but not others (Bahna & Heiner 1980). Thus the use of heat denatured milk (e.g. evaporated milk) is likely to help only cases in which the patient is sensitive to heat-labile protein. Immunoglobulins, bovine serum albumin and α-lactalbumin are the most susceptible to heat denaturation, and casein the least susceptible (Bahna & Heiner 1980). Heat treatment is discussed in more detail in chapter 16 on hypoallergenic milk formulae.

Quantity of milk   The quantity of cow's milk required to produce an adverse reaction varies from patient to patient. Some patients are highly sensitive and develop anaphylaxis after ingestion of less than 1 µg of casein, β-lactoglobulin or α-lactalbumin (Goldman *et al.* 1963). In contrast, for example, Goldman *et al.* (1983) in their study showed that 29 out of 89 children (33%) with cow's milk intolerance did not react to 100 ml of milk but did react to 200 ml or more. There is a relationship between the quantity of milk required and the time of onset of symptoms. In a sub-group of 44 patients in Goldman *et al.*'s study, the median reaction onset time in those who reacted to 100 ml milk challenges was 2 hours, but the median reaction onset time in those who required larger amounts of milk to elicit reactions was 24 hours.

areas of uncertainty   The precise relationship between the quantity of milk (or any other food for that matter) taken and the speed of onset of symptoms in those with intolerance is an important area of uncertainty. Further information on this subject might help one to understand the different mechanisms which operate in cow's milk protein or other food intolerance. For example, it is highly likely that the process requiring only micrograms of antigen to produce a response differs from that which requires large quantities. The topic is of interest in relation to the growing out of cow's milk protein intolerance, for it appears that some patients do so by acquiring increasing tolerance (Iyngkaran *et al.* 1988a), possibly accompanied by the development of increased concentrations of IgG antibodies to milk proteins (Hill *et al.* 1989). Indeed, some patients have apparently been successfully treated by oral hyposensitization – the administration of gradually increasing volumes of cow's milk (Brodribb 1944; Bahna & Heiner 1980), although this approach has never been objectively investigated.

The diet of cattle   Since it is well known that foods consumed by a nursing mother can pass via breast milk to an infant (see chapter 62), the question arises as to whether the response to cow's milk can depend on the type of food eaten by the animal. The answer is that the subject has never been systematically studied. However, in 1925, Rohrbach reported seven infants with symptoms of cow's milk protein intolerance, and in all seven the symptoms disappeared when the food or pasture of the cow were changed. Rohrbach wrote: 'I have, since early in my practice, never failed to enquire as to the feeding of the dairy herd, and have had great satisfaction in observing many a seriously sick infant become normal in a short period, if the offending food was eliminated from the diet given to the dairy cattle'.

Rohrbach believed that such events accounted for skin-test negative patients with cow's milk protein intolerance. Unfortunately it is not clear from this report exactly how the diet of the cows had been changed, although in one case an animal was prevented from grazing on a hillside and only allowed to graze on a meadowland pasture. 'Here it was evident that the cattle were getting some unusual plant on the upland pasture', deduced the author.

matters arising

This topic raises three questions.
1 Can foods eaten by cattle pass into cow's milk and there either cause sensitization or induce tolerance?
2 Human milk may contain traces of food proteins (e.g. eggs) which were consumed by the lactating mother (see chapter 62). Cows do not eat eggs. Could it be that the rather monotonous and restricted diet of cattle, compared to that of humans, results in the production of milk which is less likely than human milk to cause sensitization to proteins other than the known cow's milk proteins described above?
3 Could contaminants of cow's milk, such as antibiotics or pesticides, be responsible for adverse reactions to cow's milk? The answer to this is already known, for eczematous reactions after consumption of cow's milk which contained penicillin are well documented (Vickers *et al.* 1958).

Incidence and prevalance of cow's milk protein intolerance

Most of the published figures are flawed by being based on highly selected samples or because the diagnosis was not confirmed by challenge. The reported prevalence of intolerance to cow's milk protein varies between 0.3 and 7.5% (reviewed by Bahna & Heiner 1980). The best data comes from a prospective study of a cohort of 1749 newborns from Odense in Denmark, who were followed prospectively for the development of cow's milk protein intolerance developing in the first year of life (Høst & Halken 1990). Of 117 (6.7%) with symptoms suggestive of cow's milk protein intolerance, the diagnosis was confirmed by withdrawal and challenge in 39 infants (2.2%).

Key references 7.1   HEPPELL LMJ, CANT AJ & KILSHAW PJ (1984) Reduction in the antigenicity of whey proteins by heat treatment: a possible strategy for producing a hypoallergenic infant milk formula. *Brit J Clin Nutr* **51**:29–36. Whey protein that had been heated to 115°F was extensively denatured, and in contrast to pasteurised whey, failed to sensitize guinea-pigs for anaphylaxis. *The authors suggest that heat denaturation of whey protein may be a simple way to produce a hypoallergenic baby milk.*

7.2   HARRISON M, KILBY A, WALKER-SMITH JA, FRANCE NE & WOOD CBS (1976) Cows' milk protein intolerance: a possible association with gastroenteritis, lactose intolerance, and IgA deficiency. *Brit Med J* **1**:1501–1504. *Classic report of 25 children with cow's milk protein intolerance, 20 of whom presented initially with an illness indistinguishable from gastroenteritis. It was postulated that an acute attack of gastroenteritis, in damaging the small intestinal mucosa, allows the patient to become sensitized to cow's milk protein and thereby triggers the onset of cow's milk protein intolerance. Proof of this theory is awaited.*

7.3   WALKER-SMITH JA (1982) Cow's milk intolerance as a cause of postenteritis diarrhoea. *J Pediat Gastroenterol Nutr* **1**:163–173. *A detailed review of the hypothesized pathogenesis of cow's milk protein intolerance occurring after acute gastroenteritis. Other causes of postenteritis diarrhoea, such as carbohydrate intolerance, are also discussed.*

7.4   BÜRGIN-WOLFF A, SIGNER E, FRIESS HM, BERGER R, BIRBAUMER A & JUST M (1980) The diagnostic significance of antibodies to various cow's milk proteins (fluorescent immunosorbent test). *Eur J Pediat* **133**:17–24. In a longitudinal study of 25 children with acute gastroenteritis who had been admitted to hospital, IgG, IgA, IgM and IgE antibodies titres to cow's milk proteins remained unchanged. *These results did not support the hypothesis that increased gastrointestinal permeability to macromolecules as a result of gastroenteritis often results in the development of an antibody response (and possibly sensitization) to cow's milk protein.*

7.5   SAVILAHTI E, KUITUNEN P & VISAKORPI JK (1989) Cow's milk allergy. In Lebenthal E (ed) *Textbook of Gastroenterology and Nutrition in Infancy*, 2nd edn, pp. 473–489, Raven Press, New York. *Contains a useful review of the various antibodies to cow's milk protein found in healthy children.*

7.6   HØST A & HALKEN S (1990) A prospective study of cow milk allergy in Danish infants during the first 3 years of life. *Allergy* **45**:587–596. A cohort of 1749 newborns from Odense in Denmark were followed prospectively for the development of cow's milk protein intolerance developing in the first year of life. Of 117 (6.7%) with symptoms suggestive of cow's milk protein intolerance, the diagnosis was confirmed by withdrawal and challenge in 39 infants (2.2%). 19 infants showed immediate reactions (within 1 hour of milk intake), and 20 infants reacted later than 1 hour. Adverse reactions to other foods, particularly egg, citrus fruit and tomato developed in 21/39 (54%).

Summary 7   Of approximately 25 antigenic proteins in cow's milk, the most common to be associated with cow's milk protein intolerance are β-lactoglobulin, casein, α-lactalbumin, bovine serum albumin and bovine gamma globulin. Digestion may result in the production of additional antigens. There is marked antigenic similarity between cow's, goat's, and sheep's milk protein. Heat treatment reduces the immunological activity of some milk proteins but not others. The pathogenesis of cow's milk protein intolerance, the role of different immunological mechanisms, the role of the gut and the way that sensitization occurs are all poorly understood.

8 Cow's milk protein intolerance: clinical features I
Introduction, gastrointestinal features and irritability

Definition

Cow's milk protein intolerance has been defined (Savilahti *et al.* 1989) as a disorder in which symptoms:

1 disappear completely after withdrawal of cow's milk protein from the diet;

2 re-appear after cow's milk protein is re-introduced into the diet;

3 disappear completely after cow's milk protein is again withdrawn from the diet, and remain absent provided cow's milk protein continues to be avoided.

Further discussion of the diagnostic criteria appears in chapter 13.

Multiple symptomatology

Cow's milk protein intolerance is an heterogeneous disorder, attributable to intolerance to one or more of a variety of different proteins, and caused by several different immunological mechanisms. It is hardly surprising that there is no single symptom, or pattern of symptoms, which is pathognomonic of cow's milk protein intolerance. Most patients have multiple symptoms (Goldman *et al.* 1963). The nature of the symptoms depends to some extent on the age of the patient. For example, frank rectal bleeding and colitis (see chapter 62) are features particularly seen in early infancy (Powell 1978; Jenkins *et al.* 1984; Perisic *et al.* 1988; Iyngkaran *et al.* 1989; Wilson *et al.* 1990).

Incidence of symptoms

The incidence of different symptoms varies from one report to another. This is partly due to the different diagnostic criteria that have been employed, and also to the different age distributions of the patients studied. The widely differing incidence of symptoms also reflects the interests of the various authors. Thus gastroenterologists tend to see vomiting or diarrhoea, respiratory physicians tend to see coughing and wheezing, and dermatologists tend to see atopic eczema.

Family history

Cow's milk protein intolerance can be familial, and a history in both parent and child and multiple affected siblings are sometimes seen (Gerrard *et al.* 1963; Bahna & Heiner 1980). The mode of inheritance is unclear.

Age of onset   Most cow's milk formula-fed infants with cow's milk protein intolerance develop symptoms in the first 3 months of life. In one large study of cow's milk protein intolerance, 62% of patients had symptoms in the first month of life, and 96% developed symptoms under the age of 6 months (Goldman *et al.* 1963). The age of onset of the first symptoms in breast-fed babies depends on the age at which cow's milk is first introduced (Gerrard *et al.* 1973; Savilahti *et al.* 1989). A few breast-fed infants develop symptoms during breast-feeding, because of the presence of cow's milk protein in the mother's breast milk (Gerrard 1979).

Vomiting   Vomiting is a common symptom of cow's milk protein intolerance, and most often it occurs within the first hour after cow's milk ingestion (Goldman *et al.* 1963; Gerrard *et al.* 1973; Bahna & Heiner 1980; Savilahti *et al.* 1981; Hill & Hosking 1991). Occasionally the vomiting can be projectile, mimicking pyloric stenosis, or it can be accompanied by abdominal distension, resembling intestinal obstruction (Bahna & Heiner 1980). Rarely the vomiting may be severe and lead to dehydration and electrolyte abnormalities, especially in early infancy (Bahna & Heiner 1980). Vomiting may be the only obvious symptom of cow's milk protein intolerance (Brodribb 1944).

gastro-oesophageal reflux   In one study of infants with cow's milk protein intolerance, where vomiting was accompanied by poor weight gain, half the infants had gross gastro-oesophageal reflux demonstrated radiologically (Hill *et al.* 1984). Vomiting resolved in 'most' cases on a cow's milk-free diet, suggesting that the reflux was not the primary cause of vomiting in most cases. Unfortunately no follow-up information on this group of patients is available, and the relevance of the reflux is unclear. It has been suggested, on the highly doubtful basis of observations of cow's milk precipitins in four children with recurrent regurgitation and aspiration caused by oesophageal narrowing secondary to caustic burns or oesophageal atresia, that regurgitation and aspiration of cow's milk might be a cause of sensitization to cow's milk protein (Handelman & Nelson 1964).

Frequent loose stools   Frequent loose stools (diarrhoea) occur in 25% to 75% of patients with cow's milk protein intolerance (Goldman *et al.* 1963; Gerrard *et al.* 1973; Bahna & Heiner 1980; Savilahti *et al.* 1981; Businco *et al.* 1985; Hill & Hosking 1991). Excoriation around the anus is said to be a common associated feature (Bahna & Heiner 1980). Occasionally the loose stools may be so severe as to cause dehydration and acidosis (Casimir *et al.* 1986). The stools may be streaked with blood. In an uncommon but florid picture, infants can present with heavily bloodstained loose stools, sometimes accompanied by mucus, giving rise to the clinical description of food-allergic colitis (Powell 1978; Jenkins *et al.* 1984; Perisic *et al.* 1988; Iyngkaran *et al.* 1989; Wilson *et al.* 1990; Harrison *et al.* 1991; and see chapter 62). The presence of occult blood in the stools is common in patients with gastrointestinal features of cow's milk protein intolerance, and iron deficiency with anaemia can result (Wilson *et al.* 1964, 1974). In this context, it should be noted that feeding with cow's milk leads to increased intestinal tract blood loss in a large proportion of normal infants (Ziegler *et al.* 1990).

Malabsorption

Malabsorption as a result of cow's milk protein intolerance may mimic coeliac disease with bulky fatty stools, abdominal distension and poor weight gain (Kuitunen *et al.* 1975; Bahna & Heiner 1980). Protein-losing enteropathy may be an associated feature (Lebenthal *et al.* 1970; Walker-Smith 1988). Where there is malabsorption, proximal small bowel biopsy may show subtotal or partial villous atrophy, or just broadening of the villi with cellular infiltration of the lamina propria (Fontaine & Navarro 1975; Kuitunen *et al.* 1975; Shiner *et al.* 1975; Walker-Smith *et al.* 1978; Iyngkaran *et al.* 1988b; Walker-Smith 1988).

Poor weight gain

Because an enteropathy is a feature of cow's milk protein intolerance, it is not surprising that a fairly common consequence is some degree of poor weight gain (Kuitunen *et al.* 1975; Walker-Smith 1988).

Abdominal pain

Acute abdominal pain can be a striking symptom of cow's milk protein intolerance in subjects who are old enough to be able to describe it (Goldman *et al.* 1963; Bahna & Heiner 1980; Savilahti *et al.* 1981; Hill & Hosking 1991). Abdominal pain usually begins within an hour of cow's milk ingestion, but it can occur up to 48 hours later. Although acute abdominal pain is often accompanied by vomiting or frequent loose stools, this is not always so. The pain tends to be peri-umbilical or epigastric, and it may or may not be intermittent (Bahna & Heiner 1980). The cause of the pain is not known. In an infant recently started on cow's milk, the acute presentation of blood in the stools and apparent abdominal pain may lead to the suspicion of intussusception.

Crying, irritability

Crying, screaming and irritability are prominent and common symptoms of cow's milk protein intolerance (Goldman *et al.* 1963; Bahna & Heiner 1980; Savilahti *et al.* 1981; Hill & Hosking 1991). For parents, these features may overshadow concern about other symptoms. They may occur in conjunction with other symptoms, mainly gastrointestinal, or they may occur alone. Crying, screaming and irritability usually commence within an hour of cow's milk protein ingestion, although this is not always noted by the parents, partly because irritability from one feed can easily merge into that caused by the next feed. Crying confined to the evenings is not a symptom of cow's milk protein intolerance. The cause of the crying is not known. The usual assumption is that it is the result of pain. To what extent this represents painful hyperperistalsis of the gut or discomfort associated with vomiting or other symptoms is not known.

Feeding problems Most infants with feeding problems do not have cow's milk protein intolerance. However, poor feeding or reluctance to take milk has been reported to be a symptom of cow's milk protein intolerance (Buisseret 1978).

Key references 8.1 SAVILAHTI E, KUITUNEN P & VISAKORPI JK (1989) Cow's milk allergy. In Lebenthal E (ed) *Textbook of Gastroenterology and Nutrition in Infancy*, 2nd edn, pp. 473–489, Raven Press, New York. *Good general review.*

8.2 JENKINS HR, PINCOTT JR, SOOTHILL JF, MILLA PJ & HARRIES JT (1984) Food allergy: the major cause of infantile colitis. *Arch Dis Child* **59**:326–329. *A description of eight patients under the age of 2 years with colitis due to intolerance to cow's milk protein. Three were also intolerant to soya, and one to beef.*

8.3 WALKER-SMITH J, HARRISON M, KILBY A, PHILLIPS A & FRANCE N (1978) Cow's milk sensitive enteropathy. *Arch Dis Child* **53**:375–380. *Serial small intestinal biopsies in five infants with cow's milk protein intolerance demonstrated mucosal lesions varying in severity from a partially flat mucosa to a mild degree of partial villous atrophy.*

8.4 CASIMIR GJA, DUCHATEAU J, BRASSEUR DJ & VIS HL (1986) Life-threatening gastrointestinal symptoms in infants allergic to cow's milk. *Eur J Pediatr* **145**: 240–241. *The authors describe six infants with severe diarrhoea, dehydration and acidosis following the ingestion of cow's milk. Three needed a period of intravenous nutrition before they were able to tolerate oral feeds.*

8.5 WALKER-SMITH J (1988) *Diseases of the Small Intestine in Childhood*, 3rd edn, Butterworths, London. *Detailed review of cow's milk protein-induced enteropathy, including pathogenesis, clinical features and histological changes. It is suggested that there are two syndromes, one a primary disorder of immunological origin and a secondary disorder, a sequel of mucosal damage (e.g. caused by gastroenteritis).*

Summary 8 Cow's milk protein intolerance is an heterogeneous group of disorders, and there is no single pathognomonic symptom. Multiple symptoms are present in the majority of cases. Vomiting and frequent loose stools are the major gastrointestinal symptoms, sometimes accompanied by malabsorption, poor weight gain and occult blood loss. Crying, screaming or irritability are common symptoms in infancy, and abdominal pain can be a feature in children old enough to describe it.

9 Cow's milk protein intolerance: clinical features II
Respiratory, dermatological and anaphylaxis

Wheezing and coughing

Wheezing or coughing are common symptoms of cow's milk protein intolerance and are usually seen in combination with other symptoms such as atopic eczema or vomiting (Goldman *et al.* 1963; Gerrard *et al.* 1973; Bahna & Heiner 1980; Savilahti *et al.* 1981; Hill & Hosking 1991). It is rare for coughing or wheezing to be the sole manifestation of cow's milk protein intolerance. Although not strictly relevant to childhood, it may be worth noting that occupational asthma as a result of inhalation of bovine serum albumin powder has been reported (Joliat & Weber 1991).

Rhinitis

Sneezing, nasal congestion, and in particular a persistent mucoid nasal discharge are commonly reported features of cow's milk protein intolerance and are usually seen in combination with other symptoms such as asthma, atopic eczema or vomiting (Clein 1954; Goldman *et al.* 1963; Gerrard 1966; Gerrard *et al.* 1973; Bahna & Heiner 1980; Savilahti *et al.* 1981; Hill & Hosking 1991). It is rare for rhinitis to be the sole manifestation of cow's milk protein intolerance. For a further discussion of rhinitis and food intolerance, see chapter 69.

Stridor

The acute onset of stridor is occasionally seen within a few minutes of cow's milk ingestion (Goldman *et al.* 1963; Hill *et al.* 1984). The presence of stridor indicates angioedema of the larynx or trachea. It is usually accompanied by other features, such as perioral rash, urticaria, angioedema and wheezing. Stridor can also be a feature of anaphylactic shock. Acute severe stridor is potentially one of the most dangerous features of cow's milk protein intolerance.

Pulmonary haemosiderosis

Intolerance to cow's milk protein has been invoked as a cause of primary pulmonary haemosiderosis (Boat *et al.* 1975; Lee *et al.* 1978), but this is unproven (for a detailed discussion of childhood idiopathic pulmonary haemosiderosis see Snider 1988).

Atopic eczema

Atopic eczema is a common feature of cow's milk protein intolerance (Goldman *et al.* 1963; Gerrard *et al.* 1973; Bahna & Heiner 1980; Savilahti *et al.* 1981; Hill & Hosking 1991). The reverse association is less common; the proportion of patients with atopic eczema who have cow's milk protein intolerance is far smaller. It is an impression that the younger the patient with atopic eczema, the more likely is cow's milk protein intolerance to be present. Estimates of the incidence of cow's milk protein intolerance in atopic eczema are subject to three major sources of error. The first is that the skin lesions in some patients are only improved by the removal of several foods, and in such patients the simple exclusion of cow's milk protein alone may not help. The second problem is that estimates do not take into account the severity of the skin lesions. Food intolerance, including cow's milk protein intolerance, is far easier to detect in the less common severe generalized cases than in patients with a few tiny lesions. The more severe the lesions, the more obvious will be any improvement on an elimination diet. The final problem is that the association between cow's milk protein intolerance and atopic eczema has become so well known that simple cases where cow's milk protein is an important trigger tend increasingly to be dealt with by parents or family doctors and therefore may not become included in hospital-based research studies (Atherton 1988; Armenio *et al.* 1989).

Rash around the mouth

One of the most common features, particularly in patients with very quick reactions to cow's milk protein, is an erythematous rash around the mouth, often spreading out onto the cheeks and the chin (Bahna & Heiner 1980; Hill *et al.* 1984). The rash is often persistent rather than intermittent, so a relationship to cow's milk ingestion may not be noted by the parents.

Seborrhoeic dermatitis

Infantile seborrhoeic dermatitis is an heterogeneous entity. The skin lesions most commonly appear at the age of 4–6 weeks, and usually before the age of 6 months. Some patients improve spontaneously over a few months, but approximately 25% of affected infants are atopic and the skin lesions progress to those of atopic eczema, which may itself either disappear or persist (Yates *et al.* 1983a). This atopic fraction can be picked out by the presence of certain features (Table 9.1) and by the presence of an elevated concentration of IgE in the serum (Yates *et al.* 1983b). In this atopic fraction of patients with seborrhoeic dermatitis, a small number of cases may be attributable to cow's milk protein intolerance. The non-atopic form of

Table 9.1 Clinical features to look for in an infant with seborrhoeic dermatitis

Features which suggest that an infant with seborrhoeic dermatitis has, or will develop, atopic eczema
1 History of atopic disease in a parent or sibling
2 Dennie-Morgan crease below the eye
3 Hyperlinearity of the palms
4 Wheezing
5 Skin lesions on the forearms or shins (occurs in 20% of 'non-atopic' seborrhoeic dermatitis)

Features which suggest the patient is not atopic
1 Absence of itching
2 Absence of lesions on the face
3 Skin lesions in axillae (occurs in 20% of the 'atopic' group)
4 Eruption starts on the napkin area alone (occurs in 10% of the 'atopic' group)

seborrhoeic dermatitis is not a feature of cow's milk protein intolerance.

Napkin rash Most cases of napkin rash are not due to cow's milk protein intolerance. Nevertheless a persistent napkin rash can occasionally be a feature, if accompanied by frequent loose stools or some other symptom of cow's milk protein intolerance. An isolated napkin rash, without any other symptoms, is not a documented feature of cow's milk protein intolerance.

Urticaria Urticaria is a common feature of cow's milk protein intolerance, often accompanied by angioedema and gastrointestinal symptoms (Goldman *et al.* 1963; Gerrard *et al.* 1973; Bahna & Heiner 1980; Savilahti *et al.* 1981; Hill & Hosking 1991). Urticaria can often also result from spilling cow's milk onto the skin, particularly in patients who also have atopic eczema (Salo *et al.* 1986), in which case the urticaria usually appears within 10 min. In cases of anaphylactic shock, urticaria is often (but not always) an early feature (Goldman *et al.* 1963).

Angioedema Angioedema can be a feature of cow's milk protein intolerance, usually accompanied by urticaria and sometimes also by gastrointestinal symptoms (Goldman *et al.* 1963; Bahna & Heiner 1980; Hill & Hosking 1991). As with urticaria, angioedema can herald anaphylactic shock.

Anaphylactic shock Anaphylactic shock is a rare but dangerous feature of cow's milk protein intolerance (Rohrbach 1925; Kerley 1936; Collins Williams 1955; Goldman *et al.* 1963; David 1984; Editorial 1984; Hill *et al.* 1984). It can be *fatal* (Finkelstein 1905; Richet 1931; Kerley 1936;

Table 9.2 Associated food intolerance in 100 children with cow's milk protein intolerance[1]

Egg	40/77[2]
Orange	27/56
Soya	32/75
Chocolate	14/22
Wheat	12/88
Casein hydrolysate	11/54
Peanut	13/26
Chicken	7/75
Lamb	2/85
Beef	9/79
Fish	6/69
Tomato	5/31

[1] Source: Hill *et al.* (1984).
[2] Some parents elected to withhold or not give certain substances, hence the varying denominators.

David 1984). The symptoms usually develop within minutes of ingestion of cow's milk protein, and one drop of milk can be sufficient to cause anaphylactic shock. The usual sequence of events is the rapid and almost simultaneous onset of sneezing, generalized urticaria, angioedema, vomiting, loose stools, wheezing and hypotension. More dangerous than either of the latter two features is stridor, which is caused by laryngeal oedema and can completely obstruct the airway. A particular problem is that ingestion of cow's milk protein after a period of avoidance can cause anaphylactic shock in a child in whom previous exposure to cow's milk protein caused less serious symptoms such as diarrhoea or eczema (Goldman *et al.* 1963; David 1984).

delayed anaphylaxis

Anaphylactic shock is not confined to the first few minutes after cow's milk protein ingestion. Delayed anaphylaxis can occur several hours after milk ingestion, in one case seen locally as much as 9 hours after ingestion (David 1984). The mechanism of delayed anaphylaxis is unknown. One possibility is of a reaction to a product of digestion of cow's milk protein. Another is that profound hypotension may follow a severe gastrointestinal reaction, due to fluid loss into the gut lumen.

Acute conjunctivitis

Although poorly documented, acute conjunctivitis can be a component of a severe reaction to cow's milk protein, but it has not been described as an isolated feature after exposure to cow's milk protein.

Other food intolerance

Depending upon how patients are ascertained, a varying proportion will have intolerance to other foods. In one series of 100 children with cow's milk protein intolerance (Table 9.2), over 50% exhibited intolerance to one or more other foods (Hill *et al.* 1984). In two unpublished studies of children with cow's milk protein intolerance, four out of 52 (8%) and seven out of 36 (14%) also had intolerance to soya (Bock 1991). The practical importance of these observations is that in some patients the avoidance of cow's milk protein when accompanied by the provision of a soya-based milk formula, will not lead to improvement because of an associated soya intolerance, or, indeed, because of intolerance to other foods which are still being consumed.

Key references   9.1   GOLDMAN AS, ANDERSON DW, SELLERS WA, SAPERSTEIN S, KNIKER WT & HALPERN SR (1963) Milk allergy. I. Oral challenge with milk and isolated milk proteins in allergic children. *Pediatrics* **32**:425–443. *Classic study of presenting symptoms, and features seen after cow's milk challenge.*

9.2   HILL DJ, FORD RPK, SHELTON MJ & HOSKING CS (1984) A study of 100 infants and young children with cow's milk allergy. *Clin Rev Allergy* **2**:125–142. *Detailed clinical study of 100 cases.*

9.3   BAHNA SL & HEINER DC (1980) *Allergies to Milk*, Grune & Stratton, New York. *Major review of all aspects of cow's milk protein intolerance. More comprehensive than critical.*

9.4   HILL DJ & HOSKING CS (1991) Cow's milk allergy. In David TJ (ed) *Recent Advances in Paediatrics*, vol. 9, pp. 187–206, Churchill Livingstone, London. *Useful up-to-date review.*

9.5   GERRARD JW, MACKENZIE JWA, GOLUBOFF N, GARSON JZ & MANINGAS CS (1973) Cow's milk allergy: prevalence and manifestations in an unselected series of newborns. *Acta Paed Scand* **234** (suppl.):1–21. *Study of 787 infants, 59 of whom were found to have cow's milk protein intolerance. Useful data on timing of onset of symptoms after introduction of cow's milk into the diet.*

9.6   FINKELSTEIN H (1905) Kuhmilch als Ursache akuter Ernährungsstörungen bei Säuglingen. *Monatschr Kinderheilk* **4**:65–72. A 10-day-old infant developed 'dyspepsia', which was made worse when he was given buttermilk. Breast-feeding was recommenced at 5 weeks of age, and he thrived. At 11 weeks he was given 60 ml of 1/3 strength cow's milk, which resulted in an immediate reaction comprising pallor, collapse, profuse vomiting, loose stools and pyrexia. At 14 weeks he was given 50 ml of 1/3 strength cow's milk, with a similar but more severe immediate reaction, with the additional features of blood in the stools and spasms in the arms and legs. At 18 weeks he was given 60 ml of 1/3 strength cow's milk, with an even more severe immediate reaction. At 26 weeks of age, he was again tried on 1/3 strength diluted cow's milk. He received 10 ml, but suffered a more severe immediate reaction, but instead of recovering he deteriorated with increased fever, seizures, coma and death on the 9th day. Enterocolitis was found at necropsy. *This case is usually quoted as the first published example of death due to anaphylaxis to cow's milk protein. Such details as are available do suggest that anaphylaxis did occur, but it is not entirely clear why the child died 9 days later.*

Summary 9   The major respiratory symptoms of cow's milk protein intolerance are wheezing, coughing and rhinitis. The most dangerous respiratory symptom is acute stridor, which may be accompanied by anaphylactic shock. The major dermatological features are an erythematous rash around the mouth, atopic eczema, urticaria and angioedema. Twenty-five percent of infants with seborrhoeic dermatitis are atopic, and in a few of these the skin lesions are attributable to cow's milk protein intolerance. Anaphylactic shock is the most serious consequence of cow's milk protein intolerance, and it can be fatal. The onset of anaphylactic shock is usually within minutes of ingestion of cow's milk protein, but delayed anaphylaxis occurring as much as 9 hours later has been described. A number of patients with cow's milk protein intolerance are intolerant to one or more other foods.

10   Cow's milk protein intolerance: clinical features III
Doubtful features

Lack of data   Since most of the features listed here have not been systematically sought in double-blind challenge studies, it is not yet possible to fully exclude an association with cow's milk protein intolerance.

Large tonsils & adenoids   Leaving aside the question of how one might define enlargement of structures which are normally large in childhood, a report of six children with cow's milk-induced haemosiderosis (Boat *et al.* 1975) has been cited as evidence that enlargement of the tonsils and adenoids can be caused by cow's milk protein intolerance (Bahna & Heiner 1980). However in this study, cow's milk avoidance was combined with adenoidectomy, and the report contains no objective evidence to support the authors' contention that early use of a cow's milk protein-free diet may prevent later complications such as upper airway obstruction and cor pulmonale.

Serous otitis media   In serous or secretory otitis media, commonly called glue ear, a collection of fluid in the middle ear causes hearing loss. It has been suggested that food intolerance in general, and cow's milk protein intolerance in particular, may be a cause of serous otitis media (Bahna & Heiner 1980). The subject is examined in chapter 69.

Pneumonia   It has been reported in the USA that cow's milk protein intolerance was responsible for recurrent episodes of pneumonic consolidation (without haemosiderosis – see above) in children who also had recurrent wheezing and coughing (Lee *et al*. 1978). Many of the reported cases had major physical handicaps, and in some of these cineradiography demonstrated the presence of gastro-oesophageal reflux. It is possible that this reflux, which may itself be associated with cow's milk protein intolerance, was the cause of the severe lung involvement, by causing aspiration of vomit. It has been suggested that this disorder has become less common because doctors now swiftly deal with persistent respiratory symptoms in children by the use of a cow's milk protein-free diet (Lee *et al*. 1978). An alternative explanation is that we are now better able to identify other causes of recurrent pneumonia.

Constipation   There is an unconfirmed suggestion that constipation can be a feature of cow's milk protein intolerance. This is discussed in chapter 62.

Pyloric stenosis   The scanty evidence suggesting that pyloric stenosis can be a feature of cow's milk protein intolerance is discussed in chapter 61.

Epilepsy   Epileptic fits (see chapter 67) are described as a rare accompaniment to milk protein-induced anaphylactic shock (Goldman *et al*. 1963). There is no other objective evidence that epileptic fits are a feature of cow's milk protein intolerance.

Neurological symptoms   Lethargy, limpness and behavioural symptoms have been attributed to cow's milk protein intolerance (Bahna & Heiner 1980). Whilst all these may be part of the overall clinical picture, secondary to other major symptoms, there is no evidence that any of these vague symptoms can exist as isolated features of the condition.

Enuresis, cystitis   It has been suggested that enuresis or cystitis (see chapter 66) are features of cow's milk protein intolerance (Bahna & Heiner 1980), but this suggestion has never been objectively tested.

Thrombocytopaenia   A fall of the platelet count of about 35% occurring 3 hours after challenge with either cow's milk or egg has been described in one series (Osvath & Markus 1968), but is unconfirmed. A review of 40 cases of the thrombocytopaenia with absent radius syndrome revealed three with cow's milk protein intolerance, and a possible association between the conditions was suggested by the discovery of a fourth example of this association (Whitfield & Barr 1976). There is a single case report of congenital thrombocytopaenia which responded to withdrawal of cow's milk protein and relapsed upon re-introduction (Jones 1977). If thrombocytopaenia severe enough to cause bleeding is indeed a feature of cow's milk protein intolerance, it must be exceedingly rare.

Nephrotic syndrome

The suggested relationship between food intolerance (including cow's milk protein intolerance) and the nephrotic syndrome is discussed in chapter 66.

Sudden infant death

Professor Coombs in Cambridge has been the chief protagonist of the hypothesis that a sensitized, cow's milk formula-fed infant who is given cow's milk shortly before going to sleep, may regurgitate some stomach contents and aspirate some cow's milk protein into the lungs where it triggers an acute anaphylactic reaction and sudden death (Parish *et al.* 1960; Coombs & McLaughlin 1982; Coombs & Holgate 1990). Support for this hypothesis came from experiments in which the introduction of cow's milk into the larynx of previously sensitized animals caused fatal anaphylaxis (Devey *et al.* 1976). The hypothesis was not supported when tissue specimens from cases of sudden unexpected infant death and from those who died from other recognizable causes were compared by immunofluorescence (Valdes-Dapena & Felipe 1971). Tissues from the two groups showed no significant difference in the number of cells containing antibodies to casein, β-lactoglobulin, or α-lactalbumin. Evidence that cow's milk protein intolerance is a major cause of sudden unexpected infant death in humans is lacking, but a modified hypothesis in which anaphylaxis is responsible for a few sudden infant deaths has, like many other speculative causes, not been fully excluded.

Rheumatoid arthritis

The suggestion that juvenile rheumatoid arthritis may be associated with food intolerance is discussed in chapter 65.

Key references 10.1

LEE SK, KNIKER WT, COOK CD & HEINER DC (1978) Cow's milk-induced pulmonary disease in children. *Adv Pediat* **25**:39–57. *A review of (a) pulmonary haemosiderosis and (b) pneumonia, which the authors believed were caused by cow's milk protein intolerance. Further evidence is needed before a causal link can be accepted.*

10.2

COOMBS RRA & HOLGATE ST (1990) Allergy and cot death: with special focus on allergic sensitivity to cows' milk and anaphylaxis. *Clin Exper Allergy* **20**:359–366. *An elaboration of the hypothesis that anaphylaxis and cow's milk protein intolerance may explain some cases of sudden infant death.*

Summary 10

Enlargement of the tonsils and adenoids, serous otitis media, pneumonia, constipation, enuresis, cystitis, thrombocytopaenia, the nephrotic syndrome and juvenile rheumatoid arthritis are all highly doubtful features of cow's milk protein intolerance. These features have never been systematically sought in double-blind challenge studies, and until this is done, an association with cow's milk protein intolerance cannot be excluded. Lethargy and behavioural symptoms may be part of a more generalized reaction to cow's milk protein, but there is no evidence that these can be isolated symptoms. It is possible that intolerance to cow's milk protein may play a part in the aetiology of pyloric stenosis in a small number of cases. Epileptic fits can occur as a rare complication of anaphylactic shock caused by cow's milk, but are otherwise not caused by cow's milk protein intolerance. The hypothesis that cow's milk protein intolerance causes sudden unexpected infant death is unproven.

11   Cow's milk protein intolerance: diagnosis I
History, clinical picture and clinical profiles

History

Clues in the history which suggest cow's milk protein intolerance are as follows.

1 Symptoms occur, or are made worse, soon after ingestion of cow's milk protein. Such a history may have to be asked for, as it is not always volunteered.

2 Symptoms date from the time, or soon after the time, that breast-feeding was stopped or cow's milk protein was first introduced into the diet.

3 A family history of cow's milk protein intolerance.

4 The presence of multiple atopic disorders (e.g. atopic eczema plus asthma) in an infant under the age of 12 months.

5 The observation that spilling cow's milk onto the skin causes an urticarial reaction.

6 Multiple symptoms of cow's milk protein intolerance (e.g. gut, chest and skin symptoms – see details of individual symptoms in chapters 8 to 10).

Clinical picture

The most commonly seen clinical pictures are patients with multiple symptoms, such as:

1 the infant with a perioral rash, intermittent vomiting and irritability;

2 the infant with intermittent vomiting, frequent loose stools, irritability and poor weight gain;

Table 11.1 Three patterns of response in children with cow's milk protein intolerance[1]

Characteristic feature	Time of onset of symptoms after milk challenge
Early skin reaction	1–45 min
Early gut reaction	45 min to 20 hours
Late reaction	Over 20 hours

[1] Source: Hill *et al.* (1984).

3 the infant with persistent wheezing, frequent loose stools, atopic eczema and poor weight gain.

Less commonly seen are patients with persistent single symptoms:
1 the onset of persistent frequent loose stools following an episode of acute gastroenteritis;
2 the infant with persistent frequent loose stools or vomiting;
3 the infant with atopic eczema;
4 the infant who persistently or frequently wheezes (only rarely caused by cow's milk protein intolerance);
5 the infant who is frequently irritable or who cries or screams a lot throughout the day (only rarely caused by cow's milk protein intolerance).

It is important to emphasize that most patients with these isolated symptoms do not have cow's milk protein intolerance, but a few do, and at present the only way these can be detected is by a trial of cow's milk protein avoidance.

Clinical profiles In the previous chapter, clinical features were considered in isolation, but it is important to remember that multiple symptoms are the usual finding. The time of onset can vary. If patients with cow's milk protein intolerance are given cow's milk, then they can be divided by the time of onset of symptoms after challenge has commenced into three fairly characteristic clinical profiles. These patterns have been most clearly defined by Hill and his colleagues in Australia, and the description below is based on their observations (Hill *et al.* 1984). The three groups are shown in Table 11.1. In Hill and coworkers (1984) study of 100 children with cow's milk protein intolerance, 26 were in the early skin reaction group, 57 were in the early gut reaction group, and 17 had late reactions.

early skin reaction group In the early skin reaction group, symptoms begin to develop within 45 min of cow's milk challenge. The clinical features are shown in Table 11.2. Hill *et al.* found that almost all (24 out of 26) patients in this group had a positive skin-prick test to cow's milk.

Table 11.2 Clinical features resulting from milk challenge and presenting symptoms in children with cow's milk protein intolerance[1]

Clinical features	Presenting symptoms
Early skin reaction group	
Principal features (>50% cases)	
Rash around the mouth	Rash around the mouth or urticaria
Common features (20–50% cases)	
Angioedema	Vomiting
Urticaria	Frequent loose stools
Wheeze/cough	Irritability
Rhinitis	Wheeze/cough
Vomiting	Atopic eczema
Occasional features (<20% cases)	
Atopic eczema	Poor weight gain
Pallor	
Frequent loose stools	
Irritability	
Stridor	
Early gut reaction group	
Principal features (>50% cases)	
Vomiting	Vomiting
Frequent loose stools	Irritability
Common features (20–50% cases)	
Pallor	Frequent loose stools
Irritability	Poor weight gain
Occasional features (<20% cases)	
Rhinitis	Rash around the mouth
Rash around the mouth	Atopic eczema or urticaria
Wheeze/cough	Wheeze/cough
Atopic eczema	
Urticaria	
Angioedema	
Stridor	
Late reaction group	
Principal feature (>50% cases)	
Frequent loose stools	Wheeze/cough, frequent loose stools
Common features (20–50% cases)	
Wheeze/cough	Poor weight gain
Rhinitis	Atopic eczema
Eczema	Vomiting
Angioedema	Irritability
Occasional features (<20% cases)	
Perioral rash	
Pallor	
Vomiting	
Irritability	

[1] Source: Hill *et al.* (1984).

early gut reaction group

In the early gut reaction group, symptoms begin to develop between 45 min and 20 hours after cow's milk challenge. The clinical features are shown in Table 11.2. Hill *et al.* found that about one-third of patients in this group had a positive skin-prick test to cow's milk.

late reaction group

In the late reaction group, symptoms begin to develop about 20 hours after cow's milk protein challenge. The clinical features are shown in Table 11.2. Hill *et al.* found that about 20% of this late reaction group had a positive skin-prick test to cow's milk, and these were mostly children with atopic eczema. Almost all patients in the late reaction group presented over the age of 6 months, and as a group their age at presentation was significantly higher than that of the two other groups.

Presenting features

The clinical profiles described above are those seen when known patients with cow's milk protein intolerance are challenged with cow's milk while on a cow's milk protein-free diet. These character-istic features of the effects of milk challenge often differ from the presenting symptoms noted by the parents before the child has been placed on a cow's milk protein-free diet. The common presenting symptoms of the three major clinical profiles, as described by Hill *et al.* (1984), are shown in Table 11.2. Unfortunately these workers did not study a control population, and the difficulty with lists such as these is that they include symptoms such as irritability or coughing which must be present at sometime in almost all children. It is the persistence or frequent recurrence of normally transient symptoms which is important.

Key references 11.1

HILL DJ, FORD RPK, SHELTON MJ & HOSKING CS (1984) A study of 100 infants and young children with cow's milk allergy. *Clin Rev Allergy* **2**:125–142. *A detailed review of the features of cow's milk protein intolerance, with an analysis of 100 patients.*

11.2

HILL DJ, FIRER MA, SHELTON MJ & HOSKING CS (1986) Manifestations of milk allergy in infancy: clinical and immunologic findings. *J Pediatr* **109**:270–276. *This paper and the one above present the basis for the classification of all patients into three groups on the basis of the time of onset of symptoms after milk challenge.*

Summary 11

Features in the history which might suggest cow's milk protein intolerance comprise a relationship of symptoms to cow's milk feeds or to the onset of bottle-feeding, a family history of the disorder, the presence of multiple atopic disorders under the age of 12 months, a history of urticaria after skin contact with cow's milk, and the presence of multiple symptoms. On the basis of the timing of the onset of symptoms after a cow's milk challenge, cases can be divided into three groups who have different clinical profiles:

1 an early skin reaction group, the symptoms occurring 1–45 min after a challenge has commenced;

2 an early gut reaction group, the symptoms occurring 45 min to 20 hours after challenge;

3 a late reaction group, the symptoms occurring more than 20 hours after challenge.

The common presenting symptoms in each of these groups are not quite the same as those seen with milk challenge; for example, irritability is a very common presenting feature in the early gut reaction group, but is not seen quite so often after milk challenge.

12 Cow's milk protein intolerance: diagnosis II
Differential diagnosis and investigations

Differential diagnosis Symptoms identical to those of cow's milk protein intolerance may be caused by a wide variety of other disorders, and no single clinical feature is pathognomonic. Overdiagnosis may result in a more serious disorder being overlooked.

Lactose intolerance The gastrointestinal features of cow's milk protein intolerance may be difficult to distinguish from those caused by lactose intolerance. The two conditions may co-exist (for example after viral gastroenteritis), and both conditions improve when lactose-free casein hydrolysate or soya-based formulae are given. The detection of lactose intolerance rests on testing the stools for reducing sugars before alteration of the diet (see chapter 6).

Feeding problems A common cause of vomiting in bottle-fed young infants is underfeeding. Too small a hole in the teat leads to air swallowing, followed by regurgitation of air plus some feed, hunger, more air swallowing, and persistent vomiting. If the feeding bottle is turned upside down, the flow of milk should be a steady stream only just broken into drops. A slow drip-drip indicates too small a hole.

Other causes of vomiting Other causes of vomiting in infancy are gastro-oesophageal reflux, urinary infection (see below), pyloric stenosis, and serious infections such as meningitis or septicaemia.

Coeliac disease   The gastrointestinal features of cow's milk protein intolerance may to some extent overlap with those of coeliac disease, but confusion should not occur because the symptoms of coeliac disease do not respond to the withdrawal of cow's milk protein.

Cystic fibrosis   There is some overlap of symptoms between cystic fibrosis and cow's milk protein intolerance. Furthermore, it has been suggested recently, but not yet confirmed, that these two conditions co-exist more commonly than one might expect by chance (Hill *et al.* 1989). Where cystic fibrosis is a possibility, it must be excluded by sweat testing.

Persistent loose stools   In a child with persistent loose stools it is essential that other disorders such as infection (e.g. giardiasis), cystic fibrosis or coeliac disease are borne in mind.

Intussusception   Cow's milk protein intolerance can present acutely, particularly in early infancy, with symptoms similar to those of intussusception, with abdominal pain, vomiting and blood in the stools. Clearly in such patients the exclusion of intussusception is the priority.

Urinary infection   Vomiting and/or loose stools can be presenting features of a urinary infection, and this should be excluded by microscopy and culture of the urine in any child with unexplained vomiting or loose stools.

Colic   Misuse of the term colic is common (see chapter 61). The assumption that crying in a baby is due to intestinal colic may be dangerous, for it may delay the detection of more serious causes of irritability which include urinary infection, meningitis, intestinal obstruction, intussusception, maternal depression or fractures caused by child abuse. Having said this, it should be pointed out that persistent irritability and crying or screaming are important and common presenting features of cow's milk protein intolerance in infancy, especially if associated with other symptoms.

Persistent wheezing   It is common to see infants whose sole symptom is persistent or very frequent wheezing and coughing. If one excludes rare causes such as vascular ring, inhaled foreign body or cystic fibrosis, then most of these so-called 'happy wheezers' have early asthma or wheezing as a sequel to a viral respiratory infection (e.g. with the respiratory syncytial virus). The author has yet to see a beneficial response to cow's milk protein exclusion where persistent wheezing in infancy was the sole symptom. The only cases to respond to milk protein exclusion were those who had additional symptoms (e.g. loose stools, or a patch of atopic eczema).

Investigations   In the clinical situation, as opposed to research studies, investigations are unhelpful.

skin-prick tests   The major problem with skin-prick tests in cow's milk protein intolerance is the high proportion of patients who have negative skin tests (Hill *et al.* 1986). False positive tests are a further problem (see chapter 41).

serum IgE concentration   As far as cow's milk protein intolerance is concerned, the only value in a measurement of the serum IgE level is that an elevated level may help to detect the subgroup of infants with seborrhoeic dermatitis who are atopic, but this can be done almost as reliably on clinical criteria (Yates *et al.* 1983a, b; see Table 9.1). A few of the atopic subjects with seborrhoeic dermatitis may have cow's milk protein intolerance, whereas this is not likely in the non-atopic subjects. Otherwise measuring the serum IgE concentration is unhelpful, for an elevated IgE concentration is only present in about 50% of cases (Bahna & Heiner 1980), and there are other causes for an elevated IgE concentration, most notably atopic disease and especially atopic eczema.

RAST tests   Testing for IgE-specific antibodies (RAST test) is as unreliable as skin-prick testing (Hill *et al.* 1986; Tainio & Savilahti 1990; see chapter 43).

basophil histamine release   There is a positive correlation between the results of basophil histamine release assays and tests for circulating IgE antibodies and skin-prick tests in children with cow's milk protein intolerance (Prahl *et al.* 1988). This is entirely predictable, given that the three tests are in effect all detecting specific IgE antibody. Thus testing for basophil histamine release is likely to be just as unhelpful as skin-prick or RAST testing.

cow's milk precipitins   Testing for milk precipitins is unhelpful because of false positive and false negative results (Bahna & Heiner 1980).

eosinophil count   Seeking eosinophilia in the blood is unhelpful, as it is only present in 25–50% of cases (Bahna & Heiner 1980) and is a non-specific finding.

small bowel biopsy   A jejunal biopsy is likely to be indicated to help make a diagnosis in a child with malabsorption (see chapter 61; Walker-Smith 1988) but is not otherwise indicated in the routine diagnosis of cow's milk protein intolerance.

contrast radiography

In contrast radiography studies of three infants with gastrointestinal manifestations of cow's milk or soya protein intolerance, a number of abnormalities were reported (Richards *et al.* 1988). These included thickening of the valvulae conniventes (plicae circulares), a ribbon-like ileum, and a thickened bowel wall in the small intestine, with narrowing, thumbprinting and spasm in the large intestine. The non-specific nature of these abnormalities (Taylor 1988) means that this is not a useful diagnostic investigation in a case of suspected cow's milk protein intolerance.

Key references 12.1

HILL DJ, FIRER MA, SHELTON MJ & HOSKING CS (1986) Manifestations of milk allergy in infancy: clinical and immunologic findings. *J Pediatr* **109**:270–276. In a series of children with cow's milk protein intolerance, only 42% had a positive RAST test to cow's milk, and only 47% had a positive skin test to cow's milk.

12.2

BÜRGIN-WOLFF A, SIGNER E, FRIESS HM, BERGER R, BIRBAUMER A & JUST M (1980) The diagnostic significance of antibodies to various cow's milk proteins (fluorescent immunosorbent test). *Eur J Pediat* **133**:17–24. The authors studied IgG, IgA, IgM and IgE antibodies to cow's milk proteins in 41 newborn infants and their mothers, 398 infants and young children not suffering from gastrointestinal conditions (mainly surgical patients), 41 healthy schoolchildren, 138 healthy adults, 20 children with cow's milk protein intolerance, 26 children with coeliac disease, and 25 children with gastroenteritis. *Detailed results showing the effect of age and disease on the incidence of different classes of milk protein antibodies, and underlining the fact that the possession of antibody to cow's milk protein is not pathognomonic for cow's milk protein intolerance.*

12.3

TAINIO VM & SAVILAHTI E (1990) Value of immunologic tests in cow milk allergy. *Allergy* **45**:189–196. 34 children with symptoms suggestive of cow's milk protein intolerance were studied; 19 had a positive reaction when challenged with cow's milk protein. Measurements were made of circulating IgG, IgA, IgM and IgE antibodies to cow's milk protein, as well as C3, C4, and lymphocyte responses to phytohaemagglutinin A, concavalin A and β-lactoglobulin. Twelve out of 19 had IgE antibodies to cow's milk protein. *No single laboratory method was sufficient to discriminate between the children who reacted to cow's milk protein and those who did not.*

12.4

FONTAINE JL & NAVARRO J (1975) Small intestinal biopsy in cow's milk protein allergy in infancy. *Arch Dis Child* **50**:357–362. Small bowel biopsies were performed in 31 infants with cow's milk protein intolerance. Mucosal changes were present in all but lacked any distinctive histological features.

Summary 12

Before making a diagnosis of cow's milk protein intolerance, it is important to consider other disorders, including lactose intolerance, feeding problems, coeliac disease, cystic fibrosis, chronic infection (e.g. giardiasis), and urinary tract infection. Investigations such as skin-prick tests, RAST tests, tests for milk precipitins, and an eosinophil count are unhelpful.

13 Cow's milk protein intolerance: diagnosis III
Diagnostic criteria

Trial of milk elimination

There are two situations which require a trial period of cow's milk protein elimination. One is when the doctor suspects the diagnosis of cow's milk protein intolerance. The other is when the parent suspects the diagnosis, but the doctor does not. If both parties are to be satisfied, then the procedure must be carefully planned, to avoid doubts later, for example: 'If only the cow's milk had been withdrawn a little longer, he might have got better'.

Coincidental improvement

The disappearance of symptoms following cow's milk protein withdrawal does not prove the diagnosis. The loss of symptoms could easily be a coincidence. The risks of failing to confirm the diagnosis at this stage are:
1 incorrect labelling of the child as cow's milk intolerant, and exposing the child to unnecessary dietary restriction;
2 failure to detect the real cause of the patient's reported symptoms.

Need for challenge

The second step to make the diagnosis is to demonstrate the reappearance of symptoms after the re-introduction of cow's milk protein. This should be done immediately following a successful trial period of cow's milk protein avoidance, except in two situations.
1 Where there is a history of a previous anaphylactic reaction to cow's milk protein. Challenges in this situation are especially hazardous, and should be delayed for a period of 6–12 months. Special precautions are then required for the challenge (see below).
2 Where a short period of cow's milk protein avoidance in hospital has been successful, especially where the intolerance may have been a sequel to gastroenteritis. Challenging the infant while still in hospital, and possibly before full recovery, risks serious relapse and is likely to prolong the period in hospital. Such infants should be discharged on a cow's milk substitute formula, and brought back for challenge once recovery is quite complete, say in 2–3 months.

Goldman criteria

In 1963, Goldman and his colleagues proposed stringent minimal criteria for the diagnosis of cow's milk protein intolerance (Goldman *et al.* 1963). These are usually referred to as the Goldman criteria, and for a time their fulfilment was regarded as an essential prerequisite for the diagnosis of cow's milk protein intolerance. The Goldman criteria are as follows.

1 Symptoms subside following cow's milk protein elimination.

2 Symptoms recur within 48 hours following a challenge with up to 100 ml of cow's milk. If a reaction fails to occur, unspecified larger amounts of cow's milk are added to the diet, and if this produces symptoms then this larger volume is used in subsequent challenges.

3 Three such challenges to be positive and similar as to onset, duration and clinical features.

4 Symptoms to subside following each challenge.

late reactors

In fact, Goldman *et al.* did not rigidly adhere to their own criteria, by including in their report several patients who only produced symptoms more than 48 hours after milk challenge, and they documented three patients who only reacted 7 days after a challenge. It is clear that insisting that symptoms must occur within 48 hours of a challenge will exclude a group of late reactors.

diagnostic delay

Goldman *et al.* recorded symptoms lasting up to 14 days after a single challenge. If one allowed 7 days to permit symptoms to appear after a challenge, and a further 14 days for symptoms to disappear before the next challenge, then it is clear that to employ the Goldman criteria of three challenges would entail a delay of at least 2 months before a diagnosis could be made of cow's milk protein intolerance. Such a strategy is impractical for routine clinical use, and possibly inappropriate for research studies, because some patients will have grown out of their intolerance before the challenges are complete. Goldman *et al.* provided no evidence to support the contention that three challenges were better or more reliable than one.

modified criteria

In the author's opinion, a single challenge, preceded and followed by improvement while avoiding cow's milk protein, is the most appropriate way to make the diagnosis. The exception to this is where the outcome of a challenge is unclear because the challenge accidentally coincides with an intercurrent illness. If there is doubt about the outcome, and this can be a problem with delayed eczematous reactions, then the challenge may have to be repeated several times.

Lactose intolerance

Because soya-based and casein hydrolysate-based milk formulae are lactose-free, patients with lactose intolerance will improve on cow's milk avoidance and relapse on re-introduction of cow's milk. Thus, if lactose intolerance is to be detected it has to be sought (see chapter 6) prior to cow's milk withdrawal and challenge.

Key reference 13.1

GOLDMAN AS, ANDERSON DW, SELLERS WA, SAPERSTEIN S, KNIKER WT & HALPERN SR (1963) Milk allergy 1. Oral challenge with milk and isolated milk proteins in allergic children. *Pediatrics* **32**:425–443. *A classic and detailed report of 89 children with cow's milk protein intolerance. This paper clearly describes the hazards of anaphylactic shock during cow's milk challenge and provides a useful breakdown of the timing and duration of symptoms after milk challenge. The authors suggest that three challenges are required for the diagnosis, a cumbersome approach which is no longer generally accepted.*

Summary 13

The criteria for the diagnosis of cow's milk protein intolerance are loss of symptoms on withdrawal of cow's milk protein, followed by recurrence of symptoms on re-introduction of cow's milk, followed by loss of symptoms when cow's milk is again withdrawn. These criteria will not distinguish between cow's milk protein intolerance and lactose intolerance. If the latter is to be detected then it must be sought prior to cow's milk withdrawal and challenge. Goldman and his colleagues suggested very stringent criteria for the diagnosis of cow's milk protein intolerance (three separate periods of withdrawal and challenge), but a single withdrawal-challenge-withdrawal sequence, provided the result is clear-cut, is generally regarded as adequate.

14 Cow's milk protein intolerance: diagnosis IV
Cow's milk exclusion and challenge: procedure

General strategy

The basic procedure required to diagnose cow's milk protein intolerance is:

1 a period of avoidance (2–28 days) causing loss of symptoms;
2 recurrence of symptoms on re-introduction of cow's milk protein;
3 loss of symptoms after second withdrawal of cow's milk protein;
4 continued abatement of symptoms with continued avoidance of cow's milk protein.

This strategy must be accompanied by regular attempts to re-introduce cow's milk protein, for example yearly, to see if the patient has grown out of the intolerance. It must be remembered that the features of cow's milk intolerance seen after cow's milk protein challenge may not be the same as the presenting symptoms, and in particular new symptoms (especially anaphylactic shock) may occur.

Duration of milk exclusion   The choice of duration required for a therapeutic trial of cow's milk protein avoidance depends on the symptoms, the circumstances and the response. In general, purely gastrointestinal symptoms and irritability improve within 1–3 days of cow's milk protein withdrawal, whereas in atopic eczema improvement may not be seen for 7–14 days. For most patients in hospital with troublesome vomiting or frequent loose stools, failure to improve at all within a couple of days on clear fluids suggests the problem is not straightforward cow's milk protein intolerance. There are some other reasons why cow's milk protein avoidance may fail, and these are described below.

for out-patients   For out-patient management, a trial period of 2 weeks is adequate, unless atopic eczema is a feature in which case up to 4 weeks elimination may be required. A shorter period of elimination risks uncertainty – 'would the child have improved if the diet had been tried a bit longer?'

Failure of milk exclusion   The reasons why a trial period of cow's milk elimination may fail are as follows.

1 The patient has an alternative cause for the reported symptoms.

2 The period of elimination was too short (see above).

3 Cow's milk protein has not been fully excluded from the diet, as would be the case, for example, in a child who continued to receive butter, cheese, or foods containing whey or casein. This is more likely to happen if a dietitian's help has not been sought.

4 The patient is intolerant to other items which have not been withdrawn from the diet. If there is no improvement on cow's milk protein withdrawal and other food intolerances are suspected, the options are either to abandon a dietary approach or to eliminate additional food items.

5 The patient is intolerant to the cow's milk substitute which has been given. This is a common problem with goat's milk or sheep's milk, an occasional problem with soya-based milk formulae (see chapter 21), and an uncommon problem with casein hydrolysate milk formulae (see chapter 18).

6 Co-existing or intercurrent disease, for example the symptoms of a baby with vomiting and loose stools caused by cow's milk protein intolerance which failed to improve because of an attack of gastroenteritis.

7 The patient's symptoms are trivial and have been exaggerated, or alternatively do not exist at all and have either been imagined or fabricated by the parents. Complete fabrication of symptoms by parents is uncommon, but the field of food intolerance appears to

offer special scope to parents who are susceptible to such behaviour (Warner & Hathaway 1984; Taylor 1992).

Overdiagnosis

The flaw in the strategy outlined so far is that the milk withdrawal and challenge are conducted as open rather than double-blind procedures. Where there is doubt about the existence of symptoms either on presentation or after challenge, then admission to hospital is required to verify the presence of symptoms. If, as happens rarely, the parents claim they can observe abnormalities which are not apparent to the nursing or medical staff, then the challenge must be repeated in a double-blind manner. This can be done quite simply by the introduction of cow's milk into the child's milk substitute.

Milk challenge procedure

A challenge with cow's milk protein is done for two reasons:
1 to confirm the diagnosis;
2 to see if the patient has grown out of the intolerance.

Challenge not needed

Before performing a milk challenge to see if a child has grown out of cow's milk protein intolerance, it is important to ask the parents what has happened if the child has recently been given cow's milk or food containing cow's milk protein. This frequently happens by accident. If it has been found at home that the child can tolerate small amounts of cow's milk then a formal challenge in hospital is not required, and the parents can simply continue to increase the quantity of cow's milk given to the child.

WARNING! anaphylaxis

It is vital to remember that during cow's milk protein challenge, symptoms may appear that had not been present previously. The real worry here is anaphylactic shock. In Goldman *et al.*'s original study, three out of 89 patients developed anaphylactic shock as a new symptom during milk challenge (Goldman *et al.* 1963). In a further five patients, anaphylaxis had been noted prior to milk challenge. Any strategy for cow's milk protein challenges has to take into account the risk of anaphylaxis (Editorial, 1984). The relative dearth of data on anaphylaxis means that the recommendations below are empirical, and based on the author's personal experience.

Procedure for patients with NO history of anaphylaxis after cow's milk ingestion
skin test

Prior to the challenge procedure described below, gently rub some cow's milk onto the patient's skin with a piece of gauze or cotton wool and observe for 15 min for urticaria. If this occurs, do not proceed with the challenge, continue cow's milk protein avoidance, and repeat direct skin tests in 12 months.

safest in hospital

If possible, perform milk challenges in hospital, because of the need for resuscitation facilities should anaphylaxis occur.

drugs   Adrenaline one in 1000, an antihistamine for intravenous use (e.g. chlorpheniramine), a nebulizer and a β-2 stimulant bronchodilator respiratory solution (e.g. terbutaline), and facilities for endotracheal intubation and tracheostomy must all be available.

observations   For the first 60 min of the procedure, a nurse or doctor should be present; the patient must not be left alone. The observer is looking for signs of an adverse reaction, which are:
1 rash around the mouth;
2 urticarial rash;
3 sneezing;
4 vomiting;
5 irritability and pallor;
6 wheezing or coughing;
7 loose stools;
8 stridor;
9 collapse.
After the first 60 min, the patient should be checked half-hourly, provided a parent is present, or quarter-hourly if no parent is present. The observer needs to know that the signs above are being sought, and that it is just as important to remove the clothes and look for an urticarial rash as it is to perform the usual nursing observations of the temperature, pulse and respiration rate.

stopping challenge   If any of the above signs appear, no further cow's milk should be given, and in the event of a rash, wheezing, stridor or collapse a doctor should be summoned.

milk administration   During the challenge, apart from the cow's milk being given, the patient should remain on a cow's milk protein-free diet.
1 Place one drop of ordinary cow's milk on the patient's tongue, and observe for 15 min.
2 If no reaction, give 5 ml of cow's milk and observe for 15 min.
3 If no reaction, give 10 ml of cow's milk and observe for 15 min.
4 If no reaction, give 30 ml of cow's milk and observe for 15 min.
5 If no reaction, give cow's milk freely, and give cow's milk protein-free solids as normal at meal times. Provided this does not exceed the usual intake volume, ensure the patient has taken at least 200 ml of cow's milk.

duration of observation   It is unclear how long obervation in hospital should be continued. Our former policy was to start challenges at 0900 hours, and if there was no reaction the patient was allowed to go home at 1700 hours. However, following a case in which delayed anaphylaxis only developed 9 hours after the commencement of milk challenge (David 1984) we now maintain observation in hospital for 12 hours.

if reaction occurs   If any adverse reaction occurs, as well as stopping further cow's milk it is essential to monitor the patient very closely, as such patients are at special risk of suffering severe and possibly fatal collapse without warning. Our practice is to keep infants in hospital overnight where a challenge has had to be stopped because of an adverse reaction. Such infants require close monitoring, including the use of an apnoea alarm.

uneventful challenge   If the challenge proceeds uneventfully, cow's milk should continue to be given to the child at home. Before discharge home, the parents need to be warned that adverse reactions can still happen for a few days, and if this happens cow's milk protein may need to be withdrawn again. Follow-up in about 4–6 weeks is arranged to check the final outcome of the challenge.

Procedure for patients with previous history of anaphylaxis after cow's milk ingestion
avoid challenges   Serious consideration should be given to whether a cow's milk challenge is really necessary. If it is being done to confirm the diagnosis, it is best omitted, because the risks of misdiagnosis are likely to be outweighed by the hazards of the challenge procedure. If the challenge is being done to see if the patient has grown out of cow's milk protein intolerance, then the author's recommendations are as follows.

1 Ensure that 12 months have elapsed since the previous positive challenge or anaphylactic reaction.
2 Prior to the challenge procedure outlined above, gently rub some cow's milk onto the patient's skin with a piece of gauze or cotton wool and observe for 15 min for urticaria. If this occurs, do not proceed with the challenge, continue cow's milk protein avoidance, and repeat direct skin tests in 12 months.
3 If there is no urticarial reaction (a red flare without a weal does not count), proceed with milk challenge as described above.

Key references   14.1   WALKER-SMITH JA (1988) *Diseases of the Small Intestine in Childhood*, 3rd edn, Butterworths, London. *Review, from a gastroenterological perspective.*

14.2   DAVID TJ (1989) Hazards of challenge tests in atopic dermatitis. *Allergy* **44** (suppl. 9):101–107. *Review, with special discussion of the risk of anaphylaxis and the way in which it might be minimized.*

Summary 14   The duration required for the initial period of cow's milk avoidance depends on the symptoms and the situation. For infants in hospital with loose stools or vomiting, 48 hours (on clear fluids) is usually adequate to demonstrate improvement. For patients at home a period of 2 weeks avoidance of cow's milk protein is best, unless atopic eczema is a feature, in which case 4 weeks elimination may be required. Cow's milk elimination may fail if the patient does not have cow's milk protein intolerance, if the duration of elimination was too short, if cow's milk protein has not been fully excluded, or if the patient has co-existing or intercurrent disease. Cow's milk challenge needs to be done in hospital because of the risk of anaphylaxis. The challenge procedure, which is only undertaken if rubbing cow's milk onto the skin fails to produce urticaria, is to introduce increasing volumes of ordinary cow's milk, starting with just one drop, while observing the patient closely.

15 Cow's milk protein intolerance: management
Milk exclusion, milk substitutes and prognosis

Cow's milk exclusion   Once the diagnosis has been established, then in most cases, if treatment is to be successful, cow's milk protein needs to be completely excluded (see also chapter 73). There are some patients with cow's milk protein intolerance who are able to tolerate small but not large quantities of cow's milk protein (see chapter 70), and clearly such patients need not be on a very strict avoidance regimen. In practice, the identification of such patients is not easy. Further, there is the worry that incomplete restriction of cow's milk protein may cause important symptoms which are undetected by parents. Goldman *et al.* (1963), in their challenge studies, pointed out that the signs of some reactions (for example auscultatory findings) would have been missed had it not been for careful medical observation during the challenges. Local practice, therefore, is to recommend complete avoidance, at least initially. A further reason for strict exclusion, at least when the cow's milk protein avoidance is commenced, is that on occasions a symptom is only recognized as such after it has disappeared, following strict dietary elimination. If it becomes clear, either because of accidental or planned re-introduction of cow's milk, that a patient can tolerate small amounts of cow's milk protein without symptoms, there are no grounds for insisting on complete exclusion.

complete exclusion   Complete exclusion means the avoidance not only of cow's milk or cow's milk formulae, but also a wide range of foods which contain cow's milk or its protein components. It is fairly apparent that

Table 15.1 Foods in which it is not obvious that cow's milk protein may be present

Soya cheese
Vegetarian cheese
Margarine and low fat spreads
Some bread
Biscuits
Sausages
Rusks
'Non-milk-fat' ice-cream
Instant mashed potato
Muesli and other breakfast cereals
Packet and tinned soups
Fish fingers and fish in batter

certain products such as butter or cheese are derived from cow's milk, but for other food such as, for example, most margarines, it is not at all obvious (Table 15.1). Furthermore, cow's milk protein may be included in foodstuffs in the form of casein or whey, and although this may be clearly indicated on the list of ingredients, many people are unaware that whey and casein are derived from cow's milk. Finally, in the UK at least, there are some inconsistencies in the requirements for listing the ingredients in food. An example is chocolate, which is exempt from the usual requirements to list ingredients, so that a purchaser is likely to be unaware of the presence of cow's milk protein.

special traps

In practice, there are some common and potentially dangerous problems for those who wish to avoid completely cow's milk protein.
1 *Casein and whey.* The medical profession may be accustomed to technical names, but parents are not. It may be obvious to the reader of this book that 'caseinate' and 'whey powder' are related to casein and whey, but lay people find these names unfamiliar and confusing. Even the most diligent parent may make mistakes, and this means that these terms need very careful explanation.
2 *Soya products.* Soya products are often specifically purchased because of the need to avoid cow's milk protein. Parents and shopkeepers may assume wrongly that because a product is soya-based it is therefore cow's milk-free (Fig. 15.1). There is a case for special labelling of all soya-based products, so that there is a clear indication on the front of the packet if cow's milk protein is present.
3 *Vegetarian cheese.* This is often purchased in the mistaken belief that it is free from cow's milk protein. In fact, the term 'vegetarian cheese' simply means that it has been made with rennet of vegetable origin (David 1989a).

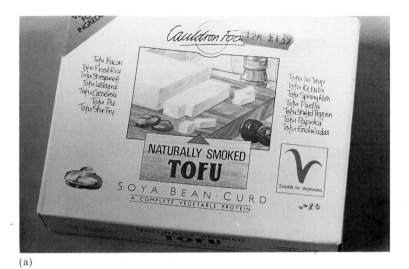

(a)

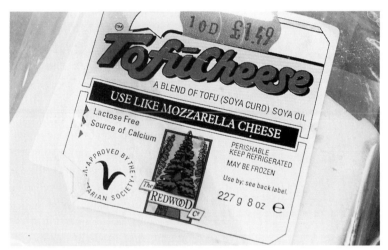

(b)

(c)

Fig. 15.1 (a) This smoked tofu, made from soya curd, and free from cow's milk protein, was regularly eaten by a 12-year-old boy with eczema, asthma and intolerance to cow's milk protein. (b) Relatives of the child purchased this cheese, also made from soya curd, having been assured by a health food shop vendor that the product was milk free. After eating two mouthfuls of a grated cheese sandwich made from this product the boy developed a severe generalized anaphylactic reaction, and he was dead within 35 minutes. (c) The list of ingredients on the back of the tofu cheese clearly indicated that the product contained cow's milk protein in the form of casein.

Dietitian   Parents cannot be expected to be aware of such details, and the parents of all patients on a cow's milk-free diet need to be referred to a dietitian if complete cow's milk exclusion is to be achieved. This includes infants who are only receiving milk, as the parents will require advice about a cow's milk-free weaning diet. In the UK, as well as giving advice, a dietitian will be able to provide an appropriate diet sheet and a list of milk-free manufactured foods which is regularly kept up to date by the British Dietetic Association.

Beef exclusion   There is no need to exclude beef just because a patient is on a cow's milk-free diet. Patients with cow's milk protein intolerance can indeed have other food intolerances, but co-existing intolerance to beef is the exception rather than the rule. In the most informative study which addressed the issue of co-existing food intolerance in children with cow's milk protein intolerance, 21 out of 39 patients had reproducible intolerance to other foods, but in only one child was this intolerance to beef (Høst & Halken 1990). (The most common foods were egg (11 out of 39), citrus fruit (9 out of 39) and tomato (5 out of 39). Thus routine beef avoidance is unwarranted, and is likely to cause needless dietary restriction in most cases.

Tolerance   Although the author recommends cow's milk challenges to be done in hospital, patients often receive cow's milk prior to such challenge, either by accident or because the parents disregard advice. In some of these cases recurrence of symptoms ensures continuation of the diet. In others the absence or minor nature of the symptoms leads parents to gradually re-introduce cow's milk. An important area of uncertainty is the question of whether repeated exposure to small quantities of food (in this case cow's milk) increases, decreases, or has no effect upon the chances of growing out of intolerance to the food.

Prognosis   There is little objective data on the prognosis. The duration of milk protein intolerance varies greatly (Bahna & Heiner 1980). Often it lasts only a few months, and in many cases it has disappeared completely by the age of 12 months. For this reason we re-challenge at the age of 12 months all patients who were diagnosed in infancy. Most patients become tolerant to cow's milk protein by the age of 5 years, although intolerance persists, occasionally into adult life, in a small number of patients (Savilahti *et al.* 1989; Bishop *et al.* 1990; Høst & Halken 1990). The severity of the symptoms seems to have no bearing on the prognosis, although in one series of patients with cow's milk protein intolerance who presented with chronic diarrhoea, one-third remained intolerant at a median age of 7 years (Businco *et al.* 1985).

Table 15.2 Types of milk and milk substitute, and their calcium content

Milk	Calcium (mg/100 ml)	Unit weight	Price[1]
Animal milk			
Human milk	34		
Cow's milk	120		
Goat's milk	130		
Sheep's milk	200		
Cow's milk formulae			
SMA White cap	56	450 g	£2.37
SMA Gold cap	44.5	450 g	£2.37
Ostermilk	35	450 g	£2.38
Ostermilk two	61	450 g	£2.38
Cow & Gate Premium	54	450 g	£2.69
Cow & Gate Plus	85	450 g	£2.60
Milumil	71	450 g	£2.52
Aptamil	59	450 g	£2.52
Milupa HN25	70	250 g	£4.21
Progress	115	450 g	£2.19
Farley's Junior	72	450 g	£2.57
Soya-based formulae			
Wysoy	60	430 g	£3.10
Cow & Gate Formula S	54	450 g	£3.08
Isomil	70	400 g	£2.99
Prosobee	60	400 g	£3.56
Ostersoy	56	450 g	£2.89
Cow's milk protein hydrolysate formulae			
Nutramigen	64	1 lb	£7.00
Pregestimil	63	1 lb	£8.01
Alfare	54	400 g	£7.27
Pepti Junior	54	400 g	£7.18
Bovine collagen, soya hydrolysate and amino acid-based formula			
Prejomin	51	400 g	£7.35

[1] Trade price. Source: Chemist & Druggist Price List (1991) **32**(10) (October). The retail price varies, but it is up to twice the trade price.

Cow's milk substitutes

Infants on a cow's milk protein-free diet require a cow's milk substitute. The choice is between a soya-based milk formula or a casein-hydrolysate milk formula (Table 15.2). Goat's and sheep's milk are inadvisable. Both have a high solute content and in an unmodified form they are unsuitable for infants under the age of 12 months (Parry 1984; Taitz & Armitage 1984; Taitz & Wardley 1985). The production of milk from goats and sheep is not subject to the same stringent health regulations as cow's milk, and both carry the risk of serious gastrointestinal infection (Taitz & Armitage 1984; Roberts 1985; Taitz & Wardley 1985). Finally, a high proportion of those with cow's milk protein intolerance are also intolerant to goat or sheep's milk, which are antigenically very similar to cow's milk.

Soya   The advantages of soya-based cow's milk formulae, which are all lactose-free, is their cheapness and reasonably acceptable flavour. The principal drawback is the possibility of associated soya intolerance. Parents using soya-based milk substitutes must be warned that other soya-based milks, such as Plamil or Granose Soya Milk, are not complete infant formulae, and are lacking in calcium, vitamins and energy.

Casein or whey hydrolysate   An alternative cow's milk substitute is a milk formula in which the protein content is hydrolysed cow's milk protein. These formulae often have a poor flavour and tend to be expensive. Animal experiments have suggested that these formulae are less antigenic than cow's milk, but intolerance, although uncommon, can occur. Protein hydrolysate formulae, and so-called hypoallergenic formulae are discussed in detail in chapters 16 to 18. If an infant with cow's milk protein intolerance is also intolerant to soya-based and protein hydrolysate-based formulae, the options are to use donated human milk (more difficult in practice nowadays because of the need to ensure that the donor is not infected with the HIV virus), a comminuted chicken-based formula (see chapter 19), a so-called elemental diet (see chapter 19), or in exceptional circumstances intravenous feeding. After early infancy, the rare cases of intolerance to all milk substitutes are dealt with by introducing milk-free solids, with added calcium supplements.

Breast-fed infants   In infants with cow's milk protein intolerance who are being breast-fed, the mother will also need to avoid cow's milk protein in her own diet.

Need for calcium   Cow's milk and cow's milk products are the major source of *calcium* in the diet of human infants. If cow's milk and its products are withdrawn from the diet, then some source of calcium is required in infancy, and possibly later. The simplest way to do this is to provide a standard soya-based or casein hydrolysate-based milk formula, which contains amounts of calcium similar to ordinary cow's milk based formulae (see Table 15.2). An alternative, in an infant old enough, is to avoid the use of any form of milk and provide a calcium supplement (Table 15.3). If this is done a vitamin supplement may also be needed, as milk formulae constitute a major source of vitamins for infants who are not fully weaned.

Table 15.3 Selected calcium supplements[1]

Supplement	Contents per tablet	Elemental calcium per tablet[2]
Calcium and ergocalciferol[3]		
Calcium sodium lactate		
(or calcium lactate 300 mg)	450 mg	1.975 mmol
Calcium phosphate	150 mg	
Calciferol	0.01 mg	
Effervescent calcium gluconate[4]		
Calcium gluconate	1000 mg	2.25 mmol
Calcium gluconate[3]		
Calcium gluconate	600 mg	1.35 mmol

[1] Numerous other calcium supplements are available, but they are not listed here as they all contain either colouring agents or preservatives or both, and the details of these additives are not published. Details of these additives can sometimes be obtained by contacting the manufacturers.
[2] 1 mmol of calcium is equal to 40.08 mg calcium.
[3] Excipients vary with manufacturer, but may include vanillin, prepared theobroma, sucrose, lactose, maize starch, stearic acid, magnesium stearate.
[4] Excipients vary with manufacturer, but may include vanillin, prepared theobroma, sucrose, lactose, maize starch, stearic acid, magnesium stearate, saccharin sodium, anhydrous citric acid, tartaric acid, sodium bicarbonate, povidone.

How much calcium is needed?
general recommendations

The amount of calcium required for infants and children is far from clear (Devlin *et al.* 1989). Formerly, the then UK Department of Health and Social Security recommended an intake of 600 mg (15 mmol) per day for children under the age of 9 years (Department of Health & Social Security, 1981). More recently, a working party of the Department of Health (in the UK) recommended a daily intake of 13.1 mmol for infants, rising to 25.0 mmol for those aged 11–18 years (Department of Health, 1991). The requirements for calcium (Table 15.4) are age-related (more needed for rapid growth during the first year of life and during the pubertal growth spurt), but are enhanced by obligatory urinary losses and incomplete intestinal absorption (Devlin *et al.* 1989).

requirements of normal children are not necessarily appropriate

Claims that normal healthy children can grow satisfactorily with far lower intakes of calcium (Walker 1972) need to be treated with caution. There are two potential traps. Firstly, those with food intolerance should not be regarded as normal healthy subjects. For example, some children with cow's milk protein intolerance will

Table 15.4 Calcium accretion rate
and requirements by age[1]

Age (years)	Accretion rate (mg/day)	Approximate requirements (mg/day)
0–1	190	300
2–7	70	150
8–10	140	250
11–18	250	500

[1] Source: Devlin *et al.* (1989).

have had some degree of malabsorption prior to cow's milk elimination, and an enteropathy has been described in children with intolerance to other foods such as soya, egg, fish, rice and chicken (Ament & Rubin 1972; Iyngkaran *et al.* 1982; Vitoria *et al.* 1982; see chapter 61). Secondly, the intake of calcium cannot be taken in isolation, without consideration of the phosphate intake and the vitamin D status. Much of the evidence suggesting that normal children need very little calcium comes from countries with a lot of sunshine (Walker 1972), and the situation may be very different in temperate areas. We have reported rickets in two children with a low calcium intake due to a cow's milk-free diet (David 1989b). Both had been kept out of the sunlight for prolonged periods because of severe atopic eczema, and a lack of vitamin D is likely to have compounded the effects of a low calcium intake. Thus, those with atopic eczema may be at special risk from a deficient calcium intake (David *et al.* 1984), as may be those from certain populations especially prone to rickets (e.g. Asians).

author's recommendations Our practice is to provide one calcium and ergocalciferol tablet (see Table 15.3) daily to children on a long-term cow's milk-free diet who are not receiving a calcium and vitamin D-containing milk substitute and:

1 who are under the age of 2 years; or
2 who are avoiding other foods as well; or
3 who have atopic eczema; or
4 who are Asian.

Mothers who are breast-feeding and who are on a diet avoiding cow's milk products may also require a calcium supplement.

Calcium supplements In practice, calcium supplements can be divided into those which contain no colouring agents or preservatives, and those that do. This is of practical importance because it is common in certain patients (for example those with atopic eczema) to attempt to avoid these additives. The only calcium supplements free from colouring agents or preservatives in the UK are calcium and ergocalciferol tablets and calcium gluconate tablets (see Table 15.3). The former are crushed or chewed, and the latter dissolved in water. Our preference is for calcium with ergocalciferol if the patient has atopic eczema, because of its ergocalciferol content and because of the risk that the child may (rightly or wrongly) be kept out of the sunlight.

intolerance to calcium supplements

Inexplicably, there appear to be a small number of children who are intolerant to calcium supplements, even to supplements which are free from colouring agents and preservatives. Studies in two such patients demonstrated adverse reactions (worsening of pre-existing atopic eczema) to the blind administration of intravenous calcium salts, implicating the calcium salts rather than an excipient in calcium tablets (Devlin & David 1990). The mechanism of such reactions is unknown.

Key references 15.1   Taitz LS & Armitage BL (1984) Goat's milk for infants and children. *Br Med J* **288**:428–429. *An editorial review of the inappropriate use and hazards of feeding goat's milk to infants and children.*

15.2   Department of Health (1991) Report on Health and Social Subjects 41. *Dietary Reference Values for Food Enery and Nutrients for the United Kingdom. Report of the Panel on Dietary Reference Values of the Committee on Medical Aspects of Food Policy*, Her Majesty's Stationery Office, London. *The old term of recommended daily amount (RDA), which was intended to refer to nutrient needs of populations rather than individuals has been scrapped. This new report introduces the concept of the reference nutrient intake (RNI), which is defined as the amount of the nutrient that is enough, or more than enough, for about 97% of people in a group. The panel set up a number of expert working groups to consider the requirements of children and adults for about 40 different nutrients, and their recommendations are accompanied by a well referenced discussion of the function, metabolism and age-related requirements for each nutrient.*

15.3   David TJ, Waddington E & Stanton RHJ (1984) Nutritional hazards of elimination diets in children with atopic eczema. *Arch Dis Child* **59**:323–325. Low intakes of calcium were discovered in 13 out of 23 children with atopic eczema on elimination diets, but in none of the 23 controls. *This study pointed out the need for continued supervision by a dietitian in any child on an elimination diet.*

15.4   Devlin J, Stanton RHJ & David TJ (1989) Calcium intake and cows' milk free diets. *Arch Dis Child* **64**:1183–1184. Predictably enough, of 20 children with atopic eczema who were on a diet with excluded cow's milk protein and a number of other foods, and in whom a milk substitute was not given, eight had a calcium intake (as assessed by 5-day diet survey) which was below the age-related requirement. Less predictably, of 26 who were on a similar diet but who were prescribed a milk substitute, three had a low calcium intake. *It is unsafe to assume that a prescription for a milk substitute will guarantee an adequate calcium intake. Some milk substitutes have a lower calcium content than cow's milk formulae, and poor palatability may mean that the child refuses to drink the milk substitute.*

15.5   Kooh SW, Fraser D, Reilly BJ, Hamilton JR, Gall DG & Bell L (1977) Rickets due to calcium deficiency. *New Engl J Med* **297**:1264–1266. *This detailed case report demonstrates that a deficient calcium intake, even in the face of adequate vitamin D intake, and in the absence of vitamin D resistance, can cause rickets.*

15.6   Walker ARP (1972) The human requirement of calcium: should low intakes be supplemented? *Amer J Clin Nutr* **22**:518–530. *This detailed review challenges the concept that a low calcium intake is harmful. The author supports his argument with data from South Africa, where a large proportion of the Bantu population have a very low intake of calcium in the diet.*

15.7   Bürgin-Wolff A, Signer E, Friess HM, Berger R, Birbaumer A & Just M (1980) The diagnostic significance of antibodies to various cow's milk proteins (fluorescent immunosorbent test). *Eur J Pediat* **133**:17–24. IgG antibodies to cow's milk proteins fell immediately after commencing cow's milk protein avoidance, and continued to fall over the next 6 to 8 months. After challenge, the antibody titre rose. *The results suggest that one might be able to use IgG antibody measurements as a way of checking adherence to a cow's milk protein-free diet. (But see also Hill et al. (1989) – in this study it appeared that those in whom tolerance developed had higher levels of IgG antibodies to milk proteins.)*

15.8   Høst A & Halken S (1990) A prospective study of cow milk allergy in Danish infants during the first 3 years of life. *Allergy* **45**:587–596. A cohort of 1749 newborns from Odense in Denmark were followed prospectively for the development of cow's milk protein intolerance developing in the first year of life. Of 117 (6.7%) with symptoms suggestive of cow's milk protein intolerance, the diagnosis was confirmed by withdrawal and challenge in 39 infants (2.2%). Patients were re-challenged every 6–12 months. Total recovery had occurred in 22 patients (56%) by 1 year, 30 patients (77%) at 2 years, and 34 out of 39 patients (87%) at 3 years. 9 out of 39 were still intolerant to other foods at 3 years. *This careful, community-based study confirms a good prognosis for most children who develop cow's milk protein intolerance in the first year of life.*

15.9   Bishop JM, Hill DJ & Hosking CS (1990) Natural history of cow milk allergy: clinical outcome. *J Pediat* **116**:862–867. Of an initial cohort of 100 children with cow's milk protein intolerance (mean age at diagnosis 16 months), 97 were reviewed after 5 years. Tolerance to cow's milk was demonstrated by challenge in 28% by 2 years of age, 56% by 4 years, and 78% by 6 years. *Not quite as secure a study as the one above, but again showing a good prognosis.*

Summary 15   In the initial period, once a diagnosis of cow's milk protein intolerance has been made, complete exclusion of cow's milk protein is required in children with cow's milk intolerance, though sooner or later many patients are able to tolerate varying quantities of cow's milk protein. The majority of patients are able to fully tolerate cow's milk by the age of 3 years. Since cow's milk protein is included in a large range of manufactured foods, and because this is often not obvious from the food label, it is best to refer all patients who require a cow's milk-free diet to a dietitian. Beef exclusion is usually unnecessary. Goat's milk or sheep's milk are unsuitable as cow's milk substitutes, and the choice lies between soya-based or casein hydrolysate-based formulae. A deficient calcium intake is the principal hazard of an unsupervised diet avoiding cow's milk, and some children not receiving a milk formula require a calcium supplement.

References to Chapters 5–15

AMENT ME & RUBIN CE (1972) Soy protein – another cause of the flat intestinal lesion. *Gastroenterology* **62**:227–234.

ARMENIO L, BRUNETTI L, COLAZZO D, CARDINALE F & MAPPA L (1989) Food hypersensitivity and atopic dermatitis: something is changing? *Allergy* **44** (suppl. 9):140–146.

ATHERTON DJ (1988) Diet and atopic eczema. *Clin Allergy* **18**:215–228.

BAHNA SL & HEINER DC (1980) *Allergies to Milk*, Grune & Stratton, New York.

BARFOOT RA, McENERY G, ERSSER RS & SEAKINS JW (1988) Diarrhoea due to breast milk: case of fucose intolerance? *Arch Dis Child* **63**:311.

BAUMER H (1988) Diarrhoea due to breast milk: a case of fucose intolerance. *Arch Dis Child* **63**:1296–1297.

BISHOP JM, HILL DJ & HOSKING CS (1990) Natural history of cow milk allergy: clinical outcome. *J Pediat* **116**:862–867.

BOAT TF, POLMAR SH, WHITMAN V, KLEINERMAN JL, STERN RC & DOERSHUK CF (1975) Hyperreactivity to cow milk in young children with pulmonary hemosiderosis and cor pulmonale secondary to nasopharyngeal obstruction. *J Pediat* **87**:23–29.

BOCK SA (1991) Oral challenge procedures. In Metcalfe DD, Sampson HA & Simon RA (eds) *Food Allergy: Adverse Reactions to Foods and Food Additives*, pp. 81–95, Blackwell Scientific Publications, Boston.

BRODRIBB HS (1944) Allergic vomiting in an infant. *Arch Dis Child* **19**:140–142.

BUISSERET PD (1978) Common manifestations of cow's milk allergy in children. *Lancet* **1**:304–305.

BUSINCO L, BENINCORI N, CANTANI A, TACCONI L & PICARAZZI A (1985) Chronic diarrhea due to cow's milk allergy. A 4- to 10-year follow-up study. *Ann Allergy* **55**:844–847.

CARRE IJ, McCRAE WM, MOWAT AP, BRUNT PW & CAMPBELL AGM (1984) Disorders of the alimentary tract. In Forfar JO & Arneil GC (eds) *Textbook of Paediatrics*, 3rd edn, pp. 415–524, Churchill Livingstone, Edinburgh.

CASIMIR GJA, DUCHATEAU J, BRASSEUR DJ & VIS HL (1986) Life-threatening gastrointestinal symptoms in infants allergic to cow's milk. *Eur J Pediat* **145**:240–241.

CLEIN NW (1954) Cow's milk allergy in infants. *Pediat Clin North Am* **4**:949–962.

COLLINS-WILLIAMS C (1955) Acute allergic reactions to cow's milk. *Ann Allergy* **13**:415–421.

COOMBS RRA & HOLGATE ST (1990) Allergy and cot death: with special focus on allergic sensitivity to cows' milk and anaphylaxis. *Clin Exper Allergy* **20**: 359–366.

COOMBS RRA & MCLAUGHLAN P (1982) The enigma of cot death: is the modified-anaphylaxis hypothesis an explanation for some cases? *Lancet* **1**: 1388–1389.

COULTATE TP (1984) *Food. The Chemistry of Its Components.* Royal Society of Chemistry, London.

COUNAHAN R & WALKER-SMITH J (1976) Stool and urinary sugars in normal neonates. *Arch Dis Child* **51**:517–520.

CRAWFORD LV & GROGAN FT (1961) Allergenicity of cow's milk proteins. IV. Relationship of goat's milk proteins as studied by serum-agar precipitation. *J Pediat* **59**:347–350.

CREMIN FM & POWER P (1985) Vitamins in bovine and human milks. In Fox PF (ed) *Developments in Dairy Chemistry – 3. Lactose and Minor Constituents*, pp. 337–398, Elsevier, London.

DAVID TJ (1984) Anaphylactic shock during elimination diets for severe atopic eczema. *Arch Dis Child* **59**:983–986.

DAVID TJ (1989a) Hazards of challenge tests in atopic dermatitis. *Allergy* **44** (suppl. 9):101–107.

DAVID TJ (1989b) Short stature in children with atopic eczema. *Acta Derm Venereol* **144** (suppl.):41–44.

DAVID TJ, WADDINGTON E & STANTON RHJ (1984) Nutritional hazards of elimination diets in children with atopic eczema. *Arch Dis Child* **59**:323–325.

DEPARTMENT OF HEALTH (1991) *Report on health and social subjects 41. Dietary Reference Values for Food Enery and Nutrients for the United Kingdom.* Her Majesty's Stationery Office, London.

DEPARTMENT OF HEALTH AND SOCIAL SECURITY (1981) *Report on health and social subjects no. 15. Recommended Daily Amounts of Food Energy and Nutrients for Groups of People in the United Kingdom.* Her Majesty's Stationery Office, London.

DEVEY ME, ANDERSON KJ, COOMBS RRA, HENSCHEL MJ & COATES ME (1976) The modified anaphylaxis hypothesis for cot death. Anaphylactic sensitisation in guinea-pigs fed cow's milk. *Clin Exp Immunol* **26**:542–548.

DEVLIN J & DAVID TJ (1990) Intolerance to oral and intravenous calcium supplements in atopic eczema. *J Roy Soc Med* **83**:497–498.

DEVLIN J, STANTON RHJ & DAVID TJ (1989) Calcium intake and cows' milk free diets. *Arch Dis Child* **64**:1183–1184.

EDITORIAL (1984) Infantile bloody diarrhoea and cow's milk allergy. *Lancet* **1**:1159–1160.

EGAN H, KIRK RS & SAWYER R (1987) *Pearson's Chemical Analysis of Foods.* 8th edn, pp. 432–473, Longman Scientific & Technical, Harlow.

FINKELSTEIN H (1905) Kuhmilch als Ursache akuter Ernährungsstörungen bei Säuglingen. *Monatschr Kinderheilk* **4**:65–72.

FLATZ G (1989) The genetic polymorphism of intestinal lactase activity in adult humans. In Scriver CR, Beaudet AL, Sly WS & Valle D (eds) *The Metabolic Basis of Inherited Disease*, 6th edn, pp. 2999–3006, McGraw Hill, New York.

FONTAINE JL & NAVARRO J (1975) Small intestinal biopsy in cow's milk protein allergy in infancy. *Arch Dis Child* **50**:357–362.

GERRARD JW (1966) Familial recurrent rhinorrhea and bronchitis due to cow's milk. *J Am Med Ass* **198**:605–607.

GERRARD JW (1979) Allergy in breast fed babies to ingredients in breast milk. *Ann Allergy* **42**:69–72.

GERRARD JW, HEINER DC, IVES EJ & HARDY LW (1963) Milk allergy. *Clin Pediat* **2**:634–641.

GERRARD JW, MACKENZIE JWA, GOLUBOFF N, GARSON JZ & MANINGAS CS (1973) Cow's milk allergy: prevalence and manifestations in an unselected series of newborns. *Acta Paed Scand* **234** (suppl.):1–21.

GITZELMANN R, STEINMANN B & VAN DEN BERGHE G (1989) Disorders of fructose metabolism. In Scriver CR, Beaudet AL, Sly WS & Valle D (eds) *The Metabolic Basis of Inherited Disease*, 6th edn, pp. 399–424, McGraw Hill, New York.

GJESING B, ØSTERBALLE O, SCHWARTZ B, WAHN U & LØWENSTEIN H (1986) Allergen-specific IgE antibodies against antigenic components in cow milk and milk substitutes. *Allergy* **41**:51–56.

GOLDMAN AS, ANDERSON DW, SELLERS WA, SAPERSTEIN S, KNIKER WT & HALPERN SR (1963) Milk allergy. I. Oral challenge with milk and isolated milk proteins in allergic children. *Pediatrics* **32**:425–443.

GRAY GM (1983) Intestinal disaccharidase deficiencies and glucose-galactose malabsorption. In Stanbury JB, Wyngaarden JB, Fredrickson DS, Goldstein JL & Brown MS (eds) *The Metabolic Basis of Inherited Disease*, 5th edn, pp. 1729–1742, McGraw Hill, New York.

GRIBBIN M, WALKER-SMITH J & WOOD C (1976) Delayed recovery following acute gastroenteritis. *Acta Paed Belgica* **29**:167–176.

GUDMAND-HOYER E (1985) Sucrose malabsorption in children: a report of thirty-one Greenlanders. *J Pediat Gastroenterol Nutr* **4**:873–877.

HADDAD ZH, KALRA V & VERMA S (1979) IgE antibodies to peptic-tryptic digets of betalactoglobulin: significance in food hypersensitivity. *Ann Allergy* **42**:368–371.

HANDELMAN NI & NELSON TL (1964) Association of milk precipitins and esophageal lesions causing aspiration. *Pediatrics* **34**:699–703.

HANSON LA & MANSSON I (1961) Immune electrophoretic studies of bovine milk and milk products. *Acta Paediat* **50**:484–490.

HARRISON CJ, PUNTIS JWL, DURBIN GM, GORNALL P & BOOTH IW (1991) Atypical allergic colitis in preterm infants. *Acta Paediat Scand* **80**:1113–1116.

HILL DJ, FIRER MA, BALL G & HOSKING CS (1989) Recovery from milk allergy in early childhood: antibody studies. *J Pediat* **114**:761–766.

HILL DJ, FIRER MA, SHELTON MJ & HOSKING CS (1986) Manifestations of milk allergy in infancy: clinical and immunologic findings. *J Pediat* **109**:270–276.

HILL DJ, FORD RPK, SHELTON MJ & HOSKING CS (1984) A study of 100 infants and young children with cow's milk allergy. *Clin Rev Allergy* **2**:125–142.

HILL DJ & HOSKING CS (1991) Cow's milk allergy. In David TJ (ed) *Recent Advances in Paediatrics*, vol. 9, pp. 187–206, Churchill Livingstone, London.

HILL LW (1939) Immunologic relationships between cow's milk and goat's milk. *J Pediat* **15**:157–162.

HILL SM, PHILLIPS AD, MEARNS M & WALKER-SMITH JA (1989) Cows' milk sensitive enteropathy in cystic fibrosis. *Arch Dis Child* **64**:1251–1255.

HØST A & HALKEN S (1990) A prospective study of cow milk allergy in Danish infants during the first 3 years of life. Clinical course in relation to clinical and immunological type of hypersensitivity reaction. *Allergy* **45**:587–596.

IYNGKARAN N, ABIDAIN Z, MENG LL & YADAV M (1982) Egg-protein-induced villous atrophy. *J Pediat Gastroenterol Nutr* **1**:29–35.

IYNGKARAN N, YADAV M, BOEY CG & LAM KL (1988a) Effect of continued feeding of cows' milk on asymptomatic infants with milk protein sensitive enteropathy. *Arch Dis Child* **63**:911–915.

IYNGKARAN N, YADAV M, BOEY CG & LAM KL (1988b) Severity and extent of upper small bowel mucosal damage in cow's milk protein-sensitive entero-pathy. *J Pediat Gastroenterol Nutr* **7**:667–674.

IYNGKARAN N, YADAV M & BOEY CG (1989) Rectal mucosa in cow's milk allergy. *Arch Dis Child* **64**:1256–1260.

JENKINS HR, PINCOTT JR, SOOTHILL JF, MILLA PJ & HARRIES JT (1984) Food allergy: the major cause of infantile colitis. *Arch Dis Child* **59**:326–329.

JOLIAT TL & WEBER RW (1991) Occupational asthma and rhinoconjunctivitis from inhalation of crystalline bovine serum albumin powder. *Ann Allergy* **66**:301–304.

JONES RHT (1977) Congenital thrombocytopenia and milk allergy. *Arch Dis Child* **52**:744–745.

JUNTUNEN K & ALI-YRKKÖ S (1983) Goat's milk for children allergic to cow's milk. *Kiel Milchwirt Forschungsber* **35**:439–440.

KERLEY CG (1936) Allergic manifestations to cow's milk. *New York J Med* **36**:1320–1322.

KERRY KR & ANDERSON CM (1964) A ward test for sugar in the faeces. *Lancet* **1**:981–982.

KITCHEN BJ (1985) Indigenous milk enzymes. In Fox PF (ed) *Developments in Dairy Chemistry – 3. Lactose and Minor Constituents*, pp. 239–279, Elsevier, London.

KUITUNEN P, VISAKORPI JK, SAVILAHTI E & PELKONEN P (1975) Malabsorption syndrome with cow's milk intolerance. Clinical findings and course in 54 cases. *Arch Dis Child* **50**:351–356.

LACTOCHEM LTD (1988) Crewe, Cheshire CW1 1QT, United Kingdom. Personal communication to author.

LEBENTHAL E, LAOR J, LEWITUS Z, MATOTH Y & FREIER S (1970) Gastrointes-tinal protein loss in allergy to cow's milk β-lacto-globulin. *Israel J Med Sci* **6**:506–510.

LEE FA (1983) *Basic Food Chemistry*, 2nd edn, pp. 363–395, Avi Publishing Company, Westport.

LEE SK, KNIKER WT, COOK CD & HEINER DC (1978) Cow's milk-induced pulmonary disease in children. *Adv Paediat* **25**:39–57.

LEVIN B, ABRAHAM JM, BURGESS EA & WALLIS PG (1970) Congenital lactose malabsorption. *Arch Dis Child* **45**:173–177.

MANUEL P & WALKER-SMITH JA (1980) Decline of hypernatraemia as a problem in gastroenteritis. *Arch Dis Child* **55**:124–127.

MCENERY G & SEAKINS JW (1988) Reply to letter from Dr H. Baumer. *Arch Dis Child* **63**:1296–1297.

MCLAUGHLAN P, ANDERSON KJ, WIDDOWSON EM & COOMBS RRA (1981) Effect of heat on the anaphylactic-sensitising capacity of cows' milk, goats' milk, and various infant formulae fed to guinea pigs. *Arch Dis Child* **56**:165–171.

OSVATH P & MARKUS M (1968) Diagnostic value of thrombopenia and eosino-philia after food ingestion in children with milk and egg allergy. *Acta Paediat Acad Sci Hung* **9**:279–284.

OSVATH P, MURANYI L, ENDRE L & HARSANYI G (1972) Investigation of the cross reaction of cow's hair and milk antigen in bronchial provocation. *Acta Allergol* **27**:355–363.

PARISH WE, BARRETT AM, COOMBS RRA & CAMPS FE (1960) Hypersensitivity to milk and sudden death in infancy. *Lancet* **2**:1106–1110.

PARRY TE (1984) Goat's milk in infants and children. *Br Med J* **288**:863.

POWELL GK (1978) Milk- and soy-induced enterocolitis of infancy. *J Pediat* **93**:553–560.

PRAHL P, KRASILNIKOFF F, STAHL SKOV P & NORN S (1988) Basophil histamine release in children with adverse reactions to cow milk. Comparison to RAST and skin prick test. *Allergy* **43**:442–448.

RICHARDS DG, SOMERS S, ISSENMAN RM & STEVENSON GW (1988) Cow's milk protein/soy protein allergy: gastrointestinal imaging. *Radiology* **167**:721–723.

RICHET C (1931) Food anaphylaxis. *J Allergy* **2**:76–84.

ROBERTS D (1985) Microbiological aspects of goat's milk. A Public Health Laboratory Service Survey. *J Hyg* **94**:31–44.

ROHRBACH HO (1925) Supervision of the dairy herd is necessary to prevent some anaphylactic symptoms in infant feeding. *Atlantic Med J* **27**:670–674.

SALO OP, MAKINEN-KILJUNEN S & JUNTUNEN K (1986) Milk causes a rapid urticarial reaction on the skin of children with atopic dermatitis and milk allergy. *Acta Derm Venereol* **66**:438–442.

SAPERSTEIN S (1960) Antigenicity of the whey proteins in evaporated cow's milk and whole goat's milk. *Ann Allergy* **18**:765–773.

SAVILAHTI E, KUITUNEN P & VISAKORPI JK (1989) Cow's milk allergy. In Lebenthal E (ed) *Textbook of Gastroenterology and Nutrition in Infancy*, 2nd edn, pp. 473–489, Raven Press, New York.

SEGAL S (1989) Disorders of galactose metabolism. In Scriver CR, Beaudet AL, Sly WS & Valle D (eds) *The Metabolic Basis of Inherited Disease*, 6th edn, pp. 453–480, McGraw Hill, New York.

SHINER M, BALLARD J, BROOK CGD & HERMAN S (1975) Intestinal biopsy in the diagnosis of cow's milk protein intolerance without acute symptoms. *Lancet* **2**:1060–1063.

SNIDER GL (1988) Case records of the Massachusetts General Hospital. Case 30 – 1988. *New Engl J Med* **319**:227–237.

SPIES JR (1971) New antigens in lactose (35546). *Proc Soc Exp Biol Med* **137**:211–214.

SWAISGOOD HE (1985) Characteristics of edible fluids of animal origin: milk. In Fennema OR (ed) *Food Chemistry*, 2nd edn, pp. 791–827, Marcel Dekker, New York.

TAINIO VM & SAVILAHTI E (1990) Value of immunologic tests in cow milk allergy. *Allergy* **45**:189–196.

TAITZ LS & ARMITAGE BL (1984) Goat's milk for infants and children. *Br Med J* **288**:428–429.

TAITZ LS & WARDLEY B (1985) Dangers of goats' milk as an infant feed. *Goats Vet Soc J* **6**:20–26.

TAYLOR DC (1992) Outlandish factitious illness. In David TJ (ed) *Recent Advances in Paediatrics*, vol. 10, pp. 63–76, Churchill Livingstone, London.

TAYLOR GA (1988) Cow's milk protein/soy protein allergy: gastrointestinal imaging. *Radiology* **167**:866.

TROUNCE JQ & WALKER-SMITH JA (1985) Sugar intolerance complicating acute gastroenteritis. *Arch Dis Child* **60**:986–990.

UUSI-RAUVA E, ALI-YRKKÖ S & ANTILA M (1970) Die Zusammensetzung der Finnischen Ziegenmilch. *Suomen Kemistilehti* **43**:178–182.

VALDES-DAPENA MA & FELIPE RP (1971) Immunofluorescent studies in crib deaths: absence of evidence of hypersensitivity to cow's milk. *Am J Clin Path* **56**:412–415.

VICKERS HR, BAGRATUNI L & ALEXANDER S (1958) Dermatitis caused by penicillin in milk. *Lancet* **1**:351–352.

VITORIA JC, CAMARERO C, SOJO A, RUIZ A & RODRIGUEZ-SORIANO J (1982) Enteropathy related to fish, rice and chicken. *Arch Dis Child* **57**:44–48.

WALKER ARP (1972) The human requirement of calcium: should low intakes be supplemented? *Am J Clin Nutr* **22**:518–530.

WALKER-SMITH JA (1988) *Diseases of the Small Intestine in Childhood*, 3rd edn, Butterworths, London.

WALKER-SMITH J, HARRISON M, KILBY A, PHILLIPS A & FRANCE N (1978) Cow's milk sensitive enteropathy. *Arch Dis Child* **53**:375–380.

WARNER JO & HATHAWAY MJ (1984) Allergic form of Meadow's syndrome (Munchausen by proxy). *Arch Dis Child* **59**:151–156.

WHISTLER RL & DANIEL JR (1985) Carbohydrates. In Fennema OR (ed) *Food Chemistry*, 2nd edn, pp. 69–137, Marcel Dekker, New York.

WHITFIELD MF & BARR DGD (1976) Cow's milk allergy in the syndrome of thrombocytopenia with absent radius. *Arch Dis Child* **51**:337–343.

WHYTE RK, HOMER R & PENNOCK CA (1978) Faecal excretion of oligosaccharides and other carbohydrates in normal neonates. *Arch Dis Child* **53**:913–915.

WILSON JF, HEINER DC & LAHEY ME (1964) Milk-induced gastrointestinal bleeding in infants with hypochromic microcytic anemia. *J Am Med Ass* **189**: 568–572.

WILSON JF, LAHEY ME & HEINER DC (1974) Studies on iron metabolism. V. Further observations on cow's milk-induced gastrointestinal bleeding in infants with iron-deficiency anaemia. *J Pediat* **84**:335–344.

WILSON NW, SELF TW & HAMBURGER RN (1990) Severe cow's milk induced colitis in an exclusively breast-fed neonate. Case report and clinical review of cow's milk allergy. *Clin Pediat* **29**:77–80.

YATES VM, KERR REI & MACKIE RM (1983a) Early diagnosis of infantile seborrhoeic dermatitis and atopic dermatitis – clinical features. *Br J Dermatol* **108**:633–638.

YATES VM, KERR REI, FRIER K, COBB SJ & MACKIE RM (1983b) Early diagnosis of infantile seborrhoeic dermatitis and atopic dermatitis – total and specific IgE levels. *Br J Dermatol* **108**:639–645.

ZIEGLER EE, FOMON SJ, NELSON SE *et al.* (1990) Cow milk feeding in infancy: further observations on blood loss from the gastrointestinal tract. *J Pediat* **116**:11–18.

Part 3 Hypoallergenic Milk Formulae

16 Heat treatment of cow's milk
Works better in guinea-pig model than in humans

Important milk proteins

There is uncertainty as to the relative immunogenicity of individual proteins in cow's milk. Judged by the percentage of positive antibody responses in patients with cow's milk protein intolerance, immune responses to β-lactoglobulin are generally seen most often, followed by casein and α-lactalbumin (Table 16.1). However in some studies casein stimulated antibody production more frequently than β-lactoglobulin (Bürgin-Wolff *et al.* 1980). This finding is supported by recent data from Otani *et al.* (1989) who were able to differentiate between the various casein subunits and found IgE antibodies to α-casein in 76% of children with cow's milk protein intolerance (Table 16.1).

The uncertainty about the relative allergenicity of individual proteins in cow's milk makes it difficult to predict the allergic potential for infant formulae based on different casein/whey ratios.

Guinea-pig model

In guinea-pigs fed either ultra heat-treated (Table 16.2) cow's milk or spray-dried whole cow's milk (reconstituted with water) for 37 days, it was found that severe anaphylactic reactions could be provoked by intravenous injection or intratracheal introduction of β-lactoglobulin (Devey *et al.* 1976; Coombs *et al.* 1978; Anderson *et al.*

Table 16.1 Allergenicity of individual cow's milk proteins as judged by incidence of antibodies in patients with a history of cow's milk protein intolerance

Protein	Bahna (1978)	Bahna & Heiner Vautrin (1980)	Moneret *et al.* (1982)	Otani *et al.* (1989)
Whey proteins				
β-lactoglobulin	82%	62–80%	46%	29%
α-lactalbumin	41%	56%	31%	6%
Bovine serum albumin	18%	52%	0%	0%
Bovine immunoglobulins	27%	—	—	12%
Casein	43%	56%	23%	—
α-casein	—	—	—	76%
β-casein	—	—	—	35%
κ-casein	—	—	—	41%

Table 16.2 Types of heat treatment for cow's milk[1]

Designation	Treatment
Raw	Unheated and untreated
Pasteurized	Heated at 72°C for 20 s
Ultra heat-treated	Heated at 140° for 1–2 s
Boiled	Heated to 100°C and allowed to cool
Evaporated	Heated to 95°C for 10 min, evaporated under reduced pressure at 50°C, autoclaved in cans at 110–115°C for 15–20 min
Sterilized	Autoclaved at 112.8–114.4°C for 20 min
Spray-dried	Heated to 105°C for 30 s, then cooled to 16°C. Heated in a preheater to 78°C then into spray-drier and raised to 167°C – drying occurs instantaneously

[1] Source: McLaughlan *et al.* (1981).

1979). In contrast, anaphylactic reactions to β-lactoglobulin could not be similarly provoked in guinea-pigs that had been drinking evaporated milks (see Table 16.2 for definitions of different types of heat treatment of milk). A subsequent study showed that commercial infant milk formulae that had received severe heat treatment during manufacture were less efficient at sensitizing guinea-pigs by mouth than mildly treated preparations (McLaughlan *et al.* 1981).

Effect of heat treatment

Whey proteins are easily denatured by heat but casein is highly resistant. The three-dimensional structure of β-lactoglobulin and α-lactalbumin becomes disorganized through cleavage of hydrophobic bonds, rearrangement of disulphide bridges, and aggregation, whereas casein has neither secondary nor tertiary structure and is not so easily modified (Kilshaw *et al.* 1982).

heated whey

Kilshaw *et al.* (1982) showed that severe heat treatment (up to 121°C for 20 min) of skimmed cow's milk resulted in extensive denaturation of whey proteins, but the milk retained its capacity to sensitize guinea-pigs for systemic anaphylaxis when administered orally. Animals drinking heated milk produced circulating antibodies to β-lactoglobulin and casein, although titres were lower than for unheated milk. In contrast, heat-treated whey failed to sensitize guinea-pigs, though it resulted in the production of trace levels of antibodies which were specific for residual casein.

Doubt about value of heat treatment

The above observations led to the suggestion that the heat treatment of whey proteins may be a simple and logical strategy for producing a hypoallergenic infant milk formula (Kilshaw *et al.* 1982; Heppell *et al.* 1984). However, double-blind placebo-controlled oral challenges gave rise to immediate hypersensitivity reactions to heat-treated whey protein in four out of five children with cow's milk protein intolerance (Ebbeling & Buckley 1989). The reason for these reactions is not known, but one possibility is a reaction to residual casein (see Lorenz *et al.* 1988), which is always present in trace amounts in commercial whey preparations.

Doubt about guinea-pig model

There are serious doubts about the validity of the guinea-pig anaphylaxis model as a tool for the prediction of allergenicity in man. An ultrafiltered whey hydrolysate that provoked no immune response in guinea-pigs (Granti *et al.* 1985; Pahud *et al.* 1985) led to immediate reactions in five infants with cow's milk protein intolerance (Businco *et al.* 1989). Studies of a heat-treated cow's milk whey in guinea-pigs suggested a loss of allergenicity (Kilshaw *et al.* 1982), but when five children with cow's milk protein intolerance were challenged with an ultrafiltered, heat-treated whey preparation, four developed immediate reactions (Ebbeling & Buckley 1989). Reports of human intolerance to casein hydrolysate milk formulae (see chapter 18) which were innocuous in the guinea-pig model (Knights & Manes 1987) further undermine confidence in the relevance to man of data obtained in this animal model.

Lack of practical application

The small proportion of patients with cow's milk protein intolerance likely to tolerate heat-treated cow's milk, such as evaporated milk, means that heat-treated milk is unlikely to be suitable as a substitute for a cow's milk infant formula. This does not exclude the possibility of further development of a heat-treated casein-free milk formula.

Key references   16.1   McLaughlan P, Anderson KJ, Widdowson EM & Coombs RRA (1981) Effect of heat on the anaphylactic-sensitising capacity of cows' milk, goats' milk, and various infant formulae fed to guinea pigs. *Arch Dis Child* **56**:165–171. *Cow's milk — fresh, boiled, and processed in different ways for the domestic market, and various infant milk formulae — were investigated for their sensitising capacity in the guinea pig after being fed for 37 days. The sensitizing capacity was considerably reduced by heat treatment. In its raw state, goat's milk proved to be as sensitizing as raw cow's milk. Boiling reduced the sensitizing capacity of goat's milk to an even greater extent than was the case with cow's milk.*

16.2   Kilshaw PJ, Heppell LMJ & Ford JE (1982) Effects of heat treatment of cows' milk and whey on the nutritional quality and antigenic properties. *Arch Dis Child* **57**:842–847. *Severe heat treatment of skimmed milk caused extensive denaturation of whey proteins, but the milk retained its capacity to sensitize guinea pigs for systemic anaphylaxis, but heated-treated diafiltered whey failed to sensitize guinea pigs. Severe heat treatment of milk destroyed all the vitamin B_{12}, and approximately 60% of the thiamin and vitamin B_6, 70% of the ascorbic acid and 30% of the folate; available lysine was reduced by*

21%. It was suggested that heat-denatured whey could form the basis for a hypoallergenic milk, and the nutritional quality preserved by removing low molecular weight nutrients before heat treatment and adding back appropriate quantities later.

16.3   HANSON LA & JOHANSSON BG (1970) Immunological studies of milk. In McKenzie HE (ed) *Milk Proteins. Chemistry and Molecular Biology*, vol. 1, pp. 45–123, Academic Press, New York. *Useful detailed review of pre-1970 literature.*

16.4   HØST A & SAMUELSSON EG (1988) Allergic reactions to raw, pasteurized, and homogenized/pasteurized cow milk: a comparison. A double-blind placebo-controlled study in milk allergic children. *Allergy* **43**:113–118. Five children aged 12–40 months with quick onset adverse reactions to cow's milk protein were challenged with raw untreated cow's milk, pasteurized cow's milk (75°C for 15 s), homogenised (at 60°C and pressure of 175 kg/cm^2) and pasteurized milk, and a casein hydrolysate formula (Nutramigen). All children reacted adversely to all three forms of cow's milk, but none reacted to the casein hydrolysate formula. *The authors conclude that homogenized cow's milk is not suitable for infants with cow's milk protein intolerance. They also suggest, without any convincing data, that the process of homogenization might even lead to an enhanced ability to evoke adverse reactions in those with cow's milk protein intolerance.*

Summary 16   Whey proteins are easily denatured by heat but casein is highly resistant. In theory, and on the basis of experiments using the guinea-pig anaphylaxis model, a milk formula based on heat-treated whey ought to be tolerated by children with cow's milk protein intolerance. In practice one small human study showed that four of five children with cow's milk protein intolerance experienced immediate allergic reactions to such a formula, casting doubt on the relevance to man of this particular animal model. Denaturation of whey by heat treatment explains why some heat-treated milks, such as evaporated milk, are occasionally tolerated by a child with cow's milk protein intolerance.

17   Protein hydrolysate formulae I: composition and types
Getting the peptide size just right

Importance of peptide size   The work of Aas (1987) on the allergens in cod suggests that the minimum size of an allergenic peptide is one with 14 amino acid residues having a molecular weight of between 1200 and 1600.

Table 17.1 Types of cow's milk protein hydrolysate formulae

Type	Manufacturer
Casein hydrolysate formulae	
Nutramigen	Mead Johnson
Pregestimil	Mead Johnson
Whey hydrolysate formulae	
Alfa-Ré	Nestlé
LHA	Nestlé
Pepti-Junior	Cow & Gate

Extent of hydrolysis

The most effective means of reducing the allergenicity of food proteins is by decreasing their molecular size by proteolysis. In theory, the smaller the molecular weight the better, but advantages of reduced allergenicity may be offset by poor palatibility. In other words, turning milk protein into amino acids would abolish allergenicity, but the resulting solution would be unpalatable and no longer resemble milk.

Milk protein hydrolysis

Enzymatic hydrolysis of casein and whey have been used to develop a number of casein or whey hydrolysate milk formulae (Table 17.1).

What is the crucial peptide size for milk protein?

Even if it were technologically feasible to produce a protein hydrolysate formula with peptides with molecular weights all below 1200, this would provide no guarantee of non-allergenicity. Small peptides could aggregate or cross-link with one another or with polysaccharides to become larger molecules, large enough to result in intolerance.

On the basis of work in guinea-pigs and rabbits, and bearing in mind the uncertain relevance of animal experiments to man (see chapter 16), Seban *et al.* (1977) suggested that the residual allergenicity of casein hydrolysate formulae may be attributed to the presence of peptides with molecular weights larger than 3850. Further animal studies using IgG antibody binding, IgG and IgM antibody responses and heterologous passive cutaneous anaphylactic tests suggested that a critical value for immunogenicity or allergenicity in milk protein hydrolysates is in the order of a molecular weight of 3500 to 5000 (Otani *et al.* 1990).

Inaccuracy of molecular weight estimation

When designing a protein hydrolysate hypoallergenic milk, much attention is given to the molecular weight distribution of the peptides. For single peptides with a known structure, the molecular weight can be accurately determined. However, for mixtures of peptides, one has to rely on chromatographic or electrophoretic methods, and a practical difficulty is that the chromatographic or electrophoretic behaviour of peptides with a molecular weight of under 10 000 does not only depend on molecular size. Each technique has its own drawbacks, making it difficult to compare molecular weight distributions obtained with different methods. Claims that peptides with a molecular weight above a certain value are *absent* should be interpreted as being *undetected* since such peptides may very well be present at levels below the detection limit. It is thought to be these undetected peptides which are responsible for some reports of intolerance to protein hydrolysate formulae (chapter 18).

Molecular weight: conclusion

In view of the above, there is no definite molecular weight above which peptides are allergenic and below which they are non-allergenic. In general there appears to be a lower limit for antigenicity for peptides with molecular weight at around 1200 to 1600. Because of the necessity for peptides to bear at least two independent IgE binding sites on the surface of a mast cell to elicit IgE-mediated reactions, a critical molecular weight value of approximately 3500 is likely to be applicable for IgE-mediated reactions. However peptides with a molecular weight between 3500 and 6000 can still be 'hypoallergenic' depending on the nature of the specific protein hydrolysate. On the other hand, products with peptides having molecular weights below 1200 may, under specific conditions, still be allergenic. Thus the peptide molecular weight distribution data of a protein hydrolysate provides only an approximate estimate of the allergenic characteristics and does not guarantee tolerance or hypoallergenicity in clinical practice (Bindels & Verwimp 1990).

Poor flavour

A practical difficulty which limits the use of protein hydrolysate milk formulae is their poor flavour. This is usually accepted by infants under 1 year of age, but with increasing age there is a reluctance to take hydrolysates.

Key references 17.1

KNIGHTS RJ & MANES JD (1987) Composition, molecular weight, and antigenicity of casein hydrolysates used in a formula for food allergic and malabsorptive infants. In Chandra RK (ed) *Food Allergy*, pp. 273–285, Nutrition Research Education Foundation, St Johns, Newfoundland. *Review of production, composition, molecular weight profiles and measurement of antigenicity of two casein hydrolysate milk formulae, Nutramigen and Pregestimil.*

17.2

BINDELS JG & VERWIMP J (1990) *Allergenic Aspects of Infant Feeding.* Nutricia Research Communications: 2. Zoetermeer, Holland, N.V. Verenigde Bedrijven Nutricia. Includes a *detailed review of relevance of peptide molecular weight.*

17.3

JOST R (1988) Physicochemical treatment of food allergens: application to cow's milk proteins. In Reinhardt E & Schmidt E (eds) *Food Allergy*, pp. 187–197,

Raven Press, New York. *Review of heat processing, proteolytic cleavage and effects on antigenicity of cow's milk proteins.*

Summary 17

Based on *in vitro* and animal studies, there appears to be a lower limit for antigenicity for peptides with molecular weight at around 1200 to 1600, although this provides no guarantee of non-allergenicity, as in theory small peptides could aggregate or cross-link with one another or with polysaccharides to become molecules large enough to result in intolerance. A minimum peptide size for non-IgE-mediated allergic responses is a molecular weight in the order of 1000 to 1800, and for IgE-mediated allergic responses it is approximately 3500.

18 Protein hydrolysate formulae II: intolerance
An occasional problem

Animal studies unhelpful

Animal models suggest that hydrolysed milk proteins do not elicit an antibody response to cow's milk proteins (Granati *et al.* 1985), and protein hydrolysate formulae have therefore been given to children with cow's milk protein intolerance. Problems with the guinea-pig model are discussed in chapter 16. In many, and perhaps most cases of cow's milk protein intolerance, these hydrolysate formulae are well tolerated (e.g. Walker-Smith *et al.* 1989; Merritt *et al.* 1990; Sampson *et al.* 1991). But it is now clear that intolerance to protein hydrolysates can occur, although the incidence of such reactions is unknown.

Casein hydrolysate intolerance

Kuitinen *et al.* (1975) reported intolerance to casein hydrolysate (Nutramigen) in three out of 17 infants with cow's milk protein intolerance. Hill *et al.* (1984) reported intolerance to casein hydrolysate in 11 out of 54 infants with cow's milk protein intolerance. Lifschitz *et al.* (1988) reported a cow's milk protein intolerant infant who developed anaphylactic shock after ingesting a casein hydrolysate formula (Nutramigen). Bock (1989) reported immediate reactions, with urticaria, vomiting and severe wheezing after ingestion of casein hydrolysate formulae (Nutramigen and Pregestimil) in a 7-month-old infant with atopic eczema, asthma and urticaria; the observations were confirmed by double-blind challenge. Saylor

& Bahna (1991) reported a 3-year-old boy with intolerance to cow's milk protein who developed severe vomiting, erythema and wheezing immediately after ingestion of a casein hydrolysate formula (Nutramigen). Because of the severity of the reaction, confirmation by double-blind challenge was not sought. Finally, there is a report of three infants with cow's milk protein intolerance who developed severe gastrointestinal reactions after ingestion of casein hydrolysate formulae (Nutramigen in two; Pregestimil in one), with loose stools, malaena and weight loss (Rosenthal *et al.* 1991).

Whey hydrolysate intolerance

Businco *et al.* (1989) reported five breast-fed infants, aged 3–8 months, who all suffered from atopic eczema, and who had experienced immediate reactions (urticaria, lip oedema or wheezing) when a cow's milk formula was first introduced into the diet. All exhibited identical reactions when given a whey hydrolysate formula (Alfa-Ré). All five had positive skin-prick tests to bovine lactoglobulin, lactalbumin, casein and Alfa-Ré. On the assumption (which is far from proven) that whey protein is more likely to provoke an allergic reaction than casein, the authors argued that casein hydrolysates may be more suitable for children with cow's milk protein intolerance. Heyman *et al.* (1990) reported a 6-month-old infant with gastrointestinal symptoms of intolerance to a formula based on hydrolysed lactalbumin, a whey protein. Ellis *et al.* (1991) reported vomiting, generalized urticaria, rhinorrhoea, wheezing and cyanosis immediately after ingestion of an hydrolysed whey protein formula (Good Start, Carnation). Confirmation by double-blind challenge was not sought.

Incidence of intolerance

The incidence of milk protein hydrolysate intolerance is not known. It is worth pointing out that intolerance was only confirmed by double-blind placebo-controlled challenge in a single case (Bock 1989).

Skin-prick tests unhelpful

As in other examples of food intolerance, skin-prick testing is unhelpful. In one study of 10 children with cow's milk protein intolerance (Sampson *et al.* 1991), all 10 had positive skin-prick tests to cow's milk protein, six had positive skin tests to Nutramigen (a casein hydrolysate formula), and five had positive skin tests to Alimentum (another casein hydrolysate formula). All 10 reacted adversely to double-blind placebo-controlled challenges with cow's milk protein, but there were no reactions to Nutramigen or Alimentum.

Prevention of atopic disease or food intolerance

The suggestion that the use of protein hydrolysate milk formulae or other types of dietary manipulation in infancy (such as prolonged breast-feeding) may prevent the development of atopic disease or food intolerance is a contentious subject which is outside the scope of this book. For recent studies, none of which are entirely satisfactory, and for reviews of the subject, the reader is referred to Savilahti *et al.* 1987; Lindfors & Enocksson 1988; Vandenplas *et al.* 1988; Chandra *et al.* 1989a, b; Zeiger *et al.* 1989; Businco & Cantani 1990; Zeiger 1990; Björkstén & Kjellman 1991; and Bousquet & Michel 1991.

Key references 18.1 Bock SA (1989) Probable allergic reaction to casein hydrolysate formula. *J Allergy Clin Immunol* **84**:272. *Misleadingly modest title. The best documented case.*

18.2 Businco L, Cantani A, Longhi MA & Giampietro PG (1989) Anaphylactic reactions to a cow's milk whey protein hydrolysate (Alfa-Ré, Nestlé) in infants with cow's milk allergy. *Ann Allergy* **62**:333–335. *Detailed study of five cases, but challenges were not blinded.*

18.3 Sampson HA, Bernhisel-Broadbent J, Yang E & Scanlon SM (1991) Safety of casein hydrolysate formula in children with cow milk allergy. *J Pediat* **118**: 520–525. Twenty-five children with cow's milk protein intolerance underwent double-blind placebo-controlled challenges with cow's milk and a new casein hydrolysate formula, Alimentum. Two patients lost their intolerance to cow's milk protein and did not react. The remaining 23 reacted to cow's milk protein, but none reacted to the casein hydrolysate. The results provided a 90% confidence that at least 90% of children with cow's milk protein intolerance who ingest Alimentum will have no reaction.

Summary 18 Although most children with cow's milk protein intolerance will tolerate protein hydrolysate milk formulae such as Nutramigen or Pregestimil, it is clear that intolerance to these formulae can occasionally occur. Neither the mechanism nor the precise incidence of milk protein hydrolysate intolerance are known.

19 Meat-based and elemental formulae
Last resorts

Lamb- and horse-based formulae A formula based on lamb (Table 19.1) was devised in Rome in the early 1970s. Businco *et al.* (1985) used this diet in 41 infants, median age 3 months, with chronic diarrhoea in whom cow's milk protein intolerance was assumed to be present. The diarrhoea subsided within a week. The presence of milk protein intolerance was tested by challenge, but only 1–7 years after the onset of

Table 19.1 Constituents per litre of
lamb-based formula[1]

Lamb meat	100 g
Precooked rice flour	70 g
Olive oil	40 g
Table salt	2 g
Calcium gluconate	0.3 g

[1] Businco *et al.* (1985).

diarrhoea. By this time, only 15 of the 40 children were unable to tolerate cow's milk protein.

further Italian data

In the report of the Italian Collaborative Study on cow's milk protein intolerance, the use of a home made diet consisting of lamb or horse meat, rice, corn oil, calcium and trace elements was described (Ventura *et al.* 1988). Whereas 27% of infants were intolerant to soya milk formulae, and 17% were intolerant to protein hydrolysate formulae (it is not clear whether this was casein or whey hydrolysate), only 8% were intolerant to the meat-based formulae. In another report, a lamb-based formula was successfully used in infants with intolerance to casein hydrolysate but specific details of the patients or the formulae were not provided (Self *et al.* 1969).

Beef-based formula

A beef-based formula, Meat Base (Gerber), had beef heart as its source of protein, and also contained beef fat, sesame oil, tapioca starch, sucrose, trace elements and vitamins (Ogle & Bullock 1980).

Chicken-based formulae

Auricchio *et al.* (1985) reported that a formula based on chicken meat was suitable for infants with chronic diarrhoea caused by intolerance to cow's milk protein, soya, or protein hydrolysate. Godard *et al.* (1989) chose chicken meat as a basis for a formula for refeeding children with protracted diarrhoea.

intractable diarrhoea

Feeds based on chicken are well-established in the management of intractable infantile diarrhoea associated with intolerance to other sources of protein. A commercially available form of puréed chicken (Comminuted Chicken – Cow & Gate) forms the basis for a number of feeds (Table 19.2). The use of such feeds, which must be initiated in hospital, is complex, and the supervision of a paediatric dietitian (Francis 1987) is mandatory.

Drawback to meat-based feeds

Drawbacks are the complexity of devising and using meat-based feeds, the lack of validation of their use in the management of food intolerance, and the possibility of intolerance to the protein content. The latter leads into the use of so-called elemental feeds, where the protein fraction is replaced by amino acids.

Table 19.2 Composition[1] of Comminuted Chicken (Cow & Gate) feeds[2]

Ingredients per 100 ml	Full-protein low-energy feed	Full-protein normal-energy feed	Full-protein high-energy feed
Comminuted Chicken	30 g	30 g	30 g
Glucose polymer	5 g	10 g	10 g
Vegetable oil emulsion[3]	nil	3 ml	6 ml
Mineral mixture[4]	0.8 g	0.8 g	1.0 g
Water	to 100 ml	to 100 ml	to 100 ml
Osmolality	159 mmol/kg	221 mmol/kg	247 mmol/kg

[1] Note that vitamins are not included in these formulae.
[2] Source: Francis (1987).
[3] Calogen or Liquigen (Scientific Hospital Supplies).
[4] Aminogran Mineral Mixture (Allen & Hanburys) or Metabolic Mineral Mixture (Scientific Hospital Supplies).

Elemental diets therapy or diagnosis

Elemental diets can either be used as therapy, to treat intolerance to other foods, or for diagnosis, where multiple food intolerance is strongly suspected. Given the lack of valid tests for the diagnosis of food intolerance or the identification of individual food triggers, the withdrawal of all normal food and drink from the diet, and the use of an elemental diet, has been regarded as an important diagnostic test for food intolerance (Galant et al. 1977; Hughes 1978; Dockhorn & Smith 1981; Van Bever et al. 1989).

Crohn's disease

Elemental diets have also been used for feeding in the management of Crohn's disease – the rationale is discussed in the section on Crohn's disease in chapter 61.

Elemental – a misnomer

In the context of infant feeding, the term elemental, although widely accepted and without a better alternative, is misused. Strictly speaking, the word implies that the contents are reduced to single elements (such as sodium, carbon, zinc and so on). In practice the designation elemental is used to describe feeds which are based on amino acids, and in which the constituents are largely non-macromolecular. The composition of the currently available manufactured elemental feeds, Vivonex and Elemental 028, are listed in Table 19.3.

Semi-elemental – even worse

The illogical use of the term elemental to describe formulae which contain amino acids, glucose polymers and oil is matched only by the term semi-elemental, which is sometimes used to describe casein or whey hydrolysate formulae containing peptides, corn syrup, starch, milk fat and various oils.

Table 19.3 'Elemental' formulae

Name	Nitrogen source	Carbohydrate	Fat
Vivonex Standard[1] (Tolerex)	Amino acids 2.1 g/100 ml	Glucose solids 23 g/100 ml	Safflower oil 0.14 g/100 ml Linoleic acid 0.26 g/100 ml
Vivonex HN[1] (Tolerex TEN)	Amino acids 4.3 g/100 ml	Glucose solids 21 g/100 ml	Safflower oil 0.09 g/100 ml
Elemental 028[2]	Amino acids 2.4 g/100 ml	Maltodextrin 14.4 g/100 ml	Arachis oil 1.3 g/100 ml
Neocate[2]	Amino acids 2.4 g/100 ml	Glucose polymer 8.4 g/100 ml	Safflower oil, coconut oil, soya oil 3.5 g/100 ml

[1] Norwich Eaton, P.O. Box 231, Norwich NY 13815, USA.
[2] Scientific Hospital Supplies Ltd, Wavertree Technology Park, Wavertree Boulevard, Liverpool L7 9PQ, UK.

Vivonex

Vivonex, known in north America as Tolerex, and reformulated in 1989, has hitherto been the most widely used elemental formula. There are numerous disadvantages, all of which apply to other elemental formulae, and which are likely to restrict use to cases where intolerance to protein or peptide-based formulae has been demonstrated or is strongly suspected. The main problems, which are likely to apply to other so-called elemental formulae, are discussed below.

Vivonex problems: flavour

The flavour of Vivonex is awful. Older children may refuse to swallow it. Much depends on how well prepared and motivated is the child, but if he or she senses that there is any choice then the chances of refusal are increased. Some children are helped by knowing that it was originally designed for use in space flight, while others are helped by giving it a nickname such as 'potato soup'. Other sources of liquid refreshment, such as tap water, must be unavailable, or they will be consumed in preference. Most children prefer Vivonex cold, a few prefer it warm, and a handful will only consume it in the form of ice lollies or crushed ice. The nasogastric route is an alternative.

added flavouring

It is possible to add flavouring and colouring agents to Vivonex and other elemental formulae, but in the management of food intolerance these ingredients are not used because of the possibility of additive intolerance. The figures given in this chapter for the composition of elemental formulae (Table 19.4) refer to unflavoured formulations.

Table 19.4 Mineral content of elemental and other formulae, compared with cow's milk and cow's milk formulae

Name of formula	Sodium mg/100 g[1] (mmol/100 ml)	Potassium mg/100 g (mmol/100 ml)	Calcium mg/100 g (mmol/100 ml)	Phosphorus mg/100 g (mmol/100 ml)
Ordinary cow's milk[2]	50 mg (2.2)	150 mg (3.8)	120 mg (3.0)	95 mg (3.1)
Range	35–90 mg	110–170 mg	110–130 mg	90–100 mg
Infant milk formulae				
Cow & Gate Premium	18 mg (0.8)	65 mg (1.7)	54 mg (1.3)	27 mg (0.9)
Milupa Milumil	24 mg (1.0)	85 mg (2.1)	71 mg (1.8)	55 mg (1.8)
Protein hydrolysate formulae				
Pregestimil	32 mg (1.4)	74 mg (1.9)	63 mg (1.6)	43 mg (1.4)
Alfa-Ré	44 mg (1.9)	90 mg (2.3)	60 mg (1.5)	37 mg (1.2)
Elemental formulae				
Vivonex (pre 1989)	85 mg (3.7)	69 mg (3.0)	66 mg (1.7)	98 mg (3.2)
Vivonex (1989 on)	47 mg (2.0)	117 mg (3.0)	56 mg (1.4)	56 mg (1.8)
Elemental 028	60 mg (2.6)	93 mg (2.4)	37.5 mg (0.9)	40 mg (1.3)
Neocate	18 mg (0.8)	59 mg (1.5)	45 mg (1.1)	34 mg (1.1)

[1] Source: Paul & Southgate (1978).

Vivonex problems: hypertonicity

practical problem

Full strength Vivonex, 32 g powder added to 100 ml water, has an osmolality of 560 mmol/kg, and this is likely to causes loose stools in an infant. The best approach is to start at a weak strength, say 8 g powder added to 100 ml water (140 mmol/kg), gradually increasing to isotonicity (16 g powder added to 100 ml water, 280 mmol/kg), and increasing the concentration further if possible.

theoretical problem

It has been shown in rats that hypertonic feeds may cause increased jejunal permeability to macromolecules (Cooper *et al.* 1978) and structural damage to jejunal microvilli (Teichberg *et al.* 1978). Evidence of increased permeability has not been sought in human infants who have received hypertonic Vivonex, and it is difficult to assess the relevance of these findings.

Vivonex problems: sodium content

Vivonex was not designed for use in infants, and the old formula (prior to 1990) had a higher sodium content than conventional cow's milk or protein hydrolysate formulae (see Table 19.4). This posed a theoretical risk of sodium overload. Hypernatraemia was sought, but not found, in a group of 37 children with atopic eczema who received Vivonex for 4 weeks or longer (Devlin *et al.* 1991).

Vivonex problems: weight loss

Severely malnourished infants with protracted diarrhoea may thrive well once feeding with an elemental formula is commenced. However, weight loss has been well documented in non-malnourished severely atopic children who have received an elemental formula for the purposes of an elimination diet. Thus, 30 out of 34 children with atopic eczema lost up to 17% of their body weight while taking Vivonex for a month (Devlin *et al.* 1991). This was sometimes accompanied by a fall in the serum albumin concentration, itself a well recognized complication of severe atopic eczema. The reasons for this weight loss in the face of an intake exceeding the recommended daily intake are not known, but poor net retention of nitrogen and a low biological value were noted in a study of a high nitrogen formulation of Vivonex in adults with Crohn's disease (Smith *et al.* 1982).

Vivonex problems: safflower oil

The fat source of Vivonex is safflower oil. There is a theoretical possibility that this contains traces of protein, which could provoke intolerance, although there is no evidence that this has ever happened. The question of whether vegetable or nut oils contain protein and are therefore capable of provoking intolerance is discussed in chapter 4.

Elemental 028

Elemental 028 is an alternative to Vivonex, although there is no published experience of its use in food intolerance. The osmolarity when made up at a one in five weight to volume dilution is 500 mmol/kg. Elemental 028 is not suitable for infants under 1 year old, because of its vitamin, mineral and trace element composition. The fat source is arachis oil, and as with the safflower oil in Vivonex there is a theoretical possibility of intolerance.

Neocate

For infants under 1 year, an alternative preparation is Neocate, which is based on an amino acid mixture supplemented by taurine and carnitine. The fat component was, until 1991, pork fat, beef fat, coconut fat and peanut oil; in 1991 this changed to safflower oil, coconut oil and soya oil. The multiplicity of fat sources again raises the theoretical possibility of intolerance.

Intolerance to elemental formulae

There are no documented reports of intolerance to elemental formulae, other than loose stools due to hyperosmolarity, and rare infants who because of severe gastrointestinal pathology are unable to tolerate any oral feeding. I am aware of an anecdotal report of one child who developed urticaria/angioedema minutes after drinking unflavoured Elemental 028, which was being given for the treatment of Crohn's disease. This and other instances of intolerance to elemental formulae, referred to by Bindels & Verwimp (1990), are not easy to explain. One possibility is the presence of trace amounts of protein, either due to a manufacturing fault, or present in the oily component (Tattrie & Yaguchi, 1973) of the formula.

Key references 19.1   Auricchio S, De Vizia B, Cucchiara S, D'Antonio AM, de Ritis G & Iaccarino E (1985) Uso di una dieta a base di pollo, crema di riso, olio, minerali e vitamine nella terapia della diarrea cronica grave del lattante dei primi tre mesi di vita da intolleranze alimentari multiple. *Riv Ital Ped* **11**:383–392. 18 infants with intractible diarrhoea due to cow's milk, soya and/or casein hydrolysate intolerance were treated with a diet consisting of chicken meat, rice flour, oil and minerals. The diet was successful in all patients, though in six only after the addition of cholestyramine. The authors also reported nine other patients with intractible diarrhoea who did not respond to this formula. *There may be a place for chicken-based formulae in infants who are intolerant to cow's milk, casein hydrolysate and soya.*

19.2   Devlin J, David TJ & Stanton RHJ (1991) Elemental diet for refractory atopic eczema. *Arch Dis Child* **66**:93–99. 37 children with refractory widespread atopic eczema were treated with an antigen avoidance regimen comprising hospitalization, exclusive feeding with Vivonex for a median duration of 30 days, and measures to reduce exposure to pet and dust mite antigens at home. After the initial period of food exclusion, food challenges were performed at intervals of 7 days. 10 out of 37 (27%) either failed to respond to the regimen or relapsed within 12 months. Improvement in the eczema was seen in 27 out of 37 (73%) patients, by discharge from hospital their disease severity score had fallen to a median of 27% of the pre-treatment figure, and only three out of 27 required topical corticosteroids. Drawbacks to the regimen were prolonged hospitalization (median 70 days), and a fall in body weight and serum albumin concentration. *As a last resort, a strict antigen avoidance regimen such as this may be associated with improvement of atopic eczema where conventional treatments have failed.*

Summary 19   It is possible, with the help of a skilled dietitian, to devise an infant formula based on meat such as chicken, lamb, beef or horse. The main drawbacks are the complexity of making and using such feeds and the risk of intolerance to the protein. Elemental formulae, which are based on a mixture of amino acids, are the most likely feeds to be tolerated in a child with food intolerance. Drawbacks comprise poor flavour, hypertonicity, and the unsuitability of composition for feeding small infants.

References to Chapters 16–19

Aas K (1987) Fish allergy and the codfish allergen model. In Brostoff J & Challacombe SJ (eds) *Food Allergy and Intolerance*, pp. 356–366, Bailliere Tindall, London.

Anderson KJ, McLaughlan P, Devey ME & Coombs RRA (1979)

Anaphylactic sensitivity of guinea-pigs drinking different preparations of cows' milk and infant formulae. *Clin Exp Immunol* **35**:454–461.

AURICCHIO S, DE VIZIA B, CUCCHIARA S, D'ANTONIO AM, DE RITIS G & IACCARINO E (1985) Uso di una dieta a base di pollo, crema di riso, olio, minerali e vitamine nella terapia della diarrea cronica grave del lattante dei primi tre mesi di vita da intolleranze alimentari multiple. *Riv Ital Ped* **11**: 383–392.

BAHNA SL (1978) Control of milk allergy: a challenge for physicians, mothers and industry. *Ann Allergy* **41**:1–12.

BAHNA SL & HEINER DC (1980) *Allergies to Milk.* Grune & Stratton, New York.

BINDELS JG & VERWIMP J (1990) *Allergenic Aspects of Infant Feeding.* Nutricia Research Communications: 2. Zoetermeer, Holland, N.V. Verenigde Bedrijven Nutricia.

BJÖRKSTÈN B & KJELLMAN NM (1991) Does breast-feeding prevent food allergy? *Allergy Proc* **12**:233–237.

BOCK SA (1989) Probable allergic reaction to casein hydrolysate formula. *J Allergy Clin Immunol* **84**:272.

BOUSQUET J & MICHEL FB (1991) Overview of the concept of prevention of allergy. *Allergy Proc* **12**:239–244.

BÜRGIN-WOLFF A, SIGNER E, FRIESS HM, BERGER R, BIRBAUMER A & JUST M (1980) The diagnostic significance of antibodies to various cow's milk proteins (fluorescent immunosorbent test). *Eur J Pediat* **133**:17–24.

BUSINCO L, BENINCORI N, CANTANI A, TACCONI L & PICARAZZI A (1985) Chronic diarrhea due to cow's milk allergy: a 4- to 10-year follow-up study. *Ann Allergy* **55**:844–847.

BUSINCO L & CANTANI A (1990) Prevention of childhood allergy by dietary manipulation. *Clin Exper Allergy* **20** (suppl. 3):9–14.

BUSINCO L, CANTANI A, LONGHI MA & GIAMPIETRO PG (1989) Anaphylactic reactions to a cow's milk whey protein hydrolysate (Alfa-Ré, Nestlé) in infants with cow's milk allergy. *Ann Allergy* **62**:333–335.

CHANDRA RK, PURI S & HAMED A (1989a) Influence of maternal diet during lactation and use of formula feeds on development of atopic eczema in high risk infants. *Br Med J* **299**:228–230.

CHANDRA RK, SINGH G & SHRIDHARA B (1989b) Effect of feeding whey hydrolysate, soy and conventional cow milk formulas on incidence of atopic disease in high risk infants. *Ann Allergy* **63**:102–106.

COOMBS RRA, DEVEY ME & ANDERSON KJ (1978) Refractoriness to anaphylactic shock after continuous feeding of cows' milk to guinea-pigs. *Clin Exp Immunol* **32**:263–271.

COOPER M, TEICHBERG S & LIFSHITZ F (1978) Alterations in rat jejunal permeability to a macromolecular tracer during a hyperosmotic load. *Lab Invest* **38**:447–454.

DEVEY ME, ANDERSON KJ, COOMBS RRA, HENSCHEL MJ & COATES ME (1976) The modified anaphylaxis hypothesis for cot death. Anaphylactic sensitisation in guinea-pigs fed cow's milk. *Clin Exp Immunol* **26**:542–548.

DEVLIN J, DAVID TJ & STANTON RHJ (1991) Elemental diet for refractory atopic eczema. *Arch Dis Child* **66**:93–99.

DOCKHORN RJ & SMITH TC (1981) Use of a chemically defined hypoallergenic diet (Vivonex) in the management of patients with suspected food allergy/ intolerance. *Ann Allergy* **47**:264–266.

EBBELING W & BUCKLEY R (1989) Double-blind, placebo-controlled challenges with heated cow milk whey protein in milk sensitive patients (abstract). *J Allergy Clin Immunol* **83**:238A.

ELLIS MH, SHORT JA & HEINER DC (1991) Anaphylaxis after ingestion of a recently introduced hydrolyzed whey protein formula. *J Pediat* **118**:74–77.

FRANCIS D (1987) *Diets for Sick Children*, 4th edn, pp. 35–38, Blackwell Scientific Publications, Oxford.

GALANT SP, FRANZ ML, WALKER P, WELLS ID & LUNDAK RL (1977) A potential diagnostic method for food allergy: clinical application and immunogenicity evaluation of an elemental diet. *Am J Clin Nutr* **30**:512–516.

GODARD C, BUSTOS M, MUNOZ M & NUSSLÉ D (1989) Value of a chicken-based formula for refeeding of children with protracted diarrhea and malnutrition in a developing country. *J Pediatr Gastroenterol Nutr* **9**:473–480.

GRANATI B, MARIONI L & RUBALTELLI FF (1985) Evaluation in guinea pigs of the allergenic capacity of two infant formulae based on hydrolyzed milk proteins. *Biol Neonate* **48**:122–124.

HEPPELL LMJ, CANT AJ & KILSHAW PJ (1984) Reduction in the antigenicity of whey proteins by heat treatment: a possible strategy for producing a hypoallergenic infant milk formula. *Br J Nutr* **51**:29–36.

HEYMAN MB, STOKER TW, RUDOLPH CD & FRICK OL (1990) Hypersensitivity reaction in an infant fed hydrolyzed lactalbumin contained in a semielemental formula. *J Pediatr Gastroenterol Nutr* **10**:253–256.

HILL DJ, FORD RPK, SHELTON MJ & HOSKING CS (1984) A study of 100 infants and young children with cow's milk allergy. *Clin Rev Allergy* **2**:125–142.

HUGHES EC (1978) Use of a chemically defined diet in the diagnosis of food sensitivities and the determination of offending foods. *Ann Allergy* **40**:393–398.

KILSHAW PJ, HEPPELL LMJ & FORD JE (1982) Effects of heat treatment of cows' milk and whey on the nutritional quality and antigenic properties. *Arch Dis Child* **57**:842–847.

KUITUNEN P, VISAKORPI JK, SAVILAHTI E & PELKONEN P (1975) Malabsorption syndrome with cow's milk intolerance: clinical findings and course in 54 cases. *Arch Dis Child* **50**:351–356.

LIFSCHITZ CH, HAWKINS HK, GUERRA C & BYRD N (1988) Anaphylactic shock due to cow's milk protein hypersensitivity in a breast-fed infant. *J Pediatr Gastroenterol Nutr* **7**:141–144.

LINDFORS A & ENOCKSSON E (1988) Development of atopic disease after early administration of cow milk formula. *Allergy* **43**:11–16.

LORENZ F, SEID M, TANGERMANN R & WAHN V (1988) Detection of casein antigen in regular and hypoallergenic formula proteins by ELISA: characterization of formula protein fractions according to their molecular weights. In Reinhardt E & Schmidt E (eds) *Food Allergy*, pp. 215–223, Raven Press, New York.

McLAUGHLAN P, ANDERSON KJ, WIDDOWSON EM & COOMBS RRA (1981) Effect of heat on the anaphylactic-sensitising capacity of cows' milk, goats' milk, and various infant formulae fed to guinea pigs. *Arch Dis Child* **56**: 165–171.

MERRITT RJ, CARTER M, HAIGHT M & EISENBERG LD (1990) Whey protein hydrolysate formula for infants with gastrointestinal intolerance to cow milk and soy protein in infant formulas. *J Pediatr Gastroenterol Nutr* **11**:78–82.

MONERET-VAUTRIN A, HUMBERT G, ALAIS C & GRILLIAT JB (1982) Données recentes sur les propriétés immunoallergologiques des protéines laitières. *Lait* **62**:396–408.

OGLE KA & BULLOCK JD (1980) Children with allergic rhinitis and/or bronchial asthma treated with elimination diet: a five-year follow-up. *Ann Allergy* **44**: 273–278.

OTANI H, DONG XY, HARA T, KOBAYASHI M, KAYAHARA H & HOSONO A (1989)

Human serum antibodies to cow milk proteins in infants and children having clinically allergic symptoms. *Milchwissenschaft* **44**:131–134.

OTANI H, DONG XY & HOSONO A (1990) Preparation of low-immunogenic peptide fragments from cow milk casein. *Milchwissenschaft* **45**:217–220.

PAHUD JJ, MONTI JC & JOST R (1985) Allergenicity of whey protein: its modification by tryptic in vitro hydrolysis of the protein. *J Pediatr Gastroenterol Nutr* **4**:408–413.

ROSENTHAL E, SCHLESINGER Y, BIRNBAUM Y, GOLDSTEIN R, BENDERLY A & FREIER S (1991) Intolerance to casein hydrolysate formula. *Acta Paediat Scand* **80**:958–960.

SAVILAHTI E, TAINIO V-M, SALMENPERA L, SIIMES MA & PERHEENTUPA J (1987) Prolonged exclusive breast feeding and heredity as determinants in infantile atopy. *Arch Dis Child* **62**:269–273.

SAMPSON HA, BERNHISEL-BROADBENT J, YANG E & SCANLON SM (1991) Safety of casein hydrolysate formula in children with cow milk allergy. *J Pediat* **118**:520–525.

SAYLOR JD & BAHNA SL (1991). Anaphylaxis to casein hydrolysate formula. *J Pediat* **118**:71–74.

SEBAN A, KONIJN AM & FREIER S (1977) Chemical and immunological properties of a protein hydrolysate formula. *Am J Clin Nutr* **30**:840–846.

SELF TW, HERSKOVIC T, CZAPEK E, CAPLAN D, SCHONBERGER T & GRYBOSKI JD (1969) Gastrointestinal protein allergy. Immunologic considerations. *J Am Med Ass* **207**:2393–2396.

SMITH JL, ARTEAGA C & HEYMSFIELD SB (1982) Increased ureagenesis and impaired nitrogen use during infusion of a synthetic amino acid formula. *New Engl J Med* **306**:1013–1018.

SWEATMAN MC, TASKER R, WARNER JO, FERGUSON MM & MITCHELL DNA (1986) Orofacial granulomatosis. Response to elemental diet and provocation by food additives. *Clin Allergy* **16**:331–338.

TATTRIE NH & YAGUCHI M (1973) Protein content of various processed edible oils. *J Inst Can Sci Technol Aliment* **6**:289–290.

TEICHBERG S, LIFSHITZ F, PERGOLIZZI R & WAPNIR RA (1978) Response of rat intestine to a hyperosmotic feeding. *Pediat Res* **12**:720–725.

VAN BEVER HP, DOCX M & STEVENS WJ (1989) Food and food additives in severe atopic dermatitis. *Allergy* **44**:588–594.

VANDENPLAS Y, DENEYER M, SACRE L & LOEB H (1988) Preliminary data on a field study with a new hypo-allergic formula. *Eur J Pediat* **148**:274–277.

VENTURA A, GRECO L, BALLI F et al. (1988) Cow's milk allergy in the first year of life. *Acta Paediatr Scand* (suppl. 348):3–14.

WALKER-SMITH JA, DIGEON B & PHILLIPS AD (1989) Evaluation of a casein and a whey hydrolysate for treatment of cow's-milk-sensitive enteropathy. *Eur J Pediatr* **149**:68–71.

ZEIGER RS (1990) Prevention of food allergy in infancy. *Ann Allergy* **65**:430–480.

ZEIGER RS, HELLER S, MELLON MH et al. (1989) Effect of combined maternal and infant food-allergen avoidance on development of atopy in early infancy: a randomized study. *J Allergy Clin Immunol* **84**:72–89.

Part 4 Soya Intolerance

20 Uses and constituents of soya beans
Sources, toxicity and flatulence factors

Soya beans
The soya bean, of which there are over 7300 species (Hapgood & Johns 1987), is a member of the Leguminosae family. Soya beans and their products are used as foodstuffs in numerous different ways. An outline is given below.

Soya oil
The seeds (beans) of soya are most widely used as the source of an edible oil, which is consumed as a salad oil, as a cooking oil, and in the production of margarine. Because of its high linolenic acid content (4 – 11%), the oil is prone to auto-oxidation and the development of rancidity. This problem has been reduced by genetic manipulation and by selective hydrogenation, bleaching and deodorization, and soya bean oil which contains less than 1% of linolenic acid is now available (Egan *et al.* 1987).

Soya flour
Soya beans may be ground into flour, which is often added to cereal flour. Soya flour, as an ingredient of cereal flour, is used extensively in the baking industry, and the majority of breads manufactured contain a small portion of soya flour. Pastries, cakes, biscuits, and baby foods also often contain soya flour. De-fatted soya flour is used in the manufacture of sausages and comminuted meats, and de-fatted soya grits (coarse particles of soya flour) are used in the manufacture of hamburgers, sausages and pie fillings.

Whole beans
Soya beans are occasionally cooked and eaten whole. Another way they can be consumed is as seedlings; for this purpose the beans are germinated in darkness so the seedling is blanched. Sometimes soya beans are fermented by *Aspergillus oryzae*, the product being used in the preparation of sauces (for example soy sauce or Worcester sauce) and in Indonesia for a kind of cake called tempe.

Soya protein
Soya beans have a high protein content. Soya protein concentrate is manufactured from de-fatted soya flour, and is used to make emulsions and to bind fat into food products (for example sausages). Soya protein isolate is extracted from de-fatted soya meal and is used in various products to fortify the protein content, for example a high protein biscuit. It is also used as a base for making soya milk, which can be turned into soya curd (tofu) or utilized in the manufacture of soya-based ice-cream.

Table 20.1 Manufactured foods which may contain soya protein[1]

Bread[2]
Biscuits[2]
Cakes[2]
Tinned or packet soup[2]
Chocolates (with chocolate or nut paste centres)
Ice cream
Dessert and trifle mixes
Sausages[2]
Black pudding[2]
Pork, steak or sausage pies[2]
Potted meats, meat paste[2]
Minced beef[3]

[1] In the UK, under the 1984 Food Labelling Regulations, where any of the foods on this list are packaged the presence of soya should be declared on the label. The exceptions to this are unwrapped food, soya present in flour, and where soya is included in a compound ingredient. Where an item (e.g. bread) is sold unwrapped, there would be no declaration of the ingredients, or of the fact that it contained soya. Soya flour is often added to wheat flour, and as with a number of other additives in flour, this does not have to be declared on the list of ingredients. Soya might not be mentioned in a list of ingredients if it is included in a 'compound' ingredient, that is to say an ingredient which is itself composed of two or more ingredients. If the compound ingredient constitutes less than 25% of the finished product, then the ingredients of the compound ingredient need not be declared. For example, for a pizza which included some sausage in the topping the label of ingredients is only obliged to list 'sausages' and not refer to the ingredients of the sausage.

[2] The presence of soya protein in these foods is due to flour which contains soya protein.

[3] This refers to non-prepacked mince, to which soya protein has been added. If minced beef is sold packed, then the labelling regulations require such mince to bear a declaration of its percentage minimum meat content.

Textured vegetable protein

The conversion of soya flour into products having a meat-like texture is carried out by converting the flour to a dough, heating it and then extruding it into atmospheric or reduced pressure. The sudden drop in pressure causes the material to expand and achieve the desired texture, the product being known as textured vegetable protein (Fox & Cameron 1986). This is either used in simulated meat products or added to meat as a meat extender.

Soya in food

Soya protein is so widely distributed in various foods (Wolf 1970; Table 20.1) that avoidance of soya in the diet (see chapter 21) is not easy.

Harmful effects of untreated soya

Soya protein is important as a replacement for cow's milk in the feeding of calves and piglets. The commercial importance of soya as an animal feed explains the large amount of research by the food industry into the toxicity and antigenicity of soya in animals.

toxicity   Early this century it was recognized that it was necessary to subject soya beans to heat treatment if they were to support the growth of rats (Osborne & Mendel 1917). The reason for the beneficial effect of heat treatment did not become apparent until Kunitz isolated a protein from raw soya beans which combines with trypsin to form an inactive complex (Kunitz 1945). Experiments where this purified protein was incorporated into the diet at a level equivalent to that present in raw soya beans demonstrated that this trypsin inhibitor was responsible for poor growth (Liener *et al.* 1949). Trypsin inhibitors from soya beans also cause hypertrophy and hypersecretion of the pancreas (Gorrill & Thomas 1967; Rackis 1974), and the consequent endogenous loss of protein is believed to impair growth (Liener 1986).

antigenicity   An immunologically-mediated intolerance to soya protein may also contribute to growth failure in animals (Smith & Sissons 1975; Barratt *et al.* 1978, 1979; Kilshaw & Sissons 1979).

implications for humans   The implications for humans is that soya beans which have been inadequately heat treated may be toxic, and there is a report of adverse reactions (e.g. abdominal pain, vomiting, diarrhoea, headache) after consumption of inadequately heat-treated soya products (Gunn *et al.* 1980). The relationship between this heat-sensitive toxin in soya beans and the toxic and heat-sensitive haemagglutinating lectins found in other beans (e.g. red kidney beans – see below) is unclear.

Haemagglutinating lectins in other legume seeds   It is well recognized that red kidney beans contain toxic haemagglutinating lectins, and ingestion of raw red kidney beans may cause severe vomiting and diarrhoea (Noah *et al.* 1980). Toxic lectins, which are destroyed by heating beans to 100°C for 10 min (Grant *et al.* 1982; Thompson *et al.* 1983), are also present in raw white kidney beans, black kidney beans, tepary beans, runner beans (seeds), winged (Goa) beans and butter (Lima) beans, but not in the seeds of the legumes lentils, peas, chick peas, mung beans, broad beans, aduki beans, pinto beans and soya beans (Grant *et al.* 1983).

Flatulence   Soya and other beans can cause the formation of gastrointestinal gas leading to flatulence, abdominal pain and loose stools (Steggerda *et al.* 1966). The gas producing factors are mainly the oligosaccharides raffinose and stachyose, and intestinal bacteria are required for the production of gas (Rackis *et al.* 1970a, b). The administration of oral antibiotics such as neomycin, by destroying anaerobic bacteria in the gut, abolishes or greatly reduces intestinal gas production after a meal of beans (Richards & Steggerda 1966). Raffinose and stachyose can pass into the stools unchanged, or they can be metabolized completely, and the susceptibility to flatulence varies greatly. This may partly depend on gastrointestinal motility, since intestinal bacteria need more time to digest these oligosaccharides than others (Rackis *et al.* 1970a).

Key references 20.1   RACKIS JJ (1974) Biological and physiological factors in soybeans. *J Am Oil Chemists' Soc* **51**:161A–174A. *A detailed review of antinutritional factors in soybeans, mainly dealing with adverse effects in animals.*

20.2   BARRATT MEJ, STRACHAN PJ & PORTER P (1979) Immunologically mediated nutritional disturbances associated with soya-protein antigens. *Proc Nutr Soc* **38**:143–150. *A review of the evidence relating to digestive disturbances in young animals attributable to immunologically-mediated inflammatory responses to soya protein within the intestinal mucosa.*

20.3   BARRATT MEJ, STRACHAN PJ & PORTER P (1978) Antibody mechanisms implicated in digestive disturbances following ingestion of soya protein in calves and piglets. *Clin Exp Immunol* **31**:305–312. Biopsy studies showed that the feeding of soya protein to young animals caused stunting of the intestinal villi and cellular infiltration of the lamina propria, changes resembling the enteropathy seen in humans with intolerance to soya.

20.4   CATSIMPOOLAS N, EKENSTAM C & MEYER EW (1969) Separation of soybean whey proteins by isoelectric focusing. *Cereal Chem* **46**:357–369. Multiple different trypsin inhibitors were demonstrated in soya bean protein by isoelectric focusing. *The best known soya-derived trypsin inhibitor is the Kunitz inhibitor, which as well as being toxic can also be antigenic in man, see* Moroz LA & Yang WH (1980) Kunitz soybean trypsin inhibitor. A specific allergen in food anaphylaxis. *New Engl J Med* **302**:1126–1128.

20.5   RACKIS JJ, HONIG DH, SESSA DJ & STEGGERDA FR (1970) Flavor and flatulence factors in soybean protein products. *J Agr Food Chem* **18**:977–982. *Includes a review of flatulence factors in soya bean products.*

Summary 20   Soya beans are widely used as a source of a number of food products which include soya oil, soya flour, soya curd (tofu) and textured vegetable protein. Consumption of unheated soya beans, which are potentially toxic, can result in acute gastrointestinal symptoms, and animals which are fed on unheated soya beans may fail to thrive. In common with other beans, soya beans contain the oligosaccharides raffinose and stachyose, which if taken in sufficient quantities may cause flatulence, abdominal pain and loose stools.

21 Soya protein intolerance
Similar to cow's milk protein intolerance

Similarity with cow's milk protein intolerance

Although less well documented, the features of intolerance to soya protein appear to be similar to those of intolerance to cow's milk protein.

Gastrointestinal features

The gastrointestinal features of soya protein intolerance are indistinguishable from those of cow's milk protein intolerance (Visakorpi 1983). Thus soya protein intolerance can cause frequent loose stools, vomiting, colitis, enteropathy and failure to thrive, intestinal blood loss and anaemia, and irritability and crying (Cook 1960; Ament & Rubin 1972; Baudon *et al.* 1976; Halpin *et al.* 1977; Goel *et al.* 1978; Powell 1978; Perkkiö *et al.* 1981; Perisic *et al.* 1988).

Respiratory features

Coughing, wheezing, asthma and rhinitis can all be features of soya protein intolerance (Fries 1971). Asthma as a result of inhalation of soya flour and dust is also well recognized (Bush & Cohen 1977; Antó *et al.* 1989; Rodrigo *et al.* 1990; Swanson *et al.* 1991).

Dermatological features

Urticaria, angioedema and atopic eczema can be features of soya protein intolerance (Matthiensen & Braun 1974; Kuroume *et al.* 1976; Skipp 1977; Burks *et al.* 1988).

Anaphylaxis

Anaphylactic shock is an uncommon but well documented feature of soya protein intolerance (Vest 1953; Cook 1960; David 1984).

Timing of reaction

As with cow's milk protein intolerance, there is some variation in the speed of onset of symptoms after challenge with soya protein. Vomiting, urticaria, angioedema and coughing or wheezing all usually occur within 2 hours of ingestion. However the onset of some adverse reactions may be delayed for 24 to 48 hours or more in the case of gastrointestinal symptoms and atopic eczema. Inhalation of soya flour has been shown to cause both immediate and delayed asthmatic reactions (Bush & Cohen 1977).

Incidence

In a prospective study of 1753 unselected infants, 632 received a soya-based milk formula in the first 6 months of life, and three developed intolerance to soya protein, an incidence of 0.5% (Halpern *et al.* 1973). However a far higher incidence of soya protein intolerance has been reported in children with preceding cow's milk protein intolerance, and the incidence of intolerance to soya protein in three series of infants with cow's milk protein intolerance was 15%

111

(Savilahti 1981), 26% (Gerrard 1973) and 43% (Hill *et al.* 1984). In unpublished studies which only included cases of intolerance proven by double-blind placebo-controlled challenges, the figures for soya protein intolerance were somewhat lower, namely 8% and 14% (Bock 1991).

Diagnosis   The diagnosis rests on clinical suspicion, followed by a trial of withdrawal and re-introduction of soya protein. As in the case of cow's milk protein intolerance, skin-prick tests (see chapter 41) or RAST tests (see chapter 43) are unhelpful.

Avoidance   Avoidance of soya protein in the diet is difficult because of the enormous range of manufactured foods which contain soya protein (see Table 20.1), and complete avoidance is unlikely to be achieved successfully without the help of a dietitian. There are a number of traps, such as the widespread use of soya protein in flour, and therefore in most breads. The use of soya in this way is not obvious to the consumer. This is partly because bread is often sold unwrapped, and therefore without any list of ingredients. It is also because soya is not likely to be declared on a list of ingredients of bread, because it is permitted to include in flour both soya and a number of other undeclared ingredients (e.g. iron salts, chalk, thiamine, nicotinic acid and a range of bleaching and improving agents – see chapter 26). In soya protein intolerant infants, the choice of milk substitute lies between a cow's milk formula (provided the child is not intolerant to cow's milk protein) or a casein or whey hydrolysate formula.

Contaminated soya products   Contamination during manufacture of soya products with cow's milk protein is a recorded cause of adverse reactions in patients with cow's milk protein intolerance (Gern *et al.* 1991).

Other forms of soya   All reports of intolerance concern soya protein. It is unknown whether soya lecithin, soya margarine or soya oil contain sufficient protein to provoke adverse reactions in those with soya protein intolerance. Only minute traces of protein were found in soya oil in one study (Tattrie & Yaguchi 1973). In one small clinical study, seven patients with intolerance to soya beans had no adverse reaction when soya oil was consumed (Bush *et al.* 1985). However in another study, some samples of soya oil, lecithin and margarine were found to contain soya protein (Porras *et al.* 1985). The implication is that these items must be excluded from the diet if soya protein needs to be completely avoided.

Other food intolerance   No figures are available for the incidence of intolerance to other foods in patients with intolerance to soya protein. Soya protein intolerance is most commonly discovered in patients with cow's milk protein intolerance, and the reverse association sometimes occurs (Whitington & Gibson 1977). On the basis of *in vitro* IgE antibody cross-reactivity, it has been suggested that subjects with intolerance to soya protein are at increased risk of being intolerant to other legumes, such as haricot beans, red kidney beans, green beans or peas (Barnett *et al.* 1987). However, there is no objective clinical data (e.g. from double-blind challenge studies) to support this claim. In a recent study of 69 children with intolerance to legumes (peanut, soya, green bean, pea and lima bean) only two patients had intolerance to two legumes (Bernhisel-Broadbent & Sampson 1989). Both had a history of anaphylaxis after peanut ingestion and a positive double-blind placebo-controlled challenge to soya.

Key references   21.1   PERKKIO M, SAVILAHTI E & KUITUNEN P (1981) Morphometric and immuno-histochemical study of jejunal biopsies from children with intestinal soya allergy. *Eur J Pediat* **137**:63–69. Jejunal biopsies of five infants with gastrointestinal features of soya protein intolerance demonstrated villous atrophy, crypt hyperplasia, an increased cell renewal rate, an inflammatory reaction in the lamina propria and an increased number of IgA and IgM containing cells.

21.2   HALPIN TC, BYRNE WJ & AMENT ME (1977) Colitis, persistent diarrhoea, and soy protein intolerance. *J Pediat* **91**:404–407. *A description of four infants with severe gastrointestinal features of soya protein intolerance.*

21.3   BUSH RK & COHEN M (1977) Immediate and late onset asthma from occupational exposure to soybean dust. *Clin Allergy* **7**:369–373. *A detailed study of a subject with asthma from occupational exposure to soya flour.*

21.4   DAVID TJ (1984) Anaphylactic shock during elimination diets for severe atopic eczema. *Arch Dis Child* **59**:983–986. *Includes a report of a near-fatal anaphylactic reaction to soya protein in a 4-year old boy with atopic eczema.*

21.5   PORRAS O, CARLSSON B, FÄLLSTRÖM SP & HANSON LÅ (1985) Detection of soy protein in soy lecithin, margarine and, occasionally, soy oil. *Int Arch Allergy Appl Immunol* **78**:30–32. Samples of soya lecithin, soya margarine and soya oil were tested for the presence of soya proteins by an inhibition technique using ELISA. Six out of seven samples of soya lecithin and all five samples of soya margarine contained soya protein at a concentration ranging from 0.1–27.2 mg/g. Of the eight samples of soya oil, three contained soya protein at a concentration which ranged from 0.11 to 3.30 mg/g. *If soya protein needs to be completely avoided, then soya lecithin, margarine and oil all must be excluded from the diet.*

21.6   BURKS AW, BROOKS JR & SAMPSON HA (1988) Allergenicity of major component proteins of soybean determined by enzyme-linked immunosorbent assay (ELISA) and immunoblotting in children with atopic dermatitis and positive soy challenges. *J Allergy Clin Immunol* **81**:1135–1142. In serum from eight children with atopic eczema and positive double-blind placebo-controlled challenges to soya, IgE and IgG specific antibodies to crude soya were elevated, but no one fraction of soya was clearly more antigenic.

Summary 21   The clinical features of intolerance to soya protein are similar to those of cow's milk protein intolerance. There is little data on the incidence of intolerance to soya protein in the general population, but there is a strong association between intolerance to cow's milk protein and soya. Estimates of the proportion of those with cow's milk protein intolerance who are also intolerant to soya protein range from 8% to 43%. The management is avoidance of all foods which contain soya protein.

References to Chapters 20 and 21

AMENT ME & RUBIN CE (1972) Soy protein – another cause of the flat intestinal lesion. *Gastroenterology* **62**:227–234.

ANTÓ JM, SUNYER J, RODRIGUEZ-ROISIN R, SUAREZ-CERVERA M & VAZQUEZ L (1989) Community outbreaks of asthma associated with inhalation of soyabean dust. *New Engl J Med* **320**:1097–1102.

BARNETT D, BONHAM B & HOWDEN MEH (1987) Allergenic cross-reactions among legume foods – an in vitro study. *J Allergy Clin Immunol* **79**:433–438.

BARRATT MEJ, STRACHAN PJ & PORTER P (1978) Antibody mechanisms implicated in digestive disturbances following ingestion of soya protein in calves and piglets. *Clin Exp Immunol* **31**:305–312.

BARRATT MEJ, STRACHAN PJ & PORTER P (1979) Immunologically mediated nutritional disturbances associated with soya-protein antigens. *Proc Nutr Soc* **38**:143–150.

BAUDON JJ, BOULESTEIX J, LAGARDERE B & FONTAINE JL (1976) Atrophie villositaire aigue par intolerance aux proteines du soja. *Arch Franc Ped* **33**: 153–160.

BERNHISEL-BROADBENT J & SAMPSON HA (1989) Cross-allergenicity in the legume botanical family in children with food hypersensitivity. *J Allergy Clin Immunol* **83**:435–440.

BOCK SA (1991) Oral challenge procedures. In Metcalfe DD, Sampson HA & Simon RA (eds) *Food Allergy: Adverse Reactions to Foods and Food Additives*, pp. 81–95, Blackwell Scientific Publications, Boston.

BURKS AW, BROOKS JR & SAMPSON HA (1988) Allergenicity of major component proteins of soybean determined by enzyme-linked immunosorbent assay (ELISA) and immunoblotting in children with atopic dermatitis and positive soy challenges. *J Allergy Clin Immunol* **81**:1135–1142.

BUSH RK & COHEN M (1977) Immediate and late onset asthma from occupational exposure to soybean dust. *Clin Allergy* **7**:369–373.

BUSH RK, TAYLOR SL, NORDLEE JA & BUSSE WW (1985) Soybean oil is not allergenic to soybean-sensitive individuals. *J Allergy Clin Immunol* **76**: 242–245.

COOK CD (1960) Probable gastrointestinal reaction to soybean. *New Engl J Med* **263**:1076–1077.

DAVID TJ (1984) Anaphylactic shock during elimination diets for severe atopic eczema. *Arch Dis Child* **59**:983–986.

EGAN H, KIRK RS & SAWYER R (1987) *Pearson's Chemical Analysis of Foods.* 8th edn, Longman Scientific & Technical, Harlow.

FOX BA & CAMERON AG (1986) *Food Science. A Chemical Approach,* 4th edn, Hodder & Stoughton, London.

FRIES JH (1971) Studies of the allergenicity of soy bean. *Ann Allergy* **29**:1–7.

GERN JE, YANG E, EVRARD HM & SAMPSON HA (1991) Allergic reactions to milk-contaminated 'non-dairy' products. *New Engl J Med* **324**:976–979.

GERRARD JW, MacKENZIE JWA, GOLUBOFF N, GARSON JZ & MANINGAS CS (1973) Cow's milk allergy: prevalence and manifestations in an unselected series of newborns. *Acta Paediat Scand* (suppl. 234):1–21.

GOEL K, LIFSHITZ F, KAN E & TEICHBERG S (1978) Monosaccharide intolerance and soy-protein hypersensitivity in an infant with diarrhea. *J Pediat* **93**: 617–619.

GORRILL ADL & THOMAS JW (1967) Body weight changes, pancreas size and enzyme activity, and proteolytic enzyme activity and protein digestion in intestinal contents from calves fed soybean and milk protein diets. *J Nutr* **92**:215–223.

GRANT G, MORE LJ, McKENZIE NH & PUSZTAI A (1982) The effect of heating on the haemagglutinating activity and nutritional properties of bean (*Phaseolus vulgaris*) seeds. *J Sci Food Agric* **33**:1324–1326.

GRANT G, MORE LJ, McKENZIE NH, STEWART JC & PUSZTAI A (1983) A survey of the nutritional and haemagglutination properties of legume seeds generally available in the UK. *Br J Nutr* **50**:207–214.

GUNN RA, TAYLOR PR & GANGAROSA EJ (1980) Gastrointestinal illness associated with consumption of a soy protein extender. *J Food Protection* **43**:525–527.

HALPERN SR, SELLARS WA, JOHNSON RB, ANDERSON DW, SAPERSTEIN S & REISCH JS (1973) Development of childhood allergy in infants fed breast, soy, or cow milk. *J Allergy Clin Immunol* **51**:139–151.

HALPIN TC, BYRNE WJ & AMENT ME (1977) Colitis, persistent diarrhea, and soy protein intolerance. *J Pediat* **91**:404–407.

HAPGOOD F & JOHNS C (1987) The prodigious soybean. *National Geographic* **172**:66–91.

HILL DJ, FORD RPK, SHELTON MJ & HOSKING CS (1984) A study of 100 infants and young children with cow's milk allergy. *Clin Rev Allergy* **2**:125–142.

KILSHAW PJ & SISSONS JW (1979) Gastrointestinal allergy to soybean protein in preruminant calves. Allergenic constituents of soybean products. *Res Vet Sci* **27**:366–371.

KUNITZ M (1945) Crystallization of a trypsin inhibitor from soybeans. *Science* **101**:688–689.

KUROUME T, OGURI M, MATSUMURA T *et al.* (1976) Milk sensitivity and soybean sensitivity in the production of eczematous manifestations in breast-fed infants with particular reference to intra-uterine sensitization. *Ann Allergy* **37**:41–46.

LIENER IE (1986) The nutritional significance of naturally occurring toxins in plant foodstuffs. In Harris JB (ed) *Natural Toxins. Animal, Plant, and Microbial,* pp. 72–94, Clarendon Press, Oxford.

LIENER IE, DEUEL HJ & FEVOLD HL (1949) The effect of supplemental methionine on the nutritive value of diets containing concentrates of the soybean trypsin inhibitor. *J Nutr* **39**:325–339.

MATTHIENSEN RP & BRAUN W (1974) Sojaprotein – ein verborgenes Allergen. *Dtsch Med Wschr* **99**:2175–2177.

NOAH ND, BENDER AE, REAIDI BG & GILBERT RJ (1980) Food poisoning from raw red kidney beans. *Br Med J* **281**:236–237.

OSBORNE TB & MENDEL LB (1917) The use of soybean as food. *J Biol Chem* **32**:369–387.

PERISIC VN, FILIPOVIC D & KOKAI G (1988) Allergic colitis with rectal bleeding in an exclusively breast-fed neonate. *Acta Paediat Scand* **77**:163–164.

PERKKIO M, SAVILAHTI E & KUITUNEN P (1981) Morphometric and immuno-histochemical study of jejunal biopsies from children with intestinal soya allergy. *Eur J Pediatr* **137**:63–69.

PORRAS O, CARLSSON B, FÄLLSTRÖM SP & HANSON LÅ (1985) Detection of soy protein in soy lecithin, margarine and, occasionally, soy oil. *Int Arch Allergy Appl Immunol* **78**:30–32.

POWELL GK (1978) Milk- and soy-induced enterocolitis of infancy. Clinical features and standardization of challenge. *J Pediat* **93**:553–560.

RACKIS JJ (1974) Biological and physiological factors in soybeans. *J Am Oil Chem Soc* **51**:161A–174A.

RACKIS JJ, HONIG DH, SESSA DJ & STEGGERDA FR (1970a) Flavor and flatulence factors in soybean protein products. *J Agr Food Chem* **18**:977–982.

RACKIS JJ, SESSA DJ, STEGGERDA FR, SHIMIZU T, ANDERSON J & PEARL SL (1970b) Soybean factors relating to gas production by intestinal bacteria. *J Food Sci* **35**:634–639.

RICHARDS EA & STEGGERDA FR (1966) Production and inhibition of gas in various regions in the intestine of the dog. *Proc Soc Exp Biol Med* **122**:573–576.

RODRIGO MJ, MORELL F, HELM RM *et al.* (1990) Identification and partial characterization of the soybean-dust allergens involved in the Barcelona asthma epidemic. *J Allergy Clin Immunol* **85**:778–784.

SAVILAHTI E (1981) Cow's milk allergy. *Allergy* **36**:73–88.

SKIPP D (1977) Possible allergic reactions to soya flour. *Brit Med J* **1**:971.

SMITH RH & SISSONS JW (1975) The effect of different feeds, including those containing soya-bean products, on the passage of digesta from the abomasum of the preruminant calf. *Br J Nutr* **33**:329–349.

STEGGERDA FR, RICHARDS EA & RACKIS JJ (1966) Effects of various soybean products on flatulence in the adult man. *Proc Soc Exp Biol Med* **121**:1235–1239.

SWANSON MC, LI JTC, WENTZ-MURTHA PE *et al.* (1991) Source of aero-allergen of soybean dust: a low molecular mass glycopeptide from soybean tela. *J Allergy Clin Immunol* **87**:783–788.

TATTRIE NH & YAGUCHI M (1973) Protein content of various processed edible oils. *J Inst Can Sci Technol Aliment* **6**:289–290.

THOMPSON LU, REA RL & JENKINS DJA (1983) Effect of heat processing on hemagglutinin activity in red kidney beans. *J Food Sci* **48**:235–236.

VEST M (1953) Nahrungsmittelallergie, insbesondere Kuhmilchallergie bei Säuglingen. *Ann Paediat* **181**:277–294.

VISAKORPI JK (1983) Milk and soybean protein allergy. *J Ped Gastroenterol Nutr* **2**(suppl.):S293–S297.

WHITINGTON PF & GIBSON R (1977) Soy protein intolerance: four patients with concomitant cow's milk intolerance. *Pediatrics* **59**:730–732.

WOLF WJ (1970) Soybean proteins: their functional, chemical, and physical properties. *J Agr Food Chem* **18**:969–976.

Part 5 Egg Intolerance

22 Composition of eggs
Water, protein, lipid and pigment

Definitions In this book a hen is taken to mean the female of the common domestic fowl, a chicken to mean the young of the common domestic fowl, and an egg to mean a hen's egg.

Egg composition The average weight of an egg produced by selectively bred strains of hens is 57 g. By weight, an egg consists of 57% white, 32% yolk and 11% shell (Egan *et al.* 1987). The major constituents of eggs are protein, lipid and water (Table 22.1).

Albumen or albumin? The main protein in egg white is album*e*n. Album*i*n is the protein found in blood. The spelling of the two is a common source of confusion.

Egg white Water comprises 88% of the egg white. The rest is mainly albumen (see Table 22.1), a mixture of some 40 different proteins (Vadehra & Nath 1973). About half the protein is ovalbumen (Table 22.2). Another major constituent is ovotransferrin, also called conalbumen, which firmly binds metallic ions such as iron. It is known that the consumption of egg inhibits the absorption of iron (Elwood 1968), although whether this is attributable to ovotransferrin is unclear. Ovomucoid is a heat-resistant glycoprotein which contributes to the gel-like structure of thick white. Avidin combines with biotin to form a stable complex incapable of absorption by the intestinal tract of man, but since cooking inactivates avidin, the consumption of eggs does not cause biotin deficiency. Ovoflavoprotein is a riboflavin-binding apoprotein (Powrie & Nakai 1986).

Egg yolk Water comprises 50% of the yolk, and 33% of the yolk is lipid, containing mainly triacylglycerol (66%), phospholipid (28%) and cholesterol (5%). The average egg contains 260 mg cholesterol (Cook & Briggs 1986).

yolk protein Although 16% of the egg yolk is comprised of protein, knowledge of the protein composition of egg yolk is scanty compared with the detailed information available about egg white proteins. Textbooks of food chemistry list phosvitins, livetins and lipovitellins as the principal classes of protein in egg yolk (see Regenstein & Regenstein 1984; Powrie & Nakai 1985 and Table 22.3). However it is clear from studies which used immunological techniques such as immuno-electrophoresis, IgE binding or immunoelectrotransfer, that egg

119

Table 22.1 The composition of albumen, yolk and whole egg[1]

Egg component	% Protein	% Lipid	% Carbohydrate
Albumen	9.7–10.6	0.03	0.4–0.9
Yolk	15.7–16.6	31.8–35.5	0.2–1.0
Whole egg	12.8–13.4	10.5–11.8	0.3–1.0

[1] Source: Powrie & Nakai (1986).

Table 22.2 Proteins in egg albumen[1]

Protein	Amount of albumen (%)	Molecular weight
Ovalbumen	54	45 000
Ovotransferrin	12	76 000
Ovomucoid	11	28 000
Ovomucin	3.5	$5.5–8.3 \times 10^6$
Lysozyme	3.4	14 300
G2 Globulin	4.0	$3.0–4.5 \times 10^4$
G3 Globulin	4.0	—
Ovoinhibitor	1.5	49 000
Ficin inhibitor	0.05	12 700
Ovoglycoprotein	1.0	24 400
Ovoflavoprotein	0.8	32 000
Ovomacroglobulin	0.5	$7.6–9.0 \times 10^5$
Avidin	0.05	68 300

[1] Source: Powrie & Nakai (1986).

Table 22.3 Proteins of egg yolk[1]

Protein	Percentage of egg white solids	Classification
Lipovitellin	16–18	Lipoprotein
Lipovitellenin	12–13	Lipoprotein
Livetins	4–10	Pseudoglobulin
Vitellin	4–15	Phosphoprotein
Vitellenin	8–9	Phosphoprotein
Phosvitin	5–6	Phosphoprotein

[1] Source: Regenstein & Regenstein (1984).

white proteins can also be detected in the yolk (Langeland 1983; Anet *et al.* 1985).

yellow colour   The yellow colour of the yolk is attributable to the presence of carotenoid pigments, mainly lutein, zeaxanthin and cryptoxanthin (Coultate 1984). The exact types and amounts of these pigments depend on the diet of the hen.

Key reference 22.1   STADELMAN WJ & COTTERILL OJ (eds) (1986) *Egg Science and Technology*, 3rd edn, Avi Publishing Company, Westport, Connecticut. *Multi-author book on the chemistry and nutritive value of eggs.*

Summary 22   The major constituents of egg white are water (88%) and protein (10%). The predominant proteins in egg white are ovalbumen, ovotransferrin and ovomucoid. The major constituents of egg yolk are water (50%), lipid (33%) and protein (16%).

23 Allergens in eggs
Ovalbumen, ovotransferrin and ovomucoid

Egg white   The major allergens in egg white have been identified as ovalbumen, ovomucoid and ovotransferrin (Bleumink & Young 1969; Langeland 1982; Hoffman 1983; Langeland & Harbitz 1983). Lysozyme and ovomucin appear to be of little or no significance as allergens (Bleumink & Young 1969; Langeland 1982; Hoffman 1983; Langeland & Aas 1987). By means of radio-immunoelectrophoresis, 10 other unnamed allergens, thought to be of minor importance, have been identified in the serum of patients with egg intolerance (Langeland 1982).

Egg yolk   Immunoelectrophoresis of egg yolk has clearly demonstrated the presence of all three major allergens of egg white (Langeland 1983a). Egg yolk contains ovotransferrin at 15% of the concentration found in egg white, but ovalbumen and ovomucin are present only in trace amounts (Langeland & Aas 1987). In practice the importance of the small amounts of egg white proteins in egg yolk is likely to be overshadowed by the difficulty of avoiding contamination by some egg white when preparing food with egg yolk. Tolerance to egg white with intolerance only to egg yolk has only been documented once (De Maat-Bleeker *et al.* 1985). Recent studies have demonstrated that the egg yolk proteins apovitellenins I and VI and phosvitin can bind IgE from the sera of egg intolerant individuals in a RAST test, and it has been postulated that these are also allergens which are responsible for some cases of egg intolerance (Walsh *et al.* 1988). There is no other evidence to suggest that the major proteins of egg yolk cause egg intolerance.

Cooking

Cooking reduces the allergenicity of eggs by 70%, but one of the major allergens in eggs, ovomucoid, is resistant to heating (Bleumink & Young 1969).

Cross-reaction — chicken

Trace quantities of ovalbumen and ovotransferrin have been detected by immunoelectrophoresis in the raw flesh of hens and chickens (Langeland 1983a). It is unclear whether this is of any clinical significance, as most children with egg intolerance can tolerate cooked chicken.

Cross-reaction — other bird's eggs

The whites of egg from turkeys, ducks, geese and seagulls all contain ovalbumen, ovomucoid and ovotransferrin, the major allergens in hens' eggs. The eggs of hens and turkeys have a similar relative potency of allergenicity, and their egg whites have a similar immunochemical identity. The immunochemical identity of proteins in the egg white of ducks and geese differs somewhat from that of hens, and they may have less potency as allergens. Seagull's egg white is the least allergenic, and bears the least immunochemical similarity with hen's eggs (Langeland 1983a).

Cross-reaction — chicken feathers

Intolerance to egg and allergy to bird feathers are common, and there is no objective data to indicate whether they co-exist more commonly than one would expect by chance. Studies which have suggested that there is an association between the two disorders have relied on skin-prick test or specific IgE antibody test results rather than information from challenges, and have often not distinguished between feathers from hens or from other birds (e.g. Bausela *et al.* 1991).

Egg & gut permeability

Ovalbumen has been used as a tracer substance in studies of gut permeability (Schloss & Worthen 1916), though it is not ideal for this purpose because of interaction with anti-ovalbumen antibodies (Dannaeus *et al.* 1979), and it has been shown to be absorbed into the blood of healthy infants and adults (Gruskay & Cooke 1955). The production of serum IgG antibodies to egg protein must be regarded as a normal immune response; such IgG antibodies are found in the newborn and simply reflect the corresponding maternal concentrations (Dannaeus *et al.* 1978).

Key references 23.1

LANGELAND T (1982) A clinical and immunological study of allergy to hen's egg white. III. Allergens in hen's egg white studied by crossed radio-immunoelectrophoresis (CRIE). *Allergy* **37**:521–530. *Identifies the important allergens.*

23.2   LANGELAND T (1983) A clinical and immunological study of allergy to hen's egg white. VI. Occurrence of proteins cross-reacting with allergens in hen's egg white as studied in egg white from turkey, duck, goose, seagull, and in hen's egg yolk, and hen and chicken sera and flesh. *Allergy* **38**:399–412. *Key study of cross-reaction between egg antigens of different birds.*

23.3   FOTHERGILL LA & FOTHERGILL JE (1971) Immunochemical comparison of ovalbumins from nine different species. *Comp Biochem Physiol* **40A**:445–451. Immunochemical comparison of egg white from hens and a wide range of birds (including golden pheasant, grouse, fulvous whistling duck, and grey lag goose) has demonstrated that in general hen's egg ovalbumen cross-reacted most strongly with the phylogenetically most closely related ovalbumen. *For information about pigeons, quail, cassowary, emu, ostrich, tinamou and green Java pea fowl see:* Miller HT & Feeney RE (1964) Immunochemical relationships of proteins of avian egg white. *Arch Biochem Biophys* **108**:117–124.

Summary 23   The major allergens in egg white are ovalbumen, ovomucoid and ovotransferrin. All three are also present in much smaller quantities in egg yolk. The eggs of turkeys, ducks and geese contain similar allergens to hen's eggs. Cooking reduces the allergenicity of eggs by 70%. Trace quantities of ovalbumen and ovotransferrin have been detected in the raw flesh of chickens, but most children with egg intolerance can tolerate cooked chicken.

24 Egg intolerance I: clinical features
Brisk reactions in infancy are common

Prevalence   The prevalence of egg intolerance is greatest in infants under the age of 12 months. After the age of 2 years it becomes much less common. Most studies of the prevalence of egg intolerance have been performed in highly selected populations which may be at increased risk for food intolerance, particularly subjects with atopic disease (Freedman & Sellars 1959; Schur *et al.* 1974; Dannaeus & Inganas 1981). Thus these studies do not provide an estimate of the prevalence in the general population. For example, a particularly large series of highly selected mainly paediatric patients with a history of food intolerance, and often with atopic eczema, were studied with double-blind placebo-controlled food challenges. In this study, egg was the most common food to provoke a positive reaction, in 143 out of 426 positive challenges (Bock *et al.* 1988).

in Finland   In a study in Finland of the prevalence of food intolerance in children aged 1–6 years, parents' reports suggested an incidence of intolerance to eggs of 6% at 1 year of age, 7% at 2 years, 9% at 3 years, falling to only 1% at 6 years (Kajosaari 1982). However, not all of these parents' reports could be confirmed by open food challenge at home, and this study did not include infants under the age of 12 months where the incidence of food intolerance in general (Bock 1987) and egg intolerance in particular are at a peak.

Clinical presentation   It is convenient to divide cases of egg intolerance into those where symptoms occur within minutes of egg ingestion, and those in whom the responses are more delayed. The former are much more common.

first exposure to egg   The most common presentation is the rapid onset of symptoms minutes after an infant is given egg for the first time in his or her life; in one series of patients with egg allergy this occurred in 57% of children (Langeland 1983b). It is unclear how such infants have become sensitized to egg (Hill 1955). It is probable that some have received small amounts of egg in a manufactured baby food, but others may have been sensitized *in utero* or via breast milk (Matsumura *et al.* 1975; Van Asperen *et al.* 1983; Cant *et al.* 1985; Gerrard & Perelmutter 1986).

Immediate reactions   The most immediate reactions consist of an erythematous rash around the mouth within seconds of eating egg, followed 1–5 min later by swelling and urticaria of the oral mucosa, around the mouth and on the face. Angioedema is common and occurs within minutes. In severe cases, urticaria may spread to the rest of the body. In some cases the features above may be accompanied by other features such as wheezing, stridor, conjunctivitis or sneezing and rhinitis. A stridor indicates angioedema of the trachea, and where there is also a hoarse voice, of the larynx. In severe cases, ingestion of egg protein may cause anaphylaxis. Vomiting may be an additional or sole symptom, and although the mechanism is not clear, it may occur within seconds of egg ingestion. Loose stools may occur, but are uncommon (Langeland 1983b).

skin contact   Children with immediate onset of urticaria and angioedema after eating egg also exhibit a local urticarial reaction if egg, especially raw egg, is applied to the skin (Court & Ng 1984). Indeed, the urticaria and swelling of the oral mucosa which occur after eating egg are probably contact reactions.

Delayed reactions
asthma   Asthma, i.e. wheezing and coughing starting more than 1 hour after egg ingestion, is uncommon. Asthma may also follow the inhalation of egg (Edwards *et al.* 1983).

atopic eczema   The ingestion of egg can undoubtedly worsen atopic eczema (Langeland 1985), but studies of the benefit of egg (and cow's milk protein) avoidance have given conflicting results (Atherton *et al.* 1978; Neild *et al.* 1986). The most common reaction in eczematous children is the rapid onset of urticaria and angioedema. Since scratching is a symptom of urticaria, it is not surprising that the eczema worsens. A controversial matter is whether egg intolerance can cause worsening of atopic eczema without causing urticaria. The author's experience is that delayed worsening of eczema following skin contact with (Benton & Barnetson 1985) or ingestion of egg does occur, but that this is overshadowed by the more common immediate reactions. An important point is that the deterioration of eczema caused by eating egg often lasts several days, far longer than immediate urticarial reactions which disappear in a few hours. It is unclear whether this persistence of symptoms is directly due to egg intolerance, or simply to a general worsening of the eczema. It is clear that patients with atopic eczema, more than any other group of patients, are especially likely to experience egg intolerance (Ford & Taylor 1982).

Other food intolerance   Little information is available about the incidence of intolerance to other foods in children with egg intolerance. One study of 84 children with egg intolerance reported that 14 (17%) had cow's milk intolerance and 14 (17%) fish intolerance, but the sample was hospital-based and highly selected, and most subjects had asthma and atopic eczema (Langeland 1983b).

Key references   24.1   LANGELAND T (1983) A clinical and immunological study of allergy to hen's egg white. I. A clinical study of egg allergy. *Clin Allergy* **13**:371–382. A description of the clinical features of 84 atopic children aged 1–15 years who had both egg intolerance and serum IgE antibodies to egg white. The patients were highly selected. *A sample of this sort will exclude the common patient who is found to be intolerant to egg in early infancy, grows out of it in a year or two, and has little or no evidence of other atopic disease.*

24.2   SCHLOSS OM (1912) A case of allergy to common foods. *Am J Dis Child* **3**:341–362. *A remarkable study of a child intolerant to eggs, almonds and oats.* Skin tests with egg white proteins showed particularly strong reactions with ovomucin. Skin tests with egg yolk, very carefully prepared so as to be free of egg white, were also positive, the activity of the egg yolk in this regard being about one-tenth as great as egg white. Six ml of the patient's serum was injected into two guinea-pigs, followed a day later by an injection of 150 mg ovomucoid. After 45 min both animals were moribund; one died. Four control animals who received normal human serum experienced no symptoms other than a slight fall in temperature after an injection with ovomucoid. The patient was treated with oral hyposensitization to ovomucoid (see next chapter).

24.3   ATHERTON DJ, SEWELL DJ, SOOTHILL JF, WELLS RS & CHILVERS CED (1978) A double-blind controlled crossover trial of an antigen-avoidance diet in atopic eczema. *Lancet* **1**:401–403. Fourteen out of 20 patients responded more favourably to avoidance of egg and cow's milk than to a control period when both foods were given. *Problems were: (a) of 36 children with atopic eczema, only 20 managed to cope with a fairly simple regimen of egg and cow's milk avoidance; (b) the period of avoidance was confused by the fact that the children were given a soya-based milk formula (to which they could have been intolerant); (c) during the period of challenge with cow's milk and egg the patients received the equivalent of one pint of milk and one egg per day, a quantity likely to be (at least for egg) well in excess of their normal intake; and (d) there was a treatment order effect; patients experienced more benefit during the first period than the second.*

24.4   NEILD VS, MARSDEN RA, BAILES JA & BLAND JM (1986) Egg and milk exclusion diets in atopic eczema. *Br J Dermatol* **114**:117–123. The results of this study are contrary to Atherton's report which stated that as many as 60% of children benefited from a diet excluding egg and cow's milk. Neild *et al.* found no significant differences between the scores for area of skin affected, itching, or consumption of steroids at the end of the trial diet compared with those at the end of the normal diet. 25% of patients appeared to benefit from egg and cow's milk avoidance; half of these were children under 8 years. *Problems were: (a) children and adults were mixed together in the same study, despite the evidence that food intolerance is far more common in children; (b) during the period of egg and cow's milk exclusion, the patients were given a soya-based milk formula, which could have made the eczema worse in subjects also intolerant to soya; and (c) half the patients were non-whites, who may have different patterns of food intolerance (Wilson 1985).*

Summary 24   Egg intolerance is most common in the first 6 months of life, and the most common presentation is the rapid onset of symptoms minutes after an infant is given egg for the first time. Reactions occurring within an hour of eating egg consist of an erythematous rash around the mouth, swelling and urticaria of the oral mucosa and angioedema of the face, sometimes with wheezing, stridor, conjunctivitis, rhinitis, vomiting, loose stools and in severe cases anaphylaxis. Those with immediate reactions also exhibit urticaria after skin contact with egg. Delayed reactions to egg may trigger asthma or a worsening of atopic eczema.

25 Egg intolerance II: management
Avoid egg and allow measles vaccination

Diagnosis   The diagnosis rests on the history. Most cases are florid, rapid-onset reactions. Most parents make the diagnosis themselves, and only seek help if the reaction is severe or they are unsure how to proceed with the child's diet. Where the suspected adverse reaction was so mild as to leave doubt as to whether egg was the cause, the simplest step is to proceed to an open challenge with egg. In the case of atopic eczema or asthma a history of repeated worsening of the condition every time the child eats egg obviously suggests egg intolerance. The only way to prove egg intolerance is by double-blind challenge.

Investigations
skin-prick tests

Skin prick tests are almost always positive in children with rapid onset symptoms of egg intolerance, but since the diagnosis is quite obvious in such subjects it is difficult to see a role for a skin test. Many children have positive skin-prick tests to egg but are able to tolerate eggs. It has been estimated that in a population with an prevalence of egg intolerance of 1%, the likelihood that a subject with a positive skin-prick test actually has clinically significant egg intolerance will be less than 3% (Sampson & Albergo 1984). The rate of false positive skin-prick tests (Bock *et al.* 1978) has been studied mostly in children with asthma and/or atopic eczema. Thus in a study of 500 children with asthma and/or atopic eczema, 20% had positive skin test reactions to egg but only one-quarter of these had egg intolerance (Ratner & Untracht 1952). The proportion of infants with atopic eczema who have positive skin-prick tests to egg is so high that one observer wrote that if the skin-prick test to egg is negative 'the chances are that what the baby has is not atopic eczema' (Hill 1955). Furthermore, a few children with genuine proven egg intolerance have persistently negative skin-prick tests (Ford & Taylor 1982). In one study of 84 children with asthma or eczema or both, 27 gave a history of egg intolerance, and all 27 had positive skin-prick tests (Aas 1978). However two patients who had outgrown their egg intolerance still had positive skin-prick tests, and a major drawback to this study is that it was based mainly on a history of food intolerance rather than upon the results of food challenges.

RAST tests

The interpretation of the results of RAST tests for egg raises similar problems to those of skin-prick tests. False negatives can occur, especially in those with reactions which occur more than 1 hour after ingestion (Wraith *et al.* 1979). A large number of false positives are seen, especially in children who have grown out of egg intolerance (Ford & Taylor 1982) or those with atopic eczema. As with skin-prick testing, studies supporting the use of RAST testing for the diagnosis of egg intolerance have generally not employed double-blind challenges to confirm the food intolerance (Aas 1978).

Table 25.1 Some manufactured foods which may contain egg

Angel cakes
Sponge cakes
Cake icing
Some bread
Most biscuits
Some sweets (e.g. truffles, soft centred sweets)
Custard
Mayonnaise
Salad cream
Meringues
Souffles
Lemon curd
Egg noodles, spaghetti
Fish in batter, fish fingers
Hollandaise sauce
Bearnaise sauce

IgG4 antibodies

Some children with egg intolerance who have no IgE antibodies to egg do possess IgG4 antibodies to ovalbumen (Nakagawa *et al.* 1986), but their significance is unclear (Lau *et al.* 1988).

Egg avoidance

Exclusion of egg from the diet requires the help of a dietitian because of the number of manufactured foods which contain egg (Table 25.1). Although manufactured foods sold packaged will have their contents stated on the label, this does not apply, for example, to sweets sold loose, some of which contain egg protein (e.g. truffles, fondant creams, Turkish delight, marshmallows). In addition, several chocolate products contain egg. In the UK this does not have to be declared on the wrapper as manufactured chocolate and cocoa products are exempt from the usual food labelling regulations (Food Labelling Regulations 1984). As well as giving advice, the dietitian should be able to provide a diet sheet, a list of egg-free manufactured foods which is regularly updated by the British Dietetic Association, and information about egg replacers. The latter tend to comprise methylcellulose, sometimes with the addition of potato starch and tapioca. For further information about egg-free diets, see chapter 74.

Oral hyposensitization

Early reports of egg intolerance described treatment with oral hyposensitization. In one case, a 13-year-old boy was given a daily pill of calcium lactate into which a minute amount of raw egg (one part in 10 000) was added, and the quantity of egg slowly increased over 6 months (Schofield 1908). In another case, an 8-year-old boy was started on 2 mg ovomucoid (in this particular child ovomucoid was the major egg allergen) three times a day, the dose being increased to 7 g/day over 3 months (Schloss 1912). After hypo-sensitization, both patients were able to tolerate egg without any adverse effects. The role of this approach, if there is one, has not been explored, and for most patients, egg intolerance is a transient problem of infancy. Practical difficulties with oral hyposensitization include uncertainty about the efficacy of this approach, the amount of work involved in preparing increasingly potent preparations, and the risk of causing anaphylactic shock.

Prognosis

In the majority of cases, egg intolerance is discovered before the age of 12 months and has disappeared by the age of 3 years. In one small hospital-based series of cases which were also atypical in their late age of presentation (over 6 months in most), only 11 out of 25 had grown out of egg intolerance in a 2-year observation period (Ford & Taylor 1982). These less encouraging results are probably explained by the age of the sample; it is likely that a later age at presentation is associated with a greater duration of egg intolerance and a lesser chance of growing out of the condition altogether. Indeed in the study referred to above, the mean age at presentation of the 11 children who grew out of egg intolerance was 15 months, whereas for the 14 who did not grow out of egg intolerance the mean age at presentation was 34 months.

Vaccination

A number of microbial vaccines, including those against influenza, yellow fever, typhus and Rocky Mountain spotted fever, are grown in chick embryo tissues. These vaccines are prepared from either infected chick embryo cultures, yolk sacs or allantoic cavities. These vaccines contain small quantities of egg protein, and anaphylaxis is a hazard in subjects with egg intolerance (Stull 1946; Hampton 1947; Ratner et al. 1952).

Measles and MMR vaccine

Formerly, measles vaccine was obtained from chick embryo cultures, and the vaccine contained traces of egg protein. Latterly, measles vaccine has been grown in chick embryo fibroblasts in vitro, and egg antigens cannot be detected by immunoelectrophoresis in these modern vaccines (Aukrust et al. 1980). However measles vaccine has been shown, also by immunoelectrophoresis, to contain trace amounts of calf serum protein (Aukrust et al. 1980), but the significance of this, if any, is unclear. The vaccine also contains neomycin or kanamycin (Juntunen-Backman et al. 1987; Walker 1991).

Measles vaccine: egg gone but problem remains

The manufacturers of measles vaccine may have removed egg protein from the product, but their continued inclusion of 'anaphylactoid or other reactions to eating eggs' as a contraindication to measles or mumps, measles and rubella (MMR) vaccination (Walker 1991) has been a potent source of confusion and anxiety. Indeed, in the context of allergy, enquiry about the risks of measles vaccine has been the single most common question the author has received from medical colleagues.

Measles vaccine: reactions

Kamin and his colleagues gave measles vaccine without incident to 22 children who had been demonstrated to have severe egg intolerance (Kamin *et al.* 1963, 1965). In addition, they wrote to over 1000 allergists throughout the world, asking for reports of allergic reactions to measles vaccine in egg intolerant children, without receiving a single positive response (Kamin *et al.* 1965). Six children, aged 12–18 months, with anaphylaxis following measles vaccination were reported from Norway, but none of these patients had a history of egg intolerance, and the cause of the adverse reactions was not identified (Aukrust *et al.* 1980). All six responded to injection of adrenaline. Skin-prick testing with the vaccine was positive in only one of the six children. Of three children from Australia who had severe allergic reactions following measles vaccination, none had a history of egg intolerance, and the cause of the adverse reaction was not identified (Van Asperen *et al.* 1981). Two other children have been reported in whom generalized urticaria, angioedema and wheezing followed MMR vaccination (Herman *et al.* 1983). Both children were alleged to have a history of egg intolerance, but this conclusion was rather doubtful in both cases, and there was no evidence to support the assumption that egg intolerance was the cause of the allergic reaction.

Measles vaccination: doubtful logic for skin testing

Several authorities have suggested that either skin-prick testing or intradermal testing could be used to identify those at risk of an allergic reaction to vaccination (Bierman *et al.* 1977; Aukrust *et al.* 1980; Herman *et al.* 1983; Juntunen-Backman *et al.* 1987). There are three flaws in this argument.

1 The assumption that a positive skin-prick test or intradermal test will predict severe allergic reactions has never been tested. Those who have used this approach have witheld the vaccine from those with a positive skin test.

2 In the largest series of cases of anaphylaxis to measles vaccine, none of the six children had a history of egg intolerance and five of the six had negative skin tests to the vaccine (Aukrust *et al.* 1980).

3 The incidence of positive skin tests to measles vaccine may be so high (e.g. six out of six subjects in one series – see Herman *et al.* 1983) as to cast doubt on the value of a positive test.

Measles vaccination: manufacturers' warnings

'Anaphylactoid or other reactions to eggs' is still given as a contraindication to measles and MMR vaccination, despite the lack of evidence of any special hazard to such subjects, and despite efforts in the past to persuade the manufacturers to remove such warnings (Katz 1978). It has been suggested that the manufacturers fear that a child who safely receives the vaccine may eat something in the next few hours which contains egg, develop a severe reaction to the food, leading the family to blame the vaccine and initiate a lawsuit (Katz 1978). In response to my own queries, two of three measles vaccine manufacturers responded that they were unwilling to guarantee the absence of traces of egg protein, and accordingly a warning had to be retained about hazards to those with severe reactions to egg. A third manufacturer commented: 'I am afraid in the present litigation orientated climate in which we find ourselves, once a statement like this has been included it is very difficult, and needs a brave man to remove it'.

Measles vaccination: recommendations

In the author's opinion, egg intolerance is not a logical reason to withhold measles or MMR vaccination. When the family doctor is unhappy to administer measles vaccination because of a history of egg intolerance, the author's practice is to offer the vaccination at hospital. There are two notes of caution.

1 Allergy to neomycin or kanamycin is a contraindication to the use of vaccines which contain the relevant antibiotic. Currently available measles and MMR vaccines contain either neomycin or kanamycin.

2 There is a remote hazard of anaphylaxis following *any* injection of any microbial vaccine, so that adrenaline and a means of injecting it should *always* be at hand when *any* vaccination is being performed.

Key references   25.1   FORD RPK & TAYLOR B (1982) Natural history of egg hypersensitivity. *Arch Dis Child* **57**:649–652. Two out of 25 patients with egg intolerance had negative skin-prick tests, and five out of 11 who grew out of egg intolerance had persistently positive skin-prick tests after egg intolerance had disappeared. Five of these 11 also had positive RAST tests after they had grown out of their egg intolerance.

25.2   LAU S, THIEMEIER M, URBANEK R, KEMENY M & WAHN U (1988) Immediate hypersensitivity to ovalbumin in children with hen's egg white allergy. *Eur J Pediat* **147**:606–608. *Neither the serum concentration of IgE, IgG1 or IgG4 antibodies to ovalbumen nor a positive histamine-release test result predicted the outcome of a challenge test with egg.*

25.3   HERMAN JJ, RADIN R & SCHNEIDERMAN R (1983) Allergic reactions to measles (rubeola) vaccine in patients hypersensitive to egg protein. *J Pediat* **102**:196–199. A report of two children with egg intolerance who experienced anaphylactic reactions when given a chick embryo measles vaccine. The authors found positive skin tests to the vaccine in six other children with egg intolerance, but safely vaccinated all six using increasing volumes of vaccine (0.05 ml increments every

20 min until the full dose had been given). There is a further report of hypo-sensitization to MMR vaccine, in a child with a positive skin-prick test to egg but negative prick test to MMR (Kletz *et al.* 1990). *There are three problems here.*

1 *It is far from clear that either child ever had egg intolerance. One child exhibited urticaria and wheezing after ingestion of a food product which contained egg white, and egg intolerance was assumed to be present. The other child developed an episode of urticaria, angioedema, wheezing and stridor whilst being breast fed. There was no history of egg exposure, and it was simply assumed that this episode must have been due to egg intolerance! In neither case was there any further historical or challenge data to support the diagnosis of egg intolerance.*

2 *The finding of positive skin tests in six out of six subjects casts doubt on the relevance of the result of the skin tests, especially considering the rarity of severe reactions to measles vaccine.*

3 *Despite positive skin tests, there were no adverse reactions to small doses of injected vaccine. There is no evidence to support giving small increments of vaccine, and tiny doses of other allergens can cause anaphylaxis in a hypersensitive subject. Until there is evidence that skin testing will predict those at risk of anaphylaxis it cannot be recommended. Giving 10 injections of a 0.05 ml dose of vaccine for fear of anaphylaxis is difficult to justify on scientific or humane grounds.*

25.4   MILLER JR, ORGEL HA & MELTZER EO (1983) The safety of egg-containing vaccines for egg-allergic patients. *J Allergy Clin Immunol* **71**:568–573. A study of 42 patients with a history of egg intolerance, although when 32 were challenged by eating upwards of four eggs (two hard-boiled, two raw) 16 had no reaction. *The authors recommended the use of intradermal skin testing, using 0.02 ml of a 1:100 dilution of the vaccine, and avoidance of vaccination in cases where intradermal testing causes a weal of greater than 5 mm, but fail to provide supporting evidence, since they withheld vaccination from subjects with strongly positive intradermal tests.*

25.5   BECK SA, WILLIAMS LW, SHIRRELL MA & BURKS AW (1991) Egg hyper-sensitivity and measles-mumps-rubella vaccine administration. *Pediatrics* **88**:913–917. Sixteen children with a history of egg intolerance, all of whom had a positive skin-prick test to egg, all had a negative skin-prick test to MMR vaccine; vaccine administration proceeded without adverse reaction. A further 12 children with atopic eczema and egg intolerance proven by blind challenge received MMR vaccination without adverse effect. In 10 of these, vaccination had been performed at the usual age of 15–18 months, before proof had been obtained of egg intolerance, but at a stage at which one can assume egg intolerance must have existed. *The authors assert that MMR vaccination is safe in egg intolerant children (I agree) and suggest that skin-prick testing is an 'adequate screening method for children with anaphylactic egg sensitivity'. This is illogical. The implication is that a positive skin-prick test would indicate a risk of adverse reaction from vaccination, but this has never been demonstrated. Before one could recommend skin-prick testing prior to MMR vaccination one would have to demonstrate that those with negative prick tests always tolerate MMR vaccination (this would require very large numbers of subjects to be tested; so far this has only been studied in very small numbers) and that at least some of those with positive prick tests do exhibit adverse reactions (a hypothesis which has never been tested).*

Summary 25   The diagnosis of egg intolerance rests mainly on the history, which is usually quite clear. Skin prick tests and RAST tests are unhelpful because of false positive and false negative results, and if the diagnosis is in doubt it can only be confirmed by double-blind challenge. The management is to exclude egg from the diet, which requires the help of a dietitian because of the wide range of food products which contain egg. Egg intolerance is not a contraindication to measles or MMR vaccination because modern measles vaccines are grown in fibroblasts and do not contain egg protein. Egg intolerance is, however, a contraindication to the injection of vaccines such as influenza or yellow fever, which do contain traces of egg protein.

References to Chapters 22–25

AAS K (1978) The diagnosis of hypersensitivity to ingested foods. Reliability of skin prick testing and the radioallergosorbent test with different materials. *Clin Allergy* **8**:39–50.

ANET J, BACK JF, BAKER RS & BARNETT D, BURLEY RW & HOWDEN MEH (1985) Allergens in the white and yolk of hen's egg. A study of IgE binding by egg proteins. *Int Arch Allergy Appl Immunol* **77**:364–371.

ATHERTON DJ, SEWELL M, SOOTHILL JF, WELLS RS & CHILVERS CED (1978) A double-blind controlled crossover trial of an antigen-avoidance diet in atopic eczema. *Lancet* **1**:401–403.

AUKRUST L, ALMELAND TL, REFSUM D & AAS K (1980) Severe hypersensitivity or intolerance reactions to measles vaccine in six children. *Allergy* **35**:581–587.

BAUSELA BA, ESTEBAN MM, ALZAMORA FM, MARCOS CP & CASAS JAO (1991) Egg protein sensitization in patients with bird feather allergy. *Allergy* **46**: 614–618.

BENTON EC & BARNETSON RC (1985) Skin reactions to foods in patients with atopic dermatitis. *Acta Derm Venereol* (suppl. 114):129–132.

BIERMAN CW, SHAPIRO GG, PIERSON WE, TAYLOR JW, FOY HM & FOX JP (1977) Safety of influenza vaccination in allergic children. *J Infect Dis* **136** (suppl.):S652–S655.

BLEUMINK E & YOUNG E (1969) Studies on the atopic allergen in hen's egg. I. Identification of the skin reactive fraction in egg-white. *Int Arch Allergy* **35**: 1–19.

BOCK SA (1987) Prospective appraisal of complaints of adverse reactions to foods in children during the first 3 years of life. *Pediatrics* **79**:683–688.

BOCK SA, LEE WY, REMIGO LK & MAY CD (1978) Studies of hypersensitivity reactions to foods in infants and children. *J Allergy Clin Immunol* **62**:327–334.

BOCK SA, SAMPSON HA, ATKINS FM *et al.* (1988) Double-blind, placebo-controlled food challenge (DBPCFC) as an office procedure: a manual. *J Allergy Clin Immunol* **82**:986–997.

CANT A, MARSDEN RA & KILSHAW PJ (1985) Egg and cows' milk hypersensitivity in exclusively breast fed infants with eczema, and detection of egg protein in breast milk. *Br Med J* **291**:932–935.

COOK F & BRIGGS GM (1986) The nutritive value of eggs. In Stadelman WJ & Cotterill OJ (eds). *Egg Science and Technology*, 3rd edn, pp.141–163, Avi Publishing Company, Westport, Connecticut.

COULTATE TP (1984) *Food – the Chemistry of Its Components*, The Royal Society of Chemistry, London.

COURT J & NG LM (1984) Danger of egg white treatment for nappy rash. *Arch Dis Child* **59**:908.

DANNAEUS A & INGANAS M (1981) A follow-up study of children with food allergy. Clinical course in relation to serum IgE- and IgG-antibody levels to milk, egg and fish. Clin Allergy **11**:533–539.

DANNAEUS A, INGANAS M, JOHANSSON SGO & FOUCARD T (1979) Intestinal uptake of ovalbumin in malabsorption and food allergy in relation to serum IgG antibody and orally administered sodium cromoglycate. *Clin Allergy* **9**: 263–270.

DANNAEUS A, JOHANSSON SGO & FOUCARD T (1978) Clinical and immunological aspects of food allergy in childhood. II. Development of allergic symptoms and humoral immune response to foods in infants of atopic mothers during the first 24 months of life. *Acta Paediat Scand* **67**:497–504.

DE MAAT-BLEEKER F, VAN DIJK AG & BERRENS L (1985) Allergy to egg yolk possibly induced by sensitisation to bird serum antigens. *Ann Allergy* **54**: 245–248.

EDWARDS JH, MCCONNOCHIE K, TROTMAN DM, COLLINS G, SAUNDERS MJ & LATHAM SM (1983) Allergy to inhaled egg material. *Clin Allergy* **13**:427–432.

EGAN H, KIRK RS & SAWYER R (1987) *Pearson's Chemical Analysis of Foods*, 8th edn, Longman Scientific & Technical, Harlow.

ELWOOD PC (1968) Iron in Flour. Part 1. Radio-active studies of the absorption by human subjects of various iron preparations from bread. *Ministry of Health Reports on Public Health and Medical Subjects*, No. 117, Her Majesty's Stationery Office, London.

FOOD LABELLING REGULATIONS (1984) SI 1984/1305, in Statutory Instruments 1984, Part II, Section II. Statutory Instrument No 1305, Her Majesty's Stationery Office, London.

FORD RPK & TAYLOR B (1982) Natural history of egg hypersensitivity. *Arch Dis Child* **57**:649–652.

FREEDMAN SS & SELLARS W (1959) Food sensitivity. A study of 150 'allergic' children. *J Allergy* **30**:42–49.

GERRARD JW & PERELMUTTER L (1986) IgE-mediated allergy to peanut, cow's milk, and egg in children with special reference to maternal diet. *Ann Allergy* **56**:351–354.

GRUSKAY FL & COOKE RE (1955) The gastrointestinal absorption of unaltered protein in normal infants and in infants recovering from diarrhea. *Pediatrics* **16**:763–769.

HAMPTON SF (1947) Anaphylactic shock in egg-sensitive individuals following vaccination with typhus vaccine. *J Lab Clin Med* **32**:109–117.

HERMAN JJ, RADIN R & SCHNEIDERMAN R (1983) Allergic reactions to measles (rubeola) vaccine in patients hypersensitive to egg protein. *J Pediat* **102**: 196–199.

HILL LW (1955) The treatment of eczema in infants and children. Part IV. *J Pediat* **47**:648–659.

HOFFMAN DR (1983) Immunochemical identification of the allergens in egg white. *J Allergy Clin Immunol* **71**:481–486.

JUNTUNEN-BACKMAN K, PELTOLA H, BACKMAN A & SALO OP (1987) Safe immunization of allergic children against measles, mumps, and rubella. *Am J Dis Child* **141**:1103–1105.

KAJOSAARI M (1982) Food allergy in Finnish children aged 1 to 6 years. *Acta Paediat Scand* **71**:815–819.

KAMIN PB, FEIN BT & BRITTON HA (1963) Live, attenuated measles vaccine. Its administration to children allergic to egg protein. *J Am Med Assoc* **185**: 647–650.

KAMIN PB, FEIN BT & BRITTON HA (1965) Use of live, attenuated measles virus vaccine in children allergic to egg protein. *J Am Med Assoc* **193**:143–144.

KATZ SL (1978) Safety of measles vaccine in egg-sensitive individuals. (Reply to letter.) *J Pediat* **92**:859.

KLETZ MR, HOLLAND CL, MENDELSON JS & BIELORY L (1990) Administration of egg-derived vaccines in patients with history of egg sensitivity. *Ann Allergy* **64**:527–529.

LANGELAND T (1982) A clinical and immunological study of allergy to hen's egg white. III. Allergens in hen's egg white studied by crossed radioimmuno-electrophoresis (CRIE). *Allergy* **37**:521–530.

LANGELAND T (1983a) A clinical and immunological study of allergy to hen's egg white. VI. Occurrence of proteins cross-reacting with allergens in hen's egg white as studied in egg white from turkey, duck, goose, seagull, and in hen's egg yolk, and hen and chicken sera and flesh. *Allergy* **38**:399–412.

LANGELAND T (1983b) A clinical and immunological study of allergy to hen's egg white. I. A clinical study of egg allergy. *Clin Allergy* **13**:371–382.

LANGELAND T (1985) Allergy to hen's egg white in atopic dermatitis. *Acta Derm Venereol* (suppl. 114):109–112.

LANGELAND T & AAS K (1987) Allergy to hen's egg white: clinical and immunological aspects. In Brostoff J & Challacombe SJ (eds) *Food Allergy and Intolerance*, pp. 367–374, Baillière Tindall, London.

LANGELAND T & HARBITZ O (1983) A clinical and immunological study of allergy to hen's egg white. V. Purification and identification of a major allergen (antigen 22) in hen's egg white. *Allergy* **38**:131–139.

LAU S, THIEMEIER M, URBANEK R, KEMENY M & WAHN U (1988) Immediate hypersensitivity to ovalbumin in children with hen's egg white allergy. *Eur J Pediat* **147**:606–608.

MATSUMURA T, KUROUME T, OGURI M et al. (1975) Egg sensitivity and eczematous manifestations in breast-fed newborns with particular reference to intrauterine sensitisation. *Ann Allergy* **35**:221–229.

NAKAGAWA T, MUKOYAMA T, BABA M, SAKAI Y, YAMASHITA N & MIYAMOTO T (1986) Egg white-specific IgE and IgG4 antibodies in atopic children. *Ann Allergy* **57**:359–362.

NEILD VS, MARSDEN RA, BAILES JA & BLAND JM (1986) Egg and milk exclusion diets in atopic eczema. *Br J Dermatol* **114**:117–123.

POWRIE WD & NAKAI S (1985) Characteristics of edible fluids of animal origin: eggs. In Fennema OR (ed) *Food Chemistry*, 2nd edn, pp. 829–855, Marcel Dekker, New York.

POWRIE WD & NAKAI S (1986) The chemistry of eggs and egg products. In Stadelman WJ & Cotterill OJ (eds) *Egg Science and Technology*, 3rd edn, pp. 97–139, Avi Publishing Company, Westport, Connecticut.

RATNER B & UNTRACHT S (1952) Egg allergy in children. *Am J Dis Child* **83**:309–316.

RATNER B, UNTRACHT S & HERTZMARK F (1952) Allergy to viral and Rickettsial vaccines. *Am J Dis Child* **83**:608–617.

REGENSTEIN JM & REGENSTEIN CE (1984) *Food Protein Chemistry. An Introduction for Food Scientists*, Academic Press, Orlando, Florida.

SAMPSON HA & ALBERGO R (1984) Comparison of results of skin tests, RAST, and double-blind, placebo-controlled food challenges in children with atopic dermatitis. *J Allergy Clin Immunol* **74**:26–33.

SCHLOSS OM (1912) A case of allergy to common foods. *Am J Dis Child* **3**:341–362.

SCHLOSS OM & WORTHEN TW (1916) The permeability of the gastro-enteric tract of infants to undigested protein. *Am J Dis Child* **11**:342–360.

SCHOFIELD AT (1908) A case of egg poisoning. *Lancet* **1**:716.

SCHUR S, HYDE JS & WYPYCH JI (1974) Egg-white sensitivity and atopic eczema. *J Allergy Clin Immunol* **54**:174–179.

STULL A (1946) Allergenic and anaphylactogenic properties of vaccines prepared from embryonic tissues of developing chicks. III. A study to determine whether chick-embryo yolk-sac vaccines contain sufficient egg proteins to cause severe systemic reactions if given to egg-sensitive individuals. *J Immunol* **53**:343–353.

VADEHRA DV & NATH KR (1933) Eggs as a source of protein. *CRC Crit Rev Food Technol* **4**:193–309.

VAN ASPEREN PP, KEMP AS & MELLIS CM (1983) Immediate food hypersensitivity reactions on the first known exposure to the food. *Arch Dis Child* **58**:253–256.

VAN ASPEREN PP, McENIERY J & KEMP AS (1981) Immediate reactions following live attenuated measles vaccine. *Med J Aust* **2**:330–331.

WALKER G (1991) *ABPI Data Sheet Compendium* 1991–92, Datapharm Publications, London.

WALSH BJ, BARNETT D, BURLEY RW, ELLIOTT C, HILL DJ & HOWDEN MEH (1988) New allergens from hen's egg white and egg yolk. In vitro study of ovomucin, apovitellenin I and VI, and phosvitin. *Int Arch Allergy Appl Immunol* **87**:81–86.

WILSON NM (1985) Food related asthma: a difference between two ethnic groups. *Arch Dis Child* **60**:861–865.

WRAITH DG, MERRETT J, ROTH A, YMAN L & MERRETT TG (1979) Recognition of food-allergic patients and their allergens by the RAST technique and clinical investigation. *Clin Allergy* **9**:25–36.

Part 6 Cereal Intolerance

26 Cereal types and constituents
Grains, gluten and gliadins

Sources of flour
The term cereal is derived from cerealia munera, the gifts of the goddess Ceres, and is used to refer to the grain itself as well as the cultivated plants. Cereals (Table 26.1) include all the cultivated grasses belonging to the Gramineae family, and they produce seeds which can be ground into flour. Pseudo-cereals are plants outside the Gramineae family with fruits and seeds that can be ground into flour to make bread (Brouk 1975).

Bread
Bread is composed of dough, yeast, water and other ingredients, which have been fermented and subsequently baked. Wheat flour may contain additional ingredients, such as caramel, bleaching and improving agents, preservatives, chalk, iron salts, thiamine, nicotinic acid, sodium bicarbonate, salt, edible oils and fats, cow's milk and milk products, sugar and non-wheat flours made from rice or soya beans (Egan *et al.* 1987).

Grain constituents
The grains (i.e. the seeds) of cereals consist of three major structures: (a) the embryo or germ of the new plant; (b) the endosperm which is the store of nutrients for the germinating plant; and (c) the protective layers of seed coat. The cells of the endosperm are packed with starch granules lying in a matrix of protein. The protein, which constitutes 7–15% of flour, is of two types. One type, about 15% of the total, consists of the residues of cytoplasmic proteins, mostly enzymes, which are soluble in water or a dilute salt solution. The remaining 85% are the storage proteins of the seed, insoluble in ordinary aqueous media and responsible for dough formation. These dough forming proteins are collectively referred to as gluten (Coultate 1984).

Table 26.1 Types of cereals and pseudo-cereals

Cereals	Pseudo-cereals
Wheat	Buckwheat
Barley	Amaranth
Oat	Chia
Rye	Quinoa
Sorghum	Water chestnut
Rice	
Corn	
Millet	

Gluten

The gluten proteins can be fractionated on the basis of their solubility in salt solution, alcohol, acid or alkali. The most soluble, the gliadins, constitute about one-third of the gluten, and a single variety of wheat may have over 40 different gliadin proteins. The remaining two-thirds are the glutenins, which dissolve poorly and which are responsible for the visco-elastic properties of dough.

Gliadins — old chemistry

The alcohol-soluble fraction of wheat gluten, which is immuno-pathogenic to patients with coeliac disease, consists of a polymorphic mixture of proline and glutamine-rich gliadin polypeptides. These have been subfractionated into α-, β-, γ- and ω subgroups on the basis of their electrophoretic mobility. Each subgroup, when fractionated by two dimensional polyacrylamide-gel electrophoresis, consists of multiple component polypeptides. Peptides from all four major gliadin sub-groups induce the intestinal lesions of coeliac disease (Ciclitira *et al.* 1984a). In contrast, the prolonged administration of gluten fails to damage the intestinal mucosa of normal subjects, so gluten is not intrinsically toxic to the intestinal mucosa (Trier 1991).

Gliadins — new chemistry

Recent studies have examined the cDNA sequence homologies of the gliadin subfractions, and of the storage proteins of barley, rye and oats, which to a variable degree share sequence homologies with wheat gliadins (reviewed by Marsh & Loft 1988). Nevertheless, the specific amino acid sequence or sequences crucial in the pathogenesis of coeliac disease have not been identified, and the molecular nature of the interaction with the intestinal mucosa has not been characterized (Trier 1991).

Gliadin dose and type

Jejunal biopsy specimens from patients with coeliac disease who had received small oral doses (100 mg to 1.5 g) of a peptic-tryptic digest of gluten demonstrated a dose-dependent response 12–84 hours after oral ingestion of a single dose of gluten (Leigh *et al.* 1985). Normal bread contains about 2.2 g gluten or 1.25 g gliadin per 30 g slice (Ciclitira *et al.* 1984a, b). It is possible that different patients with coeliac disease show unequal susceptibility to the immunopathogenic effects of gliadin. As little as 100 mg has been shown to cause damage to the jejunal mucosa in one adult with coeliac disease, although 10 mg was not harmful (Ciclitira *et al.* 1984a). The lack of further data on the effect of very small doses of gliadin is an important area of uncertainty. Could the small quantities of gluten included in certain so-called gluten-free products (see below) be harmful to certain patients with coeliac disease?

Gluten-free — a misnomer

So-called 'gluten-free' bread may, surprisingly, contain small quantities of gluten (Ciclitira *et al.* 1984b, 1985). Ciclitira *et al.*

(1984b) reported that two 'gluten-free' breads, Juvela and Rite diet, contained 0.4 mg and 0.2 mg of gliadin per standard 30 g slice. The former was given to seven adults with coeliac disease while on a gluten-free diet, and a jejunal biopsy was performed before and 1 week after regular consumption of the 'gluten-free' bread. There was no histological change in the jejunal mucosa, but the authors pointed out that this did not exclude the possibility of harm from the longer term consumption of small amounts of gluten in 'gluten-free' products, particularly in those especially sensitive to gluten (Ciclitira *et al.* 1984b, 1985).

Codex Alimentarius   The World Health Organisation Codex Alimentarius (1981) has proposed a standard for the term gluten-free. This states that gluten-free means: 'the total nitrogen content of the gluten-containing cereal grains used in the product does not exceed 0.05 g per 100 g of these grains on a dry matter basis' (equivalent to 0.3% protein).

This standard was devised in the absence of an accurate and reproducible method for measuring gluten itself. Given that studies in which as little as 100 mg of unfractionated gliadin was shown to induce jejunal mucosal injury in coeliac disease (Ciclitira *et al.* 1984a), there must be some doubt as to whether gluten-containing 'gluten-free' products are suitable for children with coeliac disease supposedly on a gluten-free diet. This highlights a major area of uncertainty. There is at present no evidence to confirm or refute the theoretical argument of possible long-term harm from very small doses of gluten. Better methods for the assay of gliadin, and the development of completely wheat-free bread may lead to a Codex Alimentarius re-definition of the term gluten-free.

Cereal type   Wheat, rye and barley are harmful in coeliac disease (Anand *et al.* 1978). However the toxicity of oats remains controversial (Anand *et al.* 1978). Four adults with coeliac disease consumed porridge oats 40–60 g per day for 1 month, while adhering to a gluten-free diet (Dissanayake *et al.* 1974). All four remained symptom free, and there was no change in jejunal histology or dissaccharidase content. It was concluded that oats are harmless to patients with coeliac disease. Packer *et al.* (1978) reported five children with coeliac disease who were apparently able to regularly consume oats for at least a year without adverse effects on the jejunal mucosa. However, since it may take years for coeliac disease to relapse after the re-introduction of gluten (see next chapter) this data does not guarantee the safety of oats. The putative safety of oats in coeliac disease, and the antigenic relationship between the gliadins in wheat, rye, barley and oats are both important areas of uncertainty.

Key references 26.1   CICLITIRA PJ, EVANS DJ, FAGG NLK, LENNOX ES & DOWLING RH (1984) Clinical testing of gliadin fractions in coeliac patients. *Clin Sci* **66**:357–364. α-, β-, γ- and ω-gliadins were separately infused into the duodenum of two adults with coeliac disease. After an intraduodenal challenge with 1000 mg, each of the four fractions induced damage in the jejunal mucosa of jejunal biopsies taken 6 hours later. A dose-response study with increasing quantities of unfractionated gliadin in one coeliac patient showed no changes after 10 mg had been given, minimal changes after 100 mg had been given, and marked changes after a further 500 mg had been given.

26.2   CICLITIRA PJ, ELLIS HJ & EVANS DJ, LENNOX (1985) A radioimmunoassay for wheat gliadin to assess the suitability of gluten free foods for patients with coeliac disease. *Clin Exp Immunol* **59**:703–708. Because of the lack of reproducible assays of gluten in foods, the authors developed a radioimmunoassay for wheat gliadin with a detection limit of 1 ng. *Nominally gluten-free foods, such as Nutregen gluten-free bread, were found to contain measureable quantities of gluten with this method. However the method failed to detect gliadin in a commercially made 'gluten-free' loaf Juvela, although there were detectable amounts of gliadin in three separate batches of bread mix from the same manufacturer. This discrepancy was unexplained.*

Summary 26   The immunopathogenic fraction of cereal flour which damages the small bowel mucosa of patients with coeliac disease is a mixture of proline and glutamine rich gliadin polypeptides. This immunopathogenic fraction is present in flour from wheat, rye and barley. There is uncertainty as to whether it is, or is not, present in oats. The specific amino acid sequence or sequences crucial to the pathogenesis of coeliac disease have not been identified. Commercially produced so-called gluten-free foods are permitted to contain, and indeed may contain, small amounts of gluten. It is unclear whether such small amounts can be harmful long term if given regularly to patients with coeliac disease.

27 Coeliac disease
Clinical features, diagnosis and management

Brief review   Coeliac disease has been reviewed extensively (see Walker-Smith 1988; Branski & Lebenthal 1989; Trier 1991), and will be only briefly described here.

History   Coeliac disease appears to have been recognized in the second century AD (Paveley 1988), although it was Gee who drew attention to the 'coeliac affection' in 1888 (Gee 1888).

banana diet   In 1924, Haas reported on the dietary treatment of 10 children with coeliac disease. The treatment was based on the avoidance of all carbohydrates, which were believed to be poorly tolerated, except sucrose which was allowed. Thus all bread, crackers and potato were avoided, and over-ripe bananas were provided as a source of sucrose. Haas appears to have been influenced by the successful treatment of a 3-year-old child with 'anorexia nervosa' with bananas, and also by the observation that town dwellers in Porto Rico who ate much bread often suffered from 'sprue', unlike the farmers who lived largely on bananas and never had sprue. On this regimen of carbohydrate avoidance and up to 16 bananas per day, eight patients with coeliac disease were cured and two who were not treated with the diet died.

starch avoidance   Andersen (1947) extended Haas' observations, and noted that provided cereal starches, bread and potatoes were witheld, patients could tolerate simple sugars as glucose, bananas or fruit.

Dutch observations   In the 1930s, a young mother's statement that her coeliac child's skin rash improved if she removed bread from the diet alerted Dicke, a paediatrician in the Hague (Dicke *et al.* 1953; Booth, 1989), leading eventually to the identification of wheat starch as the offending substance.

Definition   Coeliac disease may be defined as a disease of the proximal small intestine characterized by an abnormal small intestinal mucosa and associated with a permanent intolerance to gluten (Walker-Smith 1988).

Transient gluten intolerance   Follow-up studies of children who were diagnosed in infancy as having coeliac disease have shown that there is a category of transient intolerance to gluten (Walker-Smith 1970, 1988; Iacono *et al.* 1991). However, there are several reports of children who took as long as 5–7 years to relapse after gluten was re-introduced into the diet, so the diagnosis of transient intolerance can be difficult to establish. The possibility of late relapse means that children diagnosed as suffering from transient gluten intolerance require follow up into adult life (Walker-Smith *et al.* 1990).

Pathogenesis   Coeliac disease is currently seen as an immunological disorder in which there is a local immunological reaction to gluten. The

Table 27.1 Immunological features of coeliac disease[1]

Infiltration of gut mucosa with immunocompetent cells
Circulating antibodies to gluten
Association with HL-A antigens
Association with IgA deficiency
Immunological complications
   Hyposplenism
   Lymphoma
Associated autoimmune disorders
  Extrinsic allergic alveolitis
  Endocrine disorders
    thyroid disease
    diabetes mellitus
    Addison's disease
  Rheumatic disorders
    rheumatoid arthritis
    Sjögren syndrome
    systemic lupus erythematosus
  Dermatitis herpetiformis

[1] Mostly seen in adults rather than children with coeliac disease.

Table 27.2 Major modes of presentation of coeliac disease in childhood

Chronic diarrhoea
Failure to thrive, weight loss
Vomiting
Poor appetite
Short stature
Iron deficiency anaemia
Protuberant abdomen

pathogenesis is reviewed elsewhere by Branski & Lebenthal 1989, Marsh 1990 and Trier 1991. The principal immunological features are listed in Table 27.1. There is no association with atopic disease (Greco *et al.* 1990).

Genetics

Coeliac disease is strikingly familial (David & Ajdukiewicz 1975; Trier 1991). It is strongly associated with the class II histocompatibility antigens HLA-DR3 and HLA-DQw2 (reviewed by Trier 1991). The implication is that a disease susceptibility gene is in linkage disequilibrium with the DR subloci. There is a particularly high incidence of coeliac disease in the west of Ireland (Mylotte *et al.* 1973).

Clinical features

The symptoms most commonly begin under 1 year of age, although presentation may be delayed well into adult life. The symptoms

Dissecting microscope:	Flat ± mosaic pattern		Convolutions	Finger and leaf shaped villi
Light microscope:	'Subtotal villous atrophy'		'Partial villous atrophy'	Normal villi
Scanning electron microscope:	Crypt orifices, Grouped, Single, Hemispheres, Collars, Curvilinear ridges, Transverse lips		Convolution	Vilii, Curved base
	The various structures associated with crypt orifices leading to the formation of curvilinear ridges		Convolutions formed by thickening and increase in height of curvilinear ridges	Villi formed by cellular remodelling of convolution. There is upward growth of villus projections, the curved base remaining as a foundation

Fig. 27.1 Correlative appearances of small intestinal mucosa in coeliac disease, compared with surface ultrastructure as revealed by the scanning electron microscope. (Marsh MN (1990) *Gut* **31**:111–114.)

are all consequences of malabsorption, whether of fat leading to diarrhoea, or nutrients leading, for example, to failure to thrive, short stature or anaemia. The main modes of presentation are shown in Table 27.2. For a detailed review see Walker-Smith (1988).

Serum antibodies

Circulating IgA antigliadin, IgA antireticulin and IgA antiendomysial antibodies have a high degree of sensitivity and specificity for the diagnosis of coeliac disease (reviewed by Trier 1991). When such antibodies are present at the time of diagnosis, and when they disappear in parallel to a clinical response to a gluten-free diet, weight is added to the diagnosis. However, the diagnosis cannot be made on the presence of these antibodies alone, because of false positives, false negatives, the association of coeliac disease with IgA deficiency, and the reduced specificity in communities where other causes of enteropathy are common (Calabuig *et al.* 1990; Walker-Smith *et al.* 1990; Bürgin-Wolff *et al.* 1991). Since IgA antigliadin and IgA antiendomysial antibodies decrease in titre and may ultimately disappear in patients with coeliac disease who adhere to a gluten-free diet, serial determination of these antibodies may be useful for monitoring dietary adherence (Walker-Smith *et al.* 1990; Tosoni *et al.* 1991).

Table 27.3 Causes of a flat small intestinal mucosa in childhood

Coeliac disease
Gastroenteritis
Giardiasis
Food protein (e.g. cow's milk, soya) intolerance
Tropical sprue
Protein-calorie malnutrition
Acquired hypogammaglobulinaemia

Diagnosis

The diagnosis is based on the demonstration of an abnormal small intestinal mucosa. (usually it is flat – see Fig. 27.1) and then upon a clinical response to withdrawal of gluten from the child's diet. Although a flat small intestinal mucosa is characteristic of coeliac disease, there are a number of other causes of a flat mucosa (Table 27.3). For a detailed review see Walker-Smith (1988).

Diagnostic criteria

There is no universal agreement about the diagnostic criteria (Guandalini *et al.* 1989), which have been revised a number of times by, for example, the European Society for Paediatric Gastro-enterology (Walker-Smith *et al.* 1990). The principles are as follows.

1 *Initial diagnostic biopsy*: the characteristic small intestinal mucosal abnormalities are essential for the diagnosis of coeliac disease.

2 *Complete relief on strict gluten-free diet*: there must be complete relief of all symptoms on strict gluten-free diet, and this response should be fairly rapid, occurring within a matter of weeks rather than months.

3 *Re-biopsy on gluten-free diet*: this is required if the clinical response to gluten-free diet is equivocal, or if the patient had few symptoms initially (e.g. presenting with iron deficiency anaemia or as an asymptomatic relative of patient with coeliac disease).

4 *Gluten challenge followed by re-biopsy*: this is no longer regarded as mandatory for the diagnosis of coeliac disease. However, of transient gluten intolerance is suspected, for example where ingestion of gluten appears to cause no symptoms in a child diagnosed in early infancy, then re-introduction of gluten followed by re-biopsy is essential. This biopsy will either confirm the diagnosis of coeliac disease, or will be normal, in which case the child requires follow-up into adult life to detect those in whom several years are required before there is a late relapse.

Therapeutic trial of gluten-free diet

In a child with symptoms suggestive of coeliac disease, there may be a temptation to avoid or defer performing a jejunal biopsy and instead to employ a therapeutic trial of a gluten-free diet. The short-term advantage of sparing the child an invasive diagnostic procedure is outweighed by a number of major drawbacks.

1 Coeliac disease is a life-long and pre-malignant disorder. The need for a life-long strict gluten-free diet means that an accurate diagnosis is essential. Thus a therapeutic trial of a gluten-free diet with improvement in symptoms can only serve to delay making a firm diagnosis, for jejunal biopsy is still essential.

2 An equivocal or negative response to a therapeutic trial of a gluten-free diet always raises the questions of whether the diet was performed correctly or for long enough. The question of coeliac disease remains unsettled, and a biopsy is required.

3 In genuine coeliac disease, gluten may have to be re-introduced for some years before there is a definite change in the histological appearance of the jejunum, thus considerably delaying the final diagnosis. Thus a child who does not have coeliac disease, but who appeared to respond to a gluten-free diet, may have to be followed up for many years before coeliac disease can be excluded.

4 If the diagnosis is not coeliac disease, then a dietary trial will delay the discovery of the correct diagnosis.

Malignancy   Coeliac disease is a pre-malignant condition, and is associated with the development in adult life of a specific type of T-cell lymphoma, and carcinoma of the jejunum and oesophagus (reviewed by Trier 1991). It is unproven that strict adherence to a gluten-free diet provides protection from the development of malignancy, although a recent report suggests that it does (Holmes *et al.* 1989).

Treatment   The treatment is a life-long gluten-free diet, with medical supervision to detect and deal with non-adherence to the diet. Non-adherence to the diet is a frequent problem.

Gluten-free diet   Details of gluten-free manufactured foods can be obtained from a dietitian, and in the UK from the Coeliac Society (P.O. Box 220, High Wycombe, Buckinghamshire, HP11 4H7). The inclusion of wheat in manufactured foods is not always self-evident (Table 27.4), and the advice of a dietitian is indispensable. Gluten present in communion wafers poses a special medical and theological problem (Moriarty *et al.* 1989). Gluten is included (usually as an excipient or in the form of wheat bran fibre) in a small number of pharmaceutical preparations, such as Dimotapp LA, Nulacin and Fybranta.

Dermatitis herpetiformis   The majority (but not all) patients with dermatitis herpetiformis have a similar intestinal lesion to that found in coeliac disease. The skin lesions usually improve on a gluten-free diet (Fry *et al.* 1973; Kósnai *et al.* 1986; Hall 1987; Hall & Waldbauer 1988).

Table 27.4 Examples of manufactured foods which may contain wheat or gluten

Flour, bread, biscuits, pastry, cake
Wheat-based breakfast cereals, e.g. Weetabix
Spaghetti, macaroni, noodles and other pasta
Semolina
Sausages
Gravy made with flour
Milk shakes, Horlick's malted milks
Powdered pepper (with flour as a filler)
Rye bread
Barley, barley bread, barley drinks

Key references

27.1   WALKER-SMITH JA (1988) *Diseases of the Small Intestine in Childhood*, 3rd edn, Butterworths, London. *Includes a chapter which reviews the clinical aspects of coeliac disease.*

27.2   BRANSKI D & LEBENTHAL E (1989) Gluten-sensitive enteropathy. In Lebenthal E (ed) *Textbook of Gastroenterology and Nutrition in Infancy*, 2nd edn, pp. 1093–1106, Raven Press, New York. *Review of clinical aspects of coeliac disease.*

27.3   WALKER-SMITH JA, GUANDALINI S, SCHMITZ J, SHMERLING DH & VISAKORPI JK (1990) Revised criteria for diagnosis of coeliac disease. Report of working group of European Society of Paediatric Gastroenterology and Nutrition. *Arch Dis Child* **65**:909–911. *Recent review of diagnostic criteria, and discussion of the role of gluten challenge, re-biopsy and tests for antibodies.*

27.4   MARSH MN (1990) Grains of truth: evolutionary changes in small intestinal mucosa in response to environmental antigen challenge. *Gut* **31**:111–114. *Review of immunopathogenesis.*

27.5   TRIER JS (1991) Celiac sprue. *New Engl J Med* **325**:1709–1718. *Review of pathogenesis, clinical features, treatment and prognosis.*

Summary 27

Coeliac disease is a life-long disorder in which jejunal villous atrophy is associated with sensitivity to gluten. Complete avoidance of gluten in the diet leads to a return to normal of the intestinal morphology and function, and loss of symptoms. The principal diagnostic difficulty is to distinguish coeliac disease from other disorders which can cause flattening of the jejunal villi, and from transient intolerance to gluten. Therapeutic trials of gluten-free diets are inadvisable as they result in diagnostic delay.

28 Wheat, rye, barley and oat intolerance
Non-coeliac food intolerance

Wheat intolerance

Wheat is one of many foods capable of provoking food intolerance. In Lessof *et al.*'s description of 100 patients with food intolerance, most of whom were apparently adults, wheat was the provoking food in nine patients (Lessof *et al.* 1980). However in a series of 426 positive double-blind placebo-controlled food challenges, wheat was the positive food in only 14 instances (Bock *et al.* 1988). Unfortunately, most of the published information on wheat intolerance is rather anecdotal.

gastrointestinal

Hill (1987) has reported that of 88 children, mainly infants, with cow's milk protein intolerance, 12 out of 88 also had intolerance to wheat. The main features of the wheat intolerance in these patients were loose stools and abdominal pain, commencing within 12–72 hours after wheat ingestion, and the patients did not have histological changes in the jejunum. Jonas (1978) has reported a 16-month-old girl with loose stools, irritability and loss of appetite in whom the jejunal biopsy was normal, and in whom the symptoms abated on a wheat-free diet, relapsed on a gluten-free diet, and abated upon resumption of a wheat-free diet.

asthma

Williams *et al.* (1987) have reported a 60-year-old woman in whom placebo-controlled double-blind challenge confirmed wheat-induced asthma. Furlan *et al.* (1987) reported five adult asthmatics in whom double-blind challenge with flour resulted in a 25% or greater fall in the PEFR. Wraith (1987) has reported anecdotally on wheat-induced asthma in children and adults, and has claimed that wheat is more commonly found as a trigger of asthma in adults than children.

atopic eczema

Wheat is one of numerous foods reported to cause exacerbations of atopic eczema (Hammar 1977).

urticaria, angioedema

Wheat is one of numerous foods reported to provoke urticaria and angioedema (Kushimoto & Aoki 1985).

anaphylactic shock

A 10-week-old infant presented with loose stools and vomiting. A challenge with a 'small amount' of rusk was followed, after 2 hours, by vomiting, watery diarrhoea, bronchospasm and shock. Watery diarrhoea, due to a temporary monosaccharide intolerance, continued until he was treated with a period of bowel rest followed by regrading. He remained symptom free on a wheat-free diet, and by

149

14 months he was able to tolerate wheat without symptoms (Rudd *et al.* 1981).

exercise-induced anaphylaxis

Wheat is one of the more commonly reported foods to provoke food-provoked exercise-induced anaphylaxis (Kushimoto & Aoki 1985; Armentia *et al.* 1990).

occupational flour allergy

Occupational asthma, rhinitis and conjunctivitis due to inhalation of flour are well recognized in bakers (El Karim *et al.* 1986; Rosen 1987; Hensley *et al.* 1988; Santiago *et al.* 1988). The nature of the allergen in wheat which provokes baker's asthma is unclear (Blands *et al.* 1976; Taylor *et al.* 1987; Walsh *et al.* 1987). In an interesting study, intragastric provocation under endoscopic control with wheat flour demonstrated visible reactions (oedema, erythema, increased contraction, duodenal gastric reflux) in all seven bakers with occupational sensitivity to wheat flour (Kurek *et al.* 1990). Five subjects also experienced abdominal pain, three rhinitis, two asthma and two conjunctivitis. Of the seven patients, five had *Campylobacter pylori* infection, and it was hypothesized that flour-induced gastritis had predisposed to this infection.

Rye, barley, oat

Although reports of patients with intolerance to wheat sometimes also mention intolerance to rye, barley and oat, the incidence of intolerance to these grains, and the degree to which cross-reactivity occurs, are unknown.

Key references 28.1

WILLIAMS AJ, CHURCH SE & FINN R (1987) An unsuspected case of wheat induced asthma. *Thorax* **42**:205–206. A 60-year-old woman with a 6-year history of severe asthma noted that there was some improvement in her symptoms when, as part of an attempt to lose weight, she reduced her intake of foods which contained wheat. A strict wheat-free diet enabled her to abandon all therapy (which had included inhaled steroids), and placebo-controlled challenges with wheat 30 g/day caused a marked and progressive deterioration over 5 days.

28.2

RUDD P, MANUEL P & WALKER-SMITH J (1981) Anaphylactic shock in an infant after feeding with a wheat rusk. A transient phenomenon. *Postgrad Med J* **57**: 794–795. Report of anaphylaxis occurring after challenge with a rusk in a 2-month-old infant, whose previous vomiting and loose stools coincided with ingestion of wheat rusks.

Summary 28

Wheat can provoke gastrointestinal symptoms, asthma, urticaria, eczema or anaphylactic shock in sensitive subjects. Although poorly documented, intolerance to rye, barley and oats can also occur.

References to Chapters 26–28

ANAND BS, PIRIS J & TRUELOVE SC (1978) The role of various cereals in coeliac disease. *Quart J Med* **185**:101–110.

ANDERSEN DH (1947) Celiac syndrome. VI. The relationship of celiac disease, starch intolerance and steatorrhea. *J Pediat* **30**:564–582.

ARMENTIA A, MARTIN-SANTOS JM, BLANCO M, CARRETERO L, PUYO M & BARBER D (1990) Exercise-induced anaphylactic reaction to grain flours. *Ann Allergy* **65**:149–151.

BLANDS J, DIAMANT B, KALLÓS P, KALLÓS-DEFFNER L & LÖWENSTEIN H (1976) Flour allergy in bakers. I. Identification of allergenic fractions in flour and comparison of diagnostic methods. *Int Archs Allergy Appl Immunol* **52**: 392–406.

BOCK SA, SAMPSON HA, ATKINS FM *et al.* (1988) Double-blind, placebo-controlled food challenge (DBPCFC) as an office procedure: a manual. *J Allergy Clin Immunol* **82**:986–997.

BOOTH C (1989) History of coeliac disease. *Br Med J* **298**:527.

BRANSKI D & LEBENTHAL E (1989) Gluten-sensitive enteropathy. In Lebenthal E (ed) *Textbook of Gastroenterology and Nutrition in Infancy*, 2nd edn, pp. 1093–1106, Raven Press, New York.

BROUK B (1975) *Plants Consumed by Man*, Academic Press, London.

BÜRGIN-WOLFF A, GAZE H, HADZISELIMOVIC F *et al.* (1991) Antigliadin and antiendomysium antibody determination for coeliac disease. *Arch Dis Child* **66**:941–947.

CALABUIG M, TORREGOSA R, POLO P *et al.* (1990) Serological markers and celiac disease: a new diagnostic approach? *J Pediatr Gastroenterol Nutr* **10**: 435–442.

CICLITIRA PJ, ELLIS HJ, EVANS DJ & LENNOX ES (1985) A radioimmunoassay for wheat gliadin to assess the suitability of gluten free foods for patients with coeliac disease. *Clin Exp Immunol* **59**:703–708.

CICLITIRA PJ, ELLIS HJ & FAGG NLK (1984b) Evaluation of a gluten free product containing wheat gliadin in patients with coeliac disease. *Br Med J* **289**:83.

CICLITIRA PJ, EVANS DJ, FAGG NLK, LENNOX ES & DOWLING RH (1984a) Clinical testing of gliadin fractions in coeliac patients. *Clin Sci* **66**:357–364.

COULTATE TP (1984) *Food – the Chemistry of Its Components*, Royal Society of Chemistry, London.

DAVID TJ & AJDUKIEWICZ AB (1975) A family study of coeliac disease. *J Med Genet* **12**:79–82.

DICKE WK, WEIJERS HA & KAMER JH VAN DE (1953) Coeliac disease: the presence in wheat of a factor having a deleterious effect in cases of coeliac disease. *Acta Paediat Scand* **42**:34–42.

DISSANAYAKE AS, TRUELOVE SC & WHITEHEAD R (1974) Lack of harmful effect of oats on small-intestinal mucosa in coeliac disease. *Br Med J* **4**:189–191.

EGAN H, KIRK RS & SAWYER R (1987) *Pearson's Chemical Analysis of Foods*, 8th edn, Longman Scientific & Technical, Harlow.

EL KARIM MAA, EL RAB MOG, OMER AA & EL HAIMI YAA (1986) Respiratory and allergic disorders in workers exposed to grain and flour dusts. *Arch Environ Health* **41**:297–301.

FRY L, SEAH PP, RICHES DJ & HOFFBRAND AV (1973) Clearance of skin lesions in dermatitis herpetiformis after gluten withdrawal. *Lancet* **1**:288–291.

FURLAN J, SUSKOVIC S & RUS A (1987) The effect of food on the bronchial response in adult asthmatic patients, and the protective role of ketotifen. *Allergol Immunopathol* **15**:73–81.

GEE S (1888) On the coeliac affection. *St Bart's Hosp Rep* **24**:17–20.

GRECO L, DE SETA L, D'ADAMO G et al. (1990) Atopy and coeliac disease: bias or true relation. *Acta Paediat Scand* **79**:670–674.

GUANDALINI S, VENTURA A, ANSALDI N et al. (1989) Diagnosis of coeliac disease: time for a change? *Arch Dis Child* **64**:1320–1325.

HAAS SV (1924) The value of the banana in the treatment of celiac disease. *Am J Dis Child* **24**:421–437.

HALL RP (1987) Dietary management of dermatitis herpetiformis. *Arch Dermatol* **123**:1378a–1380a.

HALL RP & WALDBAUER GV (1988) Characterization of the mucosal immune response to dietary antigens in patients with dermatitis herpetiformis. *J Invest Dermatol* **90**:658–663.

HAMMAR H (1977) Provocation with cow's milk and cereals in atopic dermatitis. *Acta Dermatovener (Stockh)* **57**:159–163.

HENSLEY MJ, SCICCHITANO R, SAUNDERS NA et al. (1988) Seasonal variation in non-specific bronchial reactivity: a study of wheat workers with a history of wheat associated asthma. *Thorax* **43**:103–107.

HILL DJ (1987) Clinical recognition of the child with food allergy. *Ann Allergy* **59**:141–145.

HOLMES GKT, PRIOR P, LANE MR, POPE D & ALLAN RN (1989) Malignancy in coeliac disease – effect of a gluten free diet. *Gut* **30**:333–338.

IACONO G, NOCERINO A, GUANDALINI S, CARROCCIO A, CAVATAIO F & BALSAMO V (1991) Transient gluten hypersensitivity. *J Pediat Gastroenterol Nutr* **12**:400–403.

JONAS A (1978) Wheat-sensitive – but not coeliac. *Lancet* **2**:1047.

KÓSNAI I, KÁRPATI S, SAVILAHTI E, VERKASALO M, BUCSKY P & TÖRÖK E (1986) Gluten challenge in children with dermatitis herpetiformis: a clinical, morphological and immunohistological study. *Gut* **27**:1464–1470.

KUREK M, BABIC R & RING J (1990) Gastric reactibility to flour and *Campylobacter pylori* associated gastritis in patients with flour allergy (abstract). *J Allergy Clin Immunol* 1990; 85 (suppl.):274.

KUSHIMOTO H & AOKI T (1985) Masked type I wheat allergy. Relation to exercise-induced anaphylaxis. *Arch Dermatol* **121**:355–360.

LEIGH RJ, MARSH MN, CROWE P, KELLY C, GARNER V & GORDON D (1985) Studies of intestinal lymphoid tissue. IX. Dose-dependent, gluten-induced lymphoid infiltration of coeliac jejunal epithelium. *Scand J Gastroenterol* **20**:715–719.

LESSOF MH, WRAITH DG, MERRETT TG, MERRETT J & BUISSERET PD (1980) Food allergy and intolerance in 100 patients – local and systemic effects. *Quart J Med* **49**:259–271.

MARSH MN (1990) Grains of truth: evolutionary changes in small intestinal mucosa in response to environmental antigen challenge. *Gut* **31**:111–114.

MARSH MN & LOFT DE (1988) Coeliac sprue: a centennial overview 1888–1988. *Dig Dis* **6**:216–228.

MORIARTY KJ, LOFT D, MARSH MN, BROOKS ST, GORDON D & GARNER GV (1989) Holy communion wafers and celiac disease. *New Engl J Med* **321**:332.

MYLOTTE M, EGAN-MITCHELL B MCCARTHY CF & MCNICHOLL B (1973) Incidence of coeliac disease in the west of Ireland. *Br Med J* **1**:703–705.

PACKER SM, CHARLTON V, KEELING JW et al. (1978) Gluten challenge in treated coeliac disease. *Arch Dis Child* **53**:449–455.

PAVELEY WF (1988) From Aretaeus to Crosby: a history of coeliac disease. *Br Med J* **297**:1646–1648.

ROSEN JP (1987) Bakers' rhinoconjunctivitis: a case report. *New Engl Reg Allergy Proc* **8**:37–38.

RUDD P, MANUEL P & WALKER-SMITH J (1981) Anaphylactic shock in an infant after feeding with a wheat rusk. A transient phenomenon. *Postgrad Med J* **57**:794–795.

SANTIAGO AV, PAR M, VALLS JS, MARTINEZ PS, CASAJUANA AM & CALDERÓN PAG (1988) Hypersensitivity to wheat flour in bakers. *Allergol Immunopathol* **16**:309–314.

TAYLOR SL, LEMANSKE RF, BUSH RK & BUSSE WW (1987) Food allergens: structure and immunologic properties. *Ann Allergy* **59**:93–99.

TOSONI C, APOLLONIO A, CATTANEO R, SOLDATI F & RANZINI C (1991) Evaluation of a screening test for detection of IgA antigliadin antibodies in coeliac disease. *Pediatr Allergy Immunol* **2**:76–78.

TRIER JS (1991) Celiac sprue. *New Engl J Med* **325**:1709–1718.

WALKER-SMITH JA (1970) Transient gluten intolerance. *Arch Dis Child* **45**: 523–526.

WALKER-SMITH JA (1988) *Diseases of the Small Intestine in Childhood*, 3rd edn, Buttwerworths, London.

WALKER-SMITH JA, GUANDALINI S, SCHMITZ J, SHMERLING DH & VISAKORPI JK (1990) Revised criteria for diagnosis of coeliac disease. Report of working group of European Society of Paediatric Gastroenterology and Nutrition. *Arch Dis Child* **65**:909–911.

WALSH BJ, BALDO BA, BASS DJ, CLANCY R, MUSK AW & WRIGLEY CW (1987) Insoluble and soluble allergens from wheat grain and wheat dust: detection of IgE binding in inhalant and ingestion allergy. *New Engl Reg Allergy Proc* **8**:27–33.

WILLIAMS AJ, CHURCH SE & FINN R (1987) An unsuspected case of wheat induced asthma. *Thorax* **42**:205–206.

WORLD HEALTH ORGANISATION (1981) Codex standard for 'gluten-free foods' (world-wide standard). *Codex Alimentarius Commission*, Codex stan. 118–1981, pp. 9–12.

WRAITH DG (1987) Asthma. In Brostoff J & Challacombe SJ (eds). *Food Allergy and Intolerance*, pp. 486–497, Baillière Tindall, London.

Part 7 Miscellaneous Foods

29 Fish and shellfish
Quick-onset reactions, sometimes severe

Fish Fish is well recognized as a cause of quick-onset reactions, manifesting as urticaria, angioedema, asthma, vomiting, loose stools, abdominal pain, worsening of atopic eczema, and anaphylactic shock (Aas 1966a) which can be fatal (Yunginger *et al.* 1988). An enteropathy has been noted in a small number of patients who had gastrointestinal features of intolerance to other foods such as cow's milk protein (Vitoria *et al.* 1982). Extreme sensitivity to minute quantities of fish is occasionally noted, and even exposure to the fumes of fish being cooked may be enough to precipitate symptoms in certain individuals (Derbes & Krafchuk 1957; Aas 1987). Aas (1987) has reported from Norway that fish antigens could be found in house dust in most homes where fish is often eaten, and he suggested that this was a likely source for sensitization to fish.

type of fish Cod is the most frequently reported offender, but reactions to other fish such as haddock, herring, sprat, halibut, plaice, mackerel, trout and salmon are well recognized (Aas 1966b) though not proven by challenge.

cross-reaction There is a lack of useful clinical data on the cross-reactivity. In one study (de Martino *et al.* 1990), of 20 children with a history of intolerance to cod, there was a history of intolerance to sole in 11 (55%), tuna in seven (35%), and mackerel, anchovy, sardine, red mullet and salmon each in one (5%). The remaining major studies of cross-reactivity are based on skin-prick and IgE antibody test results (e.g. Tuft *et al.* 1946; Waring *et al.* 1985; de Martino *et al.* 1988) which have little bearing on clinical sensitivity.

natural history The natural history of fish intolerance has never been systematically studied. Aas reported that in a group of 50 children with fish intolerance, the intolerance to fish disappeared within 4 years in five (Aas 1966a). In three more, provocation demonstrated a reduction in the severity of symptoms after 2–3 years, and this was reported by the parents in a further 12 cases. In two cases the symptoms increased following ingestion of fish, and in the remaining patients there was no information about changes in reactivity. Although it is possible to grow out of fish intolerance, there are many occasions when, as far as one can tell, intolerance is life-long.

157

raw or cooked?   Some subjects with fish intolerance report a greater sensitivity to *raw* than to *cooked* fish. The most notable exception is that of Professor Heinz Küstner, who was intolerant to fish which had been heated to 55°C or above but not to raw fish (Prausnitz & Küstner 1921).

Shellfish   As with fish, shellfish are well recognized as a cause of quick-onset reactions, which can on rare occasions prove fatal (Yunginger *et al.* 1988). The most commonly reported shellfish to provoke intolerance are shrimp, crab, lobster, crayfish, oyster, cuttlefish, abalone and grand keyhole limpet (Daul *et al.* 1987; Shibasaki *et al.* 1989; Lehrer *et al.* 1990; Morikawa *et al.* 1990). However, few reports have included verification by double-blind challenges (Daul *et al.* 1988; Morgan *et al.* 1990). Shrimp is one of the foods reported to trigger food-provoked exercise-induced anaphylaxis (Maulitz *et al.* 1979; McNeil & Strauss 1988).

cross-reaction   The degree of cross-reaction between different shellfish, or between shellfish and other fish, is uncertain. Most data is derived from studies of skin test reactions or IgE antibodies (Tuft & Blumstein 1940; Waring *et al.* 1985; Lehrer & McCants 1987; Morgan *et al.* 1989), the presence of which cannot, of course, be taken to equate with clinical intolerance.

natural history   The natural history of shellfish intolerance has not been systematically studied. For what it is worth, one report showed relatively constant shrimp-specific IgE antibody levels during a 24-month period of study in 11 adults with shrimp intolerance (Daul *et al.* 1990).

Diagnosis   The diagnosis is usually based on the history. In the case of cod, there is a very close correlation between a history of intolerance plus a positive skin-prick test and a positive RAST test (Aas & Lundkvist 1973), but comparative data are unavailable for intolerance to other fish in childhood.

Management   As with other forms of food intolerance, the management is avoidance. Oral and parenteral hyposensitization has been attempted on a few occasions in fish intolerance (Paulsen 1961; Aas 1966a), with doubtful benefit if any and with great attendant risk.

Toxic & other reactions   Fish and shellfish are an important cause of adverse reactions due to the presence of a number of different toxins and pathogenic micro-organisms (see Table 2.3). A parasite of fish, *Anisakis*, can not only produce infection (McKerrow *et al.* 1988) but can also provoke what is possibly an allergic reaction (Kasuya *et al.* 1989). Protamine sulphate is a polypeptide derived from fish, mainly salmon, which can provoke adverse reactions which include urticaria, bronchospasm and shock (Weiler *et al.* 1990). Several mechanisms may result in these adverse reactions (Weiss *et al.* 1989). In general there does not appear to be any connection with intolerance to fish. However, there is one report of an anaphylactic reaction to protamine in a man who had worked in a fish-processing factory and was intolerant to a variety of different fish, and two other reports of an association between intolerance to fish and reactions to protamine (Caplan & Berkman 1976; Knape *et al.* 1981).

Inhalational reactions   Occupational asthma is recognized in fish and shellfish-processing workers, and is thought to be due to inhalation of antigens (Orford & Wilson 1985; Sherson *et al.* 1989).

Key references 29.1   Aas K (1966) Studies of hypersensitivity to fish. A clinical study. *Int Arch Allergy* **29**:346–363. *A clinical study of 89 children with intolerance to fish, collected during a 4-year period in Oslo, itself suggesting that the importance of fish in the diet in Norway may be associated with a higher incidence of fish intolerance.*

29.2   Aas K (1987) Fish allergy and the codfish model. In Brostoff J & Challacombe SJ (eds) *Food Allergy and Intolerance*, pp. 356–366, Ballière Tindall, London. *Review.*

Summary 29   Fish and shellfish are well recognized causes of quick-onset reactions, manifesting as urticaria, angioedema, asthma, vomiting, loose stools, abdominal pain, worsening of atopic eczema, and anaphylactic shock which can occasionally be fatal.

30 Nuts
The food most commonly reported to provoke fatal anaphylaxis

Wide variety   Nuts are edible seeds contained within a hard or brittle shell. Edible nuts include acorn, almond, beech nut, brazil nut, cashew nut, chestnut, coconut, hazel nut, oyster nut, peanut, pecan nut, pistachio nut, sunflower seed and walnut.

Peanut   Peanut is well recognized as a cause of quick-onset reactions, manifesting as urticaria, contact urticaria, angioedema, asthma, vomiting, loose stools, abdominal pain, worsening of atopic eczema, and anaphylactic shock (Fries 1982; Mathias 1983; Burks *et al.* 1989; Sampson 1990). Peanut is the food most commonly reported to cause fatal anaphylaxis (Settipane 1989; Yunginger *et al.* 1989; Assem *et al.* 1990). A number of protein constituents have been shown to be allergenic (Bush *et al.* 1989).

diagnosis   A lack of standardized peanut extracts (Bush *et al.* 1989), partly attributable to the large number of allergens in peanuts (Barnett *et al.* 1983), and a high incidence of atopic children who have positive skin-prick or RAST tests without clinical symptoms of peanut intolerance (Kemp *et al.* 1985; Kalliel *et al.* 1989; Zimmerman *et al.* 1989) are major drawbacks. The diagnosis has to be based on the history, supplemented on rare occasions where necessary by challenge.

natural history   It is uncommon to lose reactivity to peanuts, and peanut intolerance is usually life-long (Bock & Atkins 1989).

cross-reactivity   Peanut, soya, bean, pea and lentil are all members of the Leguminosae family. Cross-reactivity between peanut and other legumes has been reported (Gall *et al.* 1990), but it appears to be uncommon (Bernhisel-Broadbent & Sampson 1989).

peanut oil   Peanut oil does not usually contain detectable protein (Tattrie & Yaguchi 1973), and is therefore said to be a highly unlikely source of danger to subjects with peanut intolerance (Taylor *et al.* 1981). A study of 10 adults with peanut intolerance failed to demonstrate any adverse reactions to ingestion of peanut oil (Taylor *et al.* 1981). There is one report of a local painful and erythematous reaction, accompanied by urticaria, following injection of adrenaline in peanut oil in an adult with asthma and peanut intolerance (Chafee 1941). Furthermore, there is a recent report of two infants who developed generalized skin rashes 15 min after ingestion of 1 ml of peanut oil (Moneret-Vautrin *et al.* 1991). On data currently available, it is evident that peanut oil cannot be safely given to those with peanut intolerance. The statistical problems in assessing safety are addressed in Table 30.1, but in short, to be 99.9% sure that peanut oil is safe in 99.9% of those with peanut intolerance, one would need to test 6905 individuals with peanut intolerance.

aspirin effect   There is a single report of a 14-year-old boy known to develop angioedema of the lips and face after ingestion of peanuts, in whom

Table 30.1 Is peanut oil safe? A statistical problem

How many peanut intolerant patients have to be challenged with peanut oil before peanut oil can be declared safe for those with peanut intolerance? Are the 10 patients studied by Taylor *et al.* (1981) enough? The answer is that the number that is needed depends on the degree of certainty required. But, however many subjects are studied, for example 10 000, this is no guarantee that the 10 001 person would not react. The following calculations can be made.

If we suppose that 5% of those with peanut intolerance will react to peanut oil, the probability of one patient reacting is 0.05. The probability of one patient not reacting is 0.95.

The probability of two patients not reacting is $(0.95)^2 = 0.9025$

The probability of 58 patients not reacting is $(0.95)^{58} = 0.051$

The probability of at least one out of 58 patients reacting $= 1 - (0.95)^{58} = 0.949$

Thus, if you test 59 individuals, and none react to peanut oil, then you will be 95% certain that the incidence of reaction to peanut oil is ⩽5%.

To be 99% sure that the incidence of reaction to peanut oil is ⩽5%, one would need to test 299 individuals

$$\frac{\log 0.05}{\log 0.99} = 298.07$$

To be 99.9% sure that the incidence of reaction of peanut oil is ⩽5%, one would need to test 2995 individuals

$$\frac{\log 0.05}{\log 0.999} = 2994.322$$

One would need 459 patients to be 99% certain that the incidence of reaction to peanut oil is ⩽1%, and 6905 patients to be 99.9% sure it is ⩽0.1%.

the ingestion of peanuts 5 min after swallowing aspirin 600 mg resulted in a life-threatening anaphylactic reaction (Cant *et al.* 1984). It was postulated that the aspirin potentiated the reaction by increasing the permeability of the gastric mucosa.

management The management is avoidance of all foods which contain peanut. This is complicated by the increasing use of peanut in manufactured foods, such as vegetable burgers and cake icing (Evans *et al.* 1988; Donovan & Peters 1990), and contamination of non-peanut-containing food with peanut protein (Yunginger *et al.* 1983). For this reason, where there is a history of a severe reaction to peanut, there may be a case for instruction in the self or parental administration of injectable adrenaline (see chapter 63) to treat accidental ingestion of peanut.

inhalation Although perhaps not strictly relevant to this book, it is worth remembering that peanuts are one of the leading offenders in fatal asphyxiation resulting from inhalation of food. It has been suggested that peanuts should not be given to children under the age of 6–7 years (Stafford 1985).

Other nuts   Intolerance to other nuts, such as walnut, hazel nut, almond, pecan nut, filbert, pine nut and cashew nut are all recognized, and a fatal reaction to pecan has been reported (Bock *et al.* 1978; Atkins *et al.* 1985; Fine 1987; Boyd 1989; Nielsen 1990; Par *et al.* 1990). In a report of 12 subjects with intolerance to Brazil nuts, it was stated that five adults had been followed up for 8 years without loss of their intolerance which dated back to childhood (Arshad *et al.* 1991). In one case, an 8-year old girl, intolerance to ingested pine nuts (angioedema and urticaria) co-existed with seasonal conjunctivitis and rhinitis attributed to pine pollen (Armentia *et al.* 1990). In another poorly documented case, a flare-up of Behçet's syndrome was associated with the ingestion of walnuts (Kikuchi 1985).

cross-reactivity   The incidence of cross-reactivity between different nuts, which clearly can occur, is not known. This is an important area of uncertainty because of the potentially severe nature of adverse reactions to nuts, especially to peanuts. It would be helpful, for example, to have some objective data on the likelihood of intolerance to other nuts in children with a history of severe reactions after ingestion of peanut.

cashew nut shell oil   Cashew nuts are covered by a double-layered outer shell. Between the two layers is an oil which contains cardol and anacardic acid, which have irritant and allergic properties, and which are immunologically related to the pentadecylcatechols found in poison ivy. Faulty processing can allow cashew nuts to become contaminated by this shell oil, and in one report 54 individuals developed a poison ivy-like dermatitis after eating cashew nuts (Marks *et al.* 1984).

Key references   30.1   YUNGINGER J W, SQUILLACE D L, JONES R T & HELM R M (1989) Fatal anaphylactic reactions induced by peanuts. *Allergy Proc* **10**:249–253. *Review of four cases, one of whom was a child (an 11-year-old boy). The authors also reported a manufactured product in which peanuts are deflavoured and reflavoured and coloured to resemble pecans, almonds or walnuts. Not surprisingly the final product still contained detectable quantities of peanut protein. One danger lay in the description of these items as 'artificial walnuts' or 'artificial pecans', giving no indication of the origin of the material.*

30.2   BUSH R K, TAYLOR S L & NORDLEE J A (1989) Peanut sensitivity. *Allergy Proc* **10**:261–264. *A useful review of the chemistry of peanut proteins and peanut allergens.*

Summary 30   Peanuts are well known for their ability to provoke brisk reactions, and are responsible for more reported cases of food-provoked fatal anaphylactic shock than any other food. Other nuts can also provoke reactions, although less commonly. The degree of cross-reactivity between different nuts is uncertain. A major hazard for those who are intolerant to nuts is the increasing use of nuts in manufactured foods.

31 Pears and apples
Fructose and sorbitol may cause loose stools

Pears, apples   Some children experience loose stools after ingestion of pears, apples or the juices of these fruits (Hyams & Leichtner 1985; Kneepkens *et al.* 1989). The cause of the loose stools is not always obvious to the parents. Such patients may present with chronic diarrhoea.

fructose content   Pears and apples differ from most fruits in that they contain an excess of fructose as compared to glucose (Hardinge *et al.* 1965). Although the mechanism of intestinal fructose absorption is not fully understood, there is thought to be an energy-dependent active carrier mechanism which is facilitated by glucose (Kneepkens *et al.* 1984; Rumessen & Gudmand-Høyer 1986). A combination of high intake, a high ratio of fructose to glucose in food, and an individual's relative inability to absorb fructose lead to incomplete absorption and loose stools.

management   The diagnosis can be confirmed by measurement of the breath hydrogen response to challenges with fructose and other sugars (Rumessen & Gudmand-Høyer 1986; Kneepkens *et al.* 1989). In fructose malabsorption, ingestion of the sugar will cause a marked rise in the breath hydrogen concentration after fructose, but not after glucose or lactose. The main problem with this test is that if sufficient amounts of fructose are given then all subjects will experience malabsorption. 2 mg/kg appears to be a useful working figure (Barnes *et al.* 1983; Wales *et al.* 1989) but we lack population-based data on the quantitative capacity for absorption. The management

Table 31.1 Fructose content of fruit and other foods[1]

Food type	Fructose g/100 g edible portion	Glucose g/100 g edible portion
Fruits		
Apple	5.0	1.7
Banana	3.5	4.5
Blackberry	2.9	3.2
Blackcurrant	3.7	2.4
Cherry	7.2	4.7
Date	23.9	24.9
Fig	8.2	9.6
Gooseberry	4.1	4.4
Grape	7.3	8.2
Grapefruit	1.2	2.0
Green gage	4.0	5.5
Lemon	1.4	1.4
Loganberry	1.3	1.9
Melon	1.5	2.1
Mulberry	3.6	4.4
Orange	1.8	2.5
Peach	1.6	1.5
Pear	6.5	2.6
Pineapple	1.4	2.3
Plum	3.4	5.2
Prune	15.0	30.0
Raspberry	2.4	2.3
Redcurrant	1.9	2.3
Strawberry	2.3	2.6
Tomato	1.2	1.6
White currant	2.6	3.0
Other foods		
Potato	0.1	0.1
Honey	40.5	34.2
Royal jelly	11.3	9.8
Molasses	8.0	8.8

[1] Source: Hardinge *et al.* (1965).

is to reduce the intake of foods which contain fructose (Table 31.1). Since this means reducing the intake of fruit, a low-fructose diet may necessitate the use of supplemental vitamin C. Fructose is sometimes added to food as an aid to weight reduction (almost as sweet as sucrose – Coultate 1984) and also as a heat-stable sweetener for diabetics (metabolism independent of insulin), for example in 'diabetic chocolate'.

sorbitol   Sorbitol, which occurs naturally in pears and apples, is a further possible cause of loose stools, although the quantity of sorbitol in these fruits is generally less than that of fructose (see Hyams *et al.* 1988 and chapter 31).

oral pruritus

Apples and pears have also been reported to cause oral pruritus, as have carrot and potato, most notably during the pollen season (Tuft & Blumstein 1942; Dreborg & Foucard 1983).

Key references 31.1

WALES JKH, PRIMHAK RA, RATTENBURY J & TAYLOR CJ (1989) Isolated fructose malabsorption. *Arch Dis Child* **115**:227–229. Detailed account of fructose malabsorption which presented in infancy with screaming after feeds and diarrhoea. *This condition should be considered in any child with unexplained loose stools.*

31.2

HYAMS JS, ETIENNE NL, LEICHTNER AM & THEUER RC (1988) Carbohydrate malabsorption following fruit juice ingestion in young children. *Pediatrics* **82**: 64–68. Breath hydrogen tests were performed in 13 healthy children and seven children with chronic nonspecific diarrhoea; the results were the same for both groups. Increased breath hydrogen excretion was found after ingestion of pear juice (fructose 6.4 g/100 ml, sorbitol 2.0 g/100 ml) or 2% sorbitol solution in most subjects, after apple juice (fructose 6.4 g/100 ml, sorbitol 0.5 g/100 ml) in 50% of subjects, and after grape juice (fructose 7.5 g/100 ml, no sorbitol) in 25%. *The low proportion of subjects who reacted adversely to grape juice, despite the fact that it had the highest fructose concentration, suggests that the sorbitol content of apples and pears may contribute to the carbohydrate malabsorption that can be associated with the ingestion of these fruits and their juices.*

Summary 31

Some children poorly absorb fructose, resulting in loose stools after the ingestion of foods which contain fructose. Because of their high fructose content, the ingestion of pears or apples may cause loose stools. The sorbitol content of these fruits, although less important than fructose, may contribute to the loose stools. Fructose malabsorption should be considered in any child with unexplained loose stools, and is easily confirmed by fructose challenge and detection of a sharp rise in the excretion of hydrogen in the breath.

32   Intolerance to other foods
The list is potentially endless

Selected list of reports

This chapter provides a selected list of reports of intolerance to foods other than cow's milk, soya, egg, cereals, fish, nuts, pears, apples and food additives, all of which are discussed separately in this book. Studies which include no clinical information but simply document the presence of circulating antibodies, positive skin tests or other types of indirect information are not included. The list only comprises reports of clinically detectable adverse reactions to ingested foods. It includes observations made in adults. Most of these reports have not been validated by double-blind challenge. It also includes a few miscellaneous items which are not easily classified as foods or food additives, such as pollen, ethanol and vitamins.

Almond   Par PA, Valls JS, Pérez ML, Casajuana AM & Calderón PAG (1990) Dried fruit hypersensitivity and its correlation with pollen allergy. *Allergol Immunopathol* **18**:27–34.

Banana   Bock SA, Sampson HA & Atkins FM (1988) Double-blind, placebo-controlled food challenge (DBPCFC) as an office procedure: a manual. *J Allergy Clin Immunol* **82**:986–997.
Linaweaver WE, Saks GL & Heiner DC (1976) Anaphylactic shock following banana ingestion. *Am J Dis Child* **130**:207–209.
Tuft L & Blumstein GI (1942) Studies in food allergy. II. Sensitisation to fresh fruits: clinical and experimental observations. *J Allergy* **13**:574–582.
Wadee AA, Boting LA & Rabson AR (1990) Fruit allergy: demonstration of IgE antibodies to a 30 kd protein present in several fruits. *J Allergy Clin Immunol* **85**:801–807.

Bean   Bernhisel-Broadbent J & Sampson HA (1989) Cross-allergenicity in the legume botanical family in children with food hypersensitivity. *J Allergy Clin Immunol* **83**:435–440.
Furlan J, Suskovic S & Rus A (1987) The effect of food on the bronchial response in adult asthmatic patients, and the protective role of ketotifen. *Allergol Immunopathol* **15**:73–81.

Bean, pinto   Golbert TM, Patterson R & Pruzansky JJ (1969) Systemic allergic reactions to ingested antigens. *J Allergy* **32**:96–107.

Beef   Bock SA, Sampson HA, Atkins FM *et al.* (1988) Double-blind, placebo-controlled food challenge (DBPCFC) as an office procedure: a manual. *J Allergy Clin Immunol* **82**:986–997.

Buckwheat   Smith HL (1909) Buckwheat-poisoning. With report of a case in man. *Arch Int Med* **3**:350–359.

Cabbage   Blaiss MS, McCants ML & Lehrer SB (1987) Anaphylaxis to cabbage: detection of allergens. *Ann Allergy* **58**:248–250.

Carrot   Denton MC & Kohman E (1918) Feeding experiments with raw and boiled carrots. *J Biol Chem* **36**:249–263.
Dreborg S & Foucard T (1983) Allergy to apple, carrot and potato in children with birch pollen allergy. *Allergy* **38**:167–172.

Celery   Birnbaum J, Tafforeau M, Vervloet D, Charpin J & Charpin D (1989) Allergy to sunflower honey associated with allergy to celery. *Clin Exper Allergy* **19**:229–230.
Kauppinen K, Kousa M & Reunala T (1980) Aromatic plants – a cause of severe attacks of angio-edema and urticaria. *Contact Derm* **6**:251–254.

KIDD JM, COHEN SH, SOSMAN AJ & FINK JN (1983) Food-dependent exercise-induced anaphylaxis. *J Allergy Clin Immunol* **71**:407–411.

PAULI G, BESSOT JC, BRAUN PA *et al.* (1988) Celery allergy: clinical and biological study of 20 cases. *Ann Allergy* **60**:243–246.

PAULI G, BESSOT JC, DIETEMANN-MOLARD A, BRAUN PA & THIERRY R (1985) Celery sensitivity: clinical and immunological correlations with pollen allergy. *Clin Allergy* **15**:273–279.

SILVERSTEIN SR, FROMMER DA, DOBOZIN B & ROSEN P (1986) Celery-dependent exercise-induced anaphylaxis. *J Emergency Med* **4**:195–199.

Chamomile tea BENNER MH & LEE HJ (1973) Anaphylactic reaction to chamomile tea. *J Allergy Clin Immunol* **52**:307–308.

CASTERLINE CL (1980) Allergy to chamomile tea. *J Am Med Ass* **244**:330–331.

SUBIZA J, SUBIZA JL, HINOJOSA M *et al.* (1989) Anaphylactic reaction after the ingestion of chamomile tea: a study of cross-sensitivity with other composite pollens. *J Allergy Clin Immunol* **84**:353–358.

Cheese LESSOF MH, WRAITH DG, MERRETT TG, MERRETT J & BUISSERET PD (1980) Food allergy and intolerance in 100 patients – local and systemic effects. *Quart J Med* **49**:259–271.

Chick pea ACCIAI MC, BRUSI C, FRANCALANCI S, GOLA M & SERTOLI A (1991) Skin tests with fresh foods. *Contact Derm* **24**:67–68.

GOLBERT TM, PATTERSON R & PRUZANSKY JJ (1969) Systemic allergic reactions to ingested antigens. *J Allergy* **32**:96–107.

Chicken BOCK SA, SAMPSON HA & ATKINS FM (1988) Double-blind, placebo-controlled food challenge (DBPCFC) as an office procedure: a manual. *J Allergy Clin Immunol* **82**:986–997.

DAVID TJ (1984) Anaphylactic shock during elimination diets for severe atopic eczema. *Arch Dis Child* **59**:983–986.

LESSOF MH, WRAITH DG, MERRETT TG, MERRETT J & BUISSERET PD (1980) Food allergy and intolerance in 100 patients – local and systemic effects. *Quart J Med* **49**:259–271.

Chocolate BERNSTEIN M, DAY JH & WELSH A (1982) Double-blind food challenge in the diagnosis of food sensitivity in the adult. *J Allergy Clin Immunol* **70**:205–210.

LESSOF MH, WRAITH DG, MERRETT TG, MERRETT J & BUISSERET PD (1980) Food allergy and intolerance in 100 patients – local and systemic effects. *Quart J Med* **49**:259–271.

MASLANSKY L & WEIN G (1971) Chocolate allergy: a double-blind study. *Connecticut Med* **35**:5–9.

Coconut BERNSTEIN M, DAY JH & WELSH A (1982) Double-blind food challenge in the diagnosis of food sensitivity in the adult. *J Allergy Clin Immunol* **70**:205–210.

Corn BOCK SA, SAMPSON HA, ATKINS FM *et al.* (1988) Double-blind, placebo-controlled food challenge (DBPCFC) as an office procedure: a manual. *J Allergy Clin Immunol* **82**:986–997.

DAVID TJ (1984) Anaphylactic shock during elimination diets for severe atopic eczema. *Arch Dis Child* **59**:983–986.

LOVELESS MH (1950) Allergy for corn and its derivatives: experiments with a masked ingestion test for its diagnosis. *J Allergy* **21**:500–511.

Cottonseed   ATKINS FM, WILSON M & BOCK SA (1988) Cottonseed hypersensitivity: new concerns over an old problem. *J Allergy Clin Immunol* **82**:242–250.

BERNTON HS, COULSON EJ & STEVENS H (1949) On allergy to cottonseed oil. *J Am Med Ass* **140**:869–871.

MALANIN G & KALIMO K (1988) Angioedema and urticaria caused by cottonseed protein in whole-grain bread. *J Allergy Clin Immunol* **82**:261–264.

Ethanol   KELSO JM, KEATING MU, SQUILLACE DL, O'CONNELL EJ, YUNGINGER JW & SACHS MI (1990) Anaphylactoid reaction to ethanol. *Ann Allergy* **64**:452–454.

Grape   DOHI M, SUKO M, SUGIYAMA H et al. (1991) Food-dependent, exercise-induced anaphylaxis: a study on 11 Japanese cases. *J Allergy Clin Immunol* **87**:34–40.

TUFT L & BLUMSTEIN GI (1942) Studies in food allergy. II. Sensitisation to fresh fruits: clinical and experimental observations. *J Allergy* **13**:574–582.

Guava   WADEE AA, BOTING LA & RABSON AR (1990) Fruit allergy: demonstration of IgE antibodies to a 30 kd protein present in several fruits. *J Allergy Clin Immunol* **85**:801–807.

Gum tragacanth   BROWN EB & CREPEA SB (1947) Allergy (asthma) to ingested gum tragacanth. A case report. *J Allergy* **18**:214–215.

DANOFF D, LINCOLN L, THOMSON DMP & GOLD P (1978) 'Big Mac attack'. *New Engl J Med* **298**:1095–1096.

Honey   BIRNBAUM J, TAFFOREAU M, VERVLOET D, CHARPIN J & CHARPIN D (1989) Allergy to sunflower honey associated with allergy to celery. *Clin Exper Allergy* **19**:229–230.

BOUSQUET J, CAMPOS J & MICHEL FB (1984) Food intolerance to honey. *Allergy* **39**:73–75.

Kiwi   ANDRE F, ANDRE C, FEKNOUS M, COLIN L & CAVAGNA S (1991) Digestive permeability to different-sized molecules and to sodium cromoglycate in food allergy. *Allergy Proc* **12**:293–298.

DORÉ P, BREUIL K, MEURICE JC, VÉRON O, UNDERNER M & PATTE F (1990) Allergie au kiwi: une allergie méconnue. *Allergie Immunol* **22**:20–21.

GARCIA BE, DE LA CUESTA CG, SNATOS F, FELIU X & CÓRDOBA H (1989) A rare case of food allergy: monosensitivity to kiwi (*Actinidia chinensis*). *Allergol Immunopathol* **17**:217–218.

Lemon   BAENKLER HW & LUX G (1989) Antigen-induced histamine-release from duodenal biopsy in gastrointestinal food allergy. *Ann Allergy* **62**:449–452.

Lentil   GALL H, FORCK G, KALVERAM KJ & LERSNER-LENDERS S (1990) Soforttypallergie auf Hülsenfrüchte (Leguminosen). *Allergologie* **13**:352–355.

Limpet   CARRILLO T, DE CASTRO FR, CUEVAS M, CAMINERO J & CABRERA P (1991) Allergy to limpet. *Allergy* **46**:515–519.

Mandarin   WADEE AA, BOTING LA & RABSON AR (1990) Fruit allergy: demonstration of IgE antibodies to a 30 kd protein present in several fruits. *J Allergy Clin Immunol* **85**:801–807.

Mango DANG RWM & BELL DB (1967) Anaphylactic reaction to the ingestion of mango. Case report. *Hawaii Med J* **27**:149–150.

MIELL J, PAPOUCHADO M & MARSHALL AJ (1988) Anaphylactic reaction after eating a mango. *Br Med J* **297**:1639–1640.

RUBIN JM, SHAPIRO J, MUEHLBAUER P & GROLNICK M (1965) Shock reaction following ingestion of mango. *J Am Med Ass* **193**:147–398.

Melon ENBERG RN, LEICKLY FE, MCCULLOUGH J, BAILEY J & OWNBY DR (1987) Watermelon and ragweed share allergens. *J Allergy Clin Immunol* **79**:867–875.

ENBERG RN, MCCULLOUGH J & OWNBY DR (1988) Antibody responses in watermelon sensitivity. *J Allergy Clin Immunol* **82**:795–800.

TUFT L & BLUMSTEIN GI (1942) Studies in food allergy. II. Sensitisation to fresh fruits: clinical and experimental observations. *J Allergy* **13**:574–582.

Millet seed PARKER JL, YUNGINGER JW & SWEDLUND HA (1981) Anaphylaxis after ingestion of millet seeds. *J Allergy Clin Immunol* **67**:78–80.

Mustard DOMÍNGUEZ J, CUEVAS M, UREÑA V, MUÑOZ T & MONEO I (1990) Purification and characterization of an allergen of mustard seed. *Ann Allergy* **64**:352–357.

VIDAL C, DIAZ C, SÁEZ A, RODRIGUEZ M & IGLESIAS A (1991) Anaphylaxis to mustard. *Postgrad Med J* **67**:405–409.

Oat BERNSTEIN M, DAY JH & WELSH A (1982) Double-blind food challenge in the diagnosis of food sensitivity in the adult. *J Allergy Clin Immunol* **70**:205–210.

Orange BENDERSKY G & LUPAS JA (1960) Anaphylactoid reaction to ingestion of orange. *J Am Med Ass* **173**:255–256.

TUFT L & BLUMSTEIN GI (1942) Studies in food allergy. II. Sensitisation to fresh fruits: clinical and experimental observations. *J Allergy* **13**:574–582.

WILLIAMSON JW (1961) Anaphylactoid reaction to oranges. *J Florida Med Ass* **48**:247.

ZHU SL & YU Y (1989) Allergenicity of orange juice and orange seeds: a clinical study. *Asian Pacific J Allergy Immunol* **7**:5–8.

Parsley KAUPPINEN K, KOUSA M & REUNALA T (1980) Aromatic plants – a cause of severe attacks of angio-edema and urticaria. *Contact Derm* **6**:251–254.

Pea BOCK SA, SAMPSON HA, ATKINS FM *et al.* (1988) Double-blind, placebo-controlled food challenge (DBPCFC) as an office procedure: a manual. *J Allergy Clin Immunol* **82**:986–997.

DAVID TJ (1989) Hazards of challenge tests in atopic dermatitis. *Allergy* (suppl. 9):101–107.

GALL H, FORCK G, KALVERAM KJ & LERSNER-LENDERS S (1990) Sofort-typallergie auf Hülsenfrüchte (Leguminosen). *Allergologie* **13**:352–355.

Peach BUCHBINDER EM, BLOCH KJ, MOSS J & GUINEY TE (1983) Food-dependent, exercise-induced anaphylaxis. *J Amer Med Ass* **250**:2973–2974.

TUFT L & BLUMSTEIN GI (1942) Studies in food allergy. II. Sensitisation to fresh fruits: clinical and experimental observations. *J Allergy* **13**:574–582.

WADEE AA, BOTING LA & RABSON AR (1990) Fruit allergy: demonstration of IgE antibodies to a 30 kd protein present in several fruits. *J Allergy Clin Immunol* **85**:801–807.

Pineapple   TUFT L & BLUMSTEIN GI (1942) Studies in food allergy. II. Sensitisation to fresh fruits: clinical and experimental observations. *J Allergy* **13**:574–582.

Pollen   COHEN SH, YUNGINGER JW, ROSENBERG N & FINK JN (1979) Acute allergic reaction after composite pollen ingestion. *J Allergy Clin Immunol* **64**:270–274.
MANSFIELD LE & GOLDSTEIN GB (1981) Anaphylactic reaction after ingestion of local bee pollen. *Ann Allergy* **47**:154–156.

Pomegranate   IGEA JM, CUESTA J, CUEVAS M *et al.* (1991) Adverse reaction to pomegranate ingestion. *Allergy* **46**:472–474.

Pork   BERNSTEIN M, DAY JH & WELSH A (1982) Double-blind food challenge in the diagnosis of food sensitivity in the adult. *J Allergy Clin Immunol* **70**:205–210.
LESSOF MH, WRAITH DG, MERRETT TG, MERRETT J & BUISSERET PD (1980) Food allergy and intolerance in 100 patients – local and systemic effects. *Quart J Med* **49**:259–271.

Potato   BOCK SA, SAMPSON HA, ATKINS FM *et al.* (1988) Double-blind, placebo-controlled food challenge (DBPCFC) as an office procedure: a manual. *J Allergy Clin Immunol* **82**:986–997.
CASTELLS MC, PASCUAL C, ESTEBAN MM & OJEDA JA (1986) Allergy to white potato. *J Allergy Clin Immunol* **78**:1110–1114.
GOLBERT TM, PATTERSON R & PRUZANSKY JJ (1969) Systemic allergic reactions to ingested antigens. *J Allergy* **32**:96–107.
FURLAN J, SUSKOVIC S & RUS A (1987) The effect of food on the bronchial response in adult asthmatic patients, and the protective role of ketotifen. *Allergol Immunopathol* **15**:73–81.

Rhubarb   TROUNCE JQ & TANNER MS (1985) Eosinophilic gastroenteritis. *Arch Dis Child* **60**:1186–1188.

Rice   BOCK SA, SAMPSON HA, ATKINS FM *et al.* (1988) Double-blind, placebo-controlled food challenge (DBPCFC) as an office procedure: a manual. *J Allergy Clin Immunol* **82**:986–997.
GOLBERT TM, PATTERSON R & PRUZANSKY JJ (1969) Systemic allergic reactions to ingested antigens. *J Allergy* **32**:96–107.
STRUNK RC, PINNAS JL, JOHN TJ, HANSEN RC & BLAZOVICH JL (1978) Rice hypersensitivity associated with serum complement depression. *Clin Allergy* **8**:51–58.

Rye   BOCK SA, SAMPSON HA, ATKINS FM *et al.* (1988) Double-blind, placebo-controlled food challenge (DBPCFC) as an office procedure: a manual. *J Allergy Clin Immunol* **82**:986–997.

Sesame   KÄGI MK & WÜTHRICH B (1991) Falafel-burger anaphylaxis due to sesame seed allergy. *Lancet* **338**:582.
MALISH D, GLOVSKY MM, HOFFMAN DR, GHEKIERE L & HAWKINS JM (1981) Anaphylaxis after sesame seed ingestion. *J Allergy Clin Immunol* **67**:35–38.
UVITSKY IH (1956) Sensitivity to sesame seed. *J Allergy* **22**:377–378.

Snail   DE LA CUESTA CG, GARCÍA BE, CÓRDOBA H, DIÉGUEZ I & OEHLING A (1989) Food allergy to *Helix terrestre* (snail). *Allergol Immunopathol* **17**:337–339.

Spinach ZOHN B (1936/7) An unusual case of spinach hypersensitiveness. *J Allergy* **8**: 936–937.

Squash BOCK SA, SAMPSON HA, ATKINS FM *et al.* (1988) Double-blind, placebo-controlled food challenge (DBPCFC) as an office procedure: a manual. *J Allergy Clin Immunol* **82**:986–997.

Strawberry WADEE AA, BOTING LA & RABSON AR (1990) Fruit allergy: demonstration of IgE antibodies to a 30 kd protein present in several fruits. *J Allergy Clin Immunol* **85**:801–807.

Sunflower BERNSTEIN M, DAY JH & WELSH A (1982) Double-blind food challenge in the diagnosis of food sensitivity in the adult. *J Allergy Clin Immunol* **70**:205–210.

Tangerine GOLBERT TM, PATTERSON R & PRUZANSKY JJ (1969) Systemic allergic reactions to ingested antigens. *J Allergy* **32**:96–107.

Tapioca LOVELESS MH (1950) Allergy for corn and its derivatives: experiments with a masked ingestion test for its diagnosis. *J Allergy* **21**:500–511.

Tomato ACCIAI MC, BRUSI C, FRANCALANCI S, GOLA M & SERTOLI A (1991) Skin tests with fresh foods. *Contact Derm* **24**:67–68.
ATKINS FM, STEINBERG SS & METCALFE DD (1985) Evaluation of immediate adverse reactions to foods in adult patients. I. Correlation of demographic, laboratory, and prick skin test data with response to controlled oral food challenge. *J Allergy Clin Immunol* **75**:348–355.
BERNSTEIN M, DAY JH & WELSH A (1982) Double-blind food challenge in the diagnosis of food sensitivity in the adult. *J Allergy Clin Immunol* **70**:205–210.
FURLAN J, SUSKOVIC S & RUS A (1987) The effect of food on the bronchial response in adult asthmatic patients, and the protective role of ketotifen. *Allergol Immunopathol* **15**:73–81.

Turkey BOCK SA, SAMPSON HA, ATKINS FM *et al.* (1988) Double-blind, placebo-controlled food challenge (DBPCFC) as an office procedure: a manual. *J Allergy Clin Immunol* **82**:986–997.

Vitamins (parenteral multivitamins) BULLOCK L, ETCHASON E, FITZGERALD JF & McGUIRE WA (1990) Case report of an allergic reaction to parenteral nutrition in a paediatric patient. *J Parenteral Enteral Nutr* **14**:98–100. (**NB** The preparation, MVI Pediatric, discussed in this report, contained vitamins A, B, C, D, E, K, biotin, propylene glycol, citric acid, sodium citrate and sodium hydroxide.)
COMMITTEE ON SAFETY OF MEDICINES (1989) Parenterovite & allergic reactions. *Current Problems* (published by the Committee on Safety of Medicines) No. 24. (**NB** Parenterovite ampoules contain vitamin B group vitamins, vitamin C and metabisulphite.)

Yeast or yeast extract HIGSON N (1989) An allergy to Marmite? *Br Med J* **298**:190. (**NB** Report of lip and periorbital angioedema within 5 min of Marmite ingestion in a 15-month old child. Marmite contains yeast extract, and this case was interpreted as adverse reaction to yeast. However Marmite also contains up to 2.8 mg/g of histamine (Blackwell *et al.* 1969), which may be a more likely cause for this reaction.)
LESSOF MH, WRAITH DG, MERRETT TG, MERRETT J & BUISSERET PD (1980)

Food allergy and intolerance in 100 patients – local and systemic effects. *Quart J Med* **49**:259–271.

Key reference 32.1 Воск SA, Sampson HA, Atkins FM *et al.* (1988) Double-blind, placebo-controlled food challenge (DBPCFC) as an office procedure: a manual. *J Allergy Clin Immunol* **82**:986–997. Lists 18 foods which were shown to provoke adverse reactions under controlled conditions in studies at six centres in the USA. *The list only includes foods which are more commonly associated with intolerance.*

Summary 32 This chapter provides a source of references to reports which document intolerance to foods other than the foods which are discussed in more detail elsewhere in the book.

References to Chapters 29–32

Aas K (1966a) Studies of hypersensitivity to fish. A clinical study. *Int Arch Allergy* **29**:346–363.

Aas K (1966b) Studies of hypersensitivity to fish. Allergological and serological differentiation between various species of fish. *Int Arch Allergy* **30**:257–267.

Aas K (1987) Fish allergy and the codfish model. In Brostoff J & Challacombe SJ (eds) *Food Allergy and Intolerance*, pp. 356–366, Ballière Tindall, London.

Aas K & Lundkvist U (1973) The radioallergosorbent test with a purified allergen from codfish. *Clin Allergy* **3**:255–261.

Armentia A, Quintero A, Fernández-García A, Salvador J & Martín-Santos JM (1990) Allergy to pine pollen and pinon nuts: a review of three cases. *Ann Allergy* **64**:49–52.

Arshad SH, Malmberg E, Frapf K & Hide DW (1991) Clinical and immunological characteristics of Brazil nut allergy. *Clin Exper Allergy* **21**:373–376.

Assem ESK, Gelder CM, Spiro SG, Baderman H & Armstrong RF (1990) Anaphylaxis induced by peanuts. *Br Med J* **300**:1377–1378.

Atkins FM, Steinberg SS & Metcalfe DD (1985) Evaluation of immediate adverse reactions to foods in adult patients. I. Correlation of demographic, laboratory, and prick skin test data with response to controlled oral food challenge. *J Allergy Clin Immunol* **75**:348–355.

Barnes G, McKellar W & Lawrance S (1983) Detection of fructose malabsorption by breath hydrogen test in a child with diarrhea. *J Pediat* **103**:575–577.

Barnett D, Baldo BA & Howden MEH (1983) Multiplicity of allergens in peanuts. *J Allergy Clin Immunol* **72**:61–68.

Bernhisel-Broadbent J & Sampson HA (1989) Cross-allergenicity in the legume botanical family in children with food hypersensitivity. *J Allergy Clin Immunol* **83**:435–440.

Blackwell B, Mabbitt LA & Marley E (1969) Histamine and tyramine content of yeast products. *J Food Sci* **34**:47–51.

Bock SA, Lee WY, Remigio LK & May CD (1978) Studies of hypersensitivity reactions to foods in infants and children. *J Allergy Clin Immunol* **62**:327–334.

BOYD GK (1989) Fatal nut anaphylaxis in a 16-year-old male: case report. *Allergy Proc* **10**:255–257.

BURKS AW, WILLIAMS LW, MALLORY SB, SHIRRELL MA & WILLIAMS C (1989) Peanut protein as a major cause of adverse food reactions in patients with atopic dermatitis. *Allergy Proc* **10**:265–269.

BUSH RK, TAYLOR SL & NORDLEE JA (1989) Peanut sensitivity. *Allergy Proc* **10**:261–264.

CANT AJ, GIBSON P & DANCY M (1984) Food hypersensitivity made life threatening by ingestion of aspirin. *Br Med J* **288**:755–756.

CAPLAN SN & BERKMAN EM (1976) Protamine sulfate and fish allergy. *N Engl J Med* **295**:172.

CHAFEE FH (1941) Sensitivity to peanut oil with the report of a case. *Ann Intern Med* **15**:1116–1117.

COULTATE TP (1984) *Food. The Chemistry of Its Components*, Royal Society of Chemistry, London.

DAUL CB, MORGAN JE, HUGHES J & LEHRER SB (1988) Provocation-challenge studies in shrimp-sensitive individuals. *J Allergy Clin Immunol* **81**:1180–1186.

DAUL CB, MORGAN JE & LEHRER SB (1990) The natural history of shrimp hypersensitivity. *J Allergy Clin Immunol* **86**:88–93.

DAUL CB, MORGAN JE, WARING NP, MCCANTS ML, HUGHES J & LEHRER SB (1987) Immunologic evaluation of shrimp-allergic individuals. *J Allergy Clin Immunol* **80**:716–722.

DE MARTINO M, NOVEMBRE E, GALLI L et al. (1990) Allergy to different fish species in cod-allergic children: in vivo and in vitro studies. *J Allergy Clin Immunol* **86**:909–914.

DE MARTINO M, NOVEMBRE E, MUCCIOLI AT, MARANO E & VIERUCCI A (1988) Frequency of cutipositivities to other fish in children with allergy to cod (abstract). *New Engl Reg Allergy Proc* **9**:409.

DERBES VJ & KRAFCHUK JD (1957) Osmylogenic urticaria. *Arch Dermatol* **76**:103–104.

DONOVAN KL & PETERS J (1990) Vegetable burger allergy: all was nut as it appeared. *Br Med J* **300**:1378.

DREBORG S & FOUCARD T (1983) Allergy to apple, carrot and potato in children with birch pollen allergy. *Allergy* **38**:167–172.

EVANS S, SKEA D & DOLOVITCH J (1988) Fatal reaction to peanut antigen in almond icing. *Can Med Ass J* **139**:231–232.

FINE AJ (1987) Hypersensitivity reaction to pine nuts (Pinon nuts – pignolia). *Ann Allergy* **59**:183–184.

FRIES JH (1982) Peanuts: allergic and other untoward reactions. *Ann Allergy* **48**:220–226.

GALL H, FORCK G, KALVERAM KJ & VON LERSNER-LENDERS S (1990) Soforttypallergie auf Hülsenfrüchte (Leguminosen). *Allergologie* **13**:352–355.

HARDINGE MG, SWARNER JB & CROOKS H (1965) Carbohydrates in foods. *J Am Dietet Ass* **46**:197–204.

HYAMS JS, ETIENNE NL, LEICHTNER AM & THEUER RC (1988) Carbohydrate malabsorption following fruit juice ingestion in young children. *Pediatrics* **82**:64–68.

HYAMS JS & LEICHTNER AM (1985) Apple juice. An unappreciated cause of diarrhea. *Am J Dis Child* **139**:503–505.

KALLIEL JN, KLEIN DE & SETTIPANE GA (1989) Anaphylaxis to peanuts: clinical correlation to skin tests. *Allergy Proc* **10**:259–260.

KASUYA S, HAMANO H & IZUMI S (1989) Gastric anisakiasis with anaphylactoid reactions. *Allergy Clin Immunol News* **1**:140–141.

KEMP AS, MELLIS CM, BARNETT D, SHAROTA E & SIMPSON J (1985) Skin test, RAST and clinical reactions to peanut allergens in children. *Clin Allergy* **15**:73–78.

KIKUCHI I (1985) The effects of walnuts on Behçet's syndrome in two sisters. *J Dermatol* **12**:290–291.

KNAPE JTA, SCHULLER JL, DE HAAN P, DE JONG AP & BOVILL JG (1981) An anaphylactic reaction to protamine in a patient allergic to fish. *Anaesthesiol* **55**:324–325.

KNEEPKENS CMF, JAKOBS C & DOUWES AC (1989) Apple juice, fructose, and chronic nonspecific diarrhoea. *Eur J Pediatr* **148**:571–573.

KNEEPKENS CMF, VONK RJ & FERNANDES J (1984) Incomplete intestinal absorption of fructose. *Arch Dis Child* **59**:735–738.

LEHRER SB, IBANEZ MD, McCANTS ML, DAUL CB & MORGAN JE (1990) Characterization of water-soluble shrimp allergens released during boiling. *J Allergy Clin Immunol* **85**:1005–1013.

LEHRER SB & McCANTS ML (1987) Reactivity of IgE antibodies with crustacea and oyster allergens: evidence for common antigenic structures. *J Allergy Clin Immunol* **80**:133–139.

MARKS JG, DeMELFI T, McCARTHY MA et al. (1984) Dermatitis from cashew nuts. *J Am Acad Dermatol* **10**:627–631.

MATHIAS CGT (1983) Contact urticaria from peanut butter. *Contact Dermatitis* **9**:66–68.

MAULITZ RM, PRATT DS & SCHOCKET AL (1979) Exercise-induced anaphylactic reaction to shellfish. *J Allergy Clin Immunol* **63**:433–434.

McKERROW JH, SAKANARI J & DEARDORFF TL (1988) Anisakiasis: revenge of the sushi parasite. *New Engl J Med* **319**:1228–1229.

McNEIL D & STRAUSS RH (1988) Exercise-induced anaphylaxis related to food intake. *Ann Allergy* **61**:440–442.

MONERET-VAUTRIN DA, HATAHET R, KANNY G & AIT-DJAFER Z (1991) Allergenic peanut oil in milk formulas. *Lancet* **338**:1149.

MORGAN JE, DAUL CB & LEHRER SB (1990) The relationship among shrimp-specific IgG subclass antibodies and immediate adverse reactions to shrimp challenge. *J Allergy Clin Immunol* **86**:387–392.

MORGAN JE, O'NEIL CE, DAUL CB & LEHRER SB (1989) Species-specific shrimp allergens: RAST and RAST-inhibition studies. *J Allergy Clin Immunol* **83**:1112–1117.

MORIKAWA A, KATO M, TOKUYAMA K, KUROUME T, MINOSHIMA M & IWATA S (1990) Anaphylaxis to grand keyhole limpet (abalone-like shellfish) and abalone. *Ann Allergy* **65**:415–417.

NIELSEN NH (1990) Systemic allergic reaction to pine nuts. *Ann Allergy* **64**: 132–133.

ORFORD RR & WILSON JT (1985) Epidemiologic and immunologic studies in processors of the king crab. *Am J Indust Med* **7**:155–169.

PAR PA, VALLS JS, PÉREZ ML, CASAJUANA AM & CALDERÓN PAG (1990) Dried fruit hypersensitivity and its correlation with pollen allergy. *Allergol Immunopathol* **18**:27–34.

PAULSEN HC (1961) Alimentary allergy. Allergy to fish. *Acta Allergol* **16**:380–386.

PRAUSNITZ C & KÜSTNER H (1921) Studien über die Ueberempfindlichkeit. *Centralbl Bakt Parasitol* **86**:160–169.

RUMESSEN JJ & GUDMAND-HØYER E (1986) Absorption capacity of fructose in healthy adults. Comparison with sucrose and its constituent monosaccharides. *Gut* **27**:1161–1168.

SAMPSON HA (1990) Peanut anaphylaxis. *J Allergy Clin Immunol* **86**:1–3.

SETTIPANE GA (1989) Anaphylactic deaths in asthmatic patients. *Allergy Proc* **10**:271–274.

SHERSON D, HANSEN I & SIGSGAARD T (1989) Occupationally related respiratory symptoms in trout-processing workers. *Allergy* **44**:336–341.

SHIBASAKI M, EHARA T & TAKITA H (1989) Late anaphylactic reaction to cuttlefish. *Ann Allergy* **63**:421–422.

STAFFORD EM (1985) Flying, peanuts, and crying babies. *Pediatrics* **76**:1018.

TAYLOR SL, BUSSE WW, SACHS MI, PARKER JL & YUNGINGER JW (1981) Peanut oil is not allergenic to peanut-sensitive individuals. *J Allergy Clin Immunol* **68**:372–375.

TUFT L & BLUMSTEIN GI (1940) Studies in food allergy. I. Antigenic relationship of shellfish. *J Allergy* **11**:475–487.

TUFT L & BLUMSTEIN GI (1942) Studies in food allergy. II. Sensitisation to fresh fruits: clinical and experimental observations. *J Allergy* **13**:574–582.

TUFT L & BLUMSTEIN GI (1946) Studies in food allergy. V. Antigenic relationship among members of fish family. *J Allergy* **17**:329–339.

VITORIA JC, CAMARERO C, SOJO A, RUIZ A & RODRIGUEZ-SORIANO J (1982) Enteropathy related to fish, rice, and chicken. *Arch Dis Child* **57**:44–48.

WALES JKH, PRIMHAK RA, RATTENBURY J & TAYLOR CJ (1989) Isolated fructose malabsorption. *Arch Dis Child* **115**:227–229.

WARING NP, DAUL CB, DE SHAZO RD, McCANTS ML & LEHRER SB (1985) Hypersensitivity reactions to ingested crustacea: clinical evaluation and diagnostic studies in shrimp-sensitive individuals. *J Allergy Clin Immunol* **76**:440–445.

WEILER JM, GELLHAUS MA, CARTER JG et al. (1990) A prospective study of the risk of an immediate adverse reaction to protamine sulfate during cardiopulmonary bypass surgery. *J Allergy Clin Immunol* **85**:713–719.

WEISS ME, NYHAN D, PENG Z et al. (1989) Association of protamine IgE and IgG antibodies with life-threatening reactions to intravenous protamine. *New Engl J Med* **320**:886–892.

YUNGINGER JW, GAUERKE MB, JONES RT, DAHLBERG MJE & ACKERMAN SJ (1983) Use of radioimmunoassay to determine the nature, quantity and source of allergenic contamination of sunflower butter. *J Food Protection* **46**:625–628.

YUNGINGER JW, SQUILLACE DL, JONES RT & HELM RM (1989) Fatal anaphylactic reactions induced by peanuts. *Allergy Proc* **10**:249–253.

YUNGINGER JW, SWEENEY KG, STURNER WQ et al. (1988) Fatal food-induced anaphylaxis. *J Am Med Ass* **260**:1450–1452.

ZIMMERMAN B, FORSYTH S & GOLD M (1989) Highly atopic children: formation of IgE antibody to food protein, especially peanut. *J Allergy Clin Immunol* **83**:764–770.

Part 8 Food Additives

33 Additive types, uses and public perception
Not as dangerous as most people think

Definition A food additive is any substance intentionally added to a food, for whatever purpose. The unintentional addition of a substance is classed as contamination. Food additives can be naturally occurring or synthetic. It is a popular fallacy that substances are safe if they are naturally occurring but potentially hazardous if synthetic. This myth overlooks both the large number of toxic substances naturally occurring in, for example, plant foods (see Table 2.2 and reviewed by Harris in 1986), and the fact that most substances which provoke food intolerance are naturally occurring, such as eggs, cow's milk and nuts.

Classes of additive The principal classes of food additives are colouring agents, preservatives, flavours, and substances such as emulsifiers and stabilizers (Lindsay 1985).

History of additives The use of salt to preserve meat, sugar to preserve fruit and smoke to flavour and preserve meat and fish are all ancient practices. So too is the initially inadvertent use of sodium nitrate, present as an impurity in crude salt, to cure bacon and ham (Coltate 1984). Adulteration of food, especially wine and bread, can also be traced back to ancient times. Widespread food adulteration in England was first systematically documented in 1820 (Burnett 1985). By 1850 it was difficult to obtain bread, tea, coffee or beer that had not been seriously adulterated, and in 1857 a survey revealed that children's sweets were commonly coloured with lead chromate, lead oxide, mercuric sulphide and copper arsenite (Burnett 1985). Legislation now controls the use of additives in food, although different countries enforce their own views on what is or is not safe.

Food labelling In the UK, most manufactured foods have to carry a label with a list of most ingredients, but there are some curious exceptions. For example, under the Food Labelling Regulations 1984, chocolate and cocoa products, wine, alcoholic drinks with an alcoholic strength by volume of more than 1.2%, and unwrapped food, such as bread or confectionery, do not have to declare their ingredients. Even if bread is wrapped, there are still a whole range of permitted additives such as caramel, bleaching and improving agents, preservatives, chalk, iron salts, thiamine, nicotinic acid, sodium bicarbonate and salt

179

(Egan *et al.* 1987) which do not have to be declared. Approved additives are numbered, and the number is preceded by an E if the additive has been approved by the European Economic Community (Food Additives, HMSO, 1987).

Colouring agents

Colouring agents are used to make food more colourful, or to compensate for colour lost in processing. Naturally derived colouring agents mainly comprise curcumin, riboflavin, cochineal, chlorophyll, caramels, carbon black, carotene, annatto, canthaxanthin, calcium carbonate, iron oxide, and titanium dioxide (Food Additives, HMSO, 1987). Synthetic colouring agents are largely coal-tar dyes, which are sub-divided into azo dyes (Table 33.1) and non-azo coal-tar dyes (Table 33.2).

Preservatives

Preservatives are used to prevent deterioration of food and food poisoning caused by microbial contamination. The principal preservatives are (Food Additives, HMSO, 1987):

1 benzoic acid and related compounds, such as sodium benzoate, potassium benzoate, and esters of para-hydroxybenzoic acid (known collectively as parabens);

Table 33.1 Azo dyes

Name	Code number
Tartrazine	E102
Yellow 2G	E107
Sunset yellow FCF	E110
Carmoisine	E122
Amaranth	E123
Ponceau 4R	E124
Red 2G	E128
Brown FK	154
Chocolate brown HT	155
Black PN	E151
Pigment rubine	E180

Table 33.2 Non-azo coal-tar dyes

Name	Code number
Quinolone yellow	E104
Erythrosine	E127
Patent blue V	E131
Indigo carmine	E132
Brilliant blue FCF	133

2 sulphur dioxide and compounds which generate it such as sodium sulphite and sodium metabisulphite;

3 sorbic acid and its sodium, potassium or calcium salts;

4 propionic acid and its sodium, potassium or calcium salts;

5 sodium or potassium nitrite or nitrate;

6 biphenyl and related compounds;

7 miscellaneous substances: thiabendazole, nisin, and hexamine.

Antioxidants

Antioxidants prevent degradation of fats and fat-soluble vitamins (Lindsay 1985). The principal antioxidants are ascorbic acid, butylated hydroxyanisole (BHA), butylated hydroxytoluene (BHT), propyl gallate, and alpha-tocopherol (Food Additives, HMSO, 1987).

Emulsifiers & stabilizers

Any substance which is capable of aiding the formation of a stable mixture of two otherwise immiscible substances, for example fat and water, is called an emulsifier. A stabilizer helps to maintain an emulsion once it has formed (Taylor 1988). The principal substances in this category are the polysorbates, the alginates, compounds of sorbitan, methylcellulose, esters of fatty acids, extracts of gum (such as guar or karaya gum), and pectin (Food Additives, HMSO, 1987).

Sweeteners

There are two types of sweeteners. Intense sweeteners have a sweetness many times that of sugar, and comprise aspartame, acesulfame, saccharin and thymautin (Food Additives, HMSO, 1987). Bulk sweeteners have approximately the same sweetness as sugar, and comprise glucose, isomalt, mannitol and sorbitol (Food Additives, HMSO, 1987).

Others

Other classes of food additives comprise anticaking agents (to keep products dry), humectants (to keep products moist), firming and crisping agents, flour improvers and bleaching agents, glazing agents, flavour improvers and modifiers, propellants, sequestrants, solvents, and acids, bases and buffers (Food Additives, HMSO, 1987).

Additives in drugs

Preparations of drugs commonly contain additives such as colouring agents and preservatives. In one survey, 930 out of 2204 drug formulations contained at least one colouring agent or preservative (Pollock et al. 1989). Some form of labelling would enable people to more easily avoid preparations which contain an additive to which the subject is intolerant.

Acceptable daily intake

The term 'acceptable daily intake' (ADI), expressed on a mg/kg body weight basis, is the amount of food additive that can be taken daily in the diet, over a lifetime, without risk. The term has been introduced by the Joint Expert Committee on Food Additives (JECFA) of

The Food and Agriculture Organisation of the United Nations and the World Health Organisation (Taylor 1980; FAO/WHO 1985). It is reported that an acceptable daily intake is only allocated to substances for which the available data include either the results of adequate short-term and long-term toxicological investigations or satisfactory information on the biochemistry and metabolic fate of the compound, or both (FAO/WHO 1985). The figure for acceptable daily intake is fixed at one-hundredth of the maximum amount that can be fed to animals with toxic effects, and its applicability to humans is uncertain.

Public concern

How many people visiting a fishmonger realize that the colour of most fresh salmon is due to the presence of an artificially added colour? The flesh of wild salmon is pigmented with astaxanthin, which is obtained naturally from crustacea in their diet. Another colour, canthaxanthin, is added to the diet of farmed salmon to produce fish equivalent in colour to wild salmon (Ministry of Agriculture, Fisheries and Food 1987a). Many people are probably also unaware that titanium dioxide is added at a level of up to 400 mg/kg to Mozzarella cheese made from cow's milk, in order to give this product the same white appearance as traditional Mozzarella cheese made from buffalo milk (Ministry of Agriculture, Fisheries and Food 1987a). The scale of use of additives in food comes as a surprise to most people, and it is understandable that many should find these substances vaguely menacing.

Public misinformation and desire for natural food

Public concern about food additives is enhanced by an enormous amount of misinformation.

naturally occurring additives

Insistence on food entirely free of additives fails to take into account the fact that many additives are naturally occurring substances, such as ascorbic acid (E300), tocopherol (E306), vitamin B complex (E375) and a variety of plant pigments (Timberlake 1989).

fear of additives is not new

The public's passion for food that is natural (i.e. free from additives or extraneous ingredients) is not new. By the late 1850s, 'pure and unadulterated' had been the stock advertising slogan of those anxious to cash in on the then newly awakened fears of the public (Burnett 1985).

naturally occurring toxins

The recent obsession with food that is natural completely ignores the wide range of naturally occurring toxins (David 1990). Examples are oxalic acid in rhubarb, goitrogens in brassicas, cyanogens in almonds, tapioca and lima beans, 5-hydroxy tryptamine in bananas, psoralens in celery, peas and parsley, solanidine in potatoes, myristicin in nutmeg and carrots, and lectins in red kidney beans (Harris 1986).

misuse of natural

The desire for natural food has more recently again been exploited by food manufacturers, who have widely used the word to describe a manufactured food product, using terms such as 'finest natural ingredients', 'natural pure food', 'natural juices', 'naturally flavoured' (Ministry of Agriculture, Fisheries and Food 1987b). A survey by the trading standards departments of three local authorities in Britain in 1987 categorized 10 different types of misleading or incorrect use of the word natural to describe samples of food, and found that the word natural was misused in 357 of 451 (79%) food samples which had been purchased (Ministry of Agriculture, Fisheries and Food 1987b).

health food shops

The concept of a health food shop is misleading (David 1990). For example, a survey of 'crunchy' peanut butter showed that 11 out of 59 samples from health food producers contained over 100 µg/kg of aflatoxins, over 10 times the proposed maximum permitted level for total aflatoxins (Ministry of Agriculture, Fisheries and Food 1987c). Only one of the 26 samples from other producers contained aflatoxins in excess of 10 µg/kg, and none contained more than 50 µg/kg.

food arouses the emotions

Food arouses not only the appetite but also the emotions. Current misinformation is attributable to numerous alarmist books, uncritical coverage by the media, and misguided advice by health care professionals. The avoidance of all foods containing 'E numbers', regardless of the fact that some are naturally occurring substances such as ascorbic acid, is widespread but illogical. There is an understandable desire of parents to focus the blame on a chemical rather than to face up to other causes for their child's bad behaviour or to the fact that the cause is not known. At present one of the major problems with food additives is the level of public misinformation about the subject (David 1988).

Personal belief

There is an enormous discrepancy between the public's perception of food additive intolerance and objectively verified intolerance. When a questionnaire was offered to approximately 30 000 people in 11 388 households in the High Wycombe area, 3188 of the 18 582 responders thought that they had some sort of reaction to foods or food additives (Young et al. 1987). A check on the non-responders showed that they had almost no food-provoked symptoms. Particular attention was then paid to food additives, and it was found that 1372 of the 18 582 responders (7.4%) believed they had adverse reactions to food additives. Of the 1372, 649 attended for a detailed interview, and 132 gave a history of reproducible clinical symptoms after ingestion of food additives. Eighty-one of these completed a trial of double-blind placebo-controlled challenges with 11 food additives, but a consistent adverse reaction was found in only two subjects. One was a 50-year-old atopic man who reported headaches after ingesting colouring agents, and who reacted to challenge with annatto, which reproduced his headache at both low (1 mg) and high (10 mg) dose after 4 and 5 hours respectively. He also reacted to placebo on one occasion. The second was a 31-year-old non-atopic woman who reported abdominal pain after ingestion of foods. She had related this to ingestion of preservatives and antioxidants. Her symptoms were reproduced on challenge with annatto at low and high dose.

Controversy   So intense is the controversy which surrounds intolerance to food additives, that in the chapters describing intolerance to individual additives, rather more detail is provided about relevant studies than in the rest of the book so that the reader can more easily assess the strength or otherwise of the evidence.

Key references   33.1   TAYLOR RJ (1980) *Food Additives*, John Wiley, Chichester. *This is a good general introduction to the functional properties of food additives, and it also explains the various national and international legislative processes.*

33.2   COLTATE TP (1984) *Food – the Chemistry of its Components*. The Royal Society of Chemistry, London. *Contains excellent short chapters on food preservatives, colours and flavours.*

33.3   FENNEMA OR (1985) Food Chemistry, 2nd edn, Marcel Dekker, New York. *Contains detailed chapters on the chemistry of naturally occurring pigments, flavours and food additives.*

33.4   YOUNG E, PATEL S, STONEHAM M, RONA R & WILKINSON JD (1987) The prevalence of reaction to food additives in a survey population. *J Roy Coll Phys* **21**:241–247. *Key survey of the incidence of intolerance to food additives in a large community. Further details in text above.*

Summary 33   Food additives comprise any substance intentionally added to food, for whatever purpose. Such additives include colouring agents, preservatives, antioxidants, emulsifiers, stabilizers, sweeteners, other flavour modifiers, and a large miscellaneous group of other agents. The scale of use of additives in food comes as a surprise to most people, and it is understandable that many should find these substances vaguely menacing. Public concern about food additives is enhanced by a large amount of misinformation. Obsession with food that is natural fails to take into account naturally occurring toxins present in food.

34 Tartrazine
An occasional trigger of urticaria and asthma

Introduction

Tartrazine (E102), known as F D & C Yellow No. 5 in the USA, is a yellow colouring agent, and one of the group of azo-dyes (see Table 33.1 for complete list). It is used as a colouring agent in foods and medicines. Although best known for its use in soft drinks, tartrazine is found in a wide range of other foods (Table 34.1).

Intolerance

Possible intolerance to tartrazine was first reported in 1959, when Lockey described three urticarial reactions alleged to be due to tartrazine, which was present in tablets of dexamethasone and prednisolone (Lockey 1959). One patient was receiving steroids as treatment for a generalized skin eruption caused by 'tincture of merthiolate'. The other two patients were challenged sublingually with tartrazine in an open manner. In response, one developed tingling of the tongue and lips, and the other one 'reacted' without any description of the reaction. Since then, intolerance to tartrazine has been frequently described, and is without doubt a genuine entity, although most reports are almost as poorly substantiated as this one. The clinical features are described below.

Chronic urticaria

There have been only three double-blind placebo-controlled studies of tartrazine intolerance and chronic urticaria. All series comprised patients attending hospital or allergy clinics, and all the patients had chronic or recurrent urticaria of unknown cause lasting 2 months or more, and which had improved on a diet free of colouring agents or preservatives. In one study, using a challenge dose of 0.22 mg of tartrazine, three out of 13 (23%) adults developed an exacerbation of urticaria within 3 hours of tartrazine challenge but not after placebo (Settipane et al. 1976). In another study, using challenge doses of tartrazine from 0.5 mg rising to 150 mg, two out of 24 adults (8%) developed adverse reactions, which comprised urticaria in one, and sweating and itching in the other (Murdoch et al. 1987b). In a third

Table 34.1 Examples of foods which may contain tartrazine

Soft drinks	Marzipan
Custard powder	Jam and marmalade
Salad cream	Smoked cod and haddock
Sweets	Mustard

185

study, using a challenge dose of 0.1–1.0 mg of tartrazine, 11 of 43 (26%) children developed an exacerbation of urticaria within 4 hours of tartrazine challenge but not after placebo (Supramaniam & Warner 1986).

other studies

Other studies of tartrazine withdrawal or challenge have suggested that between 8% and 100% of subjects with chronic urticaria are intolerant to tartrazine, but, as explained in chapter 60, these studies are all seriously flawed. In view of the highly selected nature of the samples in the three sound studies mentioned above, it is not yet possible to estimate what proportion of children with chronic urticaria are intolerant to tartrazine.

good prognosis

Tartrazine intolerance, as a trigger of chronic urticaria, appears to be a transient problem. In a follow-up study in which 18 children with chronic urticaria and proven tartrazine intolerance were re-challenged between 1 and 5 years later, none exhibited tartrazine intolerance on re-challenge (Pollock & Warner 1987). In another study, none of three adults with chronic urticaria and tartrazine intolerance reacted when re-challenged 1 year later (Gibson & Clancy 1980). Finally, Kauppinen *et al.* (1984) followed up 132 children with acute or chronic urticaria of whom 13% initially reacted to food additives (reactions to individual additives were not specified). After a mean time of 3.8 years, approximately one-half of those who had initially reacted became symptom free.

Acute urticaria

The role of tartrazine in acute urticaria is unclear. It is possible that regular ingestion of tartrazine may provoke chronic or recurrent urticaria, whereas intermittent ingestion in a patient on a tartrazine-free diet may provoke acute urticaria. In the two double-blind challenge studies described above (Settipane *et al.* 1976; Supramaniam & Warner 1986), the patients were only observed for 3 or 4 hours, preventing the detection of delayed reactions if they exist. Both studies examined acute reactions to challenge, yet the patients studied all presented with chronic urticaria. The assumption implicit in both studies is that repeated administration may lead to chronic urticaria, but this has never been demonstrated. This is an important area of uncertainty because of the possibility that regular or repeated administration of a compound may lead to tolerance, as can occur in salicylate intolerance (see chapter 38).

Importance of disease activity

A major obstacle to the study of tartrazine and urticaria is that, for reasons which are unknown, when urticaria is inactive tartrazine or other chemicals such as aspirin are less likely to provoke an attack

(Warin & Smith 1982). Thus, when 12 adults with chronic urticaria who had previously reacted to tartrazine were re-challenged (Warin & Smith 1982) with 1 mg and 10 mg doses of tartrazine, the following results were obtained.

1 Five patients who had been free from urticaria for 1–7 years: no reactions to 1 mg or 10 mg tartrazine.

2 Two patients who had been free from urticaria except for 'minor episodic attacks' for 2–3 years: no reactions to 1 mg or 10 mg tartrazine.

3 Three patients who had been free from urticaria for only 3–8 weeks: no reactions to 1 mg, but all reacted to 10 mg tartrazine.

4 Two patients with active urticaria (present for 3 and 7 years): both reacted to 1 mg and 10 mg tartrazine.

What is not clear from this data is whether the state of disease inactivity and tartrazine tolerance was permanent or temporary.

Purpura

There are three reports, involving seven patients, of adults in whom tartrazine ingestion was associated with purpura (Criep 1971; Michaëlsson & Juhlin 1974; Kubba & Champion 1975). The mechanism was thought to be an allergic vasculitis.

Asthma

Settipane & Pudupakkam 1975

There have been few double-blind placebo-controlled studies of ingested tartrazine in asthma. Of 40 adult patients with aspirin intolerance, of whom 29 had asthma, nine had rhinitis without asthma, and two had urticaria (Settipane & Pudupakkam 1975). Six of the 40 reacted to double-blind challenge with 0.44 mg tartrazine but not to placebo. In three out of these six, tartrazine produced generalized itching or urticaria, and in these three patients aspirin also provoked urticaria. In the other three patients, tartrazine produced bronchospasm and a 20% or more fall in the FEV1 within 3 hours. In these latter patients, aspirin also provoked bronchospasm, except for one patient in whom aspirin provoked urticaria in addition to asthma.

Spector *et al.* 1979

Spector *et al.* performed tartrazine challenges in 277 patients with asthma, all aged over 14 years (Spector *et al.* 1979). Eleven (4%) had a positive reaction, defined as a fall of FEV1 of 20% or more within 4 hours, to the ingestion of 1–25 mg of tartrazine. All 11 patients who reacted to tartrazine also reacted similarly to aspirin, and tartrazine intolerance was not seen in patients who were not intolerant to aspirin. However, five of these 11 patients did not have a placebo challenge. Three of the six patients in whom the tartrazine challenges were double-blind also experienced rhinitis after tartrazine, and these three also experienced rhinitis after aspirin.

Vedanthan *et al.* 1977
Weber *et al.* 1979

In contrast, the studies of Vedanthan *et al.* (1977) Weber *et al.* (1979) failed to demonstrate tartrazine intolerance in asthmatics. Vedanthan *et al.* studied 54 children with asthma, 35 of whom were being treated with oral steroids (1977). Double-blind challenges with tartrazine 25 mg failed to demonstrate a fall of the FEV1 of more than two standard deviations below the response to placebo in any patient. Weber *et al.* challenged 44 adults with perennial asthma; they were described as moderately severe, which would appear to be something of an understatement as 24 were receiving prednisone up to 60 mg per day (Weber *et al.* 1979). Seven reacted, as defined by a fall in the FEV1 of 25% or more within 1 hour, to open challenge with up to 20 mg of tartrazine, but none of these seven reacted when the challenge was repeated in a double-blind manner. The drawback to these two studies was that the patients were so severely affected, in that so many received treatment with systemic steroids, that either the severity of the disease or the treatment (Rosenhall 1982) may have masked a response to tartrazine, although the Vedanthan study did manage to detect aspirin intolerance in five children. The problem of severe disease and steroid treatment also applies to another study where the ingestion of tartrazine 15 mg caused a fall in the FEV1 in only one out of 28 adult asthmatic subjects, but 82% of patients were receiving oral or inhaled steroids at the time (Tarlo & Broder 1982).

Histamine challenge

Nine children with asthma who gave a history of coughing or wheezing after orange-coloured drinks were given double-blind challenges with tartrazine 1 mg (Hariparsad *et al.* 1984). There was no change in baseline PEFR after tartrazine, but histamine sensitivity (see chapter 45) increased markedly in three children and to a lesser degree in one other. The authors of this study suggested that the estimation of bronchial reactivity by measurement of the response to histamine challenge is a more sensitive test of additive intolerance than looking for changes in the FEV1. The subject is discussed further in chapter 52 on asthma. The authors failed to explain the discrepancy between the clinical history of coughing after drinking orange-coloured drinks and the failure to demonstrate a change in lung function after tartrazine challenge. The possible explanations were:

1 measurements of FEV1 and peak expiratory flow rate can sometimes be normal in the presence of quite marked small airways obstruction (Cooper *et al.* 1977; Godfrey 1983);

2 tartrazine provokes reflex coughing rather than bronchoconstriction, akin to the effects on some patients of angiotensin converting enzyme inhibitors (Morice *et al.* 1987; Bucknall *et al.* 1988);

3 the effect of tartrazine is so minor that changes in lung function do not occur even though bronchial hyperreactivity is enhanced.

Clinical relevance

The double-blind studies described above demonstrate beyond doubt that tartrazine is capable of provoking bronchoconstriction in a few patients with asthma. Most of the studies are in adults, and it is still unclear to what extent tartrazine can provoke asthma in children. The author's personal experience is that, in contrast to the severe attacks sometimes provoked by viral respiratory infections, exposure to pets, house dust mites or pollen, he has never seen a severe attack of asthma requiring hospitalization which could be attributed to tartrazine ingestion.

tartrazine avoidance – little benefit

Where tartrazine has been shown to provoke asthma, strict avoidance has not shown to be of benefit (Tarlo & Broder 1982), although this is hardly surprising considering the multiplicity of triggers which can contribute to the pathogenesis of asthma. It is possible that the regular administration of these and related additives may result in tolerance rather than worsening of asthma. Alternatively, if intolerance does exist, it could be that the contribution of these additives to a patient's bronchoconstriction is so small that avoidance would not be expected to result in detectable benefit.

Rhinitis

It has been noted that rhinitis can be provoked by tartrazine when administered by double-blind challenge (Spector *et al.* 1979), but the clinical relevance of this observation to perennial rhinitis is doubtful.

Atopic eczema

Contrary to popular belief, there is little evidence that tartrazine can provoke worsening of atopic eczema on anything other than rare occasions. Day-to-day fluctuation in disease severity, which is a notable though unexplained feature of atopic eczema, and difficulty in objectively quantifying the disease, greatly hinder the interpretation of challenge tests in this disorder. A study of placebo-controlled additive challenges in 101 patients (only five were under 10 years of age) who suspected that foods aggravated their eczema demonstrated reproducible reactions in only eight, but data was not provided as to which additives were implicated in these eight subjects (Veien *et al.* 1987). Van Bever *et al.* (1989) reported positive blind challenges to tartrazine in two out of six children with atopic eczema, but no attempt was made to see if these reactions were reproducible, and the reactions comprised quick-onset erythematous flares and not worsening of eczema. A recent study examined tartrazine intolerance in 12 children with atopic eczema whose parents reported worsening of eczema after tartrazine ingestion, and improvement after dietary avoidance (Devlin & David 1992). Multiple double-blind placebo-controlled challenges demonstrated a reproducible and consistent worsening of eczema in association with tartrazine ingestion in only one child, and the probability of this occurring by chance in one or more patients out of 12 was 0.46.

Behaviour   The relationship between behaviour problems and food intolerance is discussed elsewhere in this book (see chapter 68). There is no evidence from double-blind challenge studies that tartrazine can provoke behaviour problems in otherwise normal children (David 1987). A major source of confusion has been the presence of atopic disease. If a food additive makes eczema or asthma worse, then concentration and behaviour may also be expected to suffer, but there is no evidence that this is anything other than an indirect effect (David 1987). Parents' reports of behaviour changes following the ingestion of tartrazine are especially unreliable. Double-blind challenges with tartrazine 250 mg were performed in hospital in 24 children whose parents gave a definite history of a purely behavioural immediate adverse reaction to tartrazine (David 1987). The patients were all on a diet avoiding tartrazine, benzoic acid and other additives, and in all the history was that any lapse of the diet caused an obvious adverse reaction within 2 hours. In no patient was any change in behaviour noted either by the parents or the nursing staff after the administration of tartrazine, benzoic acid or placebo. Twenty-two patients returned to a normal diet without problems; two parents insisted on continuing dietary restriction. In another study of 39 children whose parents also reported adverse behavioural effects of food additives, the parents were unable to detect any changes in behaviour when the additives were introduced under double-blind conditions (Pollock & Warner 1990).

Skin staining   Spilling tartrazine onto the skin or nails (Verbov 1985) causes yellow staining. This is most commonly seen when children consume liquids containing tartrazine, which tends to cause a yellow rim around the mouth and on the upper lip (David 1987). This is of no clinical importance, but it means that if double-blind challenges are to be performed tartrazine must either be given in a capsule, or if the child is too young to swallow a capsule then the contents must be dissolved and drunk through a straw (David 1987).

Dose   Although the mechanism whereby tartrazine provokes urticaria and asthma is unknown, it is clear that dosage is important, some patients reacting briskly to very low doses and others only to higher ones. Several schedules of tartrazine challenge take this into account by starting with a low dose, and then employing a higher dose if there is no response (Supramaniam & Warner 1986; Warin & Smith 1976). The two studies of urticaria referred to above used relatively low doses of tartrazine for the challenges (Settipane et al. 1976; Supramaniam & Warner 1986). The choice of these low doses (0.22 mg and 0.1–1.0 mg) appears to have been arbitrary. It has been estimated that the average daily intake of tartrazine is 9 mg in the UK (Supramaniam & Warner 1986) and 10–15 mg in the US of America (Anonymous 1980), and it is theoretically possible that the use of a higher dose might have produced a larger number of urticarial reactions. It is unclear whether there is a dose-dependent threshold for response, or whether the severity of the response depends on the dose.

Aspirin cross-sensitivity

The conventional view in the past has been that there is a common association between aspirin and tartrazine intolerance (Schlumberger 1980), but this is unproven. The idea probably arose because many of the challenge studies in adults were performed on patients with asthma who had already been selected because of the presence of aspirin intolerance. Warner's study of 43 children with chronic urticaria showed that only one of the 24 patients who reacted to food additives (including 11 who reacted to tartrazine) had a similar reaction to aspirin (Supramaniam & Warner 1986). In addition, Stevenson et al.'s study of 150 aspirin-intolerant asthmatics failed to demonstrate tartrazine intolerance as defined by a fall in FEV1 of more than 25% after double-blind ingestion of tartrazine 50 mg (Stevenson et al. 1986). Finally, in a study of 24 adults with chronic urticaria who improved on an additive-free diet, the four patients with aspirin intolerance did not experience cross-sensitivity to tartrazine (Murdoch et al. 1987b). It is doubtful whether aspirin intolerance and tartrazine intolerance do co-exist more commonly than one would expect by chance. This conclusion is supported by the fact that tartrazine and its major metabolite sulphanilic acid do not inhibit the enzyme cyclo-oxygenase (Gerber et al. 1979), a pharmacological characteristic shared by all cross-reacting, non-steroidal, anti-inflammatory drugs including aspirin (Mathison & Stevenson 1979). Interestingly, a recent study has suggested that tartrazine, sodium benzoate, monosodium glutamate and sodium metabisulphite all have a similar effect to that of aspirin and other salicylates in the inhibition of thromboxane B2 formation by noradrenaline-activated platelets (Williams et al. 1989). If confirmed, this would suggest that some food additives induce intolerance because of an aspirin-like property.

Azo dye cross-sensitivity

A commonly encountered assumption is that patients who are intolerant to one of the azo dyes (see Table 34.1) are likely to be intolerant to all of them. At present there is little objective data on this issue. The best information comes from a study of urticaria in childhood (Supramaniam & Warner 1986). Of those tested with double-blind challenges, 11 out of 43 were intolerant to tartrazine 1 mg, 10 out of 36 to sunset yellow 0.1 mg, four out of 37 to amaranth 0.1 mg and zero out of 12 to carmoisine 0.1 mg (Supramaniam & Warner 1986). Unfortunately the published data do not indicate to what extent cross-sensitivity existed between these different azo dyes. In a study of two adults with chronic urticaria and food additive intolerance, both subjects were intolerant to all four azo colours tested under blind conditions, namely tartrazine, sunset yellow, amaranth and carmoisine (Murdoch et al. 1987b).

Mechanism

The mechanism by which tartrazine provokes urticaria, asthma or atopic eczema is unknown. Evidence from animal studies and studies of isolated cell populations suggests that a pharmacological action is more likely than an immunological mechanism (Hedman & Anderson 1984; Safford & Goodwin 1984). One study demonstrated rises in plasma histamine in normal subjects after the ingestion of tartrazine 200 mg (Murdoch et al. 1987a). It remains to be established whether the pharmacological effects of large doses of tartrazine in normal subjects have any bearing on the clinical effects of normally ingested small quantities.

Tartrazine in drugs

Tartrazine is used as a colouring agent in certain drugs. In contrast to the position with foods, at present the manufacturers of drugs in the UK are under no obligation to name colouring agents on the label or data sheet. In the USA, the Food and Drug Administration have required all manufacturers to declare the presence of tartrazine on package labels since 1980 (Lee et al. 1981). There are some published lists of drugs which contain tartrazine and other possibly harmful additives (Lee et al. 1981; Aldridge et al. 1984), but these rapidly become out of date as manufacturers reformulate drugs and remove contentious additives such as tartrazine. For the patient who has to avoid tartrazine there is no option but to:
1 use products which are available as white tablets (which can be crushed for small children); or
2 contact the manufacturer to find out which additives are present. This information is freely available to doctors or pharmacists, in confidence and for an individual patient, from all drug manufacturers in the UK.

Management investigations

There are no useful laboratory investigations or skin tests for tartrazine intolerance. The diagnosis depends entirely upon the history, and the response to avoidance followed by challenge.

asthma   In patients with asthma it is part of the routine history-taking to enquire about trigger factors, which include exercise, grass pollen, house dust, pets, respiratory infections, a cold wind, laughing, and soft drinks. Where there is a history suggesting tartrazine intolerance it is reasonable to avoid tartrazine, especially during attacks. In practice it is very rare for a history to pin-point an individual additive, and it is far more common for parents to note adverse reactions to certain artificial drinks. If the history suggests intolerance to food additives, the therapeutic choice is either to avoid all additives or to try and identify which additive or additives are important by double-blind challenge. However, even where intolerance to individual additives is identified by challenges, avoidance thereafter has not been shown to be of any benefit in the management of asthma when this was studied in adults (Tarlo & Broder 1982). Although tartrazine may provoke coughing in a small number of children with asthma, it is doubtful whether it causes severe attacks. The subject is discussed further in chapter 52 on asthma.

urticaria   Tartrazine is one of several food additives of importance in chronic urticaria. The history is unhelpful, and the only useful approach is trial of an empirical diet avoiding all colouring agents and preservatives, possibly followed by a battery of double-blind challenges. Full details are given in chapter 60.

atopic eczema   The management is the same as the identification of any other food or food additive intolerance in atopic eczema; a clear history if one is lucky (rare), or the elimination of multiple items from the diet followed by re-introduction of single foods or food additives. Further details are given in chapter 56.

behavioural problems   The management of behavioural problems is complex and rarely easy. In short, tartrazine does not cause behavioural symptoms in non-atopic children, but to persuade parents who happen to believe otherwise can be a great test of a doctor's persuasiveness and tact. The subject is discussed in full in chapter 68.

Key references 34.1   STEVENSON DD, SIMON RA, LUMRY WR & MATHISON DA (1986) Adverse reactions to tartrazine. *J Allergy Clin Immunol* **78**:182–191. *This contains a helpful critique of adverse reactions to tartrazine, and contains some original data about tartrazine challenge in asthmatics with aspirin intolerance.*

34.2   SIMON RA (1986) Adverse reactions to food additives. *New Engl Regional All Proc* **7**:533–542. *A critical review by one of the authors of the paper above.*

34.3   SUPRAMANIAM G & WARNER JO (1986) Artificial food additive intolerance in patients with angio-oedema and urticaria. *Lancet* **2**:907–909. *The key reference on* *intolerance to tartrazine and other additives in children with urticaria. Discussed in detail in the text of this chapter.*

34.4   SETTIPANE GA & PUDUPAKKAM RK (1975) Aspirin intolerance. III. Subtypes, familial occurrence, and cross-reactivity with tartrazine. *J Allergy Clin Immunol* **56**:215–221. *Key reference on tartrazine intolerance in adults with asthma; discussed in the text of this chapter.*

34.5   HARIPARSAD D, WILSON N, DIXON C & SILVERMAN M (1984) Oral tartrazine challenge in childhood asthma: effect on bronchial reactivity. *Clinical Allergy* **14**:81–85. Tartrazine failed to alter the peak expiratory flow rate in nine asthmatic children, but the bronchial reactivity was enhanced after tartrazine challenge in four. *This can either be interpreted as failure to confirm the parents' observations or as evidence that changes in bronchial responsiveness are a sensitive sign of food intolerance.*

Summary 34   Tartrazine is a yellow colouring agent, and one of the group of azo dyes. It is used as a colouring agent in a wide range of foods and medicines. Double-blind placebo-controlled studies have demonstrated that tartrazine can provoke urticaria, asthma or rhinitis in a small number of subjects. The rigorous methodology of some studies in asthmatics may have underestimated the incidence of tartrazine intolerance. There is no proof that tartrazine can cause worsening of atopic eczema. The mechanism whereby tartrazine provokes atopic disease is unknown. Tartrazine intolerance can be identified by history, elimination and challenge. It is possible that repeated administration leads to tolerance, but in some individuals avoidance is necessary.

35 Benzoic acid
A rare trigger of urticaria and contact urticaria

Introduction   Benzoic acid (E210) retards the growth of bacteria and yeasts, and is used as a preservative, usually in the form of sodium benzoate (E211), potassium benzoate (E212) or calcium benzoate (E213). Esters of para-hydroxybenzoic acid, ethyl para-hydroxybenzoate (E214), sodium ethyl para-hydroxybenzoate (E215), propyl para-hydroxybenzoate (E216), sodium propyl para-hydroxybenzoate (E217), methyl para-hydroxybenzoate (E218) and sodium methyl para-hydroxybenzoate (E219) are known collectively as parabens.

Table 35.1 Foodstuffs which contain large amounts of naturally occurring benzoic acid[1]

Food	Benzoic acid (mg/kg)
Honey	
Scottish heather honey	215.8
French heather honey	143.0
Clover honey	13.2
Jam	
Cranberry	140.0
Apricot	16.4
Dried fruit	
Apricot	30.4
Prune	12.1
Other	
Strawberry	13.9
Processed cheese	23.6
Yoghurt	26.0

[1] Source: Thomas (1988).

Parabens are widely used as preservatives, especially in cosmetic and pharmaceutical preparations. It is not known to what degree if any cross-sensitivity exists within or between ingested benzoates and parabens.

Naturally occurring benzoate

Benzoates occur naturally in some foods (Table 35.1) such as cranberries and certain types of honey (Thomas 1988).

Intolerance

Sound published evidence of intolerance to ingested benzoates in childhood is scanty.

Urticaria

The only evidence from a double-blind placebo-controlled investigation of urticaria provoked by ingested benzoates in childhood comes from a study of 43 children with urticaria who had responded to an additive-free diet (Supramaniam & Warner 1986). Using a challenge dose of 100 mg of sodium benzoate, four out of 27 (15%) children developed an exacerbation of urticaria within 4 hours of sodium benzoate challenge but not after placebo. Further data from the same centre reported intolerance to sodium benzoate in seven of 34 (21%) children, but on re-challenge between 1 and 5 years later, only one of the seven had a positive reaction to challenge, suggesting that as with intolerance to tartrazine (see chapter 34), benzoic acid intolerance is a transient phenomenon (Pollock & Warner 1987). One child, an 8-year-old boy, was shown to have an urticarial reaction to tartrazine, sodium metabisulphite and sodium benzoate. On re-challenge 2 years later, he developed a mild cough and wheeze but no urticaria in response to aspirin and sodium benzoate.

need for controlled studies

The need for placebo-controlled double-blind studies with objective criteria for what constitutes a reaction is illustrated by a study from Finland (Lahti & Hannuksela 1981). In double-blind, placebo-controlled studies of reactions to challenges with 500 mg benzoic acid in 29 patients (presumably adults) with chronic urticaria, objective reactions (urticaria, angioedema, rhinitis) to benzoic acid 500 mg occurred in two (7%) but reactions to lactose placebo occurred in four (14%).

Irritant contact urticaria

Irritant contact urticaria from sodium benzoate is described in chapter 59. The symptoms consist of transient perioral erythema and minor itching and tingling in the mouth (Clemmensen & Hjorth 1982). Contact urticaria caused by parabens is reviewed elsewhere (Fisher *et al.* 1971; Bandmann 1972; Lorenzetti & Wernet 1977).

Purpura

There are two reports of adults in whom benzoate ingestion was associated with purpura (Michaëlsson & Juhlin 1974; Kubba & Champion 1975). The mechanism was thought to be an allergic vasculitis.

Asthma

There has been no double-blind placebo-controlled study of the effects of benzoates in children with asthma. Such studies as exist are on adults, and most studies are flawed. Of 272 patients (mainly adults) with asthma studied by Freedman, 30 (11%) gave a history of exacerbations occurring after ingestion of orange drinks (Freedman 1977). In an uncontrolled study, 14 of the 30 were challenged with food additives. Four experienced a fall of more than 20% in the FEV1 after 20 mg to 120 mg of sodium benzoate, occurring 10–20 min after ingestion. Tarlo and Broder (1982) performed double-blind placebo-controlled challenges in 28 adults with asthma, but only one reacted to sodium benzoate; 25 mg produced a 29% fall in the FEV1 in this subject, compared to a 9% fall after lactose placebo. Weber *et al.* found only one of 43 adults with asthma with a 25% fall of the FEV1 after double-blind challenge with a combination of sodium benzoate 250 mg and para-hydroxybenzoic acid 250 mg (Weber *et al.* 1979). When this patient was re-challenged 2 years later, he did not react. In Rosenhall's study, despite single-blind, poorly controlled challenges, only one of 504 mainly adult patients (400 with asthma, 104 with rhinitis) reacted to sodium benzoate 50 mg (Rosenhall 1982).

avoidance unhelpful

Diets avoiding tartrazine and benzoic acid appear to be unhelpful in patients where these additives have been shown to provoke asthma

(Tarlo & Broder 1982). It is possible that the regular administration of these and related additives may result in tolerance rather than a worsening of asthma.

Atopic eczema   A study of placebo-controlled additive challenges in 101 patients (only five were under 10 years of age) who suspected that foods aggravated their eczema demonstrated reproducible reactions in only eight, but data was not provided as to which additives were implicated in these eight subjects (Veien *et al.* 1987). Van Bever *et al.* (1989) reported positive blind challenges to benzoic acid in three out of six children with atopic eczema, but no attempt was made to see if these reactions were reproducible, and the reactions comprised quick-onset erythematous flares and not worsening of eczema. It remains unclear whether benzoic acid or the benzoates are capable of exacerbating atopic eczema.

Behaviour   The relationship between behavioural problems and food intolerance is discussed elsewhere in this book (see chapter 68). There is no evidence from double-blind challenge studies that benzoates can provoke behavioural problems in otherwise normal children. A major source of confusion has been the presence of co-existing atopic disease. If a food additive makes eczema or asthma worse, the concentration span and behaviour may also be expected to suffer, but there is no evidence that this is anything other than an indirect effect. Parents' reports of behaviour changes following the ingestion of benzoates are especially unreliable. Double-blind challenges with benzoic acid 250 mg were performed in hospital in 24 children whose parents gave a definite history of a purely behavioural immediate adverse reaction to tartrazine (David 1987). The patients were all on a diet avoiding tartrazine, benzoic acid and other additives, and in all the history was that any lapse of the diet caused an obvious adverse reaction within 2 hours. In no patient was any change in behaviour noted either by the parents or the nursing staff after the administration of tartrazine, benzoic acid or placebo. Twenty-two patients returned to a normal diet without problems; two parents insisted on continuing dietary restriction.

Management   The principles are the same as those for the management of tartrazine intolerance (see chapter 34).

Key references 35.1   JACOBSEN DW (1991) Adverse reactions to benzoates and parabens. In METCALFE DD, SAMPSON HA & SIMON RA (eds) *Food Allergy. Adverse Reactions to Foods and Food Additives*, pp. 276–287, Blackwell Scientific Publications, Boston. *Review.*

35.2   TARLO SM & BRODER I (1982) Tartrazine and benzoate challenge and dietary avoidance in chronic asthma. *Clin Allergy* **12**:303–312. Of 28 adults with asthma who were challenged, one responded to tartrazine and one to benzoate. Twenty-four patients completed 1-month periods of observation while first on a normal diet and then while on a tartrazine-benzoate avoidance diet. No improvement occurred during the modified diet in either patient with positive challenge tests. *Interestingly, during the period of additive avoidance, five subjects had significant worsening of peak expiratory flow rates while only two improved. The authors concluded that tartrazine and benzoate avoidance was not of value in the management of chronic asthma. It was speculated that the development of tolerance to additives, known to occur with aspirin-induced asthma, explained the failure of dietary avoidance to help patients where tartrazine or benzoate had been shown to provoke asthma while the patient was on an additive-free diet.*

35.3   SUPRAMANIAM G & WARNER JO (1986) Artificial food additive intolerance in patients with angio-oedema and urticaria. *Lancet* **2**:907–909. *The key reference on intolerance to benzoates and other additives in children with urticaria. Discussed in detail in the text above.*

Summary 35   Benzoic acid and related benzoates retard the growth of bacteria and yeasts, and are used as food preservatives. Small quantities occur naturally in certain foods such as cranberries and bilberries. Esters of para-hydroxybenzoic acid are related compounds known as parabens, and are widely used as preservatives in cosmetic and pharmaceutical preparations. Double-blind placebo-controlled studies have demonstrated that benzoates can provoke urticaria in a small number of subjects. It is unclear whether benzoates can worsen atopic eczema in some children. The mechanism whereby benzoates provoke urticaria or asthma is unknown. Benzoate intolerance can be identified by history, elimination and challenge. It is possible that repeated administration leads to tolerance, but in some individuals avoidance may be necessary.

36 Sulphite
May be important in asthma

Chemical properties   Sulphur dioxide (E220), sodium sulphite (E221), sodium bisulphite (E222), sodium metabisulphite (E223), potassium metabisulphite (E224), calcium sulphite (E226), and calcium bisulphite (E227) are widely used as food additives. Sulphite salts are water soluble, as is sulphur dioxide, which rapidly hydrates to form sulfurous acid. Sulphur dioxide, sulfurous acid, and the sulphite and bisulphite anions are readily interconvertible in aqueous solutions. The relative presence of these compounds in solution is determined primarily by the pH. Acidification will cause the liberation of sulphur dioxide (Taylor *et al.* 1986; Gunnison & Jacobsen 1987).

Naturally occurring sulphite in the body

Considerable quantities of sulphite are generated in the body by normal catabolic processing of sulphur containing amino acids and other sulphur containing compounds. Sulphite is converted to sulphate by the enzyme sulphite oxidase, and the intracellular concentrations of sulphite are low in normal individuals (Gunnison & Jacobsen 1987). It is theoretically possible that deficiency of sulphite oxidase may cause or worsen an adverse reaction to ingested sulphite, although there is little evidence for the clinical importance of this potential mechanism (Jacobsen *et al.* 1984; Walker 1985).

in food

Wine and beer cannot be made without the natural formation of sulphites. Sulphur dioxide is produced by the action of yeast during fermentation (Taylor *et al.* 1986). Sometimes further sulphur dioxide is deliberately added, initially to inhibit the growth of undesirable yeast species and later in higher concentrations to prevent secondary fermentation (Coltate 1984). It is likely that sulphur dioxide formation occurs in other food products fermented by yeasts, although this does not appear to have been studied (Taylor *et al.* 1986).

Uses of sulphites

Sulphites are widely used as food preservatives (Walker 1985; Taylor *et al.* 1986), either sprayed on to the food or by soaking the food (e.g. peeled potatoes) in sulphite solutions. The purposes of adding sulphites are:

1 to prevent non-enzymatic browning and discolouration of dried fruits, dehydrated vegetables, coconut, pectin, vinegar, grape juice and wine;

2 to inhibit enzymatic browning reactions, such as the discolouration of cut fruits, lettuce, peeled potatoes, mushrooms and grapes, or the oxidation of ascorbate in vegetables;

3 to inhibit the growth of micro-organisms;

4 to act as an antioxidant or a reducing agent;

5 to act as a bleaching agent, for example to bleach cherries for the production of maraschino cherries;

6 to inhibit the formation of nitrosamines in the kilning of barley.

Other properties

Sulphites can react with and inactivate thiamine, and for this reason sulphites in some countries cannot be legally added to foods such as meat which are considered to be important sources of thiamine (Coltate 1984; Taylor *et al.* 1986). Although sulphites are not added to food for this purpose, they have the fortuitous property of degrading certain mycotoxins and aflatoxins.

Sources of sulphite

The sources of exposure to sulphites are:
1 sulphites added to food;
2 sulphur dioxide in the atmosphere, the chief source of which is the burning of coal and oil;
3 sulphites used as preservatives in injectable and inhalable pharmaceutical preparations.

Sulphite intolerance: mechanism

Possible mechanisms of sulphite intolerance are as follows.

sulphur dioxide generation

When sulphites are dissolved in water, sulphur dioxide is liberated (the quantity depends upon the pH). Inhalation of sulphur dioxide has been shown to produce bronchoconstriction in most normal subjects (Frank et al. 1962; Snell & Luchsinger 1969). Patients with asthma develop bronchoconstriction at a lower threshold concentration than do non-asthmatic subjects, and their bronchoconstriction is of greater magnitude (Sheppard et al. 1980). The threshold for sulphur dioxide-induced bronchoconstriction in asthmatics is even lower if the subjects are exercising at the time of inhalation (Bethel et al. 1983). This response to sulphur dioxide can be prevented in both normal and asthmatic subjects by treatment with atropine, suggesting that it is mediated by parasympathetic pathways (Sheppard et al. 1980). However, the mechanism for intolerance to ingested, injected or inhaled sulphites, which only affects a proportion of asthmatics, is not fully understood (see below).

IgE mediated

There are two well documented case reports of anaphylaxis caused by exposure to sulphite in which it is possible that the mechanism was IgE mediated (Prenner & Stevens 1976; Twarog & Leung 1982). In one there was a positive skin-prick test to a 10 mg/ml sulphite solution, and this skin test reactivity could be passively transferred (Prenner & Stevens 1976). In the other there was also a positive skin-prick test to sulphite; in this case passive transfer was not possible, but incubation of the patient's leucocytes with sodium metabisulphite caused significant histamine release (Twarog & Leung 1982). Although one other patient has been found with sulphite intolerance and a positive skin test which could be passively transferred (Simon & Wasserman 1986), almost all patients with sulphite intolerance have negative skin tests (Simon 1986).

sulphite oxidase deficiency

A lower level of sulphite oxidase has been reported in the cultured fibroblasts of six patients with sulphite-provoked asthma when compared with a single control (Jacobsen *et al.* 1984; Simon 1986). It is not known whether this mechanism is of clinical importance.

Sulphite intolerance: importance of whether sulphite is in solution or encapsulated

In asthmatic subjects, there appear to be two types of sulphite intolerance. In the more common type, there is intolerance to sulphite in solution, or foods which have been sprayed with or soaked in sulphite solutions. Contact with the oral mucosa and the release of sulphur dioxide appear to be important features of this type of reaction. In the less common type of intolerance, sulphite which reaches the stomach intact (e.g. in capsules) also provokes a reaction; the mechanism is obscure (Bush *et al.* 1986; Simon 1986).

Sulphite intolerance in children with asthma

There have been only two systematic studies of sulphites in childhood asthma. In an Australian study, 29 children with asthma requiring inhaled or oral steroids were placed on a diet avoiding all colouring agents and preservatives and then challenged on one day with placebo, and on the next day with 25, 50 and 100 mg encapsulated sodium metabisulphite, followed by 5, 25 and 50 mg of the metabisulphite in a solution with 0.5% citric acid (Towns & Mellis 1984). None of the children reacted to metabisulphite in capsules, but in 19 out of 29 (66%) there was a >20% decrease in the FEV1 after ingestion of metabisulphite in solution with citric acid. These reactions mostly occurred within 1–2 min of ingestion, and in all reactions the patient complained initially of a burning sensation in the throat. All 19 patients reacting to metabisulphite were placed on a diet avoiding foods, beverages and medications known to contain high concentrations of sulphite, and reassessed 3 months later. There was no control group. Nine 'felt a subjective improvement', and in four there was a 'decrease' in bronchodilator requirement. A further study of placebo-controlled metabisulphite challenges in children with asthma documented positive challenges to metabisulphite in acid solution in eight of 51 (35%) children with asthma (Friedman & Easton 1987). The other descriptions of sulphite-induced asthma in childhood are anecdotal case reports (Kochen 1973; Sher & Schwartz 1985; Wolf & Nicklas 1985).

Sulphite intolerance in adults with asthma

Sulphite intolerance is best documented in adults with severe oral or inhaled steroid-dependent asthma. Adverse reactions in non-asthmatic subjects are exceedingly rare (Bush *et al.* 1986). Ingestion of sulphite capsules in double-blind placebo-controlled studies showed that 5% to 8% of adults with asthma had positive sulphite challenges, defined as a fall in the FEV1 of more than 25% (Simon *et al.* 1982; Buckley *et al.* 1985; Bush *et al.* 1986). A study of less severely affected adult asthmatics suggested a much lower incidence (0.8%) of intolerance to sulphite (Bush *et al.* 1986). The clinical significance of such studies is unclear, for it is uncertain what proportion of patients with positive challenges, if any, would benefit from avoidance of ingested sulphite. Furthermore, it is clear that many patients with asthma only react to sulphites in solution and not in capsule form (Delohery 1984). Nevertheless, it is recognized that a small number of asthmatics, chiefly steroid-dependent patients, are especially sensitive to the adverse effects of ingested sulphites (Baker *et al.* 1981; Stevenson & Simon 1981; Habenicht *et al.* 1983; Schwartz 1983), and respiratory arrest and death have been recorded (Simon 1986). These reports suggest that the major hazard is from restaurant food, in particular restaurant salads such as coleslaw, potato salad, guacamole (avocado dip) or lettuce itself (Bush *et al.* 1986). These salads have in the past tended to have high levels of added sulphite (Taylor *et al.* 1985; Bush *et al.* 1986; Martin *et al.* 1986), although from more recent surveys of restaurants in the USA it appears that the use of sulphites in salads is declining (Bush *et al.* 1986).

Sulphite intolerance: cross-sensitivity

Patients whose asthma is provoked by ingested sulphite do not have cross-sensitivity to ingested salicylates, benzoates, tartrazine or monosodium glutamate (Simon 1986).

Sulphite intolerance: urticaria

There are anecdotal reports of sulphited foods causing urticaria (Habenicht *et al.* 1983), but double-blind challenges of patients with urticaria have not demonstrated sulphite-provoked urticaria or angioedema (Simon 1986).

Sulphite intolerance: other symptoms

A number of symptoms have been ascribed to intolerance to ingested sulphite (Schwartz 1983; Bush *et al.* 1986). These include flushing, tingling, pruritus, dysphagia, chest pain, dizziness, urticaria and angioedema (see above), wheezing and coughing (see asthma, above), hypotension, loss of consciousness and anaphylaxis (Prenner & Stevens 1976; Twarog & Leung 1982; Tsevat *et al.* 1987).

Sulphites in pharmaceutical preparations

Sulphites are sometimes added to pharmaceutical preparations of drugs, and exposure of sulphite-intolerant patients to these medications by the intravenous, inhalational or topical (eye drops) route may provoke adverse reactions (Trautlein 1976; Dally *et al.* 1978; Koepke *et al.* 1983; Koepke *et al.* 1984; Simon 1984; Witek & Schachter 1984; Dalton-Bunnow 1985; Jamieson *et al.* 1985; Settipane 1986). Small quantities of sulphites may also reach medical preparations by their use in the processing of dextrose, starch and gelatin, but only in quantities far too small to provoke adverse reactions in even the most sensitive subjects (Dalton-Bunnow 1985).

drugs for asthma

In practice the problem is that several drugs used in the intravenous or inhalational treatment of asthma may contain sulphites, and worsening of an attack of asthma due to sulphites has been reported following the use of intravenous dexamethasone (Baker *et al.* 1981), intravenous metoclopramide (Baker *et al.* 1981), nebulized isoetharine (Twarog & Leung 1982; Koepke *et al.* 1984), a beta-2 stimulant closely related to salbutamol and terbutaline, nebulized isoproterenol (Koepke *et al.* 1983; Witek & Schachter 1984), nebulized racemic adrenaline (Koepke *et al.* 1983), and nebulized gentamicin (Dally *et al.* 1978).

Management
history

A history of worsening of pre-existing asthma after drinking artificial drinks, eating in a restaurant, or inhalation or injection of a drug containing sulphite, raise the possibility of sulphite intolerance.

investigations

Skin tests with sulphite solutions are almost always negative in subjects with sulphite intolerance (Simon 1986), and are therefore unhelpful. The only useful confirmatory test is an oral challenge with a sulphite solution, and a detailed protocol for this has been published (Simon 1987). This uses metabisulphite dissolved in an acidic solution of lemonade, with increasing doses (starting at 1 mg, increasing to 200 mg) being given every 10 min.

threshold dose

It is helpful to establish the threshold dose of sulphite that provokes asthma. For example, if a patient has a threshold dose of 10 mg, that person would need to consume 200 g of food containing 50 ppm of sulphite. If the food had 100–500 ppm of residual sulphur dioxide, consumption of 20–100 g would provoke a response (Bush *et al.* 1986). Highly sulphited foods such as dried fruits contain 2000 ppm of sulphur dioxide, and only 5 g would be required to reach the threshold (Bush *et al.* 1986). Knowledge of the threshold, in theory at least, might enable the patient to avoid only those foods with a relatively high sulphite content, making a very restrictive diet unnecessary.

avoidance

The treatment of sulphite intolerance is avoidance of foods which contain substantial quantities of sulphite. The foods which need to be avoided will vary from country to country, depending upon local legislation concerning foods to which the addition of sulphite is permitted. Foods likely to have a high content of sulphite are artificial drinks (e.g. orange squash), wine, beer, shrimps, dried fruit, salads, cider and vinegar, and prepared or restaurant food especially salads.

identification of sulphited foods

It can be difficult to identify sulphited foods in restaurants. Several makes of sulphite test strips have been produced in the USA (Wanderer & Solomons 1987; Nordlee *et al.* 1988). These rely on the formation of sulphitonitroprusside, a red product formed by the reaction of sulphite with paper strips impregnated with sodium nitroprusside, potassium hexacyanoferrate, and zinc sulphate. Although these strips may have some limited value in the detection of sulphite-treated lettuce and potatoes in restaurants, recent studies have shown a high incidence of false positive reactions with fish, meat, poultry and shrimps, and false negative reactions with dried fruit, wine and canned crab. The confusion and potential hazards caused by the false positive and false negative reactions mean that these strips are not very useful (Wanderer & Solomons 1987; Nordlee *et al.* 1988).

Key references

36.1   TAYLOR SL, HIGLEY NA & BUSH RK (1986) Sulfites in foods: uses, analytical methods, residues, fate, exposure assessment, metabolism, toxicity, and hypersensitivity. *Adv Food Chem* **30**:1–76. *Major review describing the uses and chemistry of sulphites in foods, also covering toxicity in humans.*

36.2   GUNNISON AF & JACOBSEN DW (1987) Sulfite hypersensitivity. A critical review. *CRC Crit Rev Toxicol* **17**:185–214. *A detailed review of sulphite intolerance.*

36.3   SIMON RA (1986) Sulfite sensitivity. *Ann Allergy* **56**:281–288. *Critical review of sulphite intolerance from one of the major contributors to the study of adverse reactions to sulphite.*

36.4   TAYLOR SL, BUSH RK & NORDLEE JA (1991) Sulfites. In Metcalfe DD, Sampson HA & Simon RA (eds). *Food Allergy. Adverse Reactions to Foods and Food Additives*, pp. 239–260, Blackwell, Scientific Publications, Boston. *Review.*

36.5   DELOHERY J, SIMMUL R, CASTLE WD & ALLEN DH (1984) The relationship of inhaled sulfur dioxide reactivity to ingested metabisulphite sensitivity in patients with asthma. *Am Rev Respir Dis* **130**:1027–1032. When ingested in acid solutions, which liberate significant quantities of gaseous sulphur dioxide, the preservative sodium metabisulphite provokes asthma within minutes of ingestion in a proportion of asthmatic subjects. In this study two groups of asthmatics were compared – reactors and non-reactors to metabisulphite. Patients and a group of non-asthmatic controls were separately challenged with metabisulphite, and with increasing concentrations of sulphur dioxide. To further study the site and mechanism of sulphite-provoked asthma, mouthwash and gastric challenges were also performed. The results showed: (a) that metabisulphite sensitive asthmatics were no more sensitive to inhaled sulphur dioxide than non-metabisulphite sensitive asthmatics; (b) that when metabisulphite solution was instilled via a nasogastric tube directly into the stomach, there was no reaction; (c) when metabisulphite-sensitive asthmatics swilled a metabisulphite solution around the mouth for 3 s and then discarded it and cleansed the mouth with water, brisk bronchoconstriction occurred, similar in onset and severity to that provoked by swallowing the solution. The authors concluded that the possible mechanisms were an effect in the mouth, initiating an orobronchial reflex, or variable inhalation of sulphur dioxide during swallowing or mouthwashing.

Summary 36   Sulphites are widely used as preservatives and added to certain foods and pharmaceutical preparations. In acidic solution, sulphites liberate sulphur dioxide. Virtually all asthmatics respond with bronchoconstriction when exposed to sulphur dioxide by inhalation, and many respond in a similar fashion to the ingestion of acidic solutions of sulphites. A small number of asthmatics, chiefly those who are steroid-dependent, react adversely to capsules of sulphites, but the mechanism of this response is not known.

37 Other additives
Rare triggers in urticaria and asthma

Scanty information   The information available about intolerance to these additives is scanty, and mostly anecdotal or poorly controlled. Some studies, such as those where only mixtures of food colourings were given, are impossible to interpret. Thus, for example, it is difficult to know what to make, if anything, of the observation that a capsule, which contained 10 mg each of annatto, erythrosine, ponceau, tartrazine, patent blue, sunset yellow, betanine, curcumine and quinoline yellow, provoked worsening of eczema in 25 of 101 patients (ages unstated) with chronic eczema (Veien *et al.* 1987).

Amaranth   Amaranth (E123) is a red colouring agent and one of the azo dyes.

urticaria   Double-blind challenges with amaranth were positive in four out of 37 children with chronic urticaria in one study (Supramanian & Warner 1986). Murdoch *et al.* (1987b) reported two adults with chronic urticaria in whom double-blind challenges with amaranth and other azo colours provoked adverse reactions. In an unsatisfactory study of urticaria, in which antihistamines were discontinued prior to challenges, and placebo challenges were performed before challenges with the test substances, amaranth provoked urticaria in one out of seven adults with chronic urticaria (Michaëlsson & Juhlin 1973). In a non-placebo-controlled challenge study in which the degree of blinding was unclear, amaranth provoked adverse reactions in four out of 32 adults with chronic urticaria (Thune & Granholt

1975). Lockey (1972) anecdotally reported a 53-year old man in whom ingestion of amaranth provoked urticaria and angioedema.

asthma
In a study of 45 adults with moderately severe perennial asthma, double-blind challenges with amaranth failed to provoke significant bronchoconstriction (defined as >25% fall in FEV1) in any subject (Weber *et al.* 1979).

Annatto
Annatto (E160b), also known as bixin or norbixin, is a naturally occurring yellow colouring agent, obtained from the seed coats of the annatto tree (*Bixa orellana*). In a study of 3188 adults who reported intolerance to food additives, there were two in whom double-blind placebo-controlled challenges demonstrated intolerance to annatto (Young *et al.* 1987). The symptoms were headache in one subject (who also reacted to placebo on one occasion) and abdominal pain in the other. In one uncontrolled study, annatto extract was reported to provoke urticaria in 15 of 56 patients (ages unstated) with chronic urticaria (Mikkelsen *et al.* 1978). In another uncontrolled study, it would appear from the results (which were presented rather confusingly) that annatto provoked urticaria in 10% of 112 patients with recurrent urticaria (Juhlin 1981). There is a report of an anaphylactic reaction to a breakfast cereal coloured with annatto, but challenges were not performed (Nish *et al.* 1991).

Aspartame
Aspartame, a dipeptide composed of aspartic acid and the methyl ester of phenylalanine, is a sweetener. There have been a number of reports of adverse reactions to aspartame, but few have been supported by evidence from double-blind placebo-controlled challenges.

granulomatous panniculitis
Aspartame was reported to cause granulomatous panniculitis in a 22-year-old woman, and the lesions recurred 10 days after open challenge (Novick 1985).

urticaria
Double-blind challenges confirmed reports of urticaria occurring 1–2 hours after ingestion of aspartame in two adult women aged 23 and 46 (Kulczycki 1986).

migraine
Observational reports of aspartame having provoked attacks of migraine led to a double-blind cross-over study, which compared the effect of aspartame and placebo ingestion in 40 adults who reported headaches repeatedly after consuming aspartame (Schiffman *et al.* 1987). The incidence of headache after aspartame (35%) was not significantly different from that after placebo (45%). In a further cross-over study of 25 adults with migraine, data on 14 was

excluded, but analysis of the remaining results suggested a statistically significant increase in the number of attacks of migraine while taking aspartame (Koehler & Glaros 1988). When questioned, 8% of 171 patients with migraine reported that ingestion of aspartame provoked attacks (Lipton *et al.* 1989). However, self-reported headaches (and a number of other symptoms such as dizziness, urticaria, dysphagia, diarrhoea and rhinitis) as a result of aspartame ingestion could not be confirmed in a challenge study of 12 adults (Garriga *et al.* 1991).

migraine in childhood

There is no data linking aspartame with headache or migraine in childhood.

Butylated hydroxyanisole & butylated hydroxytoluene

Butylated hydroxyanisole (E320) and butylated hydroxytoluene (E321), known as BHA and BHT, are both employed as antioxidants in foods. There is a report of urticaria associated with the regular use of a chewing gum which contained butylated hydroxytoluene (Moneret-Vautrin *et al.* 1986). The eruption subsided within a week of stopping the gum, and returned a few hours after an oral challenge. In a study of 45 adults with moderately severe perennial asthma, open challenges with a mixture of butylated hydroxyanisole and butylated hydroxytoluene resulted in a greater than 25% fall from the baseline in FEV1 in two subjects (Weber *et al.* 1979). Double-blind challenges confirmed this fall in only one of the two subjects.

Canthaxanthin

Canthaxanthin (E161g) is a carotenoid which is added to fish food to colour the flesh of trout and salmon, when it may be given to the fish with the related pigment astaxanthin. Canthaxanthin was formerly taken by mouth by humans to produce an artificial suntan, but such use led to retinal deposits, sometimes called 'gold speck maculopathy', and in some cases to impairment of vision (Reynolds 1989). In an uncontrolled challenge study of 42 patients, mainly adults, with chronic urticaria, Juhlin (1981) reported positive challenges in 14% of subjects.

Carmine

Carmine (E120), also known as cochineal, is a natural red dye extracted from the insect *Coccus cactus*. It passes through the gut unchanged, and is used as a faecal marker in a dose of 200–500 mg. Carmine is reported to have caused occupational asthma and extrinsic allergic alveolitis in adults (Burge *et al.* 1979; Dietemann-Molard *et al.* 1991).

Carmoisine

Carmoisine (E122) is a red colouring agent and one of the azo dyes. Double-blind challenges with carmoisine were negative in all 10 children with chronic urticaria in one study (Supramanian & Warner 1986), but were positive in a child with oro-facial granulomatosis (Sweatman *et al.* 1986). Murdoch *et al.* (1987b) reported two adults with chronic urticaria in whom double-blind challenges with carmoisine and other azo colours provoked adverse reactions.

Erythrosine
urticaria

Erythrosine (E127) is a red colouring agent. In a non-placebo-controlled challenge study in which the degree of blinding was unclear, erythrosine provoked adverse reactions in two out of 21 adults with chronic urticaria (Thune & Granholt 1975).

anaphylaxis

There is a single rather unconvincing report of a 40-year old woman who is said to have experienced an anaphylactic reaction to erythrosine (Bergner *et al.* 1989). The patient gave a history of itching and generalized flushing 6 hours after ingestion of an antihistamine tablet which contained, amongst 18 ingredients, erythrosine. Challenge with the tablet resulted in an anaphylactic reaction within 90 min, but oral provocation tests with erythrosine produced no adverse reactions. The authors nevertheless attributed the adverse reactions to erythrosine, on the tenuous grounds that a skin-prick test with erythrosine was positive on one occasion (but not when the patient was re-tested 6 months later).

asthma

In a study of 45 adults with moderately severe perennial asthma, double-blind challenges with erythrosine provoked significant bronchoconstriction (defined as >25% fall in FEV1) in one out of 45 subjects (Weber *et al.* 1979).

Indigo carmine
urticaria

Indigo carmine (E132) is a blue colouring agent. Double-blind challenges with indigo carmine were positive in three out of 19 children with chronic urticaria in one study (Supramanian & Warner 1986). In a non-placebo-controlled challenge study in which the degree of blinding was unclear, indigo provoked adverse reactions in three out of 21 adults with chronic urticaria (Thune & Granholt 1975).

asthma

In a study of 45 adults with moderately severe perennial asthma, double-blind challenges with indigo carmine failed to provoke significant bronchoconstriction (defined as >25% fall in FEV1) in any subject (Weber *et al.* 1979).

Monosodium glutamate
Drs Ikeda and Kwok

Monosodium glutamate (MSG) was discovered in 1910 by a Japanese chemist Ikeda when he analysed *Laminaria japonica*, a seaweed that was commonly used as a seasoning in Japanese cooking. He found that it contained glutamate, and assumed that this was the substance that enhanced the flavour of foods with which it was cooked (Swan 1982). Monosodium glutamate occurs naturally in some foods, and, for example, 100 g Camembert cheese contains as much as 1 g monosodium glutamate (Simon 1986). However the greatest exposure to monosodium glutamate occurs because of its addition to food as a flavour enhancer. Up to 6 g of monosodium glutamate may be ingested in a highly seasoned Chinese meal, a single bowl of wonton soup can contain 2.5 g, and monosodium glutamate is one of Colonel Sander's secret herbs and spices (Simon 1986). In 1968, Dr Robert Ho Man Kwok reported numbness at the back of the neck, radiating to the arms, general weakness, and palpitation whenever he ate at a Chinese restaurant. He suggested that the so-called Chinese restaurant syndrome might be attributable to the ingestion of monosodium glutamate. This was followed by a number of anecdotal reports, including one of an 18-month-old boy who screamed for 2 hours within 10 min of ingesting noodles and broth from wonton soup (Asnes 1980). This report was prefaced by a personal note from the editor of the journal, cautioning that the evidence that the infant had the Chinese restaurant syndrome was only circumstantial, but that his own wife had confirmed that the description of the symptoms was accurate and that she suffered from the same malady!

Chinese restaurant syndrome
The effects of monosodium glutamate were studied in 77 normal volunteers (Kenney & Tidball 1972). On each of 3 days the subjects received 150 ml tomato juice, which contained 5 mg monosodium glutamate on 1 day only. On the 2 placebo days the juice was adjusted to an equivalent taste by the addition of 0.8 g sodium chloride. Two hours after drinking the juice, the subjects were asked to report any symptoms, and the results are shown in Table 37.1. Twenty-five subjects reported symptoms on the day monosodium glutamate was drunk. Eleven subjects reported symptoms on one of the placebo days, but no subject reported symptoms on both placebo days. None of the reports were of the 'classical' Chinese restaurant syndrome triad of burning sensation, infraorbital pressure or tightness and substernal discomfort. Further studies showed a dose-response relationship, with a threshold for the appearance of stiffness and tightness at 2–3 g. The precise mechanism of the Chinese restaurant syndrome is uncertain.

asthma
The sole evidence supported by double-blind placebo-controlled challenge that monosodium glutamate can provoke asthma is a case report of a patient who presented with a respiratory arrest after ingestion of wonton soup which contained monosodium glutamate (Koepke & Selner 1986). Allen and colleagues described two adults with asthma and monosodium glutamate intolerance who

Table 37.1 Symptoms after ingestion of 5 g monosodium glutamate or placebo in 77 volunteers[1]

Description of sensation	Location	MSG day	Placebo days
Warmth/burning	Face	1	2
	Head	2	0
	Neck	0	1
	Shoulders	0	1
	Elsewhere	1	0
Stiffness/tightness	Face	1	0
	Neck	1	3
Weakness	Arms	0	1
	Legs	0	1
Pressure	Eyes	2	0
	Face	2	0
	Head	4	2
	Chest	4	0
Tingling	Mouth	1	0
	Jaws	1	0
	Tongue	1	2
	Teeth	2	1
	Head	2	0
	Shoulders	1	0
	Arms	1	0
Heartburn/gastric discomfort		4	1
Lightheadedness		5	0
Headache		4	2
Total symptoms		40	17

[1] Source: Kenney & Tidball (1972).

experienced life-threatening attacks which required intubation and artificial ventilation, the attacks occurring 1–12 hours after a meal in a Chinese restaurant (Allen *et al.* 1987). They also performed challenges with monosodium glutamate at a maximum dosage of 5.0 g in 32 patients with asthma, all but one of whom were adults. The patients were highly selected and either had a history of symptoms after a meal in a Chinese restaurant or of 'chemical sensitivity'. Seven patients developed asthma and symptoms of the 'Chinese restaurant syndrome' 1–2 hours after ingestion of monosodium glutamate, and six patients developed asthma alone, 6–12 hours after ingestion of monosodium glutamate. Unfortunately the authors did not employ a double-blind placebo-controlled methodology, and for this and other reasons their observations have been discredited (Ebert 1982; Garattini 1982). Furthermore, the challenge procedure included discontinuation of theophylline shortly before the challenge and then accepting any fall in the PEFR of >20% during the day as the criteria for a positive challenge. In another equally unsatisfactory study, challenges with sodium glutamate 200 mg failed to provoke asthma in 17 adults with asthma who were selected on the basis of a history suggesting adverse reaction to food additives (Genton *et al.* 1985). The question of whether or not monosodium glutamate can provoke asthma in childhood has not been systematically studied.

urticaria   Double-blind challenges with monosodium glutamate were positive in three out of 36 children with chronic urticaria in one study (Supramanian & Warner 1986).

oro-facial granulomatosis   Double-blind challenge with monosodium glutamate confirmed that this provoked oro-facial granulomatosis in an 8-year old child (Sweatman *et al.* 1986). There is a further anecdotal report of partial improvement of this disorder associated with avoidance of monosodium glutamate in a 15-year-old girl (Oliver *et al.* 1991).

Nitrite   Sodium nitrite has reported to provoke urticaria or headache under double-blind placebo-controlled conditions in five subjects (Henderson & Raskin 1972; Moneret-Vautrin *et al.* 1980).

Papain   Papain is a proteolytic enzyme derived from full-grown but unripe papaya fruit. Commercial papain also contains chymopapain,

Table 37.2 Sources of exposure to papain[1]

Domestic
Papaya fruit and juice
Digestive aids
Vitamin compounds
Meat tenderizer
Toothpaste
Cosmetics (face creams, cleansers)

Medical treatment
Insect and jelly fish stings
Chemonucleolysis
Ulcers and necrotic tissue debridement

Occupational during manufacture of
Digestive aids
Meat tenderizer
Beer
Enzyme cleaners for soft lenses

[1] Modified from: Freye (1988).

lysozyme, papaya peptidase A, lipase and other constituents (Freye 1988). As well as being found in papaya fruit, papain is used to tenderize meat, in clarifying beer, and a number of domestic, medical and occupational settings (Table 37.2). Clinical sensitivity to papain is best recognized as asthma or rhinitis in adults exposed to papain at work (e.g. Tarlo *et al.* 1978). However angioedema and asthma have been documented to occur 20–30 min after ingestion of beef steak treated with a papain-containing tenderizer in a 31-year old man (Mansfield & Bowers 1983). Intolerance to papain has also been reported to cause palatal pruritus, conjunctivitis, sneezing, abdominal pain and diarrhoea (Mansfield *et al.* 1985).

Patent blue   Patent blue (E131) is a bluish-violet colouring agent. In an unsatisfactory study of chronic urticaria in adults, in which antihistamines were discontinued prior to challenges, and placebo challenges were performed before challenges with the test substances, patent blue failed to provoke urticaria in all 19 subjects studied (Michaëlsson & Juhlin 1973). In another unsatisfactory study in which placebo challenges were always given before challenges with the test substance, none of 10 patients with asthma or rhinitis (mainly adults) had an adverse reaction to patent blue (Rosenhall 1982).

Ponceau
urticaria   Ponceau (E124), also known as new coccine, is a red colouring agent and one of the azo dyes. In an unsatisfactory study of chronic urticaria in adults, in which antihistamines were discontinued prior to challenges, and placebo challenges were performed before challenges with the test substances, ponceau provoked adverse reactions in nine out of 25 patients (Michaëlsson & Juhlin 1973). In a non-placebo-controlled challenge study in which the degree of blinding was unclear, ponceau provoked adverse reactions in five out of 86 adults with chronic urticaria (Thune & Granholt 1975).

asthma and rhinitis   In a study of 45 adults with moderately severe perennial asthma, double-blind challenges with ponceau provoked significant bronchoconstriction (defined as >25% fall in FEV1) in one out of 45 subjects (Weber *et al.* 1979). In an unsatisfactory study in which placebo challenges were always given before challenges with the test substance, none of nine patients with asthma or rhinitis (mainly adults) had an adverse reaction to ponceau (Rosenhall 1982).

Quinoline yellow   Quinoline yellow is a mixture of the mono- and disulphonic acid salts of quinophthalone. E104 describes a mixture in which disulphonic acid predominates. In an open and uncontrolled challenge study of 91 mainly adults with chronic urticaria, Juhlin (1981) reported positive challenges with quinoline yellow in 13% of subjects.

Table 37.3 Content of sorbitol occurring naturally in fruits[1]

Edible portion	Sorbitol g/100 g
Apple	1.0
Apricot	1.0
Pear	2.4
Peach	0.2
Plum	2.8
Pyracantha berry	4.0
Rowan berry	8.7

[1] Source: Hardinge *et al.* (1965).

Sorbitol

Sorbitol is a sugar alcohol which occurs naturally in certain fruits (Table 37.3), which is poorly absorbed by the small intestine, and which may therefore produce an osmotic diarrhoea (Wick *et al.* 1951). Sorbitol may contribute to loose stools resulting from eating apples or pears (Hyams & Leichtner 1985; Hyams *et al.* 1988), although fructose malabsorption appears to be a more important cause of loose stools after fruit consumption and is present in greater quantities than sorbitol in fruit (Hardinge *et al.* 1965 and see chapter 31). However, the use of sorbitol as a sweetener in 'sugar-free' products may occasionally result in loose stools and colicky abdominal pain (Hyams 1982, 1983), and for this reason the product label may carry a warning about 'stomach upsets'.

Sunset yellow urticaria

Sunset yellow (E110) is a yellow colouring agent and one of the azo dyes. Double-blind challenges with sunset yellow were positive in 10 out of 36 children with chronic urticaria in one study (Supramaniam & Warner 1986), and in a child with oro-facial granulomatosis (Sweatman *et al.* 1986). Murdoch *et al.* (1987b) reported two adults with chronic urticaria in whom double-blind challenges with sunset yellow and other azo colours provoked adverse reactions. In an unsatisfactory study of adults with chronic urticaria, in which anti-histamines were discontinued prior to challenges, and placebo challenges were performed before challenges with the test substances, sunset yellow provoked urticaria in 10 out of 27 adults (Michaëlsson & Juhlin 1973). In a non-placebo-controlled challenge study in which the degree of blinding was unclear, sunset yellow provoked adverse reactions in 13 out of 86 adults with chronic urticaria (Thune & Granholt 1975).

asthma and rhinitis

In another unsatisfactory study in which placebo challenges were always given before challenges with the test substance, five out of 30 patients with asthma or rhinitis (mainly adults) had an adverse reaction to sunset yellow (Rosenhall 1982). However, in a study of

45 adults with moderately severe perennial asthma, double-blind challenges with sunset yellow failed to provoke significant broncho-constriction (defined as >25% fall in FEV1) in any subject (Weber *et al.* 1979).

reactions in AIDS Sunset yellow was reported to be responsible for adverse reactions (nausea and fever) to Septrin (co-trimoxazole) in patients with the acquired immune deficiency syndrome (AIDS). The patients tolerated intravenous Septrin, but when the oral preparation, which contained sunset yellow, was used, three patients developed fever and nausea (Lowen *et al.* 1987). Unfortunately, challenges with sunset yellow were not performed.

Tragacanth Gum tragacanth is derived from the shrub *Astragalus gummifer*, a member of the family of Leguminosae. Chemically, gum tragacanth is a complex polysaccharide. It is used in the food industry as a stabilizer and thickening agent for salad dressings, ice creams, sweets and sauces (Brouk 1975). It has also been used as an excipient in tablets (Brown *et al.* 1947). There are anecdotal reports of urticaria, angioedema, asthma and abdominal pain following ingestion of foods which contained gum tragacanth (Gelfand 1943, 1949; Brown *et al.* 1947; Danoff *et al.* 1978).

Key references 37.1 SUPRAMANIAM G & WARNER JO (1986) Artificial food additive intolerance in patients with angio-oedema and urticaria. *Lancet* **2**:907–909. *The key reference on intolerance to additives in children with urticaria.*

37.2 ALLEN DH (1991) Monosodium glutamate. In Metcalfe DD, Sampson HA & Simon RA (eds) *Food Allergy. Adverse Reactions to Foods and Food Additives*, pp. 261–266, Blackwell Scientific Publications, Boston. *Review.*

37.3 HYAMS JS, ETIENNE NL, LEICHTNER AM & THEUER RC (1988) Carbohydrate malabsorption following fruit juice ingestion in young children. *Pediatrics* **82**: 64–68. Breath hydrogen tests were performed in 13 healthy children and seven children with chronic non-specific diarrhoea; the results were the same for both groups. Increased breath hydrogen excretion was found after ingestion of pear juice (fructose 6.4 g/100 ml, sorbitol 2.0 g/100 ml) or 2% sorbitol solution in most subjects, after apple juice (fructose 6.4 g/100 ml, sorbitol 0.5 g/100 ml) in 50% of subjects, and after grape juice (fructose 7.5 g/100 ml, no sorbitol) in 25%. *The low proportion of subjects who reacted adversely to grape juice, despite the fact that it had the highest fructose concentration, suggests that the sorbitol content of apples and pears may contribute to the carbohydrate malabsorption that can be associated with the ingestion of these fruits and their juices.*

Summary 37 Amaranth, annatto, aspartame, carmoisine, erythrosine, indigo carmine, monosodium glutamate, papain, patent blue, ponceau, and sunset yellow have been reported to cause adverse reactions, mainly urticaria, although the supporting evidence is not always strong.

Monosodium glutamate, found in the greatest quantities in Chinese restaurant food, appears to be responsible for a poorly defined syndrome of a burning sensation, a sensation of pressure and substernal tightness, and may also provoke asthma. Papain, a constituent of papaya, but also used amongst other things as a meat tenderizer, can provoke urticaria, rhinitis, conjunctivitis, abdominal pain and diarrhoea. Sorbitol, used as a sweetener, is a potential cause of loose stools and abdominal pain. Tragacanth, a stabilizer and thickening agent, has been reported anecdotally to cause adverse effects such as urticaria, asthma and abdominal pain.

References to Chapters 33–37

ALDRIDGE RD, SMITH ME & MAIN RA (1984) Dyes and preservatives in oral antihistamines. *Br J Dermatol* **110**:351–355.

ALLEN DH, DELOHERY J & BAKER G (1987) Monosodium L-glutamate-induced asthma. *J Allergy Clin Immunol* **80**:530–537.

ANONYMOUS (1980) Tartrazine: a yellow hazard. *Drug Ther Bull* **18**:53–55

ASNES RS (1980) Chinese restaurant syndrome in an infant. *Clin Pediat* **19**:705–706.

BAKER GJ, COLLETT P & ALLEN DH (1981) Bronchospasm induced by metabisulphite-containing foods and drugs. *Med J Aust* **2**:614–617.

BANDMANN H-J, CALNAN CD, CRONIN E et al. (1972) Dermatitis from applied medicaments. *Arch Derm* **106**:335–337.

BERGNER T, PRZYBILLA B & RING J (1989) Anaphylactoid reaction to the coloring agent erythrosine in an antiallergic drug. *Allergy Clin Immunol News* **1**:177–179.

BETHEL RA, EPSTEIN J, SHEPPARD D, NADEL JA & BOUSHEY HA (1983) Sulfur dioxide-induced bronchoconstriction in freely breathing, exercising, asthmatic subjects. *Am Rev Respir Dis* **128**:987–990.

BROUK B (1975) *Plants Consumed by Man*, Academic Press, London.

BROWN EB & CREPEA SB (1947) Allergy (asthma) to ingested gum tragacanth. A case report. *J Allergy* **18**:214–215.

BUCKLEY CE, SALTZMAN HA & SIEKER HO (1985) The prevalence and degree of sensitivity to ingested sulfites (abstract). *J Allergy Clin Immunol* **75**:144.

BUCKNALL CE, NEILLY JB, CARTER R, STEVENSON RD & SEMPLE PF (1988) Bronchial hyperreactivity in patients who cough after receiving angiotensin converting enzyme inhibitors. *Br Med J* **296**:86–88.

BURGE PS, O'BRIEN IM, HARRIES MG & PEPYS J (1979) Occupational asthma due to inhaled carmine. *Clin Allergy* **9**:185–189.

BURNETT J (1985) *Plenty and Want. A Social History of Diet in England from 1815 to the present day*, Methuen, London.

BUSH RK, TAYLOR SL & BUSSE W (1986) A critical evaluation of clinical trials in reactions to sulfites. *J Allergy Clin Immunol* **78**:191–202.

CLEMMENSEN O & HJORTH N (1982) Perioral contact urticaria from sorbic acid and benzoic acid in a salad dressing. *Contact Dermatitis* **8**:1–6.

COLTATE TP (1984) *Food – the Chemistry of its Components*, The Royal Society of Chemistry, London.

COOPER DM, CUTZ E & LEVISON H (1977) Occult pulmonary abnormalities in asymptomatic asthmatic children. *Chest* **71**:361–365.

CRIEP LH (1971) Allergic vascular purpura. *J Allergy Clin Immunol* **48**:7–12.

DALLY MB, KURRLE S & BRESLIN ABX (1978) Ventilatory effects of aerosol gentamicin. *Thorax* **33**:54–56.

DALTON-BUNNOW MF (1985) Review of sulfite sensitivity. *Am J Hosp Pharm* **42**:2220–2226.

DANOFF D, LINCOLN L, THOMSON DMP & GOLD P (1978) 'Big Mac attack'. *New Engl J Med* **298**:1095–1096.

DAVID TJ (1987) Reactions to dietary tartrazine. *Arch Dis Child* **62**:119–122.

DAVID TJ (1988) Food additives. *Arch Dis Child* **63**:582–583.

DAVID TJ (1990) The unhealthy nature of health foods. *Mat Child Health* **15**: 228–230.

DELOHERY J, SIMMUL R, CASTLE WD & ALLEN DH (1984) The relationship of inhaled sulfur dioxide reactivity to ingested metabisulphite sensitivity in patients with asthma. *Am Rev Respir Dis* **130**:1027–1032.

DEVLIN J & DAVID TJ (1992) Tartrazine in atopic eczema. *Arch Dis Child* **67**: 709–711.

DIETEMANN-MOLARD A, BRAUN JJ, SOHIER B & PAULI G (1991) Extrinsic allergic alveolitis secondary to carmine. *Lancet* **338**:460.

EBERT AG (1982) Chinese-restaurant asthma. *New Engl J Med* **306**:1180.

EGAN H, KIRK RS & SAWYER R (1987) *Pearson's Chemical Analysis of Foods*, 8th edn, Longman Scientific & Technical, Harlow.

FAO/WHO FOOD ADDITIVES DATA SYSTEM (1985) *FAO Food & Nutrition Paper No. 30*, 1st Revision, Publications Division, Food and Agriculture Organisation of the United Nations, Rome.

FISHER AA, PASVHER F & KANOF NB (1971) Allergic contact dermatitis due to ingredients of vehicles. *Arch Derm* **104**:286–290.

FOOD ADDITIVES. THE BALANCED APPROACH (1987) Her Majesty's Stationery Office, London.

FOOD LABELLING REGULATIONS (1984) SI 1984/1305, In *Statutory Instruments 1984, Part II, Section II. Statutory instrument No. 1305*, Her Majesty's Stationery Office, London.

FRANK DR, AMDUR MO, WORCESTER J & WHITTENBERGER JL (1962) Effects of acute controlled exposure to SO_2 on respiratory mechanics in healthy male adults. *J Appl Physiol* **17**:252–258.

FREEDMAN BJ (1977) Asthma induced by sulphur dioxide, benzoate and tartrazine contained in orange drinks. *Clin Allergy* **7**:407–415.

FREYE HB (1988) Papain anaphylaxis: a case report. *Allergy Proc* **9**:571–574.

FRIEDMAN ME & EASTON JG (1987) Prevalence of positive metabisulphite challenges in children with asthma. *Pediat Asthma Allergy Immunol* **1**:53–59.

GARATTINI S (1982) Chinese-restaurant asthma. *New Engl J Med* **306**:1181.

GARRIGA MM, BERKEBILE C & METCALFE DD (1991) A combined single-blind, double-blind, placebo-controlled study to determine the reproducibility of hypersensitivity reactions to aspartame. *J Allergy Clin Immunol* **87**:821–827.

GELFAND HH (1943) The allergenic properties of the vegetable gums. A case of asthma due to tragacanth. *J Allergy* **14**:203–219.

GELFAND HH (1949) The vegetable gums by ingestion in the etiology of allergic disorders. *J Allergy* **20**:311–321.

GENTON C, FREI PC & PECOUD A (1985) Value of oral provocation tests to aspirin and food additives in the routine investigation of asthma and chronic urticaria. *J Allergy Clin Immunol* **76**:40–45.

GERBER JG, PAYNE NA, OEIZ O, NIES AS & OATES JA (1979) Tartrazine and the prostaglandin system. *J Allergy Clin Immunol* **63**:289–294.

GIBSON A & CLANCY R (1980) Management of chronic idiopathic urticaria by the identification and exclusion of dietary factors. *Clin Allergy* **10**:699–704.

GODFREY S (1983) Childhood asthma. In Clark TJH & Godfrey S (eds) *Asthma*, 2nd edn, pp. 415–456, Chapman & Hall, London.

GUNNISON AF & JACOBSEN DW (1987) Sulfite hypersensitivity. A critical review. *CRC Crit Rev Toxicol* **17**:185–214.

HABENICHT HA, PREUSS L & LOVELL RG (1983) Sensitivity to ingested metabisulphites: cause of bronchospasm and urticaria. *Immunol Allergy Pract* **5**: 243–245.

HARDINGE MG, SWARNER JB & CROOKS H (1965) Carbohydrates in foods. *J Am Dietet Ass* **46**:197–204.

HARIPARSAD D, WILSON N, DIXON C & SILVERMAN M (1984) Oral tartrazine challenge in childhood asthma: effect on bronchial reactivity. *Clin Allergy* **14**:81–85.

HARRIS JB (1986) (ed) *Natural Toxins. Animal, Plant, and Microbial*, Clarendon Press, Oxford.

HEDMAN SE & ANDERSON RGG (1984) Release of biological mediators by tartrazine from human leukocytes and polyps. *Acta Pharmacol Toxicol* **52**:153–154.

HENDERSON WR & RASKIN NH (1972) 'Hot-dog' headache: individual susceptibility to nitrite. *Lancet* **2**:1162–1163.

HYAMS JS (1982) Chronic abdominal pain caused by sorbitol malabsorption. *J Pediat* **100**:772–773.

HYAMS JS (1983) Sorbitol intolerance: an unappreciated cause of functional gastrointestinal complaints. *Gastroenterol* **84**:30–33.

HYAMS JS, ETIENNE NL, LEICHTNER AM & THEUER RC (1988) Carbohydrate malabsorption following fruit juice ingestion in young children. *Pediatrics* **82**:64–68.

HYAMS JS & LEICHTNER AM (1985) Apple juice. An unappreciated cause of diarrhea. *Am J Dis Child* **139**:503–505.

JACOBSEN DW, SIMON RA & SINGH M (1984) Sulfite oxidase deficiency and cobalamin protection in sulfite-sensitive asthmatics (SSA) (abstract). *J Allergy Clin Immunol* **73**:135.

JAMIESON DM, GUILL MF, WRAY BB & MAY JR (1985) Metabisulphite sensitivity: case report and literature review. *Ann Allergy* **54**:115–121.

JUHLIN L (1981) Recurrent urticaria: clinical investigation of 330 patients. *Br J Dermatol* **104**:369–381.

KAUPPINEN K, JUNTUNEN K & LANKI H (1984) Urticaria in children. Retrospective evaluation and follow-up. *Allergy* **39**:469–472.

KENNEY RA & TIDBALL CS (1972) Human susceptibility to oral monosodium L-glutamate. *Am J Clin Nutr* **25**:140–146.

KOCHEN J (1973) Sulfur dioxide, a respiratory tract irritant, even if ingested. *Pediatrics* **52**:145–146.

KOEHLER SM & GLAROS A (1988) The effect of aspartame on migraine headache. *Headache* **28**:10–13.

KOEPKE JW, CHRISTOPHER KL, CHAI H & SEINER JC (1984) Dose-dependent bronchospasm from sulfites in isoetharine. *J Am Med Ass* **251**:2982–2983.

KOEPKE JW & SELNER JC (1986) Combined monosodium glutamate (MSG)/ metabisulfite (MBS) induced asthma (abstract). *J Allergy Clin Immunol* **77** (suppl.):158.

KOEPKE JW, SELNER JC & DUNHILL AL (1983) Presence of sulfur dioxide in commonly used bronchodilator solutions. *J Allergy Clin Immunol* **72**:504–508.

KUBBA R & CHAMPION RH (1975) Anaphylactoid purpura caused by tartrazine and benzoates. *Br J Dermatol* **93** (suppl.):61–62.

KULCZYCKI A (1986) Aspartame-induced urticaria. *Ann Intern Med* **104**:207–208.

KWOK RHM (1968) Chinese-restaurant syndrome. *New Engl J Med* **278**:796.

LAHTI A & HANNUKSELA M (1981) Is benzoic acid really harmful in cases of atopy and urticaria? *Lancet* **2**:1055.

LEE M, GENTRY AF, SCHWARTZ R & BAUMAN J. (1981) Tartrazine-containing drugs. *Drug Intell Clin Pharm* **15**:782–788.

LINDSAY RC (1985) Food Additives. In Fennema OR (ed) *Food Chemistry*, 2nd edn, pp. 629–687, Marcel Dekker, New York.

LIPTON RB, NEWMAN LC, COHEN JS & SOLOMON S (1989) Aspartame as a dietary trigger of headache. *Headache* **29**:90–92.

LOCKEY SD (1959) Allergic reactions due to F D & C yellow no. 5 tartrazine, an aniline dye used as a coloring and identifying agent in various steroids. *Ann Allergy* **17**:719–721.

LOCKEY SD (1972) Sensitizing properties of food additives and other commercial products. *Ann Allergy* **30**:638–641.

LORENZETTI OJ & WERNET TC (1977) Topical parabens: benefits and risks. *Dermatologica* **154**:244–250.

LOWEN NP, MOXHAM J & McMANUS T (1987) Reactions to azo dyes in patients with AIDS. *Br Med J* **295**:612.

MANSFIELD LE & BOWERS CH (1983) Systemic reaction to papain in a non-occupational setting. *J Allergy Clin Immunol* **71**:371–374.

MANSFIELD LE, TING S, HAVERLEY RW & YOO TJ (1985) The incidence and clinical implications of hypersensitivity to papain in an allergic population, confirmed by blinded oral challenge. *Ann Allergy* **55**:541–543.

MARTIN LB, NORDLEE JA & TAYLOR SL (1986) Sulfite residues in restaurant salads. *J Food Protection* **49**:126–129.

MATHISON DA & STEVENSON DD (1979) Hypersensitivity to nonsteroidal anti-inflammatory drugs: indications and methods for oral challenge. *J Allergy Clin Immunol* **64**:669–674.

MICHAËLSSON G & JUHLIN L (1973) Urticaria induced by preservatives and dye additives in food and drugs. *Br J Dermatol* **88**:525–532.

MICHAËLSSON G & JUHLIN L (1974) Purpura caused by food and drug additives. *Arch Dermatol* **109**:49–52.

MIKKELSEN H, LARSEN JC & TARDING F (1978) Hypersensitivity reactions to food colours with special reference to the natural colour annatto extract (butter colour). *Arch Toxicol* (suppl. 1):141–143.

MINISTRY OF AGRICULTURE, FISHERIES AND FOOD (1987a) *Food Advisory Committee. Final report on the review of the colouring matter in food regulations* 1973, Her Majesty's Stationery Office, London.

MINISTRY OF AGRICULTURE, FISHERIES AND FOOD (1987b) *The use of the word 'natural' and its derivatives in the labelling, advertising and presentation of food. Report of a survey by the local authorities co-ordinating body on trading standards*, Her Majesty's Stationery Office, London.

MINISTRY OF AGRICULTURE, FISHERIES AND FOOD (1987c) *Mycotoxins. The eighteenth report of the Steering Group on Food Surveillance. The working party on naturally occurring toxicants in food: sub-group on mycotoxins.* Food Surveillance Paper No.18, Her Majesty's Stationery Office, London.

MONERET-VAUTRIN DA, BENE MC & FAURE G (1986) She should not have chewed. *Lancet* **1**:617.

MONERET-VAUTRIN DA, EINHORN C & TISSERAND J (1980) Le role du nitrite de sodium dans les urticaires histaminiques d'origine alimentaire. *Ann Nutr Alim* **34**:1125–1132.

MORICE AH, LOWRY R, BROWN MJ & HIGENBOTTAM T (1987) Angiotensin-converting enzyme and the cough reflex. *Lancet* **2**:1116–1118.

MURDOCH RD, POLLOCK I & NAEEM S (1987a) Tartrazine induced histamine release in vivo in normal subjects. *J Roy Coll Phys Lond* **21**:257–261.

MURDOCH RD, POLLOCK I, YOUNG E & LESSOF MH (1987b) Food additive-induced urticaria: studies of mediator release during provocation tests. *J Roy Coll Phys Lond* **4**:262–266.

NISH WA, WHISMAN BA, GOETZ DW & RAMIREZ DA (1991) Anaphylaxis to annatto dye: a case report. *Ann Allergy* **66**:129–131.

NORDLEE JA, NAIDU SG & TAYLOR SL (1988) False positive and false negative reactions encountered in the use of sulfite test strips for the detection of sulfite-treated foods. *J Allergy Clin Immunol* **81**:537–541.

NOVICK NL (1985) Aspartame-induced granulomatous panniculitis. *Ann Intern Med* **102**:206–207.

OLIVER AJ, RICH AM, READE PC, VARIGOS GA & RADDEN BG (1991) Mono-sodium glutamate-related orofacial granulomatosis. Review and case report. *Oral Surg Oral Med Oral Pathol* **71**:560–564.

POLLOCK I & WARNER JO (1987) A follow-up study of childhood food additive intolerance. *J Roy Coll Phys Lond* **21**:248–250.

POLLOCK I & WARNER JO (1990) Effect of artificial food colours on childhood behaviour. *Arch Dis Child* **65**:74–77.

POLLOCK I, YOUNG E, STONEHAM M, SLATER N, WILKINSON JD & WARNER JO (1989) Survey of colourings and preservatives in drugs. *Br Med J* **299**:649–651.

PRENNER BM & STEVENS JJ (1976) Anaphylaxis after ingestion of sodium bisulfite. *Ann Allergy* **37**:180–182

REYNOLDS JEF (1989) (ed) *Martindale. The Extra Pharmacopoeia*, 29th edn, Pharmaceutical Press, London.

ROSENHALL L (1982) Evaluation of intolerance to analgesics, preservatives and food colorants with challenge tests. *Eur J Respir Dis* **63**:410–419.

SAFFORD RJ & GOODWIN BJF (1984) The effect of tartrazine on histamine release from rat peritoneal mast cells. *Int J Immunopharmacol* **6**:233–240.

SCHIFFMAN SS, BUCKLEY CE, SAMPSON HA *et al.* (1987) Aspartame and susceptibility to headache. *New Engl J Med* **317**:1181–1185.

SCHLUMBERGER HD (1980) Drug-induced pseudo-allergic syndrome as exemplified by acetylsalicylic acid intolerance. In Dukor P, Kallos P, Schlumberger HD & West GB (eds) *PAR. Pseudo-Allergic Reactions. Involvement of Drugs and Chemicals*, vol.1, *Genetic Aspects and Anaphylactoid Reactions*, pp. 125–203, Karger, Basel.

SCHWARTZ HJ (1983) Sensitivity to ingested metabisulphite: variations in clinical presentation. *J Allergy Clin Immunol* **71**:487–489.

SETTIPANE GA (1986) Sulfites in drugs: a new comprehensive list. *New Engl Reg Allergy Proc* **7**:543–545.

SETTIPANE GA, CHAFEE FH, POSTMAN IM *et al.* (1976) Significance of tartrazine sensitivity in chronic urticaria of unknown etiology. *J Allergy Clin Immunol* **57**:541–546.

SETTIPANE GA & PUDUPAKKAM RK (1975) Aspirin intolerance. III. Subtypes, familial occurrence, and cross-reactivity with tartrazine. *J Allergy Clin Immunol* **56**:215–221.

SHEPPARD D, WONG WS, UEHARA CF, NADEL JA & BOUSHEY HA (1980) Lower threshold and greater bronchomotor responsiveness of asthmatic subjects to sulfur dioxide. *Am Rev Respir Dis* **122**:873–878.

SHER TH & SCHWARTZ HJ (1985) Bisulfite sensitivity manifesting as an allergic reaction to aerosol therapy. *Ann Allergy* **54**:224–226.

SIMON RA (1984) Adverse reactions to drug additives. *J Allergy Clin Immunol* **74**:623–630.

SIMON RA (1986) Sulfite sensitivity. *Ann Allergy* **56**:281–288.

SIMON RA (1987) Sulfite sensitivity. *Ann Allergy* **59**:100–105.

SIMON RA, GREEN L & STEVENSON DD (1982) The incidence of ingested metabisulphite sensitivity in an asthmatic population (abstract). *J Allergy Clin Immunol* **69**:118.

SIMON RA & WASSERMAN SI (1986) IgE mediated sulfite sensitive asthma. *J Allergy Clin Immunol* **77**:157.

SNELL RE & LUCHSINGER PC (1969) Effects of sulfur dioxide on expiratory flow rates and total resistance in normal human subjects. *Arch Environ Health* **18**:693–698.

SPECTOR SL, WANGAARD CH & FARR RS (1979) Aspirin and concomitant idiosyncrasies in adult asthmatic patients. *J Allergy Clin Immunol* **64**:500–506.

STEVENSON DD & SIMON RA (1981) Sensitivity to ingested metabisulphites in asthmatic subjects. *J Allergy Clin Immunol* **68**:26–32.

STEVENSON DD, SIMON RA, LUMRY WR & MATHISON DA (1986) Adverse reactions to tartrazine. *J Allergy Clin Immunol* **78**:182–191.

SUPRAMANIAM G & WARNER JO (1986) Artificial food additive intolerance in patients with angio-oedema and urticaria. *Lancet* **2**:907–909.

SWAN GF (1982) Management of monosodium glutamate toxicity. *J Asthma* **19**:105–110.

SWEATMAN MC, TASKER R, WARNER JO, FERGUSON MM & MITCHELL DN (1986) Oro-facial granulomatosis. Response to elemental diet and provocation by food additives. *Clin Allergy* **16**:331–338.

TARLO SM & BRODER I (1982) Tartrazine and benzoate challenge and dietary avoidance in chronic asthma. *Clin Allergy* **12**:303–312.

TARLO SM, SHAIKH W, BELL B *et al.* (1978) Papain-induced allergic reactions. *Clin Allergy* **8**:207–215.

TAYLOR RJ (1980) *Food Additives*, John Wiley, Chichester.

TAYLOR SL, HIGLEY NA & BUSH RK (1986) Sulfites in foods: uses, analytical methods, residues, fate, exposure assessment, metabolism, toxicity, and hypersensitivity. *Adv Food Chem* **30**:1–76.

TAYLOR SL, MARTIN LB & NORDLEE JA (1985) Detection of sulfite residues in restaurant salads (abstract). *J Allergy Clin Immunol* **75**:198.

THOMAS B (1988) (ed) *Manual of Dietetic Practice*, Blackwell Scientific Publications, Oxford.

THUNE P & GRANHOLT A (1975) Provocation tests with antiphlogistica and food additives in recurrent urticaria. *Dermatologica* **151**:360–367.

TIMBERLAKE CF (1989) Plant pigments for colouring food. *Br Nutr Found Nutrition Bull* **14**:113–125.

TOWNS SJ & MELLIS CM (1984) Role of acetyl salicylic acid and sodium metabisulphite in chronic childhood asthma. *Pediatrics* **73**:631–637.

TRAUTLEIN J, ALLEGRA J, FIELD J & GILLIN M (1976) Paradoxic bronchospasm after inhalation of isoproterenol. *Chest* **70**:711–714.

TSEVAT J, GROSS GN & DOWLING GP (1987) Fatal asthma after ingestion of sulfite-containing wine. *Ann Int Med* **107**:263.

TWAROG FJ & LEUNG DYM (1982) Anaphylaxis to a component of isoetharine (sodium bisulfite). *J Am Med Ass* **248**:2030–2031.

VAN BEVER HP, DOCX M & STEVENS WJ (1989) Food and food additives in severe atopic dermatitis. *Allergy* **44**:588–594.

VEDANTHAN PK, MENON MM, BELL TD & BERGIN D (1977) Aspirin and tartrazine oral challenge: incidence of adverse response in chronic childhood asthma. *J Allergy Clin Immunol* **60**:8–13.

VEIEN NK, HATTEL T, JUSTESEN O & NØRHOLM A (1987) Oral challenge with food additives. *Contact Derm* **17**:100–103.

VERBOV J (1985) Topical tartrazine as an unusual cause of nail staining. *Br J Dermatol* **112**:729.

WALKER R (1985) Sulphiting agents in foods: some risk/benefit considerations. *Food Additives & Contaminants* **2**:5–24.

WANDERER AA & SOLOMONS C (1987) Detection characteristics of a commercially available sulfite detection test (SULFITEST): problems with decreased sensitivity and false negative reactions. *Ann Allergy* **58**:41–44.

WARIN RJ & SMITH RJ (1976) Challenge test battery in chronic urticaria. *Br J Dermatol* **94**:401–406.

WARIN RP & SMITH RJ (1982) Role of tartrazine in chronic urticaria. *Br Med J* **284**:1443–1444.

WEBER RW, HOFFMAN M, RAINE DA & NELSON HS (1979) Incidence of bronchoconstriction due to aspirin, azo dyes, non-azo dyes, and preservatives in a population of perennial asthmatics. *J Allergy Clin Immunol* **64**:32–37.

WILLIAMS WR, PAWLOWICZ A & DAVIES BH (1989) Aspirin-like effects of selected food additives and industrial sensitizing agents. *Clin Exper Allergy* **19**:533–537.

WITEK TJ & SCHACHTER EN (1984) Detection of sulfur dioxide in bronchodilator aerosols. *Chest* **86**:592–594.

WOLF SI & NICKLAS RA (1985) Sulfite sensitivity in a 7 year old child. *Ann Allergy* **54**:420–423.

YOUNG E, PATEL S, STONEHAM M, RONA R & WILKINSON JD (1987) The prevalence of reaction to food additives in a survey population. *J Roy Coll Phys* **21**:241–247.

Part 9 Salicylate Intolerance

38 Aspirin and salicylate intolerance
Aspirin can provoke asthma, rhinitis and urticaria

Relevance? Intolerance to the drug aspirin, acetyl salicylic acid, is well described. The topic of aspirin and salicylate intolerance is included in this book because of the widely held but unsubstantiated belief that some people are intolerant to naturally occurring salicylates in food (Truswell 1985; Loblay & Swain 1986).

Naturally occurring salicylates Salicylates occur naturally in a wide variety of plant and bacterial species (Rainsford 1984 and Table 38.1). Saligenin occurs in willow and poplar trees. Methyl salicylate (oil of wintergreen) occurs in various species, ranging from trees (e.g. birch, myrtle and beech) to grasses (e.g. wheat, rye, sugar cane), legumes (e.g. peas, beans, clover) and exotic plants (e.g. Indian liquorice, teaberry and coffee). The reason why these and other salicylates (see Table 38.1) are produced in such abundance by plants is not clear.

Aspirin One of the first synthetic drugs, aspirin was first introduced into medical therapy in 1899, and the first example of intolerance to

Table 38.1 Some naturally occurring salicylates[1]

Compound	In
Salicyl alcohol (saligenin)	Poplar, willow bark and leaves
Salicylaldehyde	*Spirea* spp., *Filipendula* spp., e.g. meadowseet, bridal wreath
Methyl salicylate	Oils of wintergreen (*Gaultheria*), birch, myrtle, beech, wheat, rye, sugar cane, tea, coffee, cloves, olives, cassia, lily of the valley, *Camellia*, *Feijoa*, *Filipendula*, *Paederia*, *Parkia*, *Phellinus*, *Polygala*, *Primula*, *Theaceae* spp., and root beer
Salicylic acid	*Mycobacterium* spp., *Pseudomonas* spp.
3-Hydroxysalicylic acid	Coliform and other bacterial spp.
6-Methyl- and various	Ponerine ants, cashew nuts, *Pentaspadon* spp.
6-*N*-alkyl salicylic acids	*Chrysanthemum* spp.
2-Hydroxyacetophenone	*Chione glabra* (West Indies)

[1] Source: Rainsford (1984).

225

aspirin, consisting of urticaria, angioedema and respiratory distress, was reported 3 years later (Schlumberger 1980).

Aspirin toxicity

The main toxic effects of aspirin in therapeutic doses are gastro-intestinal symptoms (heartburn, epigastric pain, vomiting), gastro-intestinal bleeding (occult or frank blood loss), and renal disorders (cells, casts and albumin in the urine) (Laurence & Bennett 1980). The possibility that aspirin might be a contributory cause of Reye's syndrome led in 1986 to the withdrawal of aspirin as an antipyretic in children under 12 years of age in the UK (Hurwitz *et al.* 1985; Tarlow 1986). Few children now receive aspirin in the UK, although teething gels containing choline salicylate are still permitted. These toxic effects are not discussed further in this book, and this chapter is solely concerned with intolerance to aspirin and other salicylates.

Aspirin intolerance – ? three main types

Reports of aspirin intolerance can probably be classified into three categories.
1 Aspirin intolerance in asthma: this is probably an heterogeneous entity. Some cases just have exacerbations of asthma after ingestion of aspirin, while others in addition develop pan-respiratory tract inflammation.
2 Aspirin-provoked exacerbation of chronic urticaria.
3 Possibly a further entity of aspirin-induced acute urticaria-angioedema-anaphylaxis.

Aspirin intolerance – adults asthma, rhinitis

Aspirin intolerance is best known in adults with asthma, the intolerance being recognized most often in the third or fourth decades (Szczeklik 1987). The typical patient starts to experience intense rhinitis characterized by intermittent and profuse watery rhinorrhoea. Over a period of months, chronic nasal congestion appears and examination reveals nasal polyposis. Asthma and intolerance to aspirin develop later, and the patient gives a clear history of an attack of asthma, rhinorrhoea and sometimes con-junctivitis up to an hour after ingestion of aspirin. The asthma and nasal polyps run a protracted course even if aspirin is avoided (Chafee & Settipane 1974; Settipane *et al.* 1974; Settipane & Pudupakkam 1975; Spector & Wangaard 1979). Attacks of asthma precipitated by aspirin may be severe and even life-threatening (Picado *et al.* 1989).

cross-reactivity

Other analgesics which inhibit cyclo-oxygenase may also provoke bronchoconstriction in aspirin sensitive asthmatics (Szczeklik 1987). The analgesics which have been shown to cross-react in this way are indomethacin, fenoprofen, ibuprofen, naproxen, diclofenac, noramidopyrine, mefenamic acid, flufenamic acid, phenylbutazone, and paracetamol (Szczeklik *et al.* 1977; Szczeklik 1987; Settipane & Stevenson 1989). The non-steroidal anti-inflammatory compounds dextropropoxyphene, salicylamide, benzydamine and chloroquine do not inhibit the enzyme cyclo-oxygenase and have not been reported to provoke adverse reactions in asthmatics with aspirin intolerance (Szczeklik *et al.* 1977).

aspirin may also relieve asthma

Aspirin and other cyclo-oxygenase inhibitors have been reported to relieve asthma (Kordansky *et al.* 1978; Szczeklik *et al.* 1978) and rhinitis (Brooks & Karl 1988; Kumar *et al.* 1988) on occasions. The reason for this paradoxical reaction is unknown.

Chronic urticaria

Exacerbations of chronic urticaria and angioedema can be provoked or worsened by the ingestion of aspirin in certain patients. Challenge studies have demonstrated aspirin as a trigger factor in between 20% (Moore-Robinson & Warin 1967) and 40% (James & Warin 1970; Warin & Smith 1976) of adults with chronic urticaria. The incidence of aspirin intolerance appears to be lower in children with chronic urticaria. In a study of 43 children with chronic urticaria attending an allergy clinic, only one reacted adversely to a double-blind challenge with aspirin 100 mg (Supramaniam & Warner 1986). The effect of aspirin in chronic urticaria seems to depend on the activity of the disease. Aspirin can worsen pre-existing urticaria but does not induce eruptions in symptomless periods (James & Warin 1970; Szczeklik *et al.* 1977). Szczeklik *et al.* (1977) have claimed that other analgesics which inhibit cyclo-oxygenase can also provoke urticaria in at least some of these patients, but this requires confirmation. It is possible but unusual for a single patient to develop both asthma and urticaria following the ingestion of aspirin (Stevenson *et al.* 1982). The mechanism of aspirin intolerance is probably not the same in urticaria and asthma (Ameisen & Capron 1990; Pearson & Suarez-Mendez 1990).

Aspirin intolerance — childhood asthma

It has been shown in double-blind placebo-controlled challenge studies that aspirin intolerance can occur in children with asthma, although the incidence of aspirin intolerance is far from clear (see below).

Vedanthan (1977)

In a study of asthmatic children aged 10 to 17 years using double-blind placebo-controlled challenges, aspirin 600 mg provoked a decrease of the FEV1 exceeding two standard deviations of the mean group response to placebo in five of 54 (9%) children (Vedanthan *et al.* 1977). A further patient developed urticaria and a 30% decrease in the FEV1, a drop almost meeting the criteria for a positive reaction. In four of these five children the challenges with aspirin were repeated, with equal or greater decrements in the FEV1 in all four. These four children also underwent incremental challenges (1, 5, 15, 37.5, 75, 150 and 300 mg aspirin), and positive challenges occurred at 15 mg in three and 37.5 mg in the fourth.

Schuhl & Pereyra (1979)   In this study, 32 children with chronic asthma were challenged with 500 mg aspirin (Schuhl & Pereyra 1979). No patient had a greater than 8% reduction in the PEFR, and no other reactions such as rhinorrhoea, urticaria or conjunctival inflammation were seen.

Towns & Mellis (1984)   In this study of asthmatics aged 5 to 14 years, using single-blind challenges, aspirin 150 mg provoked a 20% decrease of the PEFR in six of 29 (21%) children (Towns & Mellis 1984). A diet which avoided all food additives, colouring agents, preservatives, cow's milk protein, and foods which contained salicylates, was employed for 2 weeks with no subjective or objective benefit.

Rachelefsky (1985)   In this study, the double-blind ingestion of aspirin 300 mg provoked a fall of over 30% in the FEV1 in 14 of 50 (28%) children (mean age 13 years) with chronic asthma (Rachelefsky *et al.* 1985). In all subjects the asthma was severe enough to require prophylaxis with cromoglycate or steroids; none had nasal polyps and none gave a history of aspirin intolerance.

Hydrocortisone   Worsening of asthma following the administration of intravenous hydrocortisone has been reported in some adults with asthma and aspirin intolerance (Partridge & Gibson 1978; Szczeklik *et al.* 1985). The mechanism is unclear, but other corticosteroids such as methylprednisolone, dexamethasone and betamethasone appear to be safe in such patients (Szczeklik *et al.* 1985). This rare adverse reaction to hydrocortisone is unrelated to the more common reaction to the phosphate radical in some preparations of injectable corticosteroids which can provoke vomiting, pruritus and paraesthesiae (Little & de Wardener 1962; Barltrop & Diba 1969; Snell 1969; Novak *et al.* 1976).

Nasal polyposis   Aspirin can provoke rhinorrhoea and the development of nasal polyps (Tan & Collins-Williams 1982). Polyposis appears to be less common in aspirin intolerant children (Yunginger *et al.* 1973) than adults, although this has not been systematically studied.

Other nasal effects   The nasal effects of aspirin in patients without aspirin intolerance are less clear. In one study, aspirin 900 mg caused a statistically significantly increased nasal resistance to airflow in 17 of 25 normal adult subjects (Jones *et al.* 1985). In contrast, however, in another study intranasal aspirin did not increase nasal airways resistance, and prior administration of intranasal aspirin or oral aspirin, sodium salicylate or indomethacin significantly inhibited nasal obstruction caused by nasal challenge with a ragweed extract (McLean *et al.* 1982).

Acute urticaria Acute urticaria can be a feature of aspirin intolerance in childhood. In one study of 618 normal children aged 2–16 years, there was a history of urticaria provoked by aspirin in two (Settipane *et al.* 1980).

Laryngeal oedema Two non-asthmatic adults have been anecdotally described in whom ingestion of aspirin was followed by hoarseness of the voice and laryngeal oedema (Hillerdal & Lindholm 1984).

Anaphylaxis Anaphylactic shock is a rare feature of aspirin intolerance (Szczeklik 1987).

Refractory period In 1976, Zeiss and Lockey (1976) observed a refractory period after ingestion of aspirin. After two doses of 300 mg aspirin on consecutive days, the patient experienced rhinitis, mild wheezing, and a fall of FEV1. The third dose of 300 mg aspirin on day 3 did not provoke any adverse symptoms. The refractory period, which lasted up to 72 hours, was repeatedly confirmed, and the finding has been confirmed by others (Bianco *et al.* 1977; Pleskow *et al.* 1982; Stevenson *et al.* 1982). The mechanism is unknown.

Hyposensitization As long ago as 1922, Widal *et al.* gave small but increasing doses to an aspirin intolerant patient. Eventually the patient could tolerate aspirin 600 mg, having previously reacted to only 100 mg of aspirin (Widal *et al.* 1922). Subsequent studies have shown that most if not all aspirin intolerant asthmatics can be rendered unresponsive to the effects of aspirin by the regular administration of aspirin. The effect only lasts a few days once aspirin is stopped (Pleskow *et al.* 1982; Kowalski *et al.* 1984), although longer-term benefit has been claimed (Sweet *et al.* 1990). This phenomenon is widely referred to in the medical literature as 'desensitization', although it is probably only a manifestation of the pharmacological refractory period and not the induction of immunological tolerance, in which one would expect the effect to be much longer lasting. Patients with proven aspirin intolerance who have been treated with regular administration of aspirin are then not only able to tolerate aspirin but all analgesics with anti-cyclo-oxygenase activity such as ibuprofen, naproxen and indomethacin (Pleskow *et al.* 1982; Kowalski *et al.* 1984). Similarly, patients with aspirin intolerance can be 'hyposensitized' by the regular administration of any of these non-steroidal anti-inflammatory agents (Pleskow *et al.* 1982). Studies of 'hypo-sensitization' have generally employed incremental doses (Kowalski *et al.* 1984), but it is unclear whether this is necessary. The same phenomenon of 'hyposensitization' has been reported to occur in some patients with urticaria provoked by aspirin (Asad *et al.* 1983, 1984).

Mechanisms

The cross-reaction between aspirin and other analgesics which inhibit cyclo-oxygenase, and the results of studies of plasma prosta-glandin levels before and after challenge and hyposensitization, all point to a pharmacological rather than an immunological mechanism for aspirin intolerance and hyposensitization (Asad *et al.* 1983, 1984, 1986, 1987). No correlation has been shown between aspirin intoler-ance and the degree of bronchial hyperreactivity (Kowalski *et al.* 1985), and aspirin intolerance is not confined to severe asthmatics. The recent report of a significantly reduced mean platelet glutathione peroxidase activity in patients with asthmatic reactions to aspirin suggests abnormal oxygen/peroxide metabolism as a final common pathway in aspirin-provoked asthma (Pearson & Suarez-Mendez 1990).

Sodium salicylate

Twelve patients with asthma known to be intolerant to aspirin were challenged with aspirin (acetylsalicylic acid) and sodium salicylate (Dahl 1980). The PEFR fell by more than 20% after aspirin (10 mg in two; 100 mg in 10) in all patients, but not after ingestion of sodium salicylate in doses up to 2000 mg. The author concluded that salts of salicylic acid, such as are found to occur naturally in food, need not be avoided in patients with aspirin intolerance.

Tartrazine

As a result of evidence from technically unsound studies such as one from Helsinki (Stenius & Lemola 1976), it was originally thought that in asthma aspirin intolerance was associated with tartrazine intolerance, but double-blind placebo-controlled studies have shown that this is not the case (Vedanthan *et al.* 1977; Weber *et al.* 1979 and see chapter 34). Nevertheless, a recent study has suggested that tartrazine, sodium benzoate, monosodium glutamate and sodium metabisulphite all have a similar effect to that of aspirin in their inhibition of thromboxane B2 formation by noradrenaline-activated platelets (Williams *et al.* 1989). If confirmed, this would suggest that the mechanism of intolerance to certain food additives and aspirin might share a common pathway.

Family history

Numerous familial examples of aspirin intolerance have been described, and these have been reviewed in detail by Schlumberger (1980). The mode of inheritance is unclear.

Food intolerance There is a single case report of a 14-year-old boy who developed mild local symptoms after eating peanuts, but who developed a life-threatening reaction after ingesting peanuts in combination with aspirin (Cant *et al.* 1984). The authors suggested that aspirin may have potentiated the effect of peanuts by increasing gastrointestinal absorption of intact peanut antigen. They warned that patients with a mild intolerance to a food could suffer a dangerous reaction if they take the offending food together with aspirin. If this is true it is surprising it has not already been reported. It is possible that the cause of the headache (presumably a viral infection) may have played some part in this patient's unusual reaction, although this was not considered in the published report. Further details of this interesting case are given in the key references below.

Salicylates in food Several authors have suggested that diets constructed to exclude foods which contain salicylates may induce prolonged remission of urticaria (Gibson & Clancy 1978; Swain *et al.* 1985a, b). However surveys of the salicylate content of foods, using high performance liquid chromatography, have demonstrated that these diets were based on scanty and inaccurate information about the salicylate content of foods (South 1976a, b, 1977, 1979; Swain *et al.* 1985a). By permitting the inclusion of foodstuffs rich in salicylates, these diets were illogical.

many foods contain salicylates In one study (South 1979), all 200 plants tested contained salicylate, and salicylate was even found in tap water. In another survey of 333 food items (Table 38.2), salicylate was found in most fruits, especially berries and dried fruit (Swain *et al.* 1985a). Vegetables showed a wide range of salicylate content. Some herbs and spices were found to have very high amounts of salicylate, for example curry powder, paprika, thyme, garam masala and rosemary. Among beverages, tea was found to contain substantial amounts of salicylate. Cereals, meat, fish and dairy products contained either undetectable or very small amounts of salicylate. The authors of this survey stated that salicylates in foods can precipitate acute urticaria and exacerbate chronic urticaria, but there is as yet no evidence from double-blind studies to support this claim.

cot death The suggestions that cot deaths can be caused by salicylate intolerance (Holborow 1980, 1987) are not supported by any evidence and are inconsistent with the epidemiological data.

behavioural problems Feingold, an American allergist, claimed that behavioural problems and personality disturbances in children dramatically improved after the use of a diet which excluded all foods containing salicylates

Table 38.2 Some foods with high natural salicylate content[1]

Food	Salicylate (mg/100 g)
Curry powder	218
Paprika (hot powder)	203
Dried thyme	183
Turmeric powder	76.4
Rosemary powder	68
Garam masala powder	66.8
Oregano powder	66
Worcestershire sauce	64.3
Cumin powder	45.0
Canella powder	42.6
Mustard powder	26
Aniseed powder	22.8
Dried sage	21.7
Cayenne powder	17.6
Cinnamon powder	15.2
Sultanas	7.80
Dill	6.9
Black pepper powder	6.2
Cloves (dry)	5.74
Allspice powder	5.2
Raspberries	5.14
Redcurrants	5.06
Ginger (fresh)	4.5
Almonds	3.0
Apricot	2.58
Oranges	2.39
Tea	1.9–6.4[2]
Honey	2.5–11.2[2]
Liquorice	7.96–9.78[2]

[1] Source: Swain *et al.* (1985).
[2] Salicylate content varies in different varieties of product.

as well as avoiding all artificial food additives (Feingold 1975). Subsequent studies focussed on the possible effects of food additives on childhood behaviour (see chapter 68), and there is no objective evidence to support Feingold's assertion of a harmful behavioural effect of foods which contain salicylate.

Acetylation   Aspirin is an acetylated carboxylic acid, but choline salicylate, diflunisal, magnesium salicylate, salicylamide, salicylate with magnesium salicylate, salsalate, and sodium salicylate are all non-acetylated (Brooks & Day 1991). It appears that it is the acetylated salicylates (Morris *et al.* 1985) which provoke the features of aspirin intolerance in asthmatics (Samter & Beers 1967, 1968; Samter 1977), although the weak inhibitor of cyclo-oxygenase salsalate and choline magnesium trisalicylate has occasionally been reported to provoke asthma in subjects with aspirin intolerance (Stevenson *et al.* 1990). There are at least seven naturally occurring salicylates in foods (Rainsford 1984), but these are not acetylated and therefore intolerance is not to be expected (Samter 1977).

Management
diagnosis

The diagnosis of aspirin intolerance can only be established by aspirin challenge (Szczeklik 1987). This is normally an oral challenge, but an inhalational challenge with a solution of lysine-aspirin is an alternative method (Phillips *et al.* 1989; Patriarca *et al.* 1991; Pawlowicz *et al.* 1991). Patients with aspirin intolerance and asthma should avoid not only aspirin but also other drugs which inhibit cyclo-oxygenase and which have not been proven safe by supervised provocation. There is a study which found that the weak inhibitor of cyclo-oxygenase, choline magnesium trisalicylate, could be safely given to adult asthmatics with aspirin intolerance (Szczeklik *et al.* 1989).

hyposensitization

An option which is more likely to be needed in adults than children, because they more commonly require regular analgesics, is so-called 'hyposensitization', which can be achieved by giving four to eight incremental doses of aspirin every 2–3 hours (Szczeklik 1987; Kowalski *et al.* 1984). Careful observation in hospital is essential. Aspirin is then administered at a daily dose of, for an adult, 600 mg. At the same time the patient should be able to ingest other anti-cyclo-oxygenase analgesics without adverse effects. It is doubtful whether long term administration of aspirin in this way helps the asthma. Szczeklik states that it does not (1987), but unpublished observations suggest that the regular administration of aspirin may reduce bronchial reactivity to histamine (Kowalski *et al.* 1985) in patients with asthma and aspirin intolerance. The major clinical benefit of regular aspirin administration is reported to be relief of rhinitis (Stevenson *et al.* 1982; Stevenson 1986). If treatment is interrupted for more than 5 days then the patient must not re-start aspirin without repeating the initial 'desensitization' procedure in hospital.

Key references 38.1

SCHLUMBERGER HD (1980) Drug-induced pseudo-allergic syndrome as exemplified by acetylsalicylic acid intolerance. In Dukor P, Kallos P, Schlumberger HD & West GB (eds) *PAR. Pseudo-Allergic Reactions*, vol. 1, *Genetic Aspects and Anaphylactoid Reactions*, pp. 125–203, Karger, Basel. *Major review of aspirin intolerance.*

38.2

STEVENSON DD (1984) Diagnosis, prevention, and treatment of adverse reactions to aspirin and nonsteroidal anti-inflammatory drugs. *J Allergy Clin Immunol* **74**:617–622. *Useful review.*

38.3   VEDANTHAN PK, MENON MM, BELL TD & BERGIN D (1977) Aspirin and tartrazine oral challenge: incidence of adverse response in chronic childhood asthma. *J Allergy Clin Immunol* **60**:8–13. In a study of asthmatic children aged 10–17 years using double-blind placebo-controlled challenges, aspirin 600 mg provoked a decrease of the FEV1 exceeding two standard deviations of the mean group response to placebo in five out of 54 (9%) children. A further patient developed urticaria and a 30% decrease in the FEV1, a drop almost meeting the criteria for a positive reaction. In four of these five children the challenges with aspirin were repeated, with equal or greater decrements in the FEV1 in all four. These four children also underwent incremental challenges (1, 5, 15, 37.5, 75, 150 and 300 mg aspirin), and positive challenges occurred at 15 mg in three and 37.5 mg in the fourth. Aspirin intolerance was not associated with intolerance to tartrazine.

38.4   PLESKOW WW, STEVENSON DD, MATHISON DA, SIMON RA, SCHATZ M & ZEIGER RS (1982) Aspirin desensitisation in aspirin-sensitive asthmatic patients: clinical manifestations and characterization of the refractory period. *J Allergy Clin Immunol* **69**:11–19. *A study of aspirin 'desensitization' and refractory period in 30 aspirin intolerant asthmatics.*

38.5   CANT AJ, GIBSON P & DANCY M (1984) Food hypersensitivity made life threatening by ingestion of aspirin. *Br Med J* **288**:755–756. A 14-year old boy experienced tingling and dryness of the lips and mouth followed by swelling of the lips and face with a sensation of choking in the throat every time he ate peanuts. The signs and symptoms passed off within 5 min. He had taken aspirin on several previous occasions without ill effects. One day he took aspirin 300 mg for a headache, and 5 min later ate some cake containing peanuts. He suffered his usual reaction to peanuts and within 5 min was fully recovered. 30 min later he developed generalized pruritus, a choking sensation, and shortness of breath. On admission to hospital he was unconscious, cyanosed and covered in an urticarial rash. He was given intravenous adrenaline, aminophylline, hydrocortisone, chlorpheniramine and sodium bicarbonate, and 45 min after admission he was asymptomatic. *The authors point out that animal experiments have shown that aspirin greatly increases the absorption of substances with molecular weights of up to 70 000, and that this change in permeability may permit the development of anaphylaxis to molecules normally too large to cross the gastric mucosa.*

Summary 38   Aspirin can provoke bronchoconstriction in up to 30% of children with asthma. Administration of one or two doses of aspirin to such patients causes a refractory period of about 3 days, during which further doses of aspirin cause little or no symptoms. There is an association between asthma, aspirin intolerance and nasal polyposis. Aspirin can also provoke acute urticaria and can aggravate chronic urticaria, although the incidence of aspirin intolerance in childhood urticaria is unknown. The mechanism of aspirin intolerance in asthmatics is unknown, but other cyclo-oxygenase inhibitors such as indomethacin or ibuprofen provoke symptoms in asthmatics with aspirin intolerance. The management is to avoid aspirin. Where the patient with asthma and aspirin intolerance requires regular aspirin or other analgesics which inhibit cyclo-oxygenase (e.g. for the treatment of arthritis) then the regular administration of a daily dose of aspirin should lead to tolerance to all cyclo-oxygenase inhibitors.

References to Chapter 38

AMIESEN JC & CAPRON A (1990) Aspirin-sensitive asthma. *Clin Exper Allergy* **20**:127–129.

ASAD SI, KEMENY DM, YOULTEN LJF, FRANKLAND AW & LESSOF MH (1984) Effect of aspirin in 'aspirin sensitive' patients. *Br Med J* **288**:745–748.

ASAD SI, MURDOCH R, YOULTEN LJF & LESSOF MH (1987) Plasma level of histamine in aspirin-sensitive urticaria. *Ann Allergy* **59**:219–222.

ASAD SI, YOULTEN LJF, HOLGATE ST & LESSOF MH (1986) Clinical and biochemical aspects of 'aspirin-sensitivity'. *New Engl Reg Allergy Proc* **7**:105–108.

ASAD SI, YOULTEN LJF & LESSOF MH (1983) Specific desensitisation in 'aspirin-sensitive' urticaria; plasma prostaglandin levels and clinical manifestations. *Clin Allergy* **13**:459–466.

BARLTROP D & DIBA YT (1969) Paraesthesia after intravenous Efcortesol. *Lancet* **1**:529–530.

BIANCO S, ROBUSCHI M, PETRIGNI G & ALLEGRA L (1977) Respiratory effects due to aspirin (ASA): ASA-induced tolerance in ASA-asthmatic patients. *Bull Eur Physiopath Resp* **13**:123–124.

BROOKS PM & DAY RO (1991) Nonsteroidal antiinflammatory drugs – differences and similarities. *New Engl J Med* **324**:1716–1725.

BROOKS CD & KARL KJ (1988) Hay fever treatment with combined antihistamine and cyclooxygenase-inhibiting drugs. *J Allergy Clin Immunol* **81**:1110–1117.

CANT AJ, GIBSON P & DANCY M (1984) Food hypersensitivity made life threatening by ingestion of aspirin. *Br Med J* **288**:755–756.

CHAFEE FH & SETTIPANE GA (1974) Aspirin intolerance. I. Frequency in an allergic population. *J Allergy Clin Immunol* **53**:193–199

CHUDWIN DS, STRUB M, GOLDEN HE, FREY C, RICHMOND GW & LUSKIN AT (1986) Sensitivity to non-acetylated salicylates in a patient with asthma, nasal polyps, and rheumatoid arthritis. *Ann Allergy* **57**:133–134.

DAHL R (1980) Sodium salicylate and aspirin disease. *Allergy* **35**:155–156.

FEINGOLD BF (1975) *Why Your Child Is Hyperactive*, Random House, New York.

GIBSON AR & CLANCY RL (1978) An Australian exclusion diet. *Med J Aust* **1**:290–292.

HILLERDAL G & LINDHOLM H (1984) Laryngeal edema as the only symptom of hypersensitivity to salicylic acid and other substances. *J Laryngol Otol* **98**:547–548.

HOLBOROW PL (1980) Sudden infant death syndrome. *Am J Clin Nutr* **33**:730–731.

HOLBOROW PL (1987) Salicylate hypersensitivity and cot death. *New Zealand Med J* **100**:536.

HURWITZ ES, BARRETT MJ, BREGMAN D *et al.* (1985) Public health service study on Reye's syndrome and medications. Report of the pilot phase. *New Engl J Med* **313**:849–857.

JAMES J & WARIN RP (1970) Chronic urticaria: the effect of aspirin. *Br J Dermatol* **82**:204–205.

JONES AS, LANCER JM, MOIR AA & STEVENS JC (1985) Effect of aspirin on nasal resistance to airflow. *Br Med J* **290**:1171–1172.

KORDANSKY D, ADKINSON NF, NORMAN PS & ROSENTHAL RR (1978) Asthma improved by nonsteroidal anti-inflammatory drugs. *Ann Int Med* **88**:508–511.

KOWALSKI ML, GRZELEWSKA-RZYMOWSKA I, ROZNIECKI J & SZMIDT M (1984)

Aspirin tolerance induced in aspirin-sensitive asthmatics. *Allergy* **39**:171–178.

KOWALSKI ML, GRZELEWSKA-RZYMOWSKA I, SZMIDT M & ROZNIECKI J (1985) Bronchial hyperreactivity to histamine in aspirin sensitive asthmatics: relationship to aspirin threshold and effect of aspirin desensitisation. *Thorax* **40**:598–602.

KUMAR P, BRYAN C, HWANG D, KADOWITZ P, BUTCHER B & LEECH SH (1988) Allergic rhinitis relieved by aspirin and other nonsteroidal antinflammatory drugs. *Ann Allergy* **60**:419–422.

LAURENCE DR & BENNETT PN (1980) *Clinical Pharmacology*, 5th edn, Churchill Livingstone, Edinburgh.

LITTLE PJ & DE WARDENER HE (1962) The use of prednisolone phosphate in the diagnosis of pyelonephritis in man. *Lancet* **1**:1145–1149.

LOBLAY RH & SWAIN AR (1985) Food intolerance. In Wahlqvist ML & Truswell AS (eds) *Recent Advances in Clinical Nutrition*, vol. 2, pp. 169–177, John Libbey, London.

MCLEAN J, MATHEWS K & BANAS J (1982) Effects of aspirin on nasal responses to ragweed in atopic subjects. *J Allergy Clin Immunol* **69**:118.

MOORE-ROBINSON M & WARIN RP (1967) Effect of salicylates in urticaria. *Br Med J* **4**:262–264.

MORRIS HG, SHERMAN NA, MCQUAIN C, GOLDLUST MB, CHANG SF & HARRISON LI (1985) Effects of salsalate (nonacetylated salicylate) and aspirin on serum prostaglandins in humans. *Ther Drug Monitor* **7**:435–438.

NOVAK E, GILBERTSON TJ, SECKMAN CE, STEWART RD, DISANTO AR & STUBBS SS (1976) Anorectal pruritus after intravenous hydrocortisone sodium succinate and sodium phosphate. *Clin Pharmacol Ther* **20**:109–112.

PARTRIDGE MR & GIBSON GJ (1978) Adverse bronchial reactions to intravenous hydrocortisone in two aspirin-sensitive asthmatic patients. *Br Med J* **1**:1521–1522.

PATRIARCA G, NUCERA E, DIRIENZO V, SCHIAVINO D, PELLEGRINO S & FAIS G (1991) Nasal provocation test with lysine acetylsalicylate in aspirin-sensitive patients. *Ann Allergy* **67**:60–62.

PAWLOWICZ A, WILLIAMS WR & DAVIES BH (1991) Inhalation and nasal challenge in the diagnosis of aspirin-induced asthma. *Allergy* **46**:405–409.

PEARSON DJ & SUAREZ-MENDEZ VJ (1990) Abnormal platelet hydrogen peroxide metabolism in aspirin hypersensitivity. *Clin Exper Allergy* **20**:157–163.

PHILLIPS GD, FOORD R & HOLGATE ST (1989) Inhaled lysine-aspirin as a bronchoprovocation procedure in aspirin-sensitive asthma: its repeatability, absence of a late-phase reaction, and the role of histamine. *J Allergy Clin Immunol* **84**:232–241.

PICADO C, CASTILLO JA, MONTSERRAT JM & AGUSTI-VIDAL A (1989) Aspirin-intolerance as a precipitating factor of life-threatening attacks of asthma requiring mechanical ventilation. *Eur Respir J* **2**:127–129.

PLESKOW WW, STEVENSON DD, MATHISON DA, SIMON RA, SCHATZ M & ZEIGER RS (1982) Aspirin desensitisation in aspirin-sensitive asthmatic patients: clinical manifestations and characterization of the refractory period. *J Allergy Clin Immunol* **69**:11–19.

RACHELEFSKY GS, COULSON A, SIEGEL SC & STIEHM ER (1975) Aspirin intolerance in chronic childhood asthma: detected by oral challenge. *Pediatrics* **56**:443–448.

RAINSFORD KD (1984) *Aspirin and the Salicylates*, Butterworths, London.

SAMTER M (1977) Aspirin, salicylates, and the magic of diets. *Cutis* **20**:18, 24 & 52.

SAMTER M & BEERS RF (1967) Concerning the nature of intolerance to aspirin. *J*

Allergy **40**:281–293.

SAMTER M & BEERS RF (1968) Intolerance to aspirin. Clinical studies and consideration of its pathogenesis. *Ann Int Med* **68**:975–983.

SCHLUMBERGER HD (1980) Drug-induced pseudo-allergic syndrome as exemplified by acetylsalicylic acid intolerance. In Dukor P, Kallos P, Schlumberger HD & West GB (eds) *PAR. Pseudo-Allergic Reactions*, vol. 1, *Genetic Aspects and Anaphylactoid Reactions*, pp. 125–203, Karger, Basel.

SCHUHL JF & PEREYRA JG (1979) Oral acetylsalicylic acid (aspirin) challenge in asthmatic children. *Clin Allergy* **9**:83–88.

SETTIPANE GA, CHAFEE FH & KLEIN DE (1974) Aspirin intolerance. II. A prospective study in an atopic and normal population. *J Allergy Clin Immunol* **53**:200–204

SETTIPANE GA & PUDUPAKKAM RK (1975) Aspirin intolerance. III. Subtypes, familial occurrence, and cross-reactivity with tartrazine. *J Allergy Clin Immunol* **56**:215–221.

SETTIPANE RA, CONSTANTINE HP & SETTIPANE GA (1980) Aspirin intolerance and recurrent urticaria in normal adults and children. *Allergy* **35**:149–154.

SETTIPANE RA & STEVENSON DD (1989) Cross sensitity with acetaminophen in aspirin-sensitive subjects with asthma. *J Allergy Clin Immunol* **84**:26–33.

SNELL ES (1969) Paraesthesia after intravenous Efcortesol. *Lancet* **1**:530.

SOUTH MA (1976a) The so-called 'salicylate-free diet'. *Cutis* **18**:183.

SOUTH MA (1976b) The so-called salicylate-free diet: part II. *Cutis* **18**:332, 339.

SOUTH MA (1977) The so-called salicylate-free diet: part III. *Cutis* **19**:23, 35.

SOUTH MA (1979) The so-called salicylate-free diet: one more time. *Cutis* **24**:488, 494.

SPECTOR SL, WANGAARD CH & FARR RS (1979) Aspirin and concomitant idiosyncrasies in adult asthmatic patients. *J Allergy Clin Immunol* **64**:500–506.

STENIUS BSM & LEMOLA M (1976) Hypersensitivity to acetylsalicylic acid (ASA) and tartrazine in patients with asthma. *Clin Allergy* **6**:119–129.

STEVENSON DD (1986) Aspirin desensitization. *New Engl Reg Allergy Proc* **7**: 101–104.

STEVENSON DD, HOUGHAM AJ, SCHRANK PJ, GOLDLUST B & WILSON RR (1990) Salsalate cross-sensitivity in aspirin-sensitive patients with asthma. *J Allergy Clin Immunol* **86**:749–758.

STEVENSON DD, PLESKOW WW, CURD JG, SIMON RA & MATHISON DA (1982) Desensitisation to acetylsalicylic acid (ASA) in ASA-sensitive patients with rhinosinusitis/asthma. In Dukor P, Kallos P, Schlumberger HD & West GB (eds), *PAR. Pseudo-Allergic Reactions*, vol. 3, *Cell Mediated Reactions. Miscellaneous Topics*, pp. 133–156, Karger, Basel.

SUPRAMANIAM G & WARNER JO (1986) Artificial food additive intolerance in patients with angio-oedema and urticaria. *Lancet* **2**:907–909.

SWAIN AR, DUTTON SP & TRUSWELL AS (1985a) Salicylates in foods. *J Am Dietet Ass* **85**:950–960.

SWAIN A, SOUTTER V, LOBLAY R & TRUSWELL AS (1985b) Salicylates, oligo-antigenic diets, and behaviour. *Lancet* **2**:41–42.

SWEET JM, STEVENSON DD, SIMON RA & MATHISON DA (1990) Long-term effects of aspirin desensitization – treatment for aspirin-sensitive rhinosinusitis-asthma. *J Allergy Clin Immunol* **85**:59–65.

SZCZEKLIK A (1987) Adverse reactions to aspirin and nonsteroidal anti-inflammatory drugs. *Ann Allergy* **59**:113–118.

SZCZEKLIK A, DWORSKI R & NIZANKOWSKA E (1989) Choline magnesium tri-salicylate in patients with aspirin-induced asthma (abstract). *J Allergy Clin Immunol* **83**:178.

SzCZEKLIK A, GRYGLEWSKI RJ & CZERNIAWSKA-MYSIK G (1977) Clinical patterns of hypersensitivity to nonsteroidal anti-inflammatory drugs and their pathogenesis. *J Allergy Clin Immunol* **60**:276–284.

SzCZEKLIK A, GRYGLEWSKI RJ & NIZANKOWSKA E (1978) Asthma relieved by aspirin and by other cyclo-oxygenase inhibitors. *Thorax* **33**:664–665.

SzCZEKLIK A, NIZANKOWSKA E, CZERNIAWSKA-MYSIK G & SEK S (1985) Hydrocortisone and airflow impairment in aspirin-induced asthma. *J Allergy Clin Immunol* **76**:530–536

TAN Y & COLLINS-WILLIAMS C (1982) Aspirin-induced asthma in children. *Ann Allergy* **48**:1–5.

TARLOW M (1986) Reye's syndrome and aspirin. *Br Med J* **292**:1543–1544.

TOWNS SJ & MELLIS CM (1984) Role of acetyl salicylic acid and sodium metabisulfite in chronic childhood asthma. *Pediatrics* **73**:631–637.

TRUSWELL AS (1985) Food sensitivity. *Br Med J* **291**:951–955.

VEDANTHAN PK, MENON MM, BELL TD & BERGIN D (1977) Aspirin and tartrazine oral challenge: incidence of adverse response in chronic childhood asthma. *J Allergy Clin Immunol* **60**:8–13.

WARIN RP & SMITH RJ (1976) Challenge test battery in chronic urticaria. *Br J Dermatol* **94**:401–406.

WEBER RW, HOFFMAN M, RAINE DA & NELSON HS (1979) Incidence of bronchoconstriction due to aspirin, azo dyes, non-azo dyes, and preservatives in a population of perennial asthmatics. *J Allergy Clin Immunol* **64**:32–37.

WIDAL F, ABRAMI P & LERMOYEZ J (1922) Anaphylaxie et idiosyncrasie. *Presse Med* **30**:189–193

WILLIAMS WR, PAWLOWICZ A & DAVIES BH (1989) Aspirin-like effects of selected food additives and industrial sensitizing agents. *Clin Exper Allergy* **19**:533–537.

YUNGINGER JW, O'CONNELL EJ & LOGAN GB (1973) Aspirin-induced asthma in children. *J Pediat* **82**:218–221.

ZEISS CR & LOCKEY RF (1976) Refractory period to aspirin in a patient with aspirin-induced asthma. *J Allergy Clin Immunol* **57**:440–448.

Part 10 Investigations

39 Inherent difficulties
The impossible challenge

Multiple mechanisms   Food intolerance is an heterogeneous disorder caused by a variety of different immunological and pharmacological mechanisms. In any individual case, the precise mechanism is often not known. It is unreasonable to expect any single type of laboratory test to cover all possible mechanisms of food intolerance.

Prediction of outcome   In many situations (e.g. atopic disease), the patient wants to know whether there will be any benefit from food avoidance (e.g. not drinking milk or not eating tomatoes). Even if there were valid tests for the diagnosis of food intolerance, the outcome of avoidance measures depends on a number of other variables. Allergen avoidance may succeed for the following reasons:
1 the patient was intolerant to the item;
2 coincidental improvement;
3 placebo response.

The reasons why food avoidance may fail can be summarized as follows.
1 The patient is not intolerant to the food.
2 The period of elimination was too short, for example, where a child has an enteropathy due to food intolerance, it may take a week or more for improvement in symptoms to occur.
3 The food has been incompletely avoided. This may happen in a child supposed to be on a cow's milk protein-free diet who still continues to receive food which contains, for example casein or whey.
4 The patient is intolerant to other items which have not been avoided. For example, a child with cow's milk protein intolerance who fails to improve when given a soya-based milk to which he or she is also intolerant.
5 Co-existing or intercurrent disease, for example gastroenteritis in a child with loose stools who is trying a cow's milk free diet.
6 The patient's symptoms are trivial and have been exaggerated, or alternatively do not exist at all and have either been imagined or fabricated by the parents.

It is obviously unrealistic to expect there to be a test which can circumvent all these problems.

241

Provocation tests

A provocation test may be useful to confirm a history of allergy. An example might be a child who developed angioedema minutes after eating a rusk which contained wheat and cow's milk protein. To determine which component, if any, caused the reaction, oral challenges with individual components can be conducted. However, provocation tests cannot prove that improvement in a disease has been caused by food avoidance. For example, a child with atopic eczema is put on a diet avoiding many foods, and the eczema improves. The improvement could be a coincidence, it could be a placebo effect, or it could be due to the diet. Neither a positive nor a negative single food challenge will prove that avoidance of the food was the cause of the improvement.

Are investigations any use?

Given the near impossible nature of the challenge to find simple or reliable tests for food intolerance, the following chapters will examine various investigations, their limitations and their possible uses.

Summary 39

The heterogeneous nature of food intolerance, and the multiple reasons why allergen avoidance may succeed or fail, impose severe limitations on the usefulness of currently available tests for food intolerance.

40 Indices of diagnostic performance
How to measure usefulness

Measure of usefulness

This chapter briefly describes the various terms used to describe the potential usefulness of tests. The principle is to compare the test in question with some accepted diagnostic standard. One difficulty in the field of food intolerance is the lack of any such reliable standard. For the purposes of illustration in this chapter, we will take the skin-prick test as the test under study, and relate the results of skin testing to those of provocation tests. The following terms are used:

True positive, true negative, false positive and false negative

True positive (TP), true negative (TN), false positive (FP) and false negative (FN) are used in terms of supposed clinical relevance. In other words, a false positive skin test is associated with a negative provocation test, and a false negative skin test is associated with a positive provocation test. The implicit assumption, that provocation test results indicate a clinically relevant intolerance, is unfortunately not necessarily true (see chapter 47), and this reduces the usefulness of these terms in the context of food intolerance.

Sensitivity and specificity
Sensitivity and specificity are statistical measures of how well a diagnostic test correctly identifies confirmed cases of a disease.

sensitivity
Sensitivity is the ability of a test to identify a condition when it is really present. In the context of tests for food intolerance, if one equates a positive provocation test with clinically relevant intolerance (not necessarily true – see chapter 47) then sensitivity is defined as the number of positive provocation tests correctly identified by a positive skin test (TP) divided by the total number of positive provocation tests (TP + FN).

specificity
Specificity is the ability of a test to identify the absence of a condition when the condition really is not present. In the context of tests for food intolerance, this is defined as the number of negative provocation tests correctly identified by skin tests (TN) divided by the total number of negative provocation tests (TN + FP).

Predictive accuracy
Although determining the sensitivity and specificity of a diagnostic test allows one to evaluate how well a test can identify a known condition, the clinician is in practice concerned with something different. One needs to know how likely a patient is to have clinical food intolerance if the test is positive, and, conversely, how likely a patient is to have no intolerance if the test is negative. Predictive accuracies indicate how likely an individual is to have a disorder, given the result of the diagnostic test.

positive predictive accuracy
Positive predictive accuracy is defined as the number of positive provocation tests correctly identified by skin test divided by the total number of positive skin tests.

negative predictive accuracy
Negative predictive accuracy is defined as the number of negative provocation tests correctly identified by skin test divided by the total number of negative skin tests.

predictive accuracies depend upon prevalence of disorder
Predictive accuracies are highly dependent on the prevalence of the disorder in the population under study. For example, the higher the prevalence of a specific food intolerance in a study group, the better the positive predictive accuracy will be. Conversely, the lower the prevalence, the better the negative predictive accuracy will appear (Sampson & Albergo 1984; Sampson 1988). As Sampson & Albergo (1984) pointed out, a skin test for egg might have a positive predictive accuracy of 61% in a population with a prevalence of egg

intolerance of 37%, but if one applies the same test to a population where the prevalence of egg intolerance is only 1%, a rate more likely to be observed in a general paediatric population, the positive predictive accuracy would be 0.026. In other words, the likelihood that a patient with a positive skin test has clinically significant egg intolerance will be less than 3%.

Efficiency Efficiency is defined as the number of tested individuals correctly classified by the test as a percentage of all who were tested.

$$\text{Efficiency} = \frac{\text{TP} + \text{TN}}{\text{TP} + \text{FP} + \text{TN} + \text{FN}}$$

Key reference 40.1 METCALFE DD & SAMPSON HA (1990) (eds) Workshop on experimental methodology for clinical studies of adverse reactions to food and food additives. *J Allergy Clin Immunol* **86**:421–442. *Includes useful discussion of sensitivity/specificity analyses as applied to food intolerance.*

Summary 40 The terms true positive, false positive, true negative, false negative, sensitivity, specificity, efficiency, and positive and negative predictive accuracy are terms used to define the potential usefulness of tests. The principle is to compare the test in question with some accepted standard, and the difficulty in the field of food intolerance is the lack of any such reliable standard.

41 Skin tests
Major problems; in practice not very helpful

Principle The principle of skin tests is that the skin weal and flare reaction to an allergen demonstrates the presence of mast-cell-fixed antibody. This is mainly IgE antibody, although in theory it could also be IgG4 antibody (Bernstein, 1988). IgE is produced in plasma cells distributed primarily in lymphoid tissue in the respiratory and gastrointestinal tract, and is distributed in the circulation to all parts of the body, so that sensitization is generalized and therefore can be demonstrated by skin testing.

Antihistamines
H1-receptor antagonists Drugs with H1-receptor antagonist properties (e.g. antihistamines and tricyclic antidepressants) suppress the histamine-induced weal

and flare response of a skin test. The suppressive effect of traditional antihistamines (e.g. chlorpheniramine) may last up to a week or more (Cook *et al.* 1973). However, more recent non-sedating antihistamines have a much longer suppressive action (Almind *et al.* 1988), so that astemizole, for example, has been shown to have suppressive action for 5 months or more (Wyse 1987).

H2-receptor antagonists H2-receptor antagonists (e.g. ranitidine) partially suppress skin test reactivity (Miller & Nelson 1989).

steroids Systemic steroids do not reduce the response to skin tests, but local applications of potent topical steroids markedly suppress the skin test response (Andersson & Pipkorn 1987; Dreborg 1989).

Allergen extracts These used to comprise extracts of an allergen, diluted with phosphate-buffered saline, with 0.4% phenol added to prevent bacterial growth. However aqueous extracts are unstable, and 50% glycerol or 0.03% human serum albumin is added to prevent allergen degradation (Bousquet 1988). These extracts are suitable for prick or scratch tests, but glycerol is irritating if injected, so for intradermal testing aqueous extracts stabilized by human serum albumin are more suitable. The major problems of variable quality and biological potency of different extracts are beyond the scope of this book, and have been described elsewhere (Aas & Belin 1972; Aas *et al.* 1978; Lessof *et al.* 1980; Hillas & Wilson, 1981; Bjorksten *et al.* 1984; Bousquet 1988).

Control solutions Because of the variability of cutaneous reactivity, it is necessary to include positive and negative controls whenever performing skin tests. The negative control solution consists of the diluent used to preserve the allergen extracts. The positive control solution usually contains histamine 1–10 mg/ml (0.1 mg/ml for intradermal tests), and is mainly used to detect suppression of reactivity, for example caused by H1-receptor antagonists. It has been suggested that compound 48/80, a histamine-releasing agent (Voorhorst & Nikkels 1977), might be preferable for a positive control. The argument is that when a skin reaction to an allergen is at its peak (12–15 min after testing) the reaction to histamine has already passed its prime (maximal at 8 min); the reaction to compound 48/80 peaks at 10–12 min (Voorhorst 1980).

Scratch testing A drop of allergen solution is placed on the skin which is then scratched so as to superficially penetrate the skin. As well as providing non-specific weal reactions which are the result of trauma (Dreborg 1989), the scratch test introduces a variable amount of allergen through the skin. The test is therefore poorly standardized and produces results which are too variable for routine clinical use (Lessof 1987; Bousquet 1988).

Prick testing

A drop of allergen solution is placed on the skin which is then pricked with an hypodermic needle. Prick tests can also produce variable results, but the introduction of standardized precision needles (Lessof 1987; Adinoff *et al.* 1989) for prick testing (e.g. the Morrow Brown needle (Brown *et al.* 1981) has made the method potentially more reproducible. However, the delegation of skin testing to untrained staff, and the continued use of unstandardized hypodermic needles leads to frequent errors and poor reproducibility.

Method

A small drop of each test extract and control solution is placed on the volar aspect of the forearm (or occasionally on the back). The implication of a recent study showing that positive reactions affect the reactivity of adjacent skin (Terho *et al.* 1989) is that drops must be placed more than 4 cm apart. Using the Morrow Brown device, the needle is pressed through the drop of allergen extract into the skin at an angle of 90° to the skin, to a standard depth of 1 mm. Other devices are passed through the drop, penetrating the skin at a 45° angle, and the skin is then gently lifted to create a small break in the epidermis (Adinoff *et al.* 1989).

Result: timing

The skin-prick test induces a response that reaches a peak in 8–9 min for histamine, 10–12 min for compound 48/80, a histamine-releasing agent, and 12–15 min for allergens (Voorhorst 1980). The standard advice is to read the histamine control result at 10 min (Bernstein 1988) and the remaining skin test sites at 15 min, and to re-inspect at 25–30 min as in some patients reactions take a little longer to develop (Dreborg 1989). Late reactions can also occur, but are not usually sought as their significance is unclear; they are discussed briefly below.

Result: size

The size of the reaction, which is often oval or irregular in shape, is measured with a ruler. The largest diameter (D) and the diameter at right angles to this (d) is measured, and the reaction is expressed as $(D + d)/2$ (Mygind 1986). Weal thickness and volume can be measured using ultrasonic techniques (Serup 1984), and a further quantitative objective tool for measurement is laser doppler flowmetry which can be used to measure blood flow in a weal (Hammarlund *et al.* 1990).

Result: weal or flare?

Most authorities recommend measurement of the size of the weal alone (Mygind 1986; Dreborg 1989), but others suggest that the size of the flare should also be measured (Voorhorst 1980; Bousquet 1988).

Criteria of positivity

There is a lack of agreed definition about what constitutes a positive reaction (Lessof *et al.* 1980). Most definitions of a positive reaction are based on the absolute diameter of the weal, with arbitrary cut-off points for positivity at 1 mm, 2 mm or 3 mm (Bousquet 1988). A major difficulty is that the size of the weal depends to some extent on the potency of the extract.

Problems with interpretation

It is easier to perform the test than to interpret the results. Skin tests tell you what is going on in the skin. Trying to extrapolate from skin test results, which is the whole purpose of the exercise, is fraught with difficulties (David 1991). The numerous problems are discussed below.

False positive tests
'asymptomatic hypersensitivity'

Skin-prick test reactivity may be present in subjects with no clinical evidence of allergy or intolerance (Curran & Goldman 1961; Fontana *et al.* 1963; Lessof *et al.* 1980; Bousquet 1988). This is sometimes described as 'asymptomatic hypersensitivity' (Bock *et al.* 1977) or 'subclinical sensitization' (Morgan *et al.* 1989), implying that the test has at least detected genuine IgE antibodies, which is not always a justifiable assumption. Some patients with positive skin-prick tests do develop symptoms later (Hagy 1972), but since the test cannot identify the subset who will develop symptoms such information is of little practical value.

persistent positivity despite development of tolerance

Skin-prick test reactivity may persist after clinical evidence of intolerance has subsided. For example, in a study of children with egg intolerance, Ford & Taylor (1982) noted that five out of 11 who grew out of egg intolerance had persistently positive skin-prick tests after egg intolerance had disappeared.

persistent positivity after hyposensitization

Not strictly relevant to food intolerance, where hyposensitization is not an established approach to treatment, but skin-prick tests may remain positive after hyposensitization (Lessof *et al.* 1980).

False negative tests

Skin-prick tests may be negative in some patients with genuine allergies. For example, Eriksson performed a direct comparison between skin test and provocation tests in 403 patients with asthma or rhinitis (Eriksson 1977); 983 skin tests with a variety of inhalant antigens were negative, but in 17% of these the provocation test was positive. Similarly, Pepys reported that skin-prick tests are negative in 13 to 17% of those with rhinitis provoked by pollen (Pepys 1975).

non IgE-mediated events   Skin-prick tests mainly detect IgE antibody. However, many adverse reactions to food are not IgE mediated, in which case skin-prick tests can be expected to be negative. Taking cow's milk protein intolerance as an example, patients with quick reactions often have positive skin-prick tests to cow's milk protein, but those with delayed reactions usually have negative skin-prick tests (Hill *et al.* 1988).

H1-receptor antagonists   False negative results may be due to recent therapy with H1-receptor antagonists, though if skin testing is done properly this should be detected by lack of reaction to a histamine control.

Problems in infancy   False negative results may occur in infants and toddlers, when the weal size is much smaller than later in life (Bousquet 1988). Data on the exact effect of age are scanty, and there are no age-related guidelines for what constitutes a positive reaction.

Poor correlation   There is a poor correlation between the results of provocation tests (e.g. double-blind food challenges) and skin-prick tests. For example, of 31 children with a strongly positive (weal > 3 mm in diameter) skin-prick test to peanut, only 16 (56%) had symptoms when peanuts were administered (Bock *et al.* 1977). This poor correlation is mainly due to the high rate of false positive skin tests. Similar problems apply to testing for allergy to inhalants in asthma (Eriksson 1977).

Varying potency of extracts   There is great variation in potency between extracts of different substances and between those produced by different manufacturers, affecting both extracts of inhalants (Hillas & Wilson 1981; Eichler *et al.* 1988) and foods (Sampson 1988).

Effect of total IgE level   There is a correlation between the total serum IgE concentration and the degree of positivity of skin-prick test results (Eriksson 1989). The precise relationship varies for different allergen extracts (Eriksson 1989).

Poor reproducibility   Using the standard approach of expressing the weal size as a ratio of that produced by an allergen extract to that produced by histamine, the reproducibility of skin-prick testing is low, due to the very poor reproducibility of the histamine-induced weal (Vohlonen *et al.* 1989). To try and overcome this, some authorities have recommended skin-prick testing in duplicate (Dreborg 1989) or even octuplate (Voorhorst & van Krieken 1973).

Other problems

These include:

1 variation in skin reactivity depending upon the skin site chosen (Alexander & McConnell 1930; Bowman 1935; Galant & Maibach 1973; Adinoff *et al.* 1989);

2 placing the histamine control site too near an adjacent site (4 cm or less) may induce a non-specific weal reaction, and it is probable that a similar problem may occur between two adjacent allergens (Terho *et al.* 1989);

3 circadian variation in skin test reactivity, which is at a peak at about 2300 hours and a trough at about 1100 hours (Reinberg *et al.* 1965; Lee *et al.* 1977).

Logic of skin testing

The role for skin-prick tests in food intolerance, if any, is far from clear. The fact that skin tests are still in use reflects both the unscientific nature of allergy practice and the lack of reliable and simple tests. The results of skin tests cannot be taken alone, and standard textbooks of allergy acknowledge that 'the proper interpretation of results requires a thorough knowledge of the history and physical findings' (Patterson 1985; Bousquet 1988).

Confirmatory evidence?

The current doctrine is that a positive skin-prick test is an indication of clinical sensitivity, past, present or future, and that prick tests are worth doing to provide confirmatory evidence. From a carefully taken history, one might suspect a particular food, and the finding of a positive prick test would increase the likelihood that the food was causing symptoms. Few people, however, would be prepared to ignore a strong history of food intolerance (e.g. anaphylaxis to pea or cow's milk) in the face of a negative prick test, yet it is illogical to regard the prick test as significant only when it confirms the history and to disregard it when it fails to do so (Holt 1967).

Poor predictor

The contentious issues in clinical practice are whether a child with atopic disease or symptoms suggestive of food intolerance will benefit from attempts to avoid certain foods or food additives, but skin-prick test results are unreliable predictors of response to such measures.

Need for scepticism

Skin test results may be misleading. For example, 14 children with perennial intractable asthma who were skin test positive to house dust were admitted to hospital, with prompt relief of symptoms, but when they inhaled dust from their own homes no symptoms occurred (Long *et al.* 1958). Had only the elimination without the challenges been attempted, one might have easily concluded that house dust was the offender.

Little use in food intolerance   Skin-prick tests for food allergy are especially unreliable because of the large number of false positive and false negative reactions (Bock *et al.* 1977; Aas 1978; Lessof *et al.* 1980; Bousquet 1988; Hill *et al.* 1988; Meglio *et al.* 1988).

raw or cooked foods for testing?   Commercial food extracts (sometimes heat-treated) and fresh or frozen raw extracts may give different results (more positives with raw foods) (Ancona & Schumacher 1950; Josephson & Glaser 1963), reflecting the fact that some patients are intolerant to certain foods only when taken in a raw state (Fries & Glaser 1950; Nater & Zwartz 1967; Aas 1989; Kägi & Wüthrich 1991). In others the reverse is the case (Prausnitz & Kustner 1921).

Poor reliability   In one study (Bahna & Ghandi 1987) of 61 patients with proven food intolerance (mainly children), the reliability of skin-prick testing for cow's milk, crab, egg, fish, peanut and shrimp (using double-blind food challenges as the gold standard for comparison) was as follows:
1 sensitivity overall 58% (range 44% for cow's milk to 83% for fish);
2 specificity overall 65% (range 50% for fish to 80% for egg);
3 positive predictive accuracy 48% (range 33% for crab to 83% for fish);
4 negative predictive accuracy 74% (range 44% for cow's milk to 89% for egg).

One needs to remember that the figures for predictive accuracy depend on the prevalence of food intolerance in the population studied (see chapter 40). The figures quoted above are for a population with a very high prevalence of food intolerance; if applied to the general paediatric population, the figures for predictive accuracy would be quite different.

Intradermal testing   Intradermal testing comprises the intradermal injection of 0.01–0.05 ml of an allergen extract (Dreborg 1989). It can cause fatal anaphylaxis (Lockey *et al.* 1987), and is only performed if a preliminary skin-prick test is negative. Intradermal tests are more sensitive than skin-prick testing (Dreborg 1989), and hence also produce even more false positive reactions (Bock *et al.* 1978; Reddy *et al.* 1978). As with skin-prick testing, there is a lack of agreement as to what constitutes a positive reaction. The number of false positive reactions makes the interpretation of the results of intradermal testing even more difficult than skin-prick testing. The difficulty in the interpretation of the results, the pain of intradermal injections, and the risk of anaphylaxis mean that intradermal testing has no place in the routine investigation of IgE-mediated allergic reactions or food intolerance in childhood. There may be a place for intra-dermal testing in the investigation of drug allergy, but that is outside the scope of this book.

Late-phase reactions

In an IgE-dependent skin test reaction, the weal and flare at 10–20 min can be followed by a late-phase reaction comprising indura-tion and inflammation that begins, peaks and terminates within 1–2 days (Agarwal & Zetterstrom 1982; Frew & Kay 1988). The clinical significance of these late-phase reactions is at present unclear (Goldstein 1988), although they appear to be partly dose related and especially noted when high concentrations of allergens are used (Reshef *et al*. 1989).

Conclusion

Skin-prick testing still has its enthusiasts. They tend to be based in the speciality of allergy, where there may be a perceived need to demonstrate 'allergy expertise' or where the performance of tests is associated with a fee for service. Although skin-prick testing has a place in research studies, it is difficult to see a place for skin testing in the general diagnosis or management of intolerance to food or food additives.

Key references

41.1 BOUSQUET J (1988) In vivo methods for study of allergy: skin tests, techniques, and interpretation. In Middleton E, Reed CE, Ellis EF, Adkinson NF & Yunginger JW (eds) *Allergy. Principles and Practice*, 3rd edn, vol. 1, pp. 419–436, Mosby, St Louis. *General review.*

41.2 BOCK SA, BUCKLEY J, HOLST A & MAY CD (1977) Proper use of skin tests with food extracts in diagnosis of hypersensitivity to food in children. *Clin Allergy* **7**:375–383. This study attempted to correlate the results of skin-prick tests and double-blind food challenges in 105 children with asthma and a control group of 27 children who 'denied hypersensitivity to common allergens'. The results of the double-blind food challenges, which were only performed in two out of 20 foods studied, and were only performed in a small number of patients, were taken as the definitive evidence of food allergy. 50% of positive skin tests for egg, and 44% of tests for peanut, were associated with a negative food challenge, and were therefore false positive results, although the authors evaded this conclusion by labelling these as indicating 'asymptomatic hypersensitivity'. *The authors claimed that skin testing was useful in that it helps to select patients for the ultimate diagnostic test, double-blind food challenges, which was still considered 'essential' for the diagnosis of food allergy. It was suggested that a negative skin test was reliable, indicating absence of allergy, but there was no data to support this claim, and patients and controls with negative skin tests were not chal-lenged with foods.*

41.3 LESSOF MH, BUISSERET PD, MERRETT J, MERRETT TG & WRAITH DG (1980) Assessing the value of skin-prick tests. *Clin Allergy* **10**:115–120. *A study of skin testing with food extracts, demonstrating variable potency and specificity. False positive reactions were seen with all major extracts studied. The authors started from the premise that skin-prick tests provide 'useful information' at the*

1–3 mm reaction level. The unreliability of the method was well shown in 19 patients with fish allergy. Only 15 had a skin test reaction of 5 mm in diameter or more, and in addition there were seven patients without allergy to fish who had skin test reactions of 4 mm.

41.4   SAMPSON HA (1988) Comparative study of commercial food antigen extracts for the diagnosis of food hypersensitivity. *J Allergy Clin Immunol* **82**:718–726. The results of skin-prick testing with a battery of food extracts from three different manufacturers were compared with the results of double-blind food challenges in 87 children with atopic eczema. The positive predictive accuracy was generally poor, and varied from 0% to 79%. The negative predictive accuracies were better, and ranged from 85% to 100%. *Problem one: the main criteria of a positive food challenge was erythema occurring within a few hours of challenge, and the relationship of these immediate erythematous reactions to eczematous lesions is unknown. Problem two: the scoring system for reading skin tests results was rather unusual in that it took into account the size of the flare as well as the size of the weal.*

41.5   TERHO EO, HUSMAN K, KIVEKAS J & RIIHIMAKI H (1989) Histamine control affects the weal produced by the adjacent diluent control in skin-prick tests. *Allergy* **44**:30–32. The study showed that the normal histamine control solution enhances skin test reactivity in adjacent skin as distant as 3–4 cm. A prick test with the diluent control (glycerol saline) was three times more likely to be positive if placed within 3–4 cm of the histamine test than if it was placed 18–19 cm away from the histamine test. *If true, this study casts doubt on a large proportion of previous studies of skin tests, for conventional recommendations have been to perform skin-prick tests 2–3 cm apart.*

41.6   BERNSTEIN IL (1988) (ed) Proceedings of the task force on guidelines for standardizing old and new technologies used for the diagnosis and treatment of allergic diseases. *J Allergy Clin Immunol* **82**:487–526. *North American consensus view on allergy testing; good source on procedures but uncritical on interpretation of results or clinical value of testing.*

41.7   DREBORG S (1989) (ed) Skin tests used in type I allergy testing. Position paper. Prepared by the sub-committee on skin tests of the European Academy of Allergology and Clinical Immunology. *Allergy* **44** (suppl. 10):1–59. *Useful review of pathophysiology, methods, standardization of allergen extracts and epidemiological studies, but uncritical on interpretation of results or clinical value of testing.*

41.8   REDDY PM, NAGAYA H, PASCUAL HC *et al.* (1978) Reappraisal of intracutaneous tests in the diagnosis of reaginic allergy. *J Allergy Clin Immunol* **61**:36–41. Thirty-four patients with perennial rhinitis who had positive intradermal but negative skin-prick tests to inhalants (pollens, dust mites) were studied with RAST, leucocyte histamine release (LHR) and nasal provocation tests. None had positive RAST or LHR tests, and only one had a positive nasal provocation test. *Intradermal tests may well be positive even if skin-prick tests are negative. Intradermal tests give numerous false positive results.*

41.9   REIMANN HJ & LEWIN J (1988) Gastric mucosal reactions in patients with food allergy. *Amer J Gastroenterol* **83**:1212–1219. Double blind challenges were performed, with food allergens directly applied to the gastric mucosa via an endoscope. *Skin-prick tests were positive in only 47% of positive reactions to food challenge.*

41.10 BOCK SA & ATKINS FM (1990) Patterns of food hypersensitivity during sixteen years of double-blind, placebo-controlled food challenges. *J Pediat* **117**:561–567. Report of 1014 double-blind placebo-controlled food challenges in 480 children. Of 235 positive challenges, the skin test was positive in 92%; for those under 3 years of age the skin test was positive in only 83%. *Although there are no details of those with positive skin tests and negative food challenges, the authors comment: 'the large number of patients with asymptomatic hypersensitivity limited the accuracy of a positive skin test result alone as a predictor of clinical symptoms during food ingestion'.*

41.11 MEGLIO P, FARINELLA F, TROGOLO E, GIAMPIETRO PG, CANTANI A & BUSINCO L (1988) Immediate reactions following challenge-tests in children with atopic dermatitis. *Allergie Immunol* **20**:57–62. *Study of 20 children, which concluded that immediate reactions following food challenges cannot be predicted by skin-prick tests or RAST tests, and that, contrary to the data of Sampson & Albergo (1984), a negative skin-prick test could be misleading, and could not be taken to exclude intolerance to a food.*

41.12 MALANIN G & KALIMO K (1989) The results of skin testing with food additives and the effect of an elimination diet in chronic and recurrent urticaria and recurrent angioedema. *Clin Exper Allergy* **19**:539–543. Of 91 subjects, mainly adults, with recurrent urticaria, who were skin-prick tested with 18 food additives, 24 had at least one positive skin test. Oral provocation tests were performed in 10 out of 24, but in only one (using benzoic acid) was the result positive. All 91 patients were advised to follow an additive free diet, and 70 returned a questionnaire on the outcome. Sixteen out of 23 (70%) of those with a positive skin test reported improvement, compared to 17 out of 47 (36%) who had had negative skin tests. *The fact that positive skin test results could not be confirmed by challenge is hardly surprising, since the mechanism of additive intolerance is rarely if ever IgE-mediated. On the basis of these subjective results of dietary treatment, the authors suggested that skin testing can be used to identify those who will respond to a diet. It seems more likely that a positive skin test enhanced a placebo response to the diet by encouraging a patient to believe that additive intolerance was important.*

41.13 DREBORG S (1991) Skin test in diagnosis of food allergy. *Allergy Proc* **12**:251–254. *Recent review, which concludes that skin testing with food allergens is unreliable.*

Summary 41 The principle of scratch, prick and intradermal skin tests is that the weal and flare reaction to an allergen demonstrates the presence of mast-cell-fixed IgE antibody. The major drawbacks to skin testing are the lack of agreed criteria of positivity, the large number of false positive results, the diminished wealing capacity of the skin in infancy, the poor correlation between results of skin testing and provocation testing, the varying potency of extracts of different foods, and the fact that a number of adverse reactions to foods are not IgE mediated. Skin testing is unhelpful in the management of food intolerance.

42 Patch tests
Rarely helpful in food intolerance

Minor relevance

Patch tests are of little direct relevance to the subject of food intolerance. A brief account is given here because of:

1 contact urticaria due to foods (see chapter 59);

2 the common but poorly described procedure of testing for food intolerance by direct application of food on to the skin;

3 recent information about the additive effect of antigens applied to the skin in patch tests.

Sensitization is generalized

In contact dermatitis, sensitization affects the whole body. The principle of patch testing is that if an allergen is applied to a small area of normal skin and enough is absorbed, inflammation develops at the site of application. The allergen is usually applied as a patch test. A positive reaction may confirm that a subject has allergic contact sensitivity to the substance tested, but does not necessarily mean that the substance is the cause of the patient's dermatitis.

Procedure

Allergens are usually applied to the skin on the back, on 1 cm diameter patches of filter paper, which are either placed on an impermeable sheet or in a cup, which holds a test substance closely applied to the skin. The patches or cups are held in place with hypoallergenic adhesive tape, and left on for 48 hours. The patient returns at 48 hours, the patches are removed, and the results recorded half to 1 hour later. The patient returns again 2 days later, and a second reading taken, as reactions to some allergens often take longer than 2 days to become positive (Cronin 1980).

Recording results

Results are graded (Champion *et al.* 1992) as:

NT	not tested;
−	negative;
?+	doubtful reaction;
+	weak (non-vesicular) reaction;
++	strong (oedematous or vesicular) reaction;
+++	extreme (bullous or ulcerative) reaction;
IR	irritant reaction.

Irritant reactions   The distinction between irritant and allergic reactions may be difficult. The features of irritant reactions are sharp delineation corresponding to the margins of the test patch, no infiltration, lack of itching, and redness with a brown hue (Champion *et al.* 1992). Positive reactions of an allergic nature are red and infiltrated with minute papules or vesicles (which in severe reactions coalesce into bullae), diffuse, and extend beyond the margins of the patch.

Standard series   Since about 80% of contact sensitivities are caused by a relatively small number of allergens, most dermatology clinics employ a standard series (battery), to which can be added selected substances as may be indicated by the history.

False positive results   The causes of false positive results (Cronin 1980) are listed in Table 42.1.

False negative results   The causes of false negative results (Cronin 1980) are listed in Table 42.2.

Clinical relevance   Difficulty arises when the morphology of the positive reaction fails to differentiate between an allergic and an irritant response (Cronin 1980; Champion *et al.* 1992). This is not uncommon, and is the main reason for the misinterpretation of patch tests (Cronin 1980). Unfortunately, there are a number of different causes of positive patch test reactions – see Table 42.3.

Additive effect of allergens   McLelland and Shuster (1990) have recently pointed out that because the patch-test response is dose-related, some sensitized subjects may have negative patch tests. The frequency of such an occurrence depends upon the balance of the degree of sensitivity and the concentration of antigens used in the test. In theory, it follows that patients who are sensitized to more than one antigen, but to a degree insufficient to produce a positive patch test to one or more of them alone, would react to a combination of antigens by the simple summation of their independent sensitivity responses.

negative patch tests   McLelland and Shuster postulated that this may explain why negative responses occur with patch testing where there is a high index of clinical suspicion. They proceeded to measure the response to common allergens, applied both singly and in combination, and confirmed that the response to mixtures of allergens was indeed additive, the combined response being the sum of the individual components.

Table 42.1 Causes of false positive patch test reactions

Concentration of test substance too high
Contamination by another allergen or an irritant excluding: allergic reaction to vehicle, allergic reaction to chamber
Skin is hyper-irritable, e.g. adjacent to strong positive, plaster reaction, generalized active atopic eczema
'Rogue' positive; when test is repeated it is negative – the cause is obscure
Artefact, e.g. patient interference

Table 42.2 Causes of false negative patch test reactions

Concentration of test substance too low
Amount of test substance applied too small
Poor absorption of allergen
Steroid (in test medicament) suppression (**NB** topical steroids can also cause allergic contact dermatitis (Coopman *et al.* 1989)
Non-occlusion (insufficient absorption)
Patch test falls off
Result read too early
Refractory state, which may occur shortly after a very severe allergic reaction
Allergen altered chemically by vehicle
Allergen degradation in vehicle

Table 42.3 Interpretation of positive patch test reactions

Relevant to the present problem
Relevant to skin problems in the past
Unexplained relevance
False positive (see Table 42.1)
Cross-reaction (i.e. to structurally similar allergen)

important implications

The practical implication for contact dermatitis, as speculated by McLelland and Shuster, is that the use of single allergens may fail to detect clinically important sensitivity, and the way to overcome this might be to use mixtures of various allergens. The theoretical significance, in the context of this book, is possibly far greater, for it is the first objective confirmation of a widely held impression that the effect of allergens can be additive. Whether this applies to ingested foods is an important area of uncertainty.

Food handling

Occupational hand eczema is a type of contact dermatitis of importance to adults who handle food. In some cases skin contact with the causative food causes an immediate (i.e. within 30 min) irritation, followed by redness and wealing. In other cases the reaction is delayed, resulting in erythema and vesiculation at the site of skin contact. Certain foods seem to more commonly provoke immediate reactions (e.g. fish and shellfish), while others more commonly provoke delayed reactions (e.g. onions or garlic), but foods may also cause both types of reaction (Cronin 1980; Veien 1986). Some foods (e.g. spices) can cause both irritant as well as immediate and delayed allergic contact dermatitis (Veien 1986). A wide range of food additives can cause contact dermatitis (Cronin 1980; Fisher 1983).

Applying food to the skin

Patch tests, like skin-prick tests, tell you what is going on in the skin. Trying to extrapolate from patch test results may be misleading. Oranje et al. (1991) have suggested that the weal and flare reaction resulting from the application to the skin for 30 min of food in its natural state (e.g. whole cow's milk) may be a useful test to confirm food intolerance, and they and others (Acciai et al. 1991) have called this a SAFT test (skin application food test). However, this is simply a test for allergic contact urticaria (see chapter 59). Since there are a number of subjects in whom skin contact with a food causes an urticarial reaction, but in whom oral ingestion is not associated with any adverse effects (unpublished personal observations, anecdotal published reports, e.g. Fine 1981, and Beck personal communication), the SAFT test is of doubtful value in the general management of food intolerance, with one possible exception which is described below.

foods suspended in
dimethylsulphoxide

It has been suggested that suspension of food extracts in 90% dimethylsulphoxide may aid skin penetration and increase the accuracy of patch testing with food extracts (Breneman et al. 1989). It has been claimed that the dimethylsulphoxide food test (DIMSOFT) enables detection of all four Gell & Coombs types of hypersensitivity reaction, and that the test is accordingly more sensitive and specific than RAST testing in the diagnosis of food intolerance. These sweeping claims require confirmation.

**Skin application of food
prior to food challenges**

In practice the one situation where direct application of food to the skin may be of value is prior to a food challenge in a child in whom one fears an anaphylactic reaction (Acciai et al. 1991). An example might be a 6-month old infant with a history of a severe allergic reaction to egg. How can the parents tell that the child has outgrown the allergy without directly administering egg and risking a violent reaction? A simple answer is that if skin application of egg causes an urticarial reaction, then a diminution and disappearance of this response can probably be taken to indicate the development of tolerance, and a continuing brisk response to skin contact would constitute a deterrent to an oral challenge. This is, however, only an approximate guide, and there are a number of possible reasons why such testing may give false positive (e.g. using a raw food when the food is usually eaten cooked, such as egg or potato) or false negative (e.g. child receiving H1-histamine antagonist or topical steroids) results. A further problem is that on occasions, sufficient quantities of a food can be absorbed through the skin to cause systemic symptoms and even anaphylaxis (Court & Ng 1984; Jarmoc & Primack 1987).

Patch tests for food intolerance

Despite unconfirmed claims to the contrary (e.g. Breneman *et al.* 1989), there is no evidence that patch testing with foods is useful in the diagnosis or management of intolerance to ingested food. The possible exception is the controversial and complex topic of intolerance to ingested nickel in adult patients with contact dermatitis or recurrent vesicular hand eczema, and this is briefly discussed below.

Intolerance to ingested nickel

A number of pieces of evidence suggest that dietary nickel may, in those who exhibit contact sensitivity to nickel, exacerbate contact dermatitis or hand eczema:

1 Anecdotal reports of contact dermatitis which flared up after swallowing a coin, after eating food with a high nickel content, or after the use of metal retractors at operation (reviewed by Burrows 1989).

2 Limited data suggesting increased excretion of nickel in the urine during exacerbations of contact dermatitis, suggesting that increased absorption had occurred (reviewed by Burrows 1989).

3 Data from uncontrolled studies of low nickel diets, suggesting benefit to some patients with nickel-sensitive contact dermatitis (reviewed by Veien 1989 and Veien & Menné 1990). Nickel enters the body mainly through food items, and certain foods (e.g. tea leaves, cocoa, soya and other beans and seeds using for sprouting, sunflower seeds, oats, hazel nuts, peanuts, liquorice) have higher contents of nickel than others (Veien 1989), but there is wide fluctuation in vegetables which in turn reflects variations in the composition of soil (Scheller *et al.* 1988). In practice, it is very difficult to produce a low-nickel diet, and even more difficult to conduct a trial under double-blind conditions.

4 Data from animals and man of dermatitis following implants of metal prostheses which allowed nickel to enter the tissues (reviewed by Burrows 1989).

5 Data from a number of double-blind placebo-controlled challenge studies of oral nickel (reviewed by Burrows 1989), which suggest that large doses of about 2.5 mg or above may produce exacerbations of contact dermatitis. The clinical relevance of this data is, however, uncertain, particularly if one bears in mind that the normal daily intake is estimated to lie between 140 and 150 µg per day (Department of Health 1991). The situation is complicated even further by a report that 5 mg nickel sulphate taken once a week for 6 weeks resulted in significantly reduced patch test reactions (Sjövall *et al.* 1987).

6 Inconclusive data from studies of nickel chelating agents in subjects with nickel dermatitis (see Burrows 1989).

conclusions – nickel

Contact sensitivity to nickel can be demonstrated by patch testing. Ingested nickel in quantities well in excess of the estimated average intake may exacerbate nickel-sensitive contact dermatitis. However it appears to be very difficult to achieve a low-nickel diet, and there is no proof that such a diet is helpful to patients with contact sensitivity to nickel.

Intolerance to ingested balsam of Peru

Balsam of Peru is an important cause of contact dermatitis, and is routinely used in patch testing. Two hundred and ten, presumably adult patients, with various types of dermatitis (only 17 had positive patch tests to balsam of Peru) were challenged under double-blind placebo-controlled conditions with 1 mg of balsam of Peru (Veien *et al.* 1985). Of these, 45 reacted with a flare-up of previous symptoms to balsam of Peru, 15 reacted to placebo, and five reacted to both. These reactions were most common in those with positive patch tests to balsam of Peru (10 out of 17). Avoidance of foods suspected to contain balsams (Table 42.4) was tried in 31 patients, and this was asssociated with improvement of the dermatitis in 16. There is no data on whether children can be intolerant to oral balsam of Peru, or on whether patch testing would be a useful way to detect such intolerance. However, since 26 out of 45 who reacted to balsam of Peru challenges in the above study had negative patch tests, the prospects look poor for patch testing being a useful tool to detect intolerance to ingested balsam.

Key references 42.1

CHAMPION RH, BURTON JL & EBLING FJG (1992) (eds) *Textbook of Dermatology*, 5th edn, Blackwell Scientific Publications, Oxford. *Major textbook of dermatology, including a full review of patch testing.*

42.2

CRONIN E (1980) *Contact Dermatitis*, Churchill Livingstone, Edinburgh. *Major textbook on contact dermatitis. Very clear short description of patch testing. A 20 page chapter on foods is largely devoted to food additives.*

Table 42.4 Food items believed to contain balsams[1]

Products which contain the peel of citrus fruits (e.g. marmalade)
Products flavoured with essences (e.g. candy)
Perfumed products (e.g. perfumed teas)
Cough medicine and lozenges
Eugenol (used by dentists)
Ice cream
Cola and soft drinks
Spices
Ketchup
Sauces (e.g. chilli sauce)
Chutney
Pickled foods (e.g. pickled herring, pickled vegetables)
Baked goods
Liver paste and paté
Vermouth and bitters

[1] Source: Veien *et al.* (1985).

42.3   MᴄLᴇʟʟᴀɴᴅ J & Sʜᴜsᴛᴇʀ S (1990) Contact dermatitis with negative patch tests: the additive effect of allergens in combination. *Br J Dermatol* **122**:623–630. *Important study of the additive effect of allergens in patch testing.*

42.4   O'Nᴇɪʟ CE & Lᴇʜʀᴇʀ SB (1991) Occupational reactions to food allergens. In Metcalfe DD, Sampson HA & Simon RA (eds) *Food Allergy. Adverse Reactions to Foods and Food Additives*, pp. 207–236, Blackwell Scientific Publications, Oxford. *Review.*

42.5   Wᴇsᴛᴏɴ WL, Wᴇsᴛᴏɴ JA, Kɪɴᴏsʜɪᴛᴀ J *et al.* (1986) Prevalence of positive epicutaneous tests among infants, children, and adolescents. *Pediatrics* **78**:1070–1074. Patch tests using a standard battery of allergens (not including foods) which commonly cause contact dermatitis were performed in 314 healthy children. 20% had at least one positive result. Neomycin (8%), nickel (8%), potassium dichromate (8%) and thimerosal (3%) were the most prevalent allergens. *Important study because of the paucity of data in normal children.*

Summary 42   Patch tests are employed for the diagnosis of contact dermatitis. Interpretation of the test is hampered by false positive and false negative results, and by the difficulty which can sometimes occur in distinguishing between irritant and allergic reactions. The fact that a positive result does not on its own distinguish between a currently relevant and previously relevant allergy is a major problem. The effect of allergens on the skin is additive, and in cases of multiple allergy, testing with a single antigen may be negative. Patch testing is not helpful in the general management of food intolerance. It may be helpful to look for allergic contact urticaria by the direct application of food to the skin; a positive result does not prove food intolerance, but might deter one from performing an oral challenge in a child with a previous history of anaphylactic shock after ingestion of the food.

43 Tests for circulating antibodies
Similar drawbacks to skin-prick tests

Principle The radioallergosorbent (RAST) test is the best known of a number of laboratory procedures (Table 43.1) for the detection and measurement of circulating IgE antibody.

Method The method is to bind allergen on to a solid-phase allergosorbent, which can be a cellulose paper disc, a plastic surface, or cellulose threads. This allergosorbent is incubated with serum from the patient, allowing antibodies of all classes (primarily IgE and IgG) to bind. The allergosorbent is then washed to remove the unbound allergen, and then incubated with anti-IgE antibody which has been isotopically or enzymatically labelled. After further washing, the radioactivity bound to the disc is counted, or in the case of enzyme-labelled antibodies, a substrate is incubated to produce a coloured or fluorescent product (Dockhorn 1982; Hamilton & Adkinson, 1986; Bernstein 1988). The other methods for the detection of circulating IgE antibodies are listed in Table 43.1.

Reporting results The radioactivity, or the quantity of product generated by enzyme activity, is related to disk-bound IgE by a standard reference curve. For routine clinical use RAST results are classified as 0 (negative), 1, 2, 3 and 4 (Dockhorn 1982). Defining a cut-off point for positivity or negativity is arbitrary (Dockhorn 1982).

Theoretical advantage This type of test avoids possible confounding variables in skin testing, namely IgE affinity for mast cells, their tendency for degranulation, and skin reactivity to released mediators. Thus, in theory, the *in vitro* test should be more reliable than skin testing.

Table 43.1 Currently available methods for measurement of circulating IgE antibody

Allergosorbent	Detection system (label type)	Test name
Paper disc	Iodine 125	RAST
Plastic surface	Enzyme (fluorescent product)	FAST[1]
Plastic surface	Enzyme (visible product)	ELISA[2]
Cellulose threads	Iodine 125	MAST[3]

[1] FAST; fluorescent allergosorbent test.
[2] ELISA; enzyme linked immunosorbent test.
[3] MAST; multiple-thread allergosorbent test.

Practical drawbacks   The clinical interpretation of *in vitro* IgE antibody tests is subject to most of the same pitfalls as the interpretation of skin-prick testing. Additional problems with IgE antibody tests are:

1 high cost;

2 a very high level of total circulating IgE (e.g. in children with severe atopic eczema) may cause a false positive result;

3 a very high level of IgG antibody with the same allergen specificity as the IgE antibody can cause a false negative result;

4 for each allergen, the test differs in the degree to which it is influenced by the total serum IgE concentration;

5 *in vitro* IgE assays are slightly less sensitive than skin testing;

6 the IgE antibody concentration in the plasma varies with allergen exposure. A few patients with allergic rhinitis are RAST negative before the pollen season, but become positive after the pollen season.

Advantages   *In vitro* tests for IgE antibody are only preferable to skin testing:

1 where the patient has had a very severe reaction to the allergen in question (because of the small risk of anaphylaxis with skin testing);

2 where the patient has widespread skin disease (e.g. atopic eczema);

3 where the skin shows dermographism;

4 when H1 antihistamines cannot be discontinued.

Correlation with skin tests   The degree of correlation between RAST test results and skin-prick test results depends on the criteria used for positivity, and thus there is endless scope for manipulation of data. Thus, in one study, in which the results of these tests were compared, it was possible to find a high degree of correlation (though it varied considerably for each food tested) if one defined a positive skin-prick test as a weal 3 mm larger than the control weal and a positive RAST as grade 3 or 4 (Sampson & Albergo 1984).

Predictive accuracy   By confining their study to immediate (within 4 hours of challenge) reactions, thereby excluding the very type of case where information from a test would be most useful, by altering the RAST assay method for eight of the 28 food antigens, and by taking a RAST score of 3 or 4 and a skin test weal of 3 mm larger than the control as positive, Sampson & Albergo (1984) reported:

1 very high concordance between skin test and RAST results;

2 excellent negative predictive accuracy (82% to 100%) for both skin and RAST tests;

3 poor positive predictive accuracies for both tests.

In other words:

1 the two tests usually give similar results;

2 negative tests make food intolerance less likely but do not exclude the possibility of food intolerance;

3 the tests are poor at predicting food intolerance.

Clearly by taking a *highly selected* group of children who react immediately to *tiny* quantities of food one can obtain apparently good results with skin or RAST tests. The problem is that children who react in this way are usually quite easily identifiable from the history.

Clinical problems
incomplete history

Where the history is incomplete, the test is unlikely to help. To quote a common example, a child with widespread atopic eczema gives a history of an anaphylactic reaction to peanut. The parents want to know if it is safe to try other nuts, e.g. Brazil nuts or hazel nuts, which to the best of their knowledge have not previously been given. The severity of the reaction to peanuts is a deterrent to food challenges. The RAST test results are grade 4 positive to peanut, grade 3 positive to Brazil nut, grade 2 positive to hazel nut and grade 0 to walnut. How do these results help? Do the results imply the need for Brazil nut and hazel nut avoidance, or are these more likely to be false positive results? Can one tell the parents it is safe to give walnuts? On the basis of probability, it is likely that the child will tolerate all three types of nut, the positive RAST tests to Brazil and hazel nuts being more likely to be false positives than true positives.

real life problems

The real life common clinical problems, in which neither skin nor RAST tests are likely to be helpful, are:

1 the identification of individual food triggers in those who do not have obvious immediate adverse reactions;

2 the identification of individual food triggers in those in whom food or food additive intolerance is not IgE mediated;

3 are symptoms (e.g. wheezing) related to food ingestion or not;

4 will a disease state (e.g. atopic eczema) improve if one or more foods are avoided;

5 confirmation that food intolerance exists and identification of individual food triggers in a child who has an adverse reaction after eating a manufactured food with multiple ingredients;

6 in a child with a history of reaction to a food (e.g. a nut), the identification of intolerance to related foods (i.e. other nuts).

Clinical relevance

The clinical interpretation of *in vitro* IgE antibody tests is subject to the same caveats and pitfalls as the interpretation of skin-prick testing (Bernstein 1988) which are described in chapter 43. In a recent study (Bahna & Ghandi 1987) of 61 patients with proven food intolerance (mainly children), the reliability of RAST testing for cow's milk, crab, egg, fish, peanut and shrimp (using double-blind food challenges as the gold standard for comparison) was as follows:

1 sensitivity overall 58% (range 33% for egg to 100% for fish);

2 specificity overall 33% (range 0% for fish to 67% for cow's milk);

3 positive predictive accuracy 44% (range 14% for egg to 71% for cow's milk and fish);

4 negative predictive accuracy 67% (range 0% for fish to 80% for crab).

One needs to remember that the figures for predictive accuracy depend on the prevalence of food intolerance in the population studied (see chapter 40). The figures quoted above are for a population with a very high prevalence of food intolerance; if applied to the general paediatric population, the figures for predictive accuracy would be quite different.

Conclusion– RASTS not helpful

In short, *in vitro* tests for specific IgE antibodies (e.g. RAST tests) are of little if any practical value in the management of food intolerance (Oehling *et al.* 1981).

Key references 43.1 SAMPSON HA & ALBERGO R (1984) Comparison of results of skin tests, RAST, and double-blind, placebo-controlled food challenges in children with atopic dermatitis. *J Allergy Clin Immunol* **74**:26–33. *Despite the limitations of this study (described in the text above) this is a useful application of the terms sensitivity, specificity and predictive accuracy as applied to food intolerance, and it clearly explains how the positive predictive accuracy (e.g. of skin testing) depends upon the prevalence of the disorder (e.g. egg intolerance).*

43.2 MEGLIO P, FARINELLA F, TROGOLO E, GIAMPIETRO PG, CANTANI A & BUSINCO L (1988) Immediate reactions following challenge-tests in children with atopic dermatitis. *Allergie Immunol* **20**:57–62. A study of skin-prick tests, RAST tests and food challenges in 20 children with atopic eczema. *The results of food challenges could not be predicted from either RAST or skin-prick test results.*

43.3 REIMANN HJ & LEWIN J (1988) Gastric mucosal reactions in patients with food allergy. *Amer J Gastroenterol* **83**:1212–1219. Double-blind challenges were performed, with food allergens directly applied to the gastric mucosa via an endoscope. RAST tests were positive in only 50% of positive reactions, and false positive results were seen in 40% of negative challenges.

43.4 BJÖRKSTÉN B (1991) *In vitro* diagnostic methods in the evaluation of food hypersensitivity. In Metcalfe DD, Sampson HA & Simon RA (eds) *Food Allergy. Adverse Reactions to Foods and Food Additives*, pp. 67–80, Blackwell Scientific Publications, Oxford. *Review, which concludes that RAST testing may be of value as a research tool but that 'laboratory diagnosis cannot replace a carefully obtained case history, confirmed by appropriate food challenge'.*

43.5   ADLER BR, ASSADULLAHI T, WARNER JA & WARNER JO (1991) Evaluation of a multiple food specific IgE antibody test compared to parental perception, allergy skin tests and RAST. *Clin Exper Dermatol* **21**:683–688. Multiple food specific IgE antibody tests were performed in 67 asthmatic children randomly selected from a hospital out-patient clinic. There was poor correlation between the results for skin-prick tests and IgE antibody tests in the case of certain foods (e.g. cow's milk, soya and wheat), and the IgE antibody test results correlated poorly with food-related symptoms as perceived by parents. *The authors concluded that knowledge about food specific IgE antibodies did not reliably add to knowledge about patients' reactions to food.*

Summary 43   The radioallergosorbent (RAST) test is the best known of a number of laboratory procedures for the detection and measurement of circulating IgE antibody. This type of test avoids certain confounding variables in skin testing (e.g. variable degree of IgE affinity for mast cells), and is suitable for patients where skin testing is impractical or impossible (e.g. patient on long-acting H1 histamine antagonists, or widespread atopic eczema). The correlation of RAST test and skin-prick test results, which ought to be very high as both detect specific IgE antibodies, is rather variable, partly because of the varying criteria used to define positivity for each test. The clinical interpretation of *in vitro* IgE antibody tests is subject to the same caveats and pitfalls as the interpretation of skin-prick testing, so that, as with skin testing, tests to detect circulating IgE antibody are of little use in the management of food intolerance.

44 Total serum IgE concentration
Little value in food intolerance

Measurement   Measurement of the total serum IgE concentration requires a sensitive immunoassay, of which the most widely used is the paper radioimmunosorbent (PRIST) test. IgE concentrations are reported in international units per ml (one international unit represents 2.4 ng of IgE). The normal concentration in serum is extremely low (120–480 ng/ml).

IgE formation   IgE is produced in plasma cells which are distributed primarily in lymphoid tissue adjacent to the respiratory and gastrointestinal tracts. The highest concentration of these cells is found in tonsil and adenoid tissue (Yunginger 1988).

Table 44.1 Age-related values of total IgE serum concentration[1]

Age	Mean (I.U./ml)	+2 SD (I.U./ml)[2]
<3 months	3.2	11
4–11 months	3.8	11
12–23 months	8.3	29
2–3 years	14.4	42
4–5 years	15.3	52
6–7 years	17.8	56
8–10 years	18.0	63
11–12 years	13.0	45
13–14 years	20.9	70
15 years and over	13.2	114

[1] Source: Supraregional Assay Service. Truncated version published in Ward MA (ed) *PRU Handbook of Clinical Immunochemistry*, 2nd edn, p. 120, Protein Reference Unit, University of Sheffield.
[2] In practice it is convenient to take this as the upper limit of normal.

Ontogeny of IgE

IgE-bearing B cells are detectable in human lung tissues by the 11th week of foetal life. Although foetal synthesis of IgE is minimal, and levels in cord blood are very low, infants of atopic parents have a higher total IgE concentration in the cord blood than infants of non-atopic parents (Magnusson 1988). It has been suggested that measurement of the cord blood IgE concentration, particularly if taken with knowledge of the family history, can be used to predict the future development of atopic disease (Michel & Bousquet 1983). However, recent studies have failed to confirm a high predictive value of cord blood IgE concentrations (Lilja *et al.* 1990; Ruiz *et al.* 1990). After birth, serum IgE levels rise, along with other immunoglobulins, with maximum values in normal children appearing between the ages of 10 and 15 years (Table 44.1).

Clinical significance

Non-atopic normal individuals generally have a lower serum concentration of IgE than atopic subjects, but there is overlap between the two groups (Yunginger 1988). Thus, only about 60% of patients with allergic rhinitis and 75% of patients with asthma have elevated total serum IgE levels (Dockhorn 1982). Of the atopics, those with atopic eczema tend to have the highest serum IgE concentration. Parasitic infestation also induces a pronounced increase in serum IgE concentration.

Practical value

In the context of food intolerance, the measurement of the total serum IgE concentration is of limited practical value. Food intolerance which is not IgE-mediated will not be associated with elevated IgE concentrations, and an elevated IgE level is so non-specific (found in most atopic individuals, who are approximately a third of the population) that it is of little diagnostic value. Possible uses are as follows.

1 Helping to distinguish between atopic eczema and seborrhoeic dermatitis in infants with florid napkin rashes and scalp lesions (see Table 9.1). An elevated level would suggest a diagnosis of atopic eczema rather than seborrhoeic dermatitis.

2 A normal result might be of value in suggesting the presence of non-atopic disease (e.g. point away from a diagnosis of asthma in a child with wheezing), but this is unreliable because even those with severe atopic disease may rarely have normal serum IgE concentrations.

3 A normal result (e.g. 20 I.U./ml in a 2-year-old) might be thought to point away from IgE-mediated food intolerance, but the reasoning is false. A child might have intolerance to egg, with all of the IgE present directed against egg, but nevertheless have a normal total serum IgE concentration.

4 Screening newborns to detect potentially atopic babies and introduce some sort of interventional regimen (e.g. antigen avoidance). Problems with this are the need for special laboratory methods to detect the very low levels of IgE found in cord blood, and the lack of proof that interventional regimens are of any benefit.

An unhelpful test

Some children with food intolerance have an elevated total serum IgE concentration, but this can either be due to the production of food-specific IgE or an associated atopic disorder (e.g. eczema or asthma). Some children with food intolerance have a normal total serum IgE concentration, either because the mechanism is not IgE-mediated or because the food-specific IgE is insufficient to cause marked elevation of the total serum IgE concentration. Thus measurement of the total serum IgE concentration is of no practical value in the management of food intolerance. In trying to distinguish atopic from non-atopic subjects, the test is of limited use because of the wide range and considerable overlap (Klink *et al.* 1990).

Key references 44.1

ZETTERSTRÖM O & JOHANSSON SGO (1981) IgE concentrations measured by PRIST in serum of healthy adults and in patients with respiratory allergy. *Allergy* **36**:537–547. This study showed unusually good separation between an adult non-atopic and atopic population. *The study shows that 'normal' IgE values depend upon the selection of the reference population. In this study the reference group originated from those who in a healthy survey denied allergic symptoms. Those who had an IgE level more than one standard deviation above the mean were called back for investigation. Twelve of 14 such persons had a positive skin-prick test and were excluded.*

44.2

DOCKHORN RJ (1982) Using the RAST and PRIST with an overview of clinical significance. *Ann Allergy* **49**:1–8. 'Except in children under one year of age, measurements of total serum IgE have not contributed significantly to the diagnosis, predictive value and treatment of atopic disorders'.

44.3 KLINK M, CLINE MG, HALONEN M & BURROWS B (1990) Problems in defining normal limits for serum IgE. *J Allergy Clin Immunol* **85**:440–444. *The spread of IgE values is so wide in subjects with and without atopic disease that trying to define upper limits of normal for IgE concentration was felt to be of little value.*

44.4 YUNGINGER JW (1988) Clinical significance of IgE. In Middleton E, Reed CE, Ellis EF, Adkinson NF & Yunginger JW (eds) *Allergy. Principles and Practice*, 3rd edn, vol. 2, pp. 849–860, Mosby, St. Louis. Review of human IgE production, factors which affect IgE levels, interpretation of IgE measurements, and immuno-assays of IgE.

Summary 44   The serum concentration of IgE is very low and sensitive immuno-assays are required. Normal values vary with age and selection of the reference population. There is a wide range and a considerable overlap between non-atopic and atopic subjects. The measurement of the total serum IgE concentration is of no practical value in the management of food intolerance.

45   Provocation tests: inhalants
Important research tool

Relevance   The subject of inhalation provocation tests is relevant to this book because of the application of such tests to the study of food and food additive intolerance in children with asthma.

Purpose   The aim of provocation tests is to try to directly provoke symptoms by delivering an allergen direct to a target organ, rather than the indirect approach of skin testing. Provocation tests can also be used to measure non-specific reactivity.

Bronchial challenge tests   The two categories of test measure:
1 specific airway responsiveness;
2 non-specific airway responsiveness.

Specific airway response   In tests of specific airway responsiveness to an individual allergen, increasing concentrations of allergen are inhaled until a 20% fall in FEV1 occurs. Reactions are generally (a) early – within 30 min of inhalation, (b) late – occurs 4–8 hours after inhalation, or (c) dual – both early and late.

problems   The test suffers from many potential drawbacks. A test with pollen grains may fail to cause bronchoconstriction in pollen allergic

Table 45.1 Variables which can affect an allergen inhalation provocation test

Strength of allergen extract
Deposition in airway, which in turn is affected by particle size and the state of the asthma itself
Non-specific bronchial reactivity (see below)
Medication
The number of bronchial mast cells, their content of mediators, and their releasability

asthmatics simply because the pollen grains $(20-30\,\mu m)$ are trapped in the nose and do not reach the bronchi. Provocation with pollen extract $(1-2\,\mu m$ droplets), on the other hand, can give bronchoconstriction even in hay fever patients who are never troubled by asthma in the pollen season (Mygind 1986). There are fundamental differences between a provocation test in the laboratory and natural exposure. For example, a provocation test will expose the airway to a total allergen dose which may correspond to exposure for days or weeks during the pollen season. The response to an allergen provocation test is affected by a number of other variables (Table 45.1).

Non-specific response

Tests of non-specific airway responsiveness measure what is often called bronchial reactivity. Increasing concentrations of pharmacological agents with airway smooth muscle contractile effects, such as histamine or methacholine, are inhaled (O'Byrne & Zamel 1989). The most common variable used to express non-specific responsiveness is the concentration of drug causing a 20% fall in FEV1, as determined by interpolation between points on the dose-response curve. If variables such as respiratory infection, allergen exposure, cigarette smoking and changes in medication are avoided, then the measurement of bronchial reactivity by histamine challenge testing is highly reproducible (Hariparsad *et al.* 1983).

significance

Non-specific bronchial hyperreactivity is well recognized in asthma, although the underlying mechanism is poorly understood (Boushey *et al.* 1980). The reasons for wanting to measure non-specific bronchial responsiveness are as follows.

1 As a research tool, to help unravel the cause of asthma. If the causes of bronchial reactivity were known our understanding of asthma would be greatly increased.

2 As a research tool, to test drugs. This approach has been of limited value, because the effectiveness of a drug in blocking an acute bronchial challenge has not correlated particularly well with its effectiveness in clinical practice.

3 As a research tool and a measurement to help in the diagnosis, assessment and treatment of asthma.

4 As a research tool in the study of food intolerance in patients with asthma. Some studies have measured bronchial reactivity before and after food additive challenges in children with asthma. An increased bronchial reactivity has been taken as an objective indicator of intolerance. The relevant studies are discussed in chapter 52.

Nasal challenge tests

The introduction of the measurement of nasal airflow, rhino-manometry (Eccles 1989), and the use of semi-quantitative objective parameters such as counting sneezes, or weighing tissues after the nose has been blown, have facilitated research studies using nasal challenges (Youlten 1987; Solomon & McLean 1989). Interpretation of the results is complicated by factors which may affect the response to nasal challenge such as seasonal variation of nasal reactivity, mucociliary clearance, and the migration of basophils, mast cells and eosinophils into the nasal submucosa (Naclerio *et al.* 1988).

Conjunctival testing

A small quantity of dry pollen or diluted allergen extract is dropped into the lower conjunctival sac, and the patient is observed for lacrimation, sneezing, or injection of the conjunctivae or sclerae (Youlten 1987; Raizman 1989).

Clinical application limited

With the exception of food challenges in patients with suspected food intolerance (see next chapter), provocation tests have little place in routine clinical practice but have been important in the study of the pathophysiology and pharmacology of atopic disease. The results suffer from the same major limitation as the results of skin or IgE antibody testing, which is that a positive result from an allergen challenge by no means proves that the allergen is contributing to the patient's disease.

Key references 45.1 BOUSHEY HA, HOLTZMAN MJ, SHELLER JR & NADEL JA (1980) Bronchial hyperreactivity. *Am Rev Respir Dis* **121**:389–413. *Major review of methods of assessment, mechanisms and relationship to disease states.*

45.2 HARGREAVE FE (1987) Inhalation provocation tests. In Lessof MH, Lee TH & Kemeny DM (eds) *Allergy: An International Textbook*, pp. 289–303, Wiley, Chichester. *Summary of applications of measures of specific and non-specific bronchial responsiveness.*

45.3 SPECTOR SL (1989) (ed) *Provocative Challenge Procedures: Background and Methodology*, Futura Publishing Company, Mount Kisco, New York. *Review.*

45.4 MELILLO G, AAS K, CARTIER A *et al.* (1991) Guidelines for the standardization of bronchial provocation tests with allergens. An update by an international committee. *Allergy* **46**:321–329. *Recommendations about choice of allergen extracts, aerosol delivery systems and inhalation methods, interval required between withdrawal of drugs (e.g. different H1-receptor antagonists, corticosteroids, bronchodilators, cromoglycate) and antigen challenge, and measurement of the response.*

45.5   SOLOMON WR & MCLEAN JA (1989) Nasal provocative testing. In Spector SL (ed) *Provocative Challenge Procedures: Background and Methodology*, pp. 569–625, Futura Publishing Company, Mount Kisco, New York. *Review.*

Summary 45   The mucosa of the bronchi, nose or eyes can be directly provoked by an allergen extract. Unfortunately the response is affected by a number of variables, including a degree of non-specific reactivity. Allergen provocation is an important research tool but is of little use in clinical practice. The measurement of non-specific bronchial reactivity is useful for the study of asthma pathophysiology and pharmacology.

46   Provocation tests: food challenges I; procedure
Open challenge sufficient in most cases

Principle   The aim of a food challenge is to study the consequences of food or food additive ingestion.

Why bother?   Provocation tests are helpful either:
1 to confirm a history (parents' observations of alleged food intolerance are notoriously unreliable – see chapter 3);
2 to confirm the diagnosis, for example of cow's milk protein intolerance in infancy, where the diagnostic criteria include improvement on elimination diet and relapse on re-introduction;
3 to see if a child has grown out of a food intolerance;
4 as a research procedure.

Basic requirements   The food challenge should replicate normal food consumption in terms of dose, route and state of food. It should also be performed in such a way that the history can be verified. Thus, for example, it is no good solely looking for an immediate reaction if the parents report a delayed reaction.

Open challenges   Open food challenges are the simplest approach. The parents, doctor and the patient (if old enough) know what food is being given. An advantage is that the challenge can be made directly with the freshly prepared foodstuff concerned, rather than a freeze-dried or dehydrated preparation. The amount of food required, and the time required to wait for a reaction depend upon the history. Further details are given in chapter 14, where cow's milk challenges are described in detail.

Drawbacks   Open food challenges run the risk of bias influencing the parents' (or doctors') observations. Often this is immaterial (e.g. in cow's milk challenges to confirm a diagnosis of cow's milk protein intolerance – see chapter 14). But in some cases parental belief in food intolerance may be disproportionate, and where this is suspected there is no substitute for a double-blind placebo-controlled challenge. An open challenge may be an open invitation to the over-diagnosis of food intolerance. For example, in the UK parents widely believe that there is an association between food additives and bad behaviour, but in one series, double-blind challenges with tartrazine and benzoic acid were negative in all 24 children with a clear parental description of adverse reaction (David 1987).

Single-blind challenges   In a single-blind challenge the observer but not the patient or family know the identity of the test material. To avoid bias on the part of the observer, a double-blind challenge is required.

Double-blind challenges   The test comprises the administration of a challenge substance, which is either the item under investigation or an indistinguishable inactive (placebo) substance. Neither the child, the parents nor the observers know the identity of the administered material at the time of the challenge.

Challenge procedure: step 1
history

A detailed history is essential:
1 which food or foods are suspected;
2 what symptoms are produced;
3 how long after ingestion do the symptoms occur;
4 what is the smallest quantity of food which will produce the symptoms;
5 how frequently does the reaction occur;
6 how reproducible is the reaction, in other words, does it always happen when a food is ingested, or only on certain occasions;
7 does the reaction only occur in the presence of some additional factor, for example, does the reaction only occur if ingestion of the food is followed by exercise?

Challenge procedure: step 2
elimination diet

Suspect foods need to be avoided for approximately 2 weeks prior to challenge, on the grounds that regular administration of a food trigger could obscure a reaction to a single dose. The regular administration of salicylates to patients with salicylate intolerance quickly leads to a state of tolerance to salicylate (Kowalski *et al.* 1984). It is possible, although unproven, that a similar phenomenon can occur with foods and food additives.

clues to the relevance of food

An elimination diet (see chapters 70–75) also gives a clue as to the relevance of food intolerance. If the diet has no effect on symptoms then the common explanations are:
1 the food(s) avoided is/are irrelevant to the symptoms;
2 other foods are involved;
3 incomplete avoidance;
4 there was a genuine effect from the diet but a second pathology (e.g. infection in atopic eczema) supervened.

On the other hand if the diet does result in improvement, then the common explanations are:
1 placebo effect of diet, food intolerance irrelevant;
2 the food(s) avoided was genuinely causing symptoms.

Challenge procedure: step 3
recording results

The results should be recorded systematically, with details of the time given, the times of observation, the dose of food material given, and the nature of the symptoms observed.

Challenge procedure: step 4
preparation of foods

Dehydrated or dried powdered food is either administered in opaque white (tinted with titanium oxide) gelatin capsules containing up to 500 mg test material, or disguised in a carrier food such as milk, apple or vegetable puree, or lentil soup (Bock *et al.* 1988; Bock 1991). The procedure has been refined in north America, where a wide range of dehydrated or freeze-dried foods are easily available from camping stores.

Challenge procedure: step 5
placebos

Where capsules are used, the simplest placebos are dextrose or lactose powder. Liquid vehicles, without the addition of anything else, can be used as a placebo.

Challenge procedure: step 6
medication avoidance

Drugs which may need to be avoided before food challenge are:
1 H1-histamine antagonists – the duration of avoidance required depends on the duration of action of the drug;
2 theophylline – 12 hours;
3 cromoglycate – 12 hours.

The need for medication avoidance depends upon the circumstances. If the history is that the food provokes a reaction despite the medication, then withdrawal of treatment may not be needed. A potential drawback to withdrawing treatment is that this alone may precipitate symptoms, which may happen to coincide with either active or placebo challenge. This problem can only be avoided: (a) by not stopping the medication; or (b) by performing multiple challenges.

Challenge procedure: step 7 food administration

Food administration should start with a small quantity, less than that estimated by the parents to produce symptoms. The dose is then doubled at intervals specified by the history, so that if the reaction is said to occur after 30 min then the dose could be doubled every 45–60 min. The doubling dose is continued until the patient has obvious symptoms, or until about 10 g of dried or 100 g of untreated food have been given. In some cases, particularly those with delayed reactions, larger quantities of food may be needed (e.g. 200 ml of cow's milk per day).

Risk of anaphylactic shock

There are certain situations which carry a risk of anaphylactic shock (see chapter 63) occurring during a food challenge. These are as follows.

1 Where there is a previous history of anaphylactic shock. Great caution is needed (see procedure for cow's milk challenges, chapter 14). Is the challenge really needed? There may be a case for directly applying the food to the skin, prior to food challenge (see chapters 14 and 42). A negative reaction is no guarantee of safety, but a strongly positive reaction should make one reconsider whether the challenge is really necessary.

2 Certain foods (cow's milk, fish, nuts, egg) carry a greater risk of anaphylactic shock than others.

3 Food challenges in patients with atopic eczema who have been on elemental diets (see chapter 19) may constitute a special risk for anaphylactic shock (David 1989).

Repeat challenges

A high proportion of children with food intolerance 'grow out' of the intolerance (Bock 1982; Bock 1985; Sampson & Scanlon 1989), the exception being intolerance to peanuts which is usually life-long (Bock & Atkins 1989). This means that where a child has a positive food challenge, it may be worth repeating the challenge at 6–12-monthly intervals to detect the development of tolerance.

Problems and limitations

There are many problems and limitations. These are discussed in the next chapter.

Key references 46.1   BOCK SA, SAMPSON HA, ATKINS FM *et al.* (1988) Double-blind, placebo-controlled food challenge (DBPCFC) as an office procedure: a manual. *J Allergy Clin Immunol* **82**:986–997. *Good description of the procedure for performing double-blind food challenges, but uncritical about the numerous limitations and problems which are largely glossed over.*

46.2   BOCK SA (1991) Oral challenge procedures. In Metcalfe DD, Sampson HA & Simon RA (eds) *Food Allergy. Adverse Reactions to Foods and Food Additives*, pp. 83–112, Blackwell Scientific Publications, Oxford. *Review of the current north American approach, orientated rather more to research studies than to everyday clinical application.*

Summary 46   Food challenges are performed to confirm a history, or to see if a child has grown out of a food intolerance. The requirements (for example for blinding or placebo control) depend upon whether the test is intended to help patient management or as part of a research protocol. The challenge should replicate natural food consumption, and should be performed in such a way that the history can be validated. The procedure is to identify suspect trigger foods from the history, eliminate the suspect foods for a period, and avoid medications which could conceal a response. Very small amounts, followed by increasing quantities of suspect trigger foods, are then administered one at a time. Special caution is required because of the risk of anaphylactic shock. The numerous problems and limitations are discussed in the next chapter.

47 Provocation tests:
food challenges II; limitations
Challenges may give the wrong answer

The 'gold standard'?   The double-blind placebo-controlled challenge is regarded as the state-of-the-art technique to confirm or refute histories of adverse reactions to foods. The ability to unravel food-related problems is said to be limited only by the imagination of the physician and a clever dietitian (Bock *et al.* 1988). In fact the technique is subject to a number of potential limitations, not all of which can be overcome. These are discussed below.

Effect of dose   In some cases of food intolerance, minute quantities of food (e.g. traces of cow's milk protein) are sufficient to provoke florid and immediate symptoms. In other cases, much larger quantities of food are required to provoke a response. For example, Hill *et al.* demonstrated that whereas 8–10 g of cow's milk powder (corresponding to 60–70 ml of milk) was adequate to provoke an adverse reaction in some patients with cow's milk protein allergy, others (with late onset symptoms and particularly atopic eczema) required up to 10 times this volume of milk daily for more than 48 hours before symptoms developed (Hill *et al.* 1988).

history may not help

It is often unclear from the history what dosage of different foods is required to exclude food intolerance.

Concealing large doses is difficult

Standard capsules which contain up to 500 mg of food are suitable for validation of immediate reactions to tiny quantities of food, but concealing much larger quantities of certain foods (especially those with a strong smell, flavour or colour) can be very difficult. If capsules are not used then performing challenges which are truly double-blind (i.e. the parents don't know whether active substance or placebo is being given) at home becomes much more difficult.

Route of administration

Reactions to food occurring within the mouth (Amlot *et al.* 1985) are likely to be missed if the challenge by-passes the oral route, for example by administration of foods in a capsule (Bock *et al.* 1988) or via a nasogastric tube (Van Bever *et al.* 1989). In practice, patients whose symptoms are exclusively confined to the mouth are unusual, and where there is a history of purely oral reactions an alternative challenge procedure can be employed. In patients who are intolerant to sulphites, it is well recognized that the administration of sulphites in capsules or directly into the stomach via a nasogastric tube usually fails to provoke an adverse reaction, whereas the oral administration of solution will succeed in doing so (Delohery *et al.* 1984; Towns & Mellis 1984).

Problems with capsules

There are three main problems.
1 Capsules are unsuitable for use in children who cannot swallow large capsules, and this is a major limitation as most cases of suspected food intolerance are in infants and toddlers. Nasogastric tubes are too invasive for routine clinical use. This means adopting the much more difficult technique, that of trying to disguise one food in another carrier food.
2 It is unsatisfactory to allow patients or parents to break open capsules and swallow the contents mixed into food or drink, as the colour (e.g. tartrazine) or smell (e.g. fish) will be difficult or impossible to conceal and the challenge will no longer be blind.
3 gelatine capsules are unacceptable to strictly observant orthodox Jewish or vegetarian and vegan patients because of the animal origin of gelatine.

Raw or cooked food? Difficulties arise if a cooked food is used for testing and the patient is only sensitive to a raw food (Fries & Glaser 1950; Nater & Zwartz 1967), or vice versa (Prausnitz & Kustner 1921). Heating has been shown to reduce the sensitizing capacity of cow's milk (reviewed in chapter 16), and intolerance to raw but not cooked egg, potato and fish are well recognized. Although it is rare for these latter foods to be taken raw, the use of uncooked food items for challenges is likely to produce a number of false positive responses. The most logical but also the most time-consuming and impractical solution would be to perform all food challenges with both raw and cooked foods. The simplest solution is to choose the food in the state it is normally consumed.

Anaphylactic shock danger There is a danger of producing anaphylactic shock, even if anaphylactic shock had not occurred on previous exposure to the food. For example, in Goldman *et al.*'s classic study of cow's milk protein intolerance, anaphylactic shock had been noted prior to cow's milk challenge in five children, but another three out of 89 children developed anaphylactic shock as a new symptom after cow's milk challenge (Goldman *et al.* 1963). In a study of 80 children with atopic eczema treated with elimination diets, anaphylactic shock occurred in four out of 1862 food challenges (David 1984). The risk appears to be greatest for those who have received elemental diets (David 1989).

Effect of disease activity A food challenge performed during a quiescent phase of the disease may fail to provoke an adverse reaction. In chronic urticaria, intolerance to salicylates is confined to patients with active disease (Moore-Robinson & Warin 1967). The same phenomenon is commonly observed in atopic eczema, and is particularly noticeable when the skin lesions improve during a holiday in the sun (Turner *et al.* 1991), during which parents may note that the child can tolerate foods which are not tolerated at home.

Additive effect of triggers Although some patients react repeatedly to challenges with single foods, it is possible (but unproven) that some patients only react adversely when multiple allergens are given together. The additive effect of allergens has been best validated in patch testing (McLelland & Shuster 1990). Another mechanism is the potentiation of food intolerance by aspirin; a boy with mild urticaria after eating peanuts developed life-threatening anaphylaxis when eating peanuts after taking aspirin (Cant *et al.* 1984).

Atopic eczema Where food intolerance exists in children with atopic eczema, it is common for the patient to be intolerant to several foods. The removal of only one offending item may fail to help the patient. For the same reason it is possible that when this item is re-introduced into the diet in the form of a food challenge, the food may not provoke any detectable worsening of the dermatitis.

Other factors
In some situations, factors other than a food are necessary for positive challenges to occur. For example, in a subgroup of patients with exercise-induced anaphylaxis, symptoms only occur if exercise follows the ingestion of a particular food (Kidd *et al.* 1983). Exercise or the food alone fail to provoke symptoms.

unidentified factors
In some cases, the nature of the 'other factor' is obscure. For example, tartrazine challenges in children with asthma who are intolerant to tartrazine may fail to provoke any significant change in lung function, although histamine challenge testing may reveal enhanced bronchial reactivity (Hariparsad *et al.* 1984). It is not known what additional factors are required to produce symptoms in such patients. The point here is that a conventional double-blind challenge, using as an endpoint, for example, a 20% fall in FEV1, would fail to confirm genuine tartrazine intolerance.

Different reactions
The nature of adverse reactions to foods may alter after a period of dietary elimination, for reasons which are unclear. The most dramatic example of this phenomenon is the occurrence of anaphylactic shock after a cow's milk challenge in a child with cow's milk protein intolerance who presented with less serious symptoms such as atopic eczema or loose stools (see chapter 9).

Statistical problems
A challenge procedure may coincide with worsening of the underlying disease process so that there is a chance of the wrong inference being drawn from the result of a single challenge. There is a special risk of this happening in children with atopic eczema, a disorder characterized by unpredictable and unexplained fluctuations, and where there is no clear end point such as a 20% fall in FEV1. To reduce the risk of this, one may need to perform multiple challenges with individual foods. Chance alone may result in incorrect identification of active or placebo substance in double-blind placebo-controlled challenges, a statistical problem which has been largely overlooked in previously published studies (Pearson 1987; Devlin & David 1992).

Clinical value
Double-blind placebo-controlled food challenges are clearly the best available tool to confirm food intolerance. However it is evident that single food challenges fail to take into account any possible additive effect of allergens. They also may fail to provoke a reaction if an underlying disease (e.g. urticaria or atopic eczema) is inactive, and

unless performed with great care may fail to replicate natural exposure in which some other factor such as exercise is required to produce a positive reaction.

Key references 47.1 BOCK SA & ATKINS FM (1990) Patterns of food hypersensitivity during sixteen years of double-blind, placebo-controlled food challenges. *J Pediat* **117**:561–567. Includes a report of 12 children with a negative double-blind placebo-controlled challenge to a food in whom open challenges to larger amounts of foods produced positive reactions. *Reinforces the observations of Goldman* et al. *and Hill* et al., *made in the context of cow's milk protein intolerance, that an important group of children only react to larger quantities of food than can be given in capsules in conventional double-blind placebo-controlled challenges.*

47.2 HILL DJ & HOSKING CS (1991) Some limitations of double-blind, placebo-controlled food challenges in young children. *J Allergy Clin Immunol* **87**: 136–137.
1 *Urges caution in using double-blind challenges in infants with cow's milk protein intolerance, because of the risk of anaphylaxis, particularly with the standard doses used for testing with dried food in capsules.*
2 *Points out that delayed reactions to food are common in young children.*
3 *Points out that it is misleading to assume that food intolerance is almost excluded by a negative skin-prick test – 31% of their skin-prick test negative patients had intolerance to cow's milk protein.*

47.3 DAVID TJ (1989) Hazards of challenge tests in atopic dermatitis. *Allergy* (suppl. 9):101–107. Reviews the possible reasons why food challenge tests may give the wrong result, and discusses anaphylactic shock. *The main danger of challenge tests is arriving at the wrong result. The possible pitfalls are outlined.*

Summary 47 The double-blind placebo-controlled food challenge is the best currently available technique for confirming or refuting a diagnosis of intolerance to a food. The major potential limitations are:
1 an inadequate dose may fail to provoke symptoms, and it may be very difficult or impossible to conceal large doses of food;
2 by bypassing the mouth, encapsulated foods may fail to provoke an adverse reaction;
3 infants and small children are unlikely to be able to swallow capsules;
4 the food should be given in the state it is normally consumed – a raw food may provoke an adverse reaction when the cooked food will not, and the reverse can also happen;
5 there is a danger that a food challenge following a period of elimination may produce new symptoms not originally present, for example anaphylactic shock;
6 a challenge performed in a quiescent phase of a disease, or when the disease is in remission, may fail to provoke an adverse reaction;
7 the effect of allergens may be additive, and challenge with a single food trigger on its own may fail to provoke a reaction;

8 where other factors (not always identifiable) are required, a challenge may fail to provoke symptoms in the absence of the other factor (e.g. in food-plus-exercise-provoked anaphylaxis);

9 a single food and placebo challenge may give a misleading result because of a chance deterioration which coincides with active or placebo challenge – only repeated challenges can deal with this problem.

48 Other types of food challenge
Observation and biopsy of mucosal surfaces

Oral mucosal challenge

Swelling of the lips, and tingling or irritation of the mouth or tongue are commonly reported features of immediate (within minutes) reactions to foods, often followed by other more generalized symptoms such as urticaria, asthma, vomiting, abdominal pain or anaphylactic shock. Patients with food intolerance commonly make use of these oral symptoms, spitting out and avoiding further consumption of a food which provokes the symptom. The importance of these oral symptoms in the context of this chapter is that oral challenges with encapsulated material will not reproduce these symptoms (Lessof *et al.* 1987). Where oral symptoms predominate, challenges should not bypass the oral mucosa.

procedure

Amlot *et al.* used 2 ml of a lyophilized egg or milk solution at 10 mg/ml (Amlot *et al.* 1985), placed in the lower labio-gingival trough, and recorded oral irritation, oral mucosal blebs, throat tightness and lip swelling occurring within 15 min of challenge.

clinical relevance

Apart from a small study in a highly selected very atopic group of adults, many of whom had notable oral symptoms after food ingestion (Amlot *et al.* 1985), buccal provocation tests have not been validated, and their use in children with suspected food intolerance has not been studied. Clearly this method cannot be used where reactions only occur to larger amounts of food than can be administered in this way.

Gastric mucosal challenge

In this procedure, an allergen is applied directly to the gastric mucosa via an endoscope, and the mucosa is then observed for signs of a reaction (Reimann & Lewin 1988). An example of a scoring system is:

0   no reaction;
1   swelling, hyperaemia;
2   petechial haemorrhage;
3   superficial haemorrhage;
4   frank haemorrhage.

mucosal biopsy

In addition, it is possible to take biopsies of the gastric mucosa to study the histological changes and measure the tissue concentration of mediators of inflammation such as histamine (Reimann *et al.* 1985).

gastric mucosal reactions

Reimann & Lewin (1988) studied 30 adults with food intolerance proven by double-blind oral food challenge, and who mainly had abdominal pain, vomiting or diarrhoea, with gastric provocation under endoscopic control. The food provocations were performed double-blind. The gastric mucosa was macroscopically normal prior to testing in all patients, but after allergen contact all patients developed mucosal reactions comprising swelling and haemorrhage.

histological changes

Histology of the gastric mucosal biopsies in the above study showed mucosal erosion and depletion of mast cell histamine content. Prior to challenge lymphocyte counts in the mucosa were elevated, but there was very little increase after food challenge.

clinical relevance

Patients challenged in this way all developed symptoms (mainly gastrointestinal – abdominal pain, diarrhoea, vomiting, colic, flatulence), but 10 healthy volunteers studied in the same way did not develop symptoms, visible mucosal changes or histological changes. It is not known whether this will prove a useful tool in the assessment of children with food intolerance; at present it remains an interesting research procedure.

Rectal challenges

The standard test to confirm a diagnosis of coeliac disease is the jejunal biopsy (see chapter 27). However, it has recently been reported that rectal challenge with gluten is a simple, safe and reliable test of gluten intolerance, both as a screening test for untreated coeliac disease and also as a confirmatory test in patients with treated coeliac disease (Loft *et al.* 1990). Rectal biopsy was performed before and 6 hours after a rectal challenge with 2 g of a peptic-tryptic digest of gluten, and the total intraepithelial lymphocytes overlying a test area of muscularis mucosae quantified by computerized image analysis. A post-challenge lymphocyte index of 10% above the pre-challenge value was used to indicate a diagnosis of coeliac disease (sensitivity 90%, specificity 91%, 95% confidence intervals 78–93%).

possible uses   Rectal gluten challenge requires further validation, but offers the prospect of a simple screening test for gluten intolerance in those with suspected coeliac disease. It may also provide a simpler alternative to the longer and potentially more unpleasant oral gluten challenge and jejunal biopsy (Loft *et al.* 1990).

Key references 48.1   AMLOT PL, URBANEK R, YOULTEN LJF, KEMENY M & LESSOF MH (1985) Type I allergy to egg and milk proteins: comparison of skin prick tests with nasal, buccal and gastric provocation tests. *Int Arch Allergy Appl Immunol* **77**:171–173. This study compared the effects of giving antigen by different routes in 15 highly selected very atopic adults with food intolerance, using prick tests, nasal drops, buccal mucosal challenge and swallowed capsules. In these cases, objective evidence of response was obtained almost as readily with nasal challenge – as indicated by repeated sneezing or a 50% increase in nasal airways resistance – as with skin tests. Larger concentrations of allergen were required to elicit a buccal mucosal response, as shown by measurable lip swelling; and a gastric response either required considerably larger quantities of antigen or did not occur at all (but the end point was clinical symptoms, such as nausea or abdominal pain, rather than direct inspection of the gastric mucosa). *In this highly selected group of patients with oral allergy symptoms, the order of tissue sensitivity was prick tests > nasal > buccal > gastric. These observations are only likely to apply to this selected subset of patients with immediate onset IgE-mediated reactions to food.*

48.2   REIMANN HJ & LEWIN J (1988) Gastric mucosal reactions in patients with food allergy. *Amer J Gastroenterol* **83**:1212–1219. Gastric biopsies taken 10 min after direct application of allergen to gastric mucosa demonstrated mast cell degranulation and histamine release. Symptoms occurred 10 min to 24 hours after challenge.

48.3   LOFT DE, MARSH MN & CROWE PT (1990) Rectal gluten challenge and diagnosis of coeliac disease. *Lancet* **335**:1293–1295. Study of 44 adult patients who were referred for jejunal biopsy, showing that rectal gluten challenge is a simple, safe and reliable test of gluten intolerance in adults with coeliac disease. *Whether children will prefer the trauma of rectal biopsy to that of jejunal biopsy remains to be determined.*

Summary 48   Buccal mucosal provocation tests with food extracts may be of value in those with prominent oral symptoms, but are unlikely to be generally applicable to children with suspected food intolerance. The observation by endoscopy and biopsy of macroscopic and microscopic changes in the gastric mucosa within hours of direct mucosal challenge in patients with gastrointestinal symptoms of food intolerance is an interesting research tool, but invasive and not yet generally applicable. Rectal gluten challenge for suspected gluten intolerance requires further validation, but offers the prospect of a simple screening test for gluten intolerance in the context of coeliac disease. It may also provide a simpler alternative to the longer and potentially more unpleasant oral gluten challenge.

49 Miscellaneous other tests
Counting eosinophils and measuring basophil histamine release

Eosinophil counts

Circulating eosinophils are seen in low numbers in the blood of healthy subjects. Counting eosinophils on a blood film as a percentage of 100 white cells is subject to two built-in forms of error – influence of the total white cell count, and sampling errors. The upper limit of normal is said to be 4%. A more reliable figure is obtained if eosinophils are specially stained and then counted in a counting chamber. The normal value for an absolute eosinophil count in children is said to be 240 cells/mm^3 (Cunningham 1975). There is a moderate degree of age and sex dependence, with higher values exhibited by boys and with peaks in the age range of 4–8 years (Cunningham 1975).

Tissue distribution

Although counting eosinophils in blood is the best available method for assessing host response characterized by eosinophilia, these circulating cells reflect only those that are trafficking between the site of production, bone marrow, and the tissues. The greatest density of eosinophils outside the bone marrow occur in the gastrointestinal tract, the lungs and the uterus. The density of eosinophils is lower in the skin, but the large mass of skin makes it the chief repository of tissue eosinophils (Nutman *et al.* 1988).

Disease associations

As with an elevated total serum IgE concentration, the major associations of increased circulating eosinophils are allergic disease and parasitic helminth infections. There are, however, a large number of other disorders associated with peripheral blood eosinophilia, and these are reviewed elsewhere (Nutman *et al.* 1988).

Eosinophilia and atopy

Eosinophils are a hallmark of IgE-mediated allergic diseases. Tissue eosinophils in the target organs in atopic subjects are sometimes degranulated, and it is believed that eosinophil products, particularly granule-associated basic proteins and membrane-derived lipids may be directly responsible for tissue damage and inflammation (Mygind 1986). The degree of eosinophilia in blood only appears to give information about the severity of inflammation and the size of the organ affected. Thus patients with eczema or asthma tend to have higher eosinophil counts than those with rhinitis. Unfortunately, eosinophilia gives no information about whether the disorder has any allergic basis or not, and eosinophil counts cannot be used to indicate the presence or absence of food intolerance.

Leucocyte histamine release Where a subject is allergic to an allergen (e.g. grass pollen), the addition of the allergen to the blood or washed leucocytes of the subject results in the release of histamine from the basophils, which are the only cells in human peripheral blood that contain histamine. The release of histamine is triggered by interaction between the allergen and specific IgE antibody fixed to the basophil (Bernstein 1988). The serum of allergic individuals also contains blocking IgG antibodies that can also react with the allergen, so to avoid this interference histamine release measurements are made with washed leucocytes.

drawbacks A drawback to the method is that in about 10% to 15% of patients with a convincing history of a specific allergy and positive skin tests, the leucocytes fail to release histamine. Cells from patients with urticaria frequently do not release histamine (Bernstein 1988). A further problem is that the test must be performed within a relatively short time after the sample of blood has been obtained, compared with tests for specific IgE antibodies where samples can be stored and processed at a central laboratory.

advantages The advantage of histamine release assays are that they are not dependent on coupling of the allergens to discs, and with washed leucocyte preparations there is no competition between IgG and IgE for binding sites, so that IgG cannot interfere with the assay. A new glass microfilter-based method of binding histamine, based on the fact that glass microfilters bind histamine with high affinity and selectivity, has enabled the automated assay of very small samples (25 μl) of blood (Nolte *et al.* 1990; Østergaard *et al.* 1990).

clinical application The limitations described above mean that histamine release is not yet applicable as an aid to routine clinical allergy diagnosis, and remains a research tool (Bernstein 1988). Since the test is ultimately dependent on allergen specific IgE, it is unlikely to be helpful in the investigation of patients with food intolerance, a heterogeneous disorder not necessarily IgE-mediated.

Target tissue histamine release As a result of a study in 24 adults with food intolerance, it was suggested that measurement of histamine release in duodenal biopsy specimens after incubation with suspect foods may be a method to diagnose gastrointestinal food intolerance (Baenkler & Lux 1989). However this cumbersome and invasive approach requires further confirmation before it could be considered anything other than a research tool.

Key references   49.1   KAY AB (1990) (ed) *Eosinophils, Allergy and Asthma*, Blackwell Scientific Publications, Oxford. Comprises 20 chapters, which succinctly review eosinophil biology, including the molecular biology of eosinophil major basic protein, the nature of receptors for immunoglobulins, and interaction between eosinophils and platelet activating factor.

49.2   NOLTE H, STORM K & SCHIØTZ PO (1990) Diagnostic value of a glass fibre-based histamine analysis for allergy testing in children. *Allergy* **45**:213–223. This study compares the results of skin-prick testing, RAST testing, bronchial provocation testing and basophil histamine release in 124 children with asthma. On the basis of these results, which showed a close correlation between RAST and basophil histamine release, the authors suggest that the latter is a reliable diagnostic test in children. *Problems:*
1 *the 'gold standard' was bronchial provocation, which as explained in chapter 47 is itself of uncertain reliability;*
2 *the study excluded an unstated number of cases who did not have 'responding basophils', artificially boosting the potential usefulness of the technique;*
3 *no mention is made of the need for freshly obtained samples.*

49.3   LAU S & WAHN U (1989) Relationship of histamine release and other in vitro methods to oral provocation test in hen's egg allergic patients. In Harms HK & Wahn U (eds) *Food Allergy in Infancy and Childhood*, pp. 138–145, Springer Verlag, London. Of 27 children with a history of egg intolerance, 17 reacted to a challenge with up to 1 g of ovalbumin, and 10 did not. Of the 17 with a positive challenge test, 12 showed significant histamine release while five did not. Of the 10 with negative provocation tests, six had significant histamine release. *Studies of specific IgE, IgG1 and IgG4 antibodies showed that these tests were almost as useless as leucocyte histamine release.*

Summary 49   The number of circulating eosinophils is best estimated in a counting chamber. The eosinophil count depicts the severity of the allergic inflammation and the size of the organs involved. Eosinophil counts cannot be used to indicate the presence or absence of food intolerance. In an allergic subject, the addition of the allergen to the subject's washed leucocytes results in basophil histamine release, triggered by interaction between the allergen and specific IgE antibody fixed to the basophil. Problems include failure to release histamine in up to 15% of patients with genuine allergies and some patients with urticaria, and a need to perform the test on freshly taken blood. Basophil histamine release is currently a research tool; it is unlikely to be any more use than other tests which detect specific IgE antibodies such as prick tests or RAST tests.

References to Chapters 39–49

AAS K (1978) The diagnosis of hypersensitivity to ingested foods. Reliability of skin-prick testing and the radioallergosorbent test with different materials. *Clin Allergy* **8**:39–50.

AAS K (1989) Biochemical characteristics of food allergens. In Harms HK & Wahn U (eds) *Food Allergy in Infancy and Childhood*, pp. 1–12, Springer, Berlin.

AAS K, BACKMAN A, BELIN L & WEEKE B (1978) Standardization of allergen extracts with appropriate methods. The combined use of skin-prick testing and radio-allergosorbent tests. *Allergy* **33**:130–137.

AAS K & BELIN L (1972) Standardization of diagnostic work in allergy. *Acta Allergol* **27**:439–468.

ACCIAI MC, BRUSI C, FRANCALANCI S, GOLA M & SERTOLI A (1991) Skin tests with fresh foods. *Contact Derm* **24**:67–68.

ADINOFF AD, ROSLONIEC DM, McCALL LL & NELSON HS (1989) A comparison of six epicutaneous devices in the performance of immediate hypersensitivity skin testing. *J Allergy Clin Immunol* **84**:168–174.

AGARWAL K & ZETTERSTROM O (1982) Diagnostic significance of late cutaneous allergic responses and their correlation with radioallergosorbent test. *Clin Allergy* **12**:489–497.

ALEXANDER HL & McCONNELL FS (1930) The variability of skin reactions in allergy. *J Allergy* **2**:23–33.

ALMIND M, DIRKSEN A, NIELSEN NH & SVENDSEN (1988) Duration of the inhibitory activity on histamine-induced skin weals of sedative and non-sedative antihistamines. *Allergy* **43**:593–596.

AMLOT PL, URBANEK R, YOULTEN LJF, KEMENY M & LESSOF MH (1985) Type I allergy to egg and milk proteins: comparison of skin-prick tests with nasal, buccal and gastric provocation tests. *Int Arch Allergy Appl Immunol* **77**:171–173.

ANCONA GR & SCHUMACHER IC (1950) The use of raw foods as skin testing material in allergic disorders. *Calif Med* **73**:473–475.

ANDERSSON M & PIPKORN U (1987) Inhibition of the dermal immediate allergic reaction through prolonged treatment with topical glucocorticosteroids. *J Allergy Clin Immunol* **79**:345–349.

BAENKLER HW & LUX G (1989) Antigen-induced histamine-release from duodenal biopsy in gastrointestinal food allergy. *Ann Allergy* **62**:449–452.

BAHNA SL & GANDHI MD (1987) Reliability of skin testing and RAST in diagnosis of food allergy. In Chandra RK (ed) *Food Allergy*, pp. 139–147, Nutrition Research Education Foundation, St. John's, Newfoundland.

BERNSTEIN IL (1988) (ed) Proceedings of the task force on guidelines for standardizing old and new technologies used for the diagnosis and treatment of allergic diseases. *J Allergy Clin Immunol* **82**:487–526.

BJORKSTEN F, HAAHTELA T, BACKMAN A & SUONIEMI I (1984) Assay of the biologic activity of allergen skin test preparations. *J Allergy Clin Immunol* **73**:324–331.

BOCK SA (1982) The natural history of food sensitivity. *J Allergy Clin Immunol* **69**:173–177.

BOCK SA (1985) Natural history of severe reactions to foods in young children. *J Pediat* **107**:676–680.

BOCK SA (1991) Oral challenge procedures. In Metcalfe DD, Sampson HA &

Simon RA (eds) *Food Allergy. Adverse Reactions to Foods and Food Additives*, pp. 83–112, Blackwell Scientific Publications, Oxford.

BOCK SA & ATKINS FM (1989) The natural history of peanut allergy. *J Allergy Clin Immunol* **83**:900–904.

BOCK SA, BUCKLEY J, HOLST A & MAY CD (1977) Proper use of skin tests with food extracts in diagnosis of hypersensitivity to food in children. *Clin Allergy* **7**:375–383.

BOCK SA, LEE WY, REMIGIO L, HOLST A & MAY CD (1978) Appraisal of skin tests with food extracts for diagnosis of food hypersensitivity. *Clin Allergy* **8**:559–564.

BOCK SA, SAMPSON HA, ATKINS FM *et al.* (1988) Double-blind, placebo-controlled food challenge (DBPCFC) as an office procedure: a manual. *J Allergy Clin Immunol* **82**:986–997.

BOUSHEY HA, HOLTZMAN MJ, SHELLER JR & NADEL JA (1980) Bronchial hyperreactivity. *Am Rev Respir Dis* **121**:389–413.

BOUSQUET J (1988) In vivo methods for study of allergy: skin tests, techniques, and interpretation. In Middleton E, Reed CE, Ellis EF, Adkinson NF & Yunginger JW (eds) *Allergy. Principles and Practice*, 3rd edn, vol. 1, pp. 419–436, Mosby, St Louis.

BOWMAN KL (1935) Pertinent factors influencing comparative skin tests on the arm. *J Allergy* **7**:39–53.

BRENEMAN JC, SWEENEY M & ROBERT A (1989) Patch tests demonstrating immune (antibody and cell-mediated) reactions to foods. *Ann Allergy* **62**: 461–469.

BROWN HM, SU S & THANTREY N (1981) Prick testing for allergen, standardization by using a precision needle. *Clin Allergy* **11**:95–98.

BURROWS D (1989) Mischievous metals – chromate, cobalt, nickel and mercury. *Clin Exper Dermatol* **14**:266–272.

CANT AJ, GIBSON P & DANCY M (1984) Food hypersensitivity made life threatening by ingestion of aspirin. *Br Med J* **288**:755–756.

CHAMPION RH, BURTON JL & EBLING FJG (1992) (eds) *Textbook of Dermatology*, 5th edn, Blackwell Scientific Publications, Oxford.

COOPMAN S, DEGREEF H & DOOMS-GOOSSENS A (1989) Identification of cross-reaction patterns in allergic contact dermatitis from topical corticosteroids. *Br J Dermatol* **121**:27–34.

COURT J & NG LM (1984) Danger of egg white treatment for nappy rash. *Arch Dis Child* **59**:908.

CRONIN E (1980) *Contact Dermatitis*, Churchill Livingstone, Edinburgh.

CUNNINGHAM AS (1975) Eosinophil counts: age and sex differences. *J Pediat* **87**:426–427.

CURRAN WS & GOLDMAN G (1961) The incidence of immediately reacting allergy skin tests in a 'normal' adult population. *Ann Intern Med* **55**:777–783.

DAVID TJ (1984) Anaphylactic shock during elimination diets for severe atopic eczema. *Arch Dis Child* **59**:983–986.

DAVID TJ (1987) Reactions to dietary tartrazine. *Arch Dis Child* **62**:119–122.

DAVID TJ (1989) Hazards of challenge tests in atopic dermatitis. *Allergy* (suppl. 9):101–107.

DAVID TJ (1991) Conventional allergy tests. *Arch Dis Child* **66**:281–282.

DEVLIN J & DAVID TJ (1992) Tartrazine in atopic eczema. *Arch Dis Child* **67**:709–711.

DELOHERY J, SIMMUL R, CASTLE WD & ALLEN DH (1984) The relationship of inhaled sulfur dioxide reactivity to ingested metabisulphite sensitivity in patients with asthma. *Amer Rev Respir Dis* **130**:1027–1032.

DEPARTMENT OF HEALTH (1991) Report on Health and Social Subjects 41. *Dietary Reference Values for Food Energy and Nutrients for the United Kingdom*, Report of the Panel on Dietary Reference Values of the Committee on Medical Aspects of Food Policy, Her Majesty's Stationery Office, London.

DOCKHORN RJ (1982) Using the RAST and PRIST with an overview of clinical significance. *Ann Allergy* **49**:1–8.

DREBORG S (1989) (ed) Skin tests used in type I allergy testing. Position paper. Prepared by the sub-committee on skin tests of the European Academy of Allergology and Clinical Immunology. *Allergy* **44** (suppl. 10):1–59.

ECCLES R (1989) Rhinomanometry and nasal challenge. In Mackay IS (ed) *Rhinitis. Mechanisms and Management*, pp. 53–67, Royal Society of Medicine, London.

EICHLER I, GOTZ M, JARISCH, EICHLER HG & MOSS R (1988) Reproducibility of skin prick testing with allergen extracts from different manufacturers. *Allergy* **43**:458–463.

ERIKSSON NE (1977) Diagnosis of reaginic allergy with house dust, animal dander and pollen allergens. II. A comparison between skin tests and provocation tests. *Int Arch Allergy Appl Immunol* **53**:341–348.

ERIKSSON NE (1989) Total IgE influences the relationship between skin test and RAST. *Ann Allergy* **63**:65–69.

FINE AJ (1981) Hypersensitivity reaction to kiwi fruit (Chinese gooseberry, *Actinidia chinensis*). *J Allergy Clin Immunol* **68**:235–237.

FISHER AA (1983) Contact dermatitis from food additives. *Immunol Allergy Prac* **5**:316–322.

FONTANA VJ, WITTIG H & HOLT LE (1963) Observations on the specificity of the skin test. The incidence of positive skin tests in allergic and nonallergic children. *J Allergy* **34**:348–353.

FORD RPK & TAYLOR B (1982) Natural history of egg hypersensitivity. *Arch Dis Child* **57**:649–652.

FREW AJ & KAY AB (1988) The pattern of human late-phase skin reactions to extracts of aeroallergens. *J Allergy Clin Immunol* **81**:1117–1121.

FRIES JH & GLAZER I (1950) Studies on the antigenicity of banana, raw and dehydrated. *J Allergy* **21**:169–175.

GALANT SP & MAIBACH HI (1973) Reproducibility of allergy epicutaneous test techniques. *J Allergy Clin Immunol* **51**:245–250.

GOLDMAN AS, ANDERSON DW, SELLERS WA, SAPERSTEIN S, KNIKER WT & HALPERN SR (1963) Milk allergy. I. Oral challenge with milk and isolated milk proteins in allergic children. *Pediatrics* **32**:425–443.

HAGY GW & SETTIPANE GA (1972) Prognosis of positive allergy skin tests in an asymptomatic population. A three year follow-up of college students. *J Allergy Clin Immunol* **48**:200–211.

HAMILTON RG & ADKINSON NF (1986) Serological methods for the assessment and management of IgE-mediated diseases. *Clin Immunol Newsletter* **7**:10–14.

HAMMARLUND A, OLSSON P & PIPKORN U (1990) Blood flow in histamine- and allergen-induced weal and flare responses, effects of an H1 antagonist, α-adrenoceptor agonist and a topical glucocorticoid. *Allergy* **45**:64–70.

HARGREAVE FE (1987) Inhalation provocation tests. In Lessof MH, Lee TH & Kemeny DM (eds) *Allergy: An International Textbook*, pp. 289–303, Wiley, Chichester.

HARIPARSAD D, WILSON N, DIXON C & SILVERMAN M (1983) Reproducibility of histamine challenge tests in asthmatic children. *Thorax* **38**:258–260.

HARIPARSAD D, WILSON N, DIXON C & SILVERMAN M (1984) Oral tartrazine challenge in childhood asthma: effect on bronchial reactivity. *Clin Allergy*

14:81–85.

HILL DJ, BALL G & HOSKING CS (1988) Clinical manifestations of cow's milk allergy in childhood. I. Associations with in-vitro cellular immune responses. *Clin Allergy* **18**:469–479.

HILL DJ, DUKE AM, HOSKING CS & HUDSON IL (1988) Clinical manifestations of cow's milk allergy in childhood. II. The diagnostic value of skin tests and RAST. *Clin Allergy* **18**:481–490.

HILLAS JL & WILSON JD (1981) Variation in potency of extracts used for allergy skin tests. *New Zealand Med J* **94**:2–4.

HOLT LE (1967) A nonallergist looks at allergy. *New Engl J Med* **276**:1449–1454.

JARMOC LM & PRIMACK WA (1987) Anaphylaxis to cutaneous exposure to milk protein in a diaper rash ointment. *Clin Pediat* **26**:154–155.

JOSEPHSON BM & GLASER J (1963) A comparison of skin-testing with natural foods and commercial extracts. *Ann Allergy* **21**:33–40.

JUTO P & STRANNEGÅRD Ö (1979) T lymphocytes and blood eosinophils in early infancy in relation to heredity for allergy and type of feeding. *J Allergy Clin Immunol* **64**:38–42.

KÄGI MK & WÜTHRICH B (1991) Falafel-burger anaphylaxis due to sesame seed allergy. *Lancet* **338**:582.

KLINK M, CLINE MG, HALONEN M & BURROWS B (1990) Problems in defining normal limits for serum IgE. *J Allergy Clin Immunol* **85**:440–444.

KOWALSKI ML, GRZELEWSKA-RZYMOWSKA I, ROZNIECKI J & SZMIDT M (1984) Aspirin tolerance induced in aspirin-sensitive asthmatics. *Allergy* **39**:171–178.

LEE RE, SMOLENSKY MH, LEACH CS & MCGOVERN JP (1977) Circadian rhythms in the cutaneous reactivity to histamine and selected antigens, including phase relationship to urinary cortisol excretion. *Ann Allergy* **38**:231–236.

LESSOF MH (1987) Skin tests. In Lessof MH, Lee TH & Kemeny DM (eds) *Allergy: An International Textbook*, pp. 281–287, Wiley, Chichester.

LESSOF MH, BUISSERET PD, MERRETT J, MERRETT TG & WRAITH DG (1980) Assessing the value of skin prick tests. *Clin Allergy* **10**:115–120.

LESSOF MH, KEMENY DM & AMLOT PL (1987) The investigation of food intolerance. In Chandra RK (ed) *Food Allergy*, pp. 7–17, Nutrition Research Education Foundation, St. John's, Newfoundland.

LILJA G, JOHANSSON SGO, KUSOFFSKY E & ÖMAN H (1990) IgE levels in cord blood and at 4–5 days of age: relation to clinical symptoms of atopic disease up to 18 months of age. *Allergy* **45**:436–444.

LOCKEY RF, BENEDICT LM, TURKELTAUB PC & BUKANTZ SC (1987) Fatalities from immunotherapy (IT) and skin testing (ST). *J Allergy Clin Immunol* **79**:660–677.

LOFT DE, MARSH MN & CROWE PT (1990) Rectal gluten challenge and diagnosis of coeliac disease. *Lancet* **335**:1293–1295.

LONG RT, LAMONT JH, WHIPPLE B, BANDLER L, BLOM GE, BURGIN I & JESSNER L (1958) A psychosomatic study of allergic and emotional factors in children with asthma. *Am J Psychol* **114**:890–899.

MAGNUSSON CGM (1988) Cord serum IgE in relation to family history and as predictor of atopic disease in early infancy. *Allergy* **43**:241–251.

MCLELLAND J & SHUSTER S (1990) Contact dermatitis with negative patch tests: the additive effect of allergens in combination. *Br J Dermatol* **122**:623–630.

MEGLIO P, FARINELLA F, TROGOLO E, GIAMPIETRO PG, CANTANI A & BUSINCO L (1988) Immediate reactions following challenge-tests in children with atopic dermatitis. *Allergie Immunol* **20**:57–62.

MICHEL FB & BOUSQUET J (1983) Neonatal predictive tests of the 'high allergic risk' newborn. In Kerr JW & Ganderton MA (eds) *Proceedings of the XI*

International Congress of Allergology and Clinical Immunology, pp. 135–138, Macmillan, London.

MILLER J & NELSON HS (1989) Suppression of immediate skin tests by ranitidine. *J Allergy Clin Immunol* **84**:895–899.

MORGAN JE, DAUL CB, HUGHES J, McCANTS M & LEHRER SB (1989) Food specific skin-test reactivity in atopic subjects. *Clin Exper Allergy* **19**:431–435.

MYGIND N (1986) *Essential Allergy*, p. 119–123, Blackwell Scientific Publications, Oxford.

NACLERIO RM, NORMAN PS & FISH JE (1988) In vivo methods for study of allergy: mucosal tests, techniques, and interpretation. In Middleton E, Reed CE, Ellis EF, Adkinson NF & Yunginger JW (eds) *Allergy. Principles and Practice*, 3rd edn, vol. 1, pp. 437–460, Mosby, St Louis.

NATER JP & ZWARTZ JA (1967) Atopic allergic reactions due to raw potato. *J Allergy* **40**:202–206.

NOLTE H, STORM K & SCHIØTZ PO (1990) Diagnostic value of a glass fibre-based histamine analysis for allergy testing in children. *Allergy* **45**:213–223.

NUTMAN TB, OTTESEN EA & COHEN SG (1988) Eosinophilia and eosinophil-related disorders. In Middleton E, Reed CE, Ellis EF, Adkinson NF & Yunginger JW (eds) *Allergy. Principles and Practice*, 3rd edn, vol. 2, pp. 861–890, Mosby, St Louis.

O'BYRNE PM & ZAMEL Z (1989) Airway challenges with inhaled constrictor mediators. In Spector SL (ed) *Provocative Challenge Procedures: Background and Methodology*, pp. 277–291, Futura Publishing Company, Mount Kisco, New York.

OEHLING A, MARTIN-GIL D, ANTEPARA I, DOMÍNGUEZ MA & SUBIRÁ ML (1981) The reliability of the RAST in food allergy. *Allergol Immunopathol* **9**:217–222.

ORANJE AP, AARSEN RSR, MULDER PGH & LIEFAARD G (1991) Immediate contact reactions to cow's milk and egg in atopic children. *Acta Derm Venereol* **71**:263–266.

ØSTERGAARD PA, EBBESEN F, NOLTE H & SKOV PS (1990) Basophil histamine release in the diagnosis of house dust mite and dander allergy of asthmatic children. Comparison between prick test, RAST, basophil histamine release and bronchial provocation. *Allergy* **45**:231–235.

PATTERSON R (1985) (ed) *Allergic Diseases. Diagnosis and Management*, 3rd edn, Lippincott, Philadelphia.

PEARSON DJ (1987) Problems with terminology and with study design in food sensitivity. In Dobbing J (ed) *Food Intolerance*, pp. 1–13, Baillère Tindall, London.

PEPYS J (1975) Skin testing. *Br J Hosp Med* **14**:412–417.

PRAUSNITZ C & KUSTNER H (1921) Studien uber die Ueberempfindlichkeit. *Centralblatt Bakteriol Parasitol* **86**:160–169.

RAIZMAN MB (1989) Conjunctival challenge. In Spector SL (ed) *Provocative Challenge Procedures: Background and Methodology*, pp. 627–637, Futura Publishing Company, Mount Kisco, New York.

RAO KS, MENON PK, HILMAN BC, SEBASTIAN CS & BAIRNSFATHER L (1988) Duration of the suppressive effect of tricyclic antidepressants on histamine-induced wheal-and-flare reactions in human skin. *J Allergy Clin Immunol* **82**:752–757.

REDDY PM, NAGAYA H, PASCUAL HC *et al.* (1978) Reappraisal of intracutaneous tests in the diagnosis of reaginic allergy. *J Allergy Clin Immunol* **61**:36–41.

REIMANN HJ & LEWIN J (1988) Gastric mucosal reactions in patients with food allergy. *Am J Gastroenterol* **83**:1212–1219.

REIMANN HJ, RING J, ULTSCH B & WENDT P (1985) Intragastric provocation under endoscopic control (IPEC) in food allergy: mast cell and histamine changes in gastric mucosa. *Clin Allergy* **15**:195–202.

REINBERG A, SIDI E & GHATA J (1965) Circadian reactivity rhythms of human skin to histamine or allergen and the adrenal cycle. *J Allergy* **36**:273–283.

RESHEF A, KAGEY-SOBOTKA A, ADKINSON NF, LICHTENSTEIN LM & NORMAN PS (1989) The pattern and kinetics in human skin of erythema and mediators during the acute and late-phase response (LPR). *J Allergy Clin Immunol* **84**:678–687.

RUIZ RGG, PRICE JF, RICHARDS D & KEMENY DM (1990) Lack of relation between IgE in neonatal period and later atopy. *Lancet* **335**:808.

SAMPSON HA (1988) Comparative study of commercial food antigen extracts for the diagnosis of food hypersensitivity. *J Allergy Clin Immunol* **82**:718–726.

SAMPSON HA & ALBERGO R (1984) Comparison of results of skin tests, RAST, and double-blind, placebo-controlled food challenges in children with atopic dermatitis. *J Allergy Clin Immunol* **74**:26–33.

SAMPSON HA & SCANLON SM (1989) Natural history of food hypersensitivity in children with atopic dermatitis. *J Pediat* **115**:23–27.

SCHELLER R, STRAHLMANN B & SCHWEDT G (1988) Lebensmittelchemische und − technologische Aspekte zur nickelarmen Ernährung bei endogen bedingten allergischen Kontaktekzemen. *Hautarzt* **39**:491–497.

SERUP J (1984) Diameter, thickness, area and volume of skin-prick histamine weals. Measurement of skin thickness by 15 MHz A-mode ultrasound. *Allergy* **39**:359–364.

SJÖVALL P, CHRISTENSEN OB & MÖLLER H (1987) Oral hyposensitization in nickel allergy. *J Am Acad Dermatol* **17**:774–778.

SOLOMON WR & MCLEAN JA (1989) Nasal provocative testing. In Spector SL (ed) *Provocative Challenge Procedures: Background and Methodology*, pp. 569–625, Futura Publishing Company, Mount Kisco, New York.

TERHO EO, HUSMAN K, KIVEKAS J & RIIHIMAKI H (1989) Histamine control affects the weal produced by the adjacent diluent control in skin prick tests. *Allergy* **44**:30–32.

TOWNS SJ & MELLIS CM (1984) Role of acetyl salicylic acid and sodium metabisulphite in chronic childhood asthma. *Pediatrics* **73**:631–637.

TURNER MA, DEVLIN J & DAVID TJ (1991) Holidays and atopic eczema. *Arch Dis Child* **66**:212–215.

VAN BEVER HP, DOCX M & STEVENS WJ (1989) Food and food additives in severe atopic dermatitis. *Allergy* **44**:588–594.

VEIEN NK (1986) Why test with environmental agents? A review of recent studies concerning the value of routine testing in dermatologic practice. *Sem Dermatol* **5**:231–242.

VEIEN NK (1989) Systemically induced eczema in adults. *Acta Derm Venereol (Stockh)* (suppl. 147):1–58.

VEIEN NK, HATTEL T, JUSTESEN O & NØRHOLM N (1985) Oral challenge with balsam of Peru. *Contact Derm* **12**:104–107.

VEIEN NK & MENNÉ T (1989) Nickel contact allergy and a nickel-restricted diet. *Sem Dermatol* **9**:197–205.

VOHLONEN I, TERHO EO, KOIVIKKO A, VANTO T, HOLMEN A & HEINONEN OP (1989) Reproducibility of the skin prick test. *Allergy* **44**:525–531.

VOORHORST R (1980) Perfection of skin test technique. *Allergy* **35**:247–261.

VOORHORST R & NIKKELS AH (1977) Atopic skin test re-evaluated. IV. The use of compound 48/80 in routine skin testing. *Ann Allergy* **38**:255–262.

WYSE DM (1987) Astemizole: prolonged suppression of skin tests to ragweed and histamine in ragweed-sensitive patients. *Clin Invest Med* **10** (suppl. 4 B):B48.

YOULTEN L (1987) Nasal and conjunctival provocation testing. In Lessof MH, Lee TH & Kemeny DM (eds) *Allergy: An International Textbook*, pp. 305–310, Wiley, Chichester.

YUNGINGER JW (1988) Clinical significance of IgE. In Middleton E, Reed CE, Ellis EF, Adkinson NF & Yunginger JW (eds) *Allergy. Principles and Practice*, 3rd edn, vol. 2, pp. 849–860, Mosby, St Louis.

Part 11 Asthma

50 Triggers of asthma
Food only one item in a large list

Definition   Asthma lacks a precise definition, but it can be described as a disease characterized by wide variations over short periods of time in resistance to flow in intrapulmonary airways (Scadding 1983).

Pathophysiology   Obstruction to airflow is caused primarily by one or more of the following:
1 contraction of bronchial wall smooth muscle;
2 mucus in the bronchial lumen;
3 thickening of the bronchial mucosa;
4 oedema of the bronchial mucosa.

Active expiration, to counteract the above, causes increased pleural pressure, and results in compression and narrowing of the airways (Pride 1983).

Triggers   Exposure to various triggers can provoke or worsen asthma in certain patients. Some triggers, most notably allergens and occupational sensitizing agents, in addition to causing airway smooth muscle contraction, also cause an increase in the responsiveness of the airway smooth muscle – bronchial hyperreactivity (reviewed by Chung 1990). In contrast, other stimuli such as cold air, exercise or inhaled irritants, cause mainly airway smooth muscle contraction with little or no increase of bronchial reactivity (Cockroft 1987).

infections   Viral respiratory infections can provoke asthma in some patients (Gregg 1983; Li & O'Conell 1987), and are the most common triggers in infants and young children.

exercise   The mechanism of exercise-induced asthma is complex and not yet entirely clear (Anderson 1988), but a standard exercise test provokes asthma in about 90% of children with asthma who are old enough to co-operate with the test (Godfrey 1983a). Certain forms of exercise (e.g. running or cycling) are more likely to provoke asthma than others (e.g. swimming).

cold   Exposure to cold air (Strauss *et al.* 1977; Reisman *et al.* 1987) and possibly the consumption of ice cold drinks (Wilson *et al.* 1985) can provoke asthma in some patients.

| weather changes | Asthma can be provoked in some patients by changes in weather (Packe & Ayres 1985; Khot *et al.* 1988). The reasons for this are unknown, but possible explanations include changes in temperature, humidity, wind, rainfall, barometric pressure and the release of aeroallergens such as fungal spores (Salvaggio *et al.* 1971). |

| air pollution | Atmospheric pollution (Meltzer *et al.* 1987) by cigarette smoke (Halken *et al.* 1991), sulphur dioxide (Harries *et al.* 1981 and see chapter 36) and possibly exposure to other substances such as chlorine can provoke asthma in some patients (Mustchin & Pickering 1979; Lopez & Salvaggio 1983). |

| pollens, spores | The inhalation of pollen, fungal spores and miscellaneous other allergens derived from plants, animals or insects, can provoke asthma in some patients (Solomon & Mathews 1983). |

| house-dust mites | Exposure to house-dust mites can provoke asthma in some patients. The house-dust mite antigens are contained in the mite faeces (Tovey *et al.* 1981; Platts-Mills & de Weck 1989). |

| animals | Exposure to household pets and other animals (e.g. horses) can provoke asthma in some patients (Vanto & Koivikko 1983). |

| psychological | Emotional factors, including anxiety, stress and conditioning, although important (Mrazek 1988), were overvalued in the past as causes of asthma. This led, for example, to children with asthma being separated from their parents and sent to boarding schools (Apley & Mackeith 1968; Morrison Smith 1970). |

| laughing, crying | Laughing (Gayrard 1978) and crying (Weinstein 1984) can both provoke asthma in some patients. Both triggers probably act by causing hyperventilation. |

| gastro-oesophageal reflux | Gastro-oesophageal reflux can provoke asthma (Wilson *et al.* 1985) but the importance of reflux in childhood asthma is unclear. |

| food | Food and food additives can provoke asthma in some patients. This is discussed in the following chapters. |

Importance of triggers   Do trigger factors just make pre-existing asthma worse, or are they the major cause of asthma? In most patients, the importance of trigger factors is unclear. It is unknown whether the complete avoidance of all potential triggers, were this possible (which it plainly is not), would abolish asthma or merely cause improvement. Improvement of asthma following the removal of household pets is a poorly documented but occasionally striking phenomenon (Cockroft 1987).

alpine resorts

Observations of children with unusually severe asthma who were sent to alpine resorts, where the exposure to house-dust mites (and pets) is greatly reduced, are that somewhere between one- and two-thirds became completely asymptomatic and could discontinue all therapy (Morrison Smith 1981, 1983; Boner *et al.* 1985). Return home was followed by relapse in many patients, and death occurred in a few who remained off treatment (David 1987). In the past it was believed that this improvement was due to separation from parents and 'family tension' (Apley & Mackeith 1968), but nowadays it is thought more likely that the benefit is due to the avoidance of inhaled allergens (Morrison Smith 1970; Spieksma *et al.* 1971; Vervloet *et al.* 1979; Boner *et al.* 1985; Charpin *et al.* 1988).

identification and avoidance are difficult

In practice, the major difficulties comprise the identification of triggers and achieving their complete avoidance.

Timing of symptoms

The timing of symptoms depends on the nature of the trigger. In the case of allergic triggers, both early and late reactions are recognized (Mygind 1986). Early reactions to allergen inhalation occur 5–10 min after allergen inhalation, and reach a maximum after 20–30 min. Late reactions occur 4–8 hours after allergen inhalation, and are much more prolonged.

Identification of triggers

A careful history is the most useful tool (Bock 1983). Examples of helpful clues are given in Table 50.1.

Investigations

The role of investigations and their limitations are discussed fully in chapters 39 to 49. In short, simple investigations such as skin-prick tests or RAST tests are unhelpful. For example, a positive skin or RAST test to cats will give no indication as to whether avoidance of cats will help the asthma or not. Negative tests may be equally misleading. Provocation tests (see chapters 46 and 47), which employ the direct inhalation of suspect items such as house-dust mite antigens, pollen and so on, can be performed in a few centres, but again a positive result cannot be taken to indicate that antigen avoidance measures will help the patient.

Avoidance is not easy

Viral infections, pollens and mould spores are ubiquitous and avoidance is virtually impossible. The feasibility and efficacy of simple house-dust mite avoidance measures are controversial (Burr *et al.* 1976; Korsgaard 1983), and the benefit, if any, of semi-permeable mattress covers, (Owen *et al.* 1990) acaricides (Green *et al.* 1989;

Table 50.1 Clues in the history which may help to identify or exclude specific triggers

Timing of attacks	Trigger	References
Interpretation usually straightforward		
During bedmaking	House-dust mites	Tovey *et al.* (1981) Murray *et al.* (1983)
When family have a cold	Viral infections	Gregg (1983) Li & O'Connell (1987)
During or after running	Exercise	Anderson (1988)
Whenever staying with friends who have a dog	Dog	Vanto & Koivikko (1983)
After drinking cow's milk	Cow's milk protein	Hill & Hosking (1991)
Interpretation more complex		
At night	? House-dust mites ? Feather bedding ? Circadian rhythm	Clark (1985) & Mackay *et al.* (1991)
Seasonal July Autumn	? Grass pollen (UK) ? House-dust mites ? Moulds ? Colder air ? Viral infections	Britton *et al.* (1988)
After drinking orange squash	? Colouring agent ? Preservative ? Coldness of drink	
Never while on holiday abroad	? Absence of pets ? Absence of dust mites ? Psychological ? Different food	Turner *et al.* (1991)

Reiser *et al.* 1990) and domestic air cleaning devices such as mechanical filters, negative ion generators and electrostatic precipitators (Nelson *et al.* 1988) is uncertain. The best evidence for the benefit of house-dust mite avoidance comes from a study in which patients slept in a mite-free controlled environment in hospital (Platts-Mills *et al.* 1982). Avoidance of pets is possible but often unpopular.

Treatment   The treatment of asthma comprises a combination of drug therapy and, where possible or relevant, avoidance of triggers. Even with the most enthusiastic approach to the identification and avoidance of triggers, it is exceptionally rare for this alone to be sufficient treatment. While it makes sense to attempt to avoid easily identifiable triggers, it is unrealistic to expect to control most cases of childhood asthma simply by avoidance of trigger factors.

Key references 50.1 KHOT A, BURN R, EVANS N, LENNEY W & STORR J (1988) Biometeorological triggers in childhood asthma. *Clin Allergy* **18**:351–358. The relationship between childhood asthma admissions and biometeorological factors was investigated in Brighton over a 16-month period. No relationship was found with many commonly suspected precipitants such as wind speed, wind direction, wind chill, average temperature, maximum temperature drop, and humidity. There were statistically significant associations with rainfall, low barometric pressure, and counts of coloured basidiospores and green algae. There was also a significant day-of-week variation, with more admissions at the weekends and progressively fewer during the week, suggesting that social factors may be important determinants of admission.

50.2 VANTO T & KOIVIKKO A (1983) Dog hypersensitivity in asthmatic children. *Acta Paediat Scand* **72**:571–575. Provocation testing with dog dander was positive in 84 out of 203 (41%) unselected asthmatic children, skin-prick tests were positive in 113 (56%), and RAST tests were positive (grade 1 or more) in 140 (69%). *The authors equated 'allergy' with a positive test, thereby attaching far greater importance to these tests than is justifiable. In fact 'dog allergy' was not significantly associated with past or present exposure to dogs at home. Rising or steadily high levels of IgE antibodies to dog dander were observed even in subjects who avoided dogs. Scientifically very weak information, but the best there is. It is remarkable that we still have no idea what proportion of children with asthma will benefit from strict avoidance of household pets.*

50.3 MYGIND N (1986) *Essential Allergy*, pp. 163–278; Blackwell Scientific Publications, Oxford. *Although this book is about allergy, it contains 33 very clearly written chapters reviewing all aspects of the management of asthma (except the role of allergy, which is rather neglected).*

50.4 DOLOVICH J, ZIMMERMAN B & HARGREAVE FE (1983) Allergy in asthma. In Clark TJH & Godfrey S (eds) *Asthma*, 2nd edn, pp. 132–159, Chapman Hall, London. *Good general review of allergy in asthma, though neglects food intolerance.*

Summary 50 Exposure to various triggers can provoke or worsen asthma in certain patients. Apart from food (dealt with in the next chapter), these triggers comprise viral infections, exercise, cold air or cold drinks, weather changes, air pollution, pollens, spores, house-dust mites, animals, psychological factors, laughing, crying and gastro-oesophageal reflux. The history is the most useful tool in the identification of these triggers, and investigations such as skin or RAST tests are unhelpful. Avoidance of triggers is at best extremely difficult (e.g. house-dust mites) and often impossible (e.g. viral infections). Few if any cases of childhood asthma can be satisfactorily controlled solely by the identification and avoidance of triggers.

51 Food intolerance and asthma
An uncommon problem

An uncommon problem
Food is only one of many items which can provoke or worsen asthma (see previous chapter), and is an uncommon trigger of asthma in childhood (Bock 1983). In one careful study of children with asthma (Novembre *et al.* 1988), food provoked asthma in only eight of 140 (6%). Food additives are discussed separately in the next chapter.

Multiple symptoms
It is uncommon for asthma to be the sole manifestation of food intolerance (Novembre *et al.* 1987). Food-provoked asthma is almost always accompanied by other symptoms (e.g. cutaneous or gastro-intestinal). Thus in one study, of eight children with food-provoked asthma, an offending food provoked other disorders in all eight, these being urticaria in six, rhinitis in two, and eczema in one (Novembre *et al.* 1988). In another study of 11 children with food-provoked asthma, the relevant food provoked other disorders in all 11, eczema in eight, urticaria in seven, vomiting, loose stools or abdominal pain in four, and rhinitis in three (May 1976). Similarly, where other atopic disorders co-exist with asthma, the incidence of food intolerance is about four times higher than in children who have asthma alone (Novembre *et al.* 1988).

History
A history that a food has already been observed to provoke asthma is almost always present in food-provoked asthma (Onorato *et al.* 1986). It is rare for food-provoked asthma to escape the parents' attention, and in most cases the parents take steps to avoid the offending food without seeking medical advice (Hill 1948). Referral related to food intolerance usually occurs for one of the following reasons:

1 the parents seek some sort of confirmatory test;
2 the parents, having spotted one food trigger wonder if there could be others (this is unlikely if the parents have not already noticed them);
3 the parents seek dietary supervision, to ensure that a food trigger has been fully excluded and the diet is safe;
4 a health care professional wishes to seek food triggers for a child with asthma or discount/disprove food triggers.

positive history or other atopic disease
Where a child has asthma without accompanying atopic disorders and without a history of food intolerance, the chances of discovering food intolerance contributing to asthma are minimal.

the problem with parents' histories

The major difficulty with parents' histories of food intolerance (see chapter 3) is that they are often unreliable. In a study of 38 children with asthma in whom the parents reported that one or more foods provoked asthmatic symptoms, double-blind challenges confirmed the parents' histories in only 11 out of the 38 children and only 14 out of 70 challenges (May 1976).

Timing of symptoms

Food-provoked asthmatic reactions are usually early reactions and occur 5–10 min after allergen ingestion, reaching a maximum after 20–30 min. In one series of 38 children with asthma, late reactions to food, occurring within 24 hours, were specifically sought but not found (May 1976). There are, however, anecdotal reports of late reactions and chronic asthma in adults following ingestion of single foods (Furlan *et al.* 1987; Williams *et al.* 1987). It is possible that where a food is given very frequently, repeated reactions may merge into chronic asthma. The best example of late reactions is that of infants with cow's milk protein intolerance, discussed below (and see chapter 11). It is also possible that exposure to a food may not directly provoke detectable symptoms but may instead cause increased bronchial reactivity, rendering the bronchi more likely to respond to some other stimulus (Hargreave *et al.* 1981). This attractive but unproven possibility is discussed below (see chapter 52).

Food triggers

The most commonly incriminated food triggers in asthma are cow's milk protein, egg, peanuts, wheat, corn and fish (May 1976; Onorato *et al.* 1986; Novembre *et al.* 1988), but any food capable of causing an immediate allergic reaction could in theory trigger asthma in a susceptible subject. Inhalation of traces of food can provoke asthma (Feinberg & Aries 1932; Horesh 1943; Pearson 1966), but this route is mainly a problem in adults with occupational asthma due to, for example, wheat (Hensley *et al.* 1988), castor beans (Thorpe *et al.* 1988), egg (Edwards *et al.* 1983), crab (Orford & Wilson 1985) or soya (Bush *et al.* 1988).

tyramine?

In a study of 36 adults with asthma who reported respiratory symptoms after ingestion of chocolate, wine or cheese, three experienced a 15% or greater fall in FEV1 after placebo-controlled challenge with tyramine 5–50 mg (Huwyler & Wüthrich 1991). Treatment with a diet which excluded foods believed to be rich in tyramine (wine, cheese, fish, chocolate, beans, liver, avocado, sausage, pickled cabbage and raspberries) was associated with improvement of the asthma in all three subjects. The relevance of these observations, which require confirmation, is uncertain.

Reproducibility

It is unclear whether the dose of food which is required to produce a reaction remains constant in an individual patient. It is stated (without supporting evidence) that over a short period of time (days or weeks) a double-blind challenge will be reproducible within a range of 1–2 g of a particular food (Bock 1983). There are, however, some exceptions.

1 It is an anecdotal and unconfirmed observation that while patients are 'growing-out' of food intolerance the dose of food required to provoke asthma gets progressively larger (Bock 1983).

2 In patients with food-dependent exercise-induced anaphylaxis, of which asthma is a common feature, (see chapter 58), attacks only occur when the exercise follows within a couple of hours of the ingestion of specific foods.

3 Some parents have claimed that specific foods only provoke asthma at certain times of the year, coinciding with high pollen counts (Bock 1983). The suggestion that allergens may be additive in this way has never been objectively demonstrated in asthma.

4 It has been suggested that food triggers may only produce symptoms in asthma in the presence of other triggers, such as a viral infection, exercise or laughter (Wilson 1985) but there is no evidence to support this claim.

Key references 51.1 MAY CD (1976) Objective clinical and laboratory studies of immediate hypersensitivity reactions to foods in asthmatic children. *J Allergy Clin Immunol* **58**:500–515. A history of food-provoked attacks was obtained in 38 children with asthma. Symptoms were evoked in double-blind challenges in only 11 out of 38 children and 14 out of 70 challenges, and were chiefly gastrointestinal, even though asthma was the common presenting complaint. All reactions occurred within an hour of food ingestion, and none were delayed. Peanut was responsible for eight, egg for five and cow's milk for one.

51.2 ONORATO J, MERLAND N, TERRAL C, MICHEL FB & BOUSQUET J (1986) Placebo-controlled double-blind food challenge in asthma. *J Allergy Clin Immunol* **78**:1139–1146. Of 300 patients with asthma aged between 7 months and 80 years, 25 had either a history of food provoking attacks, or a positive skin prick test or RAST test to one or more of six foods. Double-blind food challenges were performed in 20. Food challenge caused asthma in six and other symptoms in five. All six patients with asthma and food intolerance were under 15 years and all had a current or past history of atopic eczema. On re-challenge after pre-treatment with oral sodium cromoglycate, 300 mg 30 min before the food challenge, the asthmatic response was blocked in four of five subjects tested.

51.3 NOVEMBRE E, MARTINO M & VIERUCCI A (1988) Foods and respiratory allergy. *J Allergy Clin Immunol* **81**:1059–1065. In a study of 140 children with asthma, of eight children with food-provoked asthma, the offending food provoked other disorders such as urticaria, rhinitis or eczema, in all eight. The food triggers were egg (four), cow's milk (three) and walnut (one).

51.4 WILSON NM (1985) Food related asthma: a difference between two ethnic groups. *Arch Dis Child* **60**:861–865. A postal questionnaire (91 children) and a personal interview (78 children) were used in hospital attenders with asthma to investigate adverse reactions to food. Adverse reactions to ice, fizzy drinks, fried food and nuts, but not orange squash, milk, chocolate or eggs, were more commonly reported by Asian than non-Asian children. The results of histamine challenge tests, referred in the discussion section but not actually provided in any detail, suggested that the ingestion of oil but not potato could enhance bronchial reactivity. The author addresses the discrepancy between a lack of change in PEFR or FEV and enhanced bronchial reactivity after food challenge. The explanation given was that foods or additives on their own do not provoke symptoms unless some additional factor (such as exercise, pollen exposure or viral infection) is present, and that challenge tests in the laboratory may be misleading. *Clearly this may be true. But it does not fully explain the consistent inability of studies from the same centre to fail to reproduce objective evidence of adverse reactions to additives when others (e.g. May 1976) have managed to do so when testing foods. The omission of the key information on methods and results of histamine challenges, and the insertion of a brief outline in the discussion section of the paper, are major problems for the reader.*

51.5   VAN METRE TE, ANDERSON AS, BARNARD JH *et al.* (1968) A controlled study of the effects on manifestations of chronic asthma of a rigid elimination diet based on Rowe's cereal-free diet 1, 2, 3. *J Allergy* **41**:195–208. This study tested the contention that chronic asthma due to food allergy is common and can be detected by observing improvement after introduction of a diet. Eighteen children and adults were studied, and given two diets. One included foods commonly reported to cause asthma, including cereal, cow's milk, eggs and seafood. The other consisted of foods reported to cause asthma only very rarely. The symptom and medication scores were not significantly different for the two diets. *The results casted doubt on the then fashionable hypothesis in the US that chronic refractory asthma was usually due to food intolerance.*

51.6   CHIARAMONTE LT & ALTMAN D (1991) Food sensitivity in asthma: perception and reality. *J Asthma* **28**:5–9. *Review.*

Summary 51   Food is an uncommon trigger of asthma in childhood, and it is rare for food to provoke severe attacks of asthma. When food does provoke asthma it often provokes other symptoms as well, such as urticaria, eczema, rhinitis, or gastrointestinal symptoms. The chances of a child with asthma having food intolerance are much greater if the child has other atopic disorders. In most cases of food-provoked asthma, symptoms occur within 30 min of ingestion, and late reactions are unusual. It is possible that frequent or continuous administration of a food trigger may give rise to chronic asthma. A relationship between a food and asthma is almost always detected by parents. Unfortunately their observations are not always reliable, and in one study double-blind challenges failed to confirm food intolerance in about two-thirds of cases. Where a child has asthma without accompanying atopic disorders and without a history of food intolerance, the chances of discovering food intolerance contributing to asthma are minimal.

52 Food additives and salicylates
Sulphite and aspirin may be important

Source of confusion The lack of agreement about the role of food additives in childhood asthma is fuelled by the paucity of valid objective data. It is a common but poorly documented observation that orange squash, lemon and barley water, and similar soft drinks which rely heavily for their appearance and flavour upon artificial ingredients, can precipitate coughing and wheezing in some children with asthma (Steinman & Weinberg 1986; David 1988). But even if parents' observations are accurate, bearing in mind that they often are not (May 1976), it is far from easy to unravel the causative ingredient. Reactions may be caused by tartrazine (Settipane et al. 1975), sodium benzoate (Freedman 1977), cola (Wilson et al. 1982), sodium metabisulphite or other sulphites (Towns & Mellis 1984; Steinman & Weinberg 1986), the cold temperature of the drink (Wilson et al. 1985) or even the patient's belief that the drink will provoke symptoms (Mrazek 1988).

Food additives are discussed in detail in chapters 33 to 37, and salicylates in chapter 38.

Sulphites There have been only two systematic studies of sulphites in childhood asthma. In an Australian study, 29 children with asthma requiring inhaled or oral steroids were placed on a diet avoiding all colouring agents and preservatives and then challenged on one day with placebo, and on the next day with 25, 50 and 100 mg encapsulated sodium metabisulphite, followed by 5, 25 and 50 mg of the metabisulphite in a solution with 0.5% citric acid (Towns & Mellis 1984). None of the children reacted to metabisulphite in capsules, but in 19 out of 29 (66%) there was a >20% decrease in the FEV1 after ingestion of metabisulphite in solution with citric acid. These reactions mostly occurred within 1–2 min of ingestion, and in all reactions the patient complained initially of a burning sensation in the throat. All 19 patients reacting to metabisulphite were placed on a diet avoiding foods, beverages and medications known to contain high concentrations of sulphite, and reassessed 3 months later. There was no control group. Nine 'felt a subjective improvement', and in four there was a 'decrease' in bronchodilator requirement. A further study of placebo-controlled metabisulphite challenges in children with asthma documented positive challenges to metabisulphite in acid solution in eight of 51 (35%) children with asthma (Friedman & Easton 1987). The other descriptions of sulphite-induced asthma in childhood are anecdotal case reports (Kochen 1973; Sher & Schwartz 1985; Wolf & Nicklas 1985). Sulphites probably provoke asthma more frequently than any other food additive. As with other additives, with the exception of monosodium glutamate, it appears that sulphites tend to provoke mild rather than severe symptoms. Although it is logical for subjects who are intolerant to avoid sulphites, this does not appear to have any overall beneficial effect on asthma (Towns & Mellis 1984). Sulphite intolerance in adults with asthma is discussed in chapter 36.

Tartrazine
negative results from
challenge studies

Although tartrazine is the most notorious additive to provoke asthma, the objective evidence that it can do so in children is weak. Vedanthan *et al.* (1977) studied 54 children with asthma, 35 of whom were being treated with oral steroids. Double-blind challenges with tartrazine 25 mg failed to demonstrate a fall of the FEV1 of more than two standard deviations below the response to placebo in any patient. A drawback to this study is that the patients were severely affected, in that many received treatment with systemic steroids, so that the treatment could have masked a response to tartrazine. This argument is, however, undermined by the fact that the same study did permit the detection of other triggers, and demonstrated aspirin intolerance in five children.

enhanced bronchial reactivity

In another study, nine children with asthma were given a double-blind challenge with tartrazine 1 mg (Hariparsad *et al.* 1984). All gave a history of cough or wheeze after orange-coloured drinks. There was no change in PEFR after tartrazine, but histamine sensitivity increased markedly in three patients and to a lesser degree in a fourth. The authors of this study suggested that the estimation of bronchial reactivity by measurement of the response to histamine challenge might be a more sensitive test than looking for changes in the FEV1. However the authors failed to explain the discrepancy between the clinical history of coughing and wheezing after drinking orange-coloured drinks and the inability to demonstrate a change in lung function after tartrazine challenge. This is in marked contrast to the usual observation that provocation with inhaled cat or pollen extracts, for example, cause both a fall in the FEV1 and an increase in bronchial reactivity (Cockroft *et al.* 1987). A possible explanation is that tartrazine only provokes asthma when combined with another trigger (e.g. exercise) but if this were true one would expect the parents to have noticed this. Another albeit improbable explanation is that measurements of PEFR and FEV1 can on occasions be normal in the presence of quite marked small airways obstruction (Cooper *et al.* 1977; Godfrey 1983b). Nevertheless, the authors' complete failure to reproduce symptoms or signs with tartrazine challenge can hardly be taken as confirmation of the parents' observations.

avoidance does not help the underlying asthma

Where tartrazine has been shown to provoke asthma, strict avoidance has not shown to be of benefit to the underlying asthma (Tarlo & Broder 1982). This is hardly surprising considering the multiplicity of triggers which can contribute to the pathogenesis of asthma.

Benzoic acid

There has been no double-blind placebo-controlled study of the effects of benzoates in children with asthma (see chapter 35). Most studies on adults have been flawed, and the two sound studies showed that intolerance to benzoates was rare in adults with asthma, positive challenges occurring in one out of 28 patients in one study (Tarlo & Broder 1982) and one out of 43 patients in another study (Weber *et al.* 1979). It is possible that intolerance to benzoates occurs in a small proportion of children with asthma, but it is unlikely that it provokes severe symptoms.

Monosodium glutamate
one definite case

The sole evidence supported by double-blind placebo-controlled challenge that monosodium glutamate can provoke asthma is a case report of a patient who presented with a respiratory arrest after ingestion of wonton soup which contained monosodium glutamate (Koepke & Selner 1986).

lack of good data in adults

Allen and colleagues described two adults with asthma who experienced life-threatening attacks which required intubation and artificial ventilation, the attacks occurring 1–12 hours after a meal in a Chinese restaurant (Allen *et al.* 1987). They also performed challenges with monosodium glutamate at a maximum dosage of 5.0 g in 32 patients with asthma, all but one of whom were adults. The patients were highly selected and either had a history of symptoms after a meal in a Chinese restaurant or of 'chemical sensitivity'. Seven patients developed asthma and symptoms of the 'Chinese restaurant syndrome' (see chapter 37) 1–2 hours after ingestion of monosodium glutamate, and six patients developed asthma alone, 6–12 hours after ingestion of monosodium glutamate. Unfortunately the authors did not employ a double-blind placebo-controlled methodology, and for this and other reasons their observations have been discredited (Ebert 1982; Garattini 1982). Furthermore, the challenge procedure included discontinuation of theophylline shortly before the challenge and then accepting any fall in the PEFR of >20% during the day as the criteria for a positive challenge.

negative data

In another unsatisfactory study, challenges with sodium glutamate 200 mg failed to provoke asthma in 17 adults with asthma who were selected on the basis of a history suggesting adverse reaction to food additives (Genton *et al.* 1985).

lack of data in childhood

The question of whether or not monosodium glutamate can provoke asthma in childhood has not been systematically studied.

Salicylates

It is clear that aspirin may provoke bronchoconstriction in some children with asthma, although the incidence of aspirin intolerance in asthmatic subjects is unclear. Estimates range from 0% to 28% (Rachelefsky *et al.* 1975; Vedanthan *et al.* 1977; Schuhl & Pereyra 1979; Towns & Mellis 1984). However avoidance of aspirin in subjects with aspirin intolerance appears to have no effect on the severity of the underlying asthma (Towns & Mellis 1984). The subject, which is discussed further in chapter 38, is somewhat academic, since aspirin is no longer recommended as an analgesic in childhood because of evidence that it may be a contributory cause of Reye's syndrome (Tarlow 1986). Naturally occurring salicylates are widely distributed in foodstuffs of plant origin, but there is no objective evidence that these can provoke adverse reactions (see chapter 38).

Cola

The evidence incriminating cola drinks comprises a study of 10 asthmatic children who gave a history of cough and wheeze after consumption of cola drinks (Wilson *et al.* 1982). 'Blind' challenges with water and soda water each containing saccharin, and with Pepsi Cola, had no significant effect on the PEFR. Non-specific airway reactivity (as shown by sensitivity to inhaled histamine) increased after challenge with Pepsi Cola in six children, after challenge with soda water in two children, and after still water in none. The blindness of the study rests on one believing that children were unable to distinguish between the taste of Pepsi Cola and fizzy water containing five drops of saccharin solution, an issue which was never tested. The other difficulty with this study is that the authors stressed that most of the children gave a history that coughing and wheezing came on immediately after a cola drink, yet in none was there any change in PEFR after drinking cola. This discrepancy between history and the negative results of direct challenge, and the fact that two patients demonstrated enhanced histamine sensitivity after drinking fizzy water, undermines the hypothesis that cola drinks can adversely affect children with asthma.

Other additives

No double-blind placebo-controlled challenge studies of other food additives have been reported in children with asthma. However, in a study of 45 adults with perennial asthma, open challenges with a mixture of azo dyes (amaranth, ponceau and sunset yellow) produced a significant fall in the FEV1 in four of 43 patients tested (Weber *et al.* 1977). Double-blind placebo-controlled challenges of these four patients, using single dyes, were positive in only one patient who reacted to ponceau. Open challenges with a mixture of non-azo dyes (brilliant blue, erythrosine and indigotin) produced a significant fall in the FEV1 in three of 42 patients tested. Double-blind placebo-controlled challenges of two of these three patients, using single dyes, were positive in only one patient who reacted to erythrosine. Finally, open challenges with a mixture of butylated hydroxyanisole and butylated hydroxytoluene were negative in all 43 patients tested.

Key references 52.1   WEBER RW, HOFFMAN M, RAINE DA & NELSON HS (1979) Incidence of bronchoconstriction due to aspirin, azo dyes, non-azo dyes, and preservatives in a population of perennial asthmatics. *J Allergy Clin Immunol* **64**:32–37. In 45 adults with perennial asthma, open challenges were followed by double-blind placebo-controlled challenges of most of those who reacted positively on open challenge, with the exception of aspirin where double-blind challenges were not performed. Double-blind challenges were positive in only three instances; one each with erythrosine, ponceau and a mixture of sodium benzoate and para-hydroxybenzoic acid. Seven patients reacted to tartrazine on open challenge, but none when tested double-blind. *These findings confirm that aspirin intolerance is relatively common but suggest that reactions to colouring agents and pre-servatives are an uncommon cause of clinically significant bronchoconstriction in moderately severe perennial asthmatics.*

52.2   GENTON C, FREI PC & PÉCOUD A (1985) Value of oral provocation tests to aspirin and food additives in the routine investigation of asthma and chronic urticaria. *J Allergy Clin Immunol* **76**:40–45. Seventeen adults with asthma whose case history suggested aspirin or food additive intolerance were challenged with aspirin, sodium benzoate, sulphur dioxide, potassium sorbate, sodium glutamate, tartrazine and glafenine (an analgesic used on the continent of Europe). Positive challenges, as defined by a 20% decrease in PEFR, were found in nine out of the 17 subjects, but in none were the reactions 'serious'.

Summary 52   Aspirin and the sulphites are fairly common potential triggers in children with asthma. The azo dyes tartrazine and ponceau, the non-azo dye eythrosine, the benzoate preservatives and monosodium glutamate are rare potential triggers. The suggestion that cola is a trigger is unproven, and this requires further investigation. Reactions to colouring agents or preservatives (other than sulphites) are an uncommon and over-rated cause of clinically significant broncho-constriction in children with asthma.

53 Management of asthma
Food avoidance rarely helpful

General management The general management of asthma comprises establishing the correct diagnosis and treatment with bronchodilators and prophylactic agents, a subject well reviewed elsewhere (Mygind 1986; Ellis 1988; Shapiro 1992).

History The most important step is to obtain a careful history. Parents' observations of potential triggers are essential, notwithstanding the lack of reliability where foods and food additives are concerned. It is most important to establish whether the parents beliefs about triggers come from their own observations (important), skin tests or RAST tests (unhelpful – see chapters 41 and 43) or information from the media (often unreliable). When a parent says a child is, for example, 'allergic to milk', it is essential to probe further and establish the basis for this conclusion.

Trigger avoidance
unavoidable triggers Viral infections, exercise, cold air, laughing and crying are largely unavoidable.

inhalant triggers House-dust mites, pollen and moulds are ubiquitous, and exposure to pets is very common. Deciding when any of these are important to an individual patient, or how to attempt to reduce exposure, are contentious subjects which are studiously avoided or glossed over in reviews of the subject (e.g. Evans *et al.* 1988; Kay 1988; Salvaggio & Lopez 1992).

need for trigger avoidance The need to avoid trigger factors depends partly on the severity of the asthma, and partly on the relative importance to the patient of the trigger concerned. There is little sense in insisting on the removal of a much loved family pet in the presence of very mild symptoms requiring little treatment. On the other hand, in the face of troublesome or severe asthma, it does make sense to try to identify and reduce exposure to avoidable triggers.

food and food additives Intolerance to food and food additives are uncommon contributory causes of clinically significant bronchoconstriction (Bock 1983). Possible indications for food avoidance in asthma are discussed below.

Investigations Skin tests and RAST tests are unhelpful in pinpointing which patients will benefit from trigger avoidance, and are unhelpful in the

309

identification of which triggers should be avoided (David 1991). These tests are discussed in more detail in chapters 41 and 43, but in short a positive skin or RAST test is a poor predictor that the patient will benefit from avoidance. A blinded challenge procedure can be employed to confirm intolerance to an individual food or food additive, but avoidance of the food is no guarantee that the management of the asthma will be any easier.

A positive history   A history that ingestion of a specific food is followed by coughing or wheezing is a helpful pointer (Editorial 1991), remembering, of course, that mechanisms other than asthma could cause these symptoms after the ingestion of food, e.g. aspiration or tracheo-oesophageal fistula. The faster the onset of symptoms after ingestion of food, the more reliable is the history (Editorial 1991). Where the relationship between food and attack is obvious, the parents are likely to have instituted avoidance measures (Hill 1948). The doctor's main task is to check the nutritional adequacy of the diet, often with the help of a dietitian, and ensure that the family know how to completely avoid the trigger food. Such patients are uncommon and do not usually pose a problem. As explained above, the adverse reaction to the food is likely to comprise non-respiratory symptoms as well as asthma.

No clear history   In practice, the problem is a more general one of whether food intolerance could be contributing to chronic asthma in a child. If adverse reactions to foods have already been noted (whether urticarial, gastrointestinal or respiratory) this would raise the possibility that others have been overlooked, and should prompt an extra careful history to look for possible triggers. If no consistent adverse reactions to foods have been noted, then it is highly unlikely that food is playing an important part in the child's asthma. If one wished to pursue food intolerance further (usually at the request of parents who are insistent), then the only option is to try an empirical elimination diet (see chapters 70 to 75) for a short period (no more than a week should be necessary to establish success or failure). This may need to be performed in hospital, for unless there are uncontrolled symptoms which can be monitored, it involves withdrawing prophylactic medication (which would otherwise mask any possible benefit). Personal experience is that in the absence of any history suggesting food intolerance, empirical elimination diets (including elemental diets) are unhelpful in the management of asthma. In patients with a history of food-provoked respiratory symptoms, empirical elimination diets may help identify further food triggers, but the avoidance of these tends to be associated with only minimal benefit to the overall management of the asthma (e.g. the patient has still required the same dose of inhaled or oral steroids). The greatest value of such diets may be in helping a family to appreciate that food intolerance is not responsible for their child's asthma.

Multiple symptoms in infants The other clue to food intolerance (particularly cow's milk protein intolerance) is where there are associated features, such as trouble-some atopic eczema or frequent loose stools. Such associated symptoms should raise the possibility of food intolerance, and in infants with multiple symptoms, a trial of some sort of elimination diet (see chapters 70 to 75) should be considered. This particularly applies to infants under 2 years of age, where a combination of persistent wheezing, atopic eczema and frequent loose stools should suggest the possibility of cow's milk protein intolerance.

Food additives Artificial drinks and other foods which contain certain food addi-tives, especially sulphites, can provoke coughing and wheezing in a small number of children with asthma. The evidence suggests that such additives in general provoke mild symptoms rather than severe attacks, and that careful avoidance of all food additives is most unlikely to help the underlying asthma. If a food additive trigger has been identified, then the one time when avoidance is perhaps most useful is during an acute attack.

Key references 53.1 BOCK SA (1983) Food-related asthma and basic nutrition. *J Asthma* **20**:377–381. *A helpful discussion about food intolerance and asthma from a centre which has made an important contribution to our understanding of food intolerance in childhood by the use of double-blind placebo-controlled food challenges.*

53.2 SHEFFER AL (1991) (ed) Guidelines for the diagnosis and management of asthma. National Heart, Lung, and Blood Institute, National Asthma Education Program expert panel report. *J Allergy Clin Immunol* **88** (suppl.):425–534. *Review of diagnosis, drug treatment and allergen avoidance.*

Summary 53 The management of asthma comprises making the diagnosis and the institution of bronchodilator therapy, if necessary accompanied by prophylactic treatment. The identification of triggers and attempts to avoid them are difficult, of uncertain benefit, and not generally applied except in severe cases. In the absence of any history that foods provoke symptoms, food intolerance is most unlikely to be an important contributory factor. The one exception is the infant with multiple symptoms other than asthma, in whom food intolerance (especially cow's milk protein) should be considered. The incidence of food additive intolerance in asthma is generally over-rated, with the exception of sulphites which commonly cause a mild worsening of symptoms.

References to Chapters 50–53

ALLEN DH, DELOHERY J & BAKER G (1987) Monosodium L-glutamate-induced asthma. *J Allergy Clin Immunol* **80**:530–537.

ANDERSON SD (1988) Exercise-induced asthma. In Middleton E, Reed CE, Ellis EF, Adkinson NF & Yunginger JW (eds) *Allergy. Principles and Practice*, 3rd edn, pp. 1156–1175, Mosby, St Louis.

APLEY J & MACKEITH R (1968) *The Child and His Symptoms. A Comprehensive Approach*, 2nd edn, pp. 36–47, Blackwell Scientific Publications, Oxford.

BOCK SA (1983) Food-related asthma and basic nutrition. *J Asthma* **20**:377–381.

BONER AL, NIERO E, ANTOLINI I, VALLETTA EA & GABURRO D (1985) Pulmonary function and bronchial hyperreactivity in asthmatic children with house dust mite allergy during prolonged stay in the Italian alps (Misurina, 1756 m). *Ann Allergy* **54**:42–45.

BRITTON J, CHINN S, BURNEY, PAPACOSTA AO & TATTERSFIELD A (1988) Seasonal variation in bronchial reactivity in a community population. *J Allergy Clin Immunol* **82**:134–139.

BURR ML, ST. LEGER AS & NEALE E (1976) Anti-mite measures in mite-sensitive adult asthma. A controlled trial. *Lancet* **1**:333–335.

BUSH RK, SCHROECKENSTEIN D, MEIER-DAVIS S, BALMES J & REMPEL D (1988) Soybean flour asthma: detection of allergens by immunoblotting. *J Allergy Clin Immunol* **82**:251–255.

CHARPIN D, KLEISBAUER J-P, LANTEAUME A *et al.* (1988) Asthma and allergy to house-dust mites in populations living in high altitudes. *Chest* **93**:758–761.

CHUNG KF (1990) Mediators of bronchial hyperresponsiveness. *Clin Exper Allergy* **20**:453–458.

CLARK TJH (1985) The circadian rhythm of asthma. *Br J Dis Chest* **79**:115–124.

COCKROFT DW (1987) Airway hyperresponsiveness: therapeutic implications. *Ann Allergy* **59**:405–414.

COCKROFT DW, RUFFIN RE, DOLOVICH J & HARGREAVE FE (1977) Allergen-induced increase in non-allergic bronchial reactivity. *Clin Allergy* **7**:503–513.

COOPER DM, CUTZ E & LEVISON H (1977) Occult pulmonary abnormalities in asymptomatic asthmatic children. *Chest* **71**:361–365.

DAVID TJ (1987) Steroid scare. *Arch Dis Child* **62**:876–878.

DAVID TJ (1988) Food additives. *Arch Dis Child* **63**:582–583.

DAVID TJ (1991) Conventional allergy tests. *Arch Dis Child* **66**:281–282.

DELOHERY J, SIMMUL R, CASTLE WD & ALLEN DH (1984) The relationship of inhaled sulfur dioxide reactivity to ingested metabisulphite sensitivity in patients with asthma. *Am Rev Respir Dis* **130**:1027–1032.

EBERT AG (1982) Chinese-restaurant asthma. *New Engl J Med* **306**:1180.

EDITORIAL (1991) Food hypersensitivity and asthma. *J Asthma* **28**:1–3.

EDWARDS JH, McCONNOCHIE K, TROTMAN DM, COLLINS G, SAUNDERS MJ & LATHAM SM (1983) Allergy to inhaled egg material. *Clin Allergy* **13**:427–432.

ELLIS EF (1988) Asthma in infancy and childhood. In Middleton E, Reed CE, Ellis EF, Adkinson NF & Yunginger JW (eds) *Allergy. Principles and Practice*, 3rd edn, pp. 1037–1062, Mosby, St Louis.

EVANS R, SUMMERS RJ & NEWILL CA (1988) Allergic reactions caused by exposure to animals. In Lichtenstein LM & Fauci AS (eds) *Current Therapy in Allergy, Immunology, and Rheumatology-3*, pp. 5–7, Decker, Toronto.

FEINBERG SM & ARIES PL (1932) Asthma from food odors. *J Am Med Ass* **98**:2280–2281.

FREEDMAN BJ (1977) Asthma induced by sulphur dioxide, benzoate and tartrazine contained in orange drinks. *Clin Allergy* **7**:407–415.

FRIEDMAN ME & EASTON JG (1987) Prevalence of positive metabisulphite challenges in children with asthma. *Pediat Asthma Allergy Immunol* **1**:53–59.

FURLAN J, SUSKOVIC S & RUS A (1987) The effect of food on the bronchial response in adult asthmatic patients, and the protective role of ketotifen. *Allergol Immunopathol* **15**:73–81.

GARATTINI S (1982) Chinese-restaurant asthma. *New Engl J Med* **306**:1181.

GAYRARD P (1978) Should asthmatic patients laugh? *Lancet* **2**:1105–1106.

GENTON C, FREI PC & PECOUD A (1985) Value of oral provocation tests to aspirin and food additives in the routine investigation of asthma and chronic urticaria. *J Allergy Clin Immunol* **76**:40–45.

GODFREY S (1983a) Exercise-induced asthma. In Clark TJH & Godfrey S (eds) *Asthma*, 2nd edn, pp. 57–78, Chapman Hall, London.

GODFREY S (1983b) Childhood asthma. In Clark TJH & Godfrey S (eds) *Asthma*, 2nd edn, pp. 415–456, Chapman Hall, London.

GREEN WF, NICHOLAS NR, SALOME CM & WOOLCOCK AJ (1989) Reduction of house dust mites and mite allergens: effects of spraying carpets and blankets with Allersearch DMS, and acaricide combined with an allergen reducing agent. *Clin Exper Allergy* **19**:203–207.

GREGG I (1983) The role of infection. In Clark TJH & Godfrey S (eds) *Asthma*, 2nd edn, pp. 160–183, Chapman Hall, London.

HALKEN S, HØST A, HUSBY S, HANSEN LG, ØSTERBALLE O & NYBOE J (1991) Recurrent wheezing in relation to environmental risk factors in infancy. A prospective study of 276 infants. *Allergy* **46**:507–514.

HARGREAVE FE, RYAN G, THOMSON NC *et al.* (1981) Bronchial responsiveness to histamine or methacholine in asthma: measurement and clinical significance. *J Allergy Clin Immunol* **68**:347–355.

HARIPARSAD D, WILSON N, DIXON C & SILVERMAN M (1984) Oral tartrazine challenge in childhood asthma: effect on bronchial reactivity. *Clin Allergy* **14**:81–85.

HARRIES MG, PARKES PEG, LESSOF MH & ORR TSC (1981) Role of bronchial irritant receptors in asthma. *Lancet* **1**:5–7.

HENSLEY MJ, SCICCHITANO R, SAUNDERS NA *et al.* (1988) Seasonal variation in non-specific bronchial reactivity: a study of wheat workers with a history of wheat associated asthma. *Thorax* **43**:103–107.

HILL DJ & HOSKING CS (1991) Cow's milk allergy. In David TJ (ed) *Recent Advances in Paediatrics*, vol. 9, pp. 187–206, Churchill Livingstone, London.

HILL LW (1948) Food sensitivity in 100 asthmatic children. *New Engl J Med* **238**:657–659.

HORESH AJ (1943) Allergy to food odors. Its relation to the management of infantile eczema. *J Allergy* **14**:335–339.

HUWYLER T & WÜTHRICH B (1991) Tyramine-induced asthma. *Allergy Clin Immunol News* **3**:14–15.

KAY AB (1988) Asthma provoked by exposure to allergens. In Lichtenstein LM & Fauci AS (eds) *Current Therapy in Allergy, Immunology, and Rheumatology-3*, pp. 21–25, Decker, Toronto.

KHOT A, BURN R, EVANS N, LENNEY W & STORR J (1988) Biometeorological triggers in childhood asthma. *Clin Allergy* **18**:351–358.

KOCHEN J (1973) Sulfur dioxide, a respiratory tract irritant, even if ingested. *Pediatrics* **52**:145–146.

KOEPKE JW & SELNER JC (1986) Combined monosodium glutamate (MSG)/ metabisulfite (MBS) induced asthma (abstract). *J Allergy Clin Immunol* **77** (suppl.):158.

KORSGAARD J (1983) Preventive measures in mite asthma. A controlled trial. *Allergy* **38**:93–102.

LI JTC & O'CONNELL EJ (1987) Viral infections and asthma. *Ann Allergy* **59**:321–333.

LOPEZ M & SALVAGGIO JE (1983) Climate-weather-pollution. In Middleton E, Reed CE & Ellis EF (eds) *Allergy. Principles and Practice*, 2nd edn, vol. 2, pp. 1203–1214, Mosby, St Louis.

MACKAY TW, FITZPATRICK MF & DOUGLAS NJ (1991) Non-adrenergic, non-cholinergic nervous system and overnight airway calibre in asthmatic and normal subjects. *Lancet* **338**:1289–1292.

MAULITZ RM, PRATT DS & SCHOCKET AL (1979) Exercise-induced anaphylactic reaction to shellfish. *J Allergy Clin Immunol* **63**:433–434.

MAY CD (1976) Objective clinical and laboratory studies of immediate hypersensitivity reactions to foods in asthmatic children. *J Allergy Clin Immunol* **58**:500–515.

MELTZER EO, ORGEL HA, WELCH MJ & KEMP JP (1987) Nonpharmacologic approaches to the management of asthma. In Tinkelman DG, Falliers CJ & Naspitz CK (eds) *Child Asthma. Pathophysiology and Treatment*, pp. 281–326, Marcel Dekker, New York.

MORRISON SMITH J (1970) The treatment of asthmatic children away from home. *Publ Hlth Lond* **84**:286–290.

MORRISON SMITH J (1981) The use of high altitude treatment for childhood asthma. *Practitioner* **225**:1663–1666.

MORRISON SMITH J (1983) The recent history of the treatment of asthma: a personal view. *Thorax* **38**:244–253.

MRAZEK DA (1988) Asthma: psychiatric considerations, evaluation, and management. In Middleton E, Reed CE, Ellis EF, Adkinson NF & Yunginger JW (eds) *Allergy. Principles and Practice*, 3rd edn, pp. 1176–1196, Mosby, St Louis.

MURRAY AB, FERGUSON AC & MORRISON BJ (1983) Diagnosis of house dust mite allergy in asthmatic children: what constitutes a positive history? *J Allergy Clin Immunol* **71**:21–28.

MUSTCHIN CP & PICKERING CAC (1979) 'Coughing water': bronchial hyper-reactivity induced by swimming in a chlorinated pool. *Thorax* **34**:682–683.

MYGIND N (1986) *Essential Allergy*, Blackwell Scientific Publications, Oxford.

NELSON HS, HIRSCH SR, OHMAN JL, PLATTS-MILLS TAE, REED CE & SOLOMON WR (1988) Recommendations for the use of residential air-cleaning devices in the treatment of allergic respiratory diseases. *J Allergy Clin Immunol* **82**:661–669.

NOVEMBRE E, MARTINO M & VIERUCCI A (1988) Foods and respiratory allergy. *J Allergy Clin Immunol* **81**:1059–1065.

NOVEMBRE E, VENERUSO G, SABATINI C, BONAZZA P, BERNARDINI R & VIERUCCI A (1987) Incidenza dell'asma da allergia alimentare in eta pediatrica. *Ped Med Chir* **9**:399–404.

ONORATO J, MERLAND N, TERRAL C, MICHEL FB & BOUSQUET J (1986) Placebo-controlled double-blind food challenge in asthma. *J Allergy Clin Immunol* **78**:1139–1146.

ORFORD RR & WILSON JT (1985) Epidemiologic and immunologic studies in processors of the king crab. *Am J Indust Med* **7**:155–169.

OWEN S, MORGANSTERN M, HEPWORTH J & WOODCOCK A (1990) Control of house dust mite antigen in bedding. *Lancet* **1**:396–397.

PACKE GE & AYRES JG (1985) Asthma outbreak during a thunderstorm. *Lancet* **2**:199–204.

PEARSON RSB (1966) Potato sensitivity, an occupational allergy in housewives. *Acta Allergol* **21**:507–514.

PLATTS-MILLS TAE & DE WECK AL (1989) Dust mite allergens and asthma – a worldwide problem. *J Allergy Clin Immunol* **83**:416–427.

PLATTS-MILLS TAE, TOVEY ER, MITCHELL EB, MOSZORO H, NOCK P & WILKINS SR (1982) Reduction of bronchial hyperreactivity during prolonged allergen avoidance. *Lancet* **2**:675–678.

PRIDE NB (1983) Physiology. In Clark TJH & Godfrey S (eds) *Asthma*, 2nd edn, pp. 12–56, Chapman Hall, London.

RACHELEFSKY GS, COULSON A, SIEGEL SC & STIEHM ER (1975) Aspirin intolerance in chronic childhood asthma: detected by oral challenge. *Pediatrics* **56**:443–448.

REISER J, INGRAM D, MITCHELL EB & WARNER JO (1990) House dust mite allergen levels and an anti-mite mattress spray (natamycin) in the treatment of childhood asthma. *Clin Exper Allergy* **20**:561–567.

REISMAN J, MAPPA L, DE BENEDICTIS F, MCLAUGHLIN J & LEVISON H (1987) Cold air challenge in children with asthma. *Pediat Pulmonol* **3**:251–254.

SALVAGGIO J, SEABURY J & SCHOENHARDT EA (1971) New Orleans asthma. V. Relationship between Charity Hospital asthma admission rates, semiquantitative pollen and fungal spore counts, and total particulate aerometric sampling data. *J Allergy Clin Immunol* **48**:96–114.

SALVAGGIO JE & LOPEZ M (1992) Asthma provoked by exposure to allergens. In Lichtenstein LM & Fauci AS (eds) *Current Therapy in Allergy, Immunology, and Rheumatology*, 4th edn, pp. 22–25, Decker, St Louis.

SCADDING JG (1983) Definition and clinical categories of asthma. In Clark TJH & Godfrey S (eds) *Asthma*, 2nd edn, pp. 1–11, Chapman Hall, London.

SCHUHL JF & PEREYRA JG (1979) Oral acetylsalicylic acid (aspirin) challenge in asthmatic children. *Clin Allergy* **9**:83–88.

SETTIPANE GA & PUDUPAKKAM RK (1975) Aspirin intolerance. III. Subtypes, familial occurrence, and cross-reactivity with tartrazine. *J Allergy Clin Immunol* **56**:215–221.

SHAPIRO GG (1992) Childhood asthma. In Lichtenstein LM & Fauci AS (eds) *Current Therapy in Allergy, Immunology, and Rheumatology*, 4th edn, pp. 32–38, Decker, St Louis.

SHER TH & SCHWARTZ HJ (1985) Bisulfite sensitivity manifesting as an allergic reaction to aerosol therapy. *Ann Allergy* **54**:224–226.

SOLOMON WR & MATHEWS KP (1983) Aerobiology and inhalant allergens. In Middleton E, Reed CE & Ellis EF (eds) *Allergy. Principles and Practice*, 2nd edn, vol. 2, pp. 1143–1202, Mosby, St Louis.

SPIEKSMA FTM, ZUIDEMA P & LEUPEN MJ (1971) High altitude and house-dust mites. *Br Med J* **1**:82–84.

STEINMAN HA & WEINBERG EG (1986) The effects of soft-drink preservatives on asthmatic children. *S Afr Med J* **70**:404–406.

STRAUSS RH, MCFADDEN ER, INGRAM RH & JAEGER JJ (1977) Enhancement of exercise-induced asthma by cold air. *New Engl J Med* **297**:743–747.

TARLO SM & BRODER I (1982) Tartrazine and benzoate challenge and dietary avoidance in chronic asthma. *Clin Allergy* **12**:303–312.

TARLOW M (1986) Reye's syndrome and aspirin. *Br Med J* **292**:1543–1544.

THORPE SC, KEMENY DM, PANZANI R & LESSOF MH (1988) Allergy to castor bean. I. Its relationship to sensitisation to common inhalant allergens (atopy). *J Allergy Clin Immunol* **82**:62–66.

TOVEY ER, CHAPMAN MD, WELLS CW & PLATTS-MILLS TAE (1981) The distribution of dust mite allergen in the houses of patients with asthma. *Am*

Rev Respir Dis **124**:630–635.

TOWNS SJ & MELLIS CM (1984) Role of acetyl salicylic acid and sodium metabisulphite in chronic childhood asthma. *Pediatrics* **73**:631–637.

TURNER MA, DEVLIN J & DAVID TJ (1991) Holidays and atopic eczema. *Arch Dis Child* **66**:212–215.

VANTO T & KOIVIKKO A (1983) Dog hypersensitivity in asthmatic children. *Acta Paediat Scand* **72**:571–575.

VEDANTHAN PK, MENON MM, BELL TD & BERGIN D (1977) Aspirin and tartrazine oral challenge: incidence of adverse response in chronic childhood asthma. *J Allergy Clin Immunol* **60**:8–13.

VERVLOET D, BONGRAND P, ARNAUD A, BOUTIN C & CHARPIN J (1979) Donnees objectives cliniques et immunologiques observees au cours d'une cure d'altitude a Briancon chez des infants asthmatiques allergiques a la poussiere de maison et a dermatopahagoides. *Rev Fr Mal Resp* **7**:19–27.

WEBER RW, HOFFMAN M, RAINE DA & NELSON HS (1979) Incidence of bronchoconstriction due to aspirin, azo dyes, non-azo dyes, and preservatives in a population of perennial asthmatics. *J Allergy Clin Immunol* **64**:32–37.

WEINSTEIN AG (1984) Crying-induced bronchospasm in childhood asthma. *J Asthma* **21**:161–165.

WILLIAMS AJ, CHURCH SE & FINN R (1987) An unsuspected case of wheat induced asthma. *Thorax* **42**:205–206.

WILSON NM (1985) Food related asthma: a difference between two ethnic groups. *Arch Dis Child* **60**:861–865.

WILSON NM, CHARETTE L, THOMSON AH & SILVERMAN M (1985) Gastro-oesophageal reflux and childhood asthma: the acid test. *Thorax* **40**:592–597.

WILSON NM, DIXON C & SILVERMAN M (1985) Increased bronchial responsiveness caused by ingestion of ice. *Eur J Respir Dis* **66**:25–30.

WILSON N, VICKERS H, TAYLOR G & SILVERMAN M (1982) Objective test for food sensitivity in asthmatic children: increased bronchial reactivity after cola drinks. *Br Med J* **284**:1226–1228.

WOLF SI & NICKLAS RA (1985) Sulfite sensitivity in a 7 year old child. *Ann Allergy* **54**:420–423.

Part 12 Atopic Eczema

54 Triggers of atopic eczema
Food is only one item in a large list

Definition

Eczema is a pattern of inflammatory response of the skin. The principal clinical features of eczema are erythema, minute vesicles, and pruritus. The terms dermatitis and eczema are synonymous.

Classification of eczema

The British classification of eczema includes the principal forms of eczema (and also, by convention, certain conditions which do not necessarily show the histological changes of eczema at all stages) (Table 54.1 and Burton 1992). Two or more forms of eczema may co-exist in the same patient, simultaneously or consecutively. Atopic eczema is the type usually found in childhood.

Atopic eczema – definition

Atopic eczema is the characteristic clinical type of eczema associated with other atopic disorders, such as asthma or hay fever. There is a lack of an agreed precise definition, and atopic eczema is known by a number of other names (e.g. Besnier's prurigo, neurodermatitis) in different countries. Attempts have been made to devise a list of major and minor diagnostic criteria (Hanifin & Rajka 1980), but the list is imprecise, huge and impractical (Table 54.2).

Atopic eczema – aetiology

The fundamental defect is unknown (Champion & Parish 1992). A history of atopic disease in a first degree relative is present in almost all cases of atopic eczema in childhood, to such an extent that the absence of a family history should alert one to the possibility of an alternative diagnosis. Although an array of abnormal immunological parameters has been found in patients with atopic eczema (reviewed by Rajka 1989), their significance remains unclear (Chapel & Haeney 1988).

Role of food intolerance
one of many triggers

There is no evidence that food intolerance causes atopic eczema. It is, however, one of a number of triggers (Table 54.3) which can exacerbate pre-existing eczema.

erythematous reactions

There is proof that in selected children with atopic eczema, the administration of certain foods in doses of 8 g or less can provoke an immediate (within 2 hours) itchy erythematous macular rash, accompanied by a significant rise in the plasma histamine concentration (Sampson & Jolie 1984; Sampson & McCaskill 1985; Burks *et al.* 1988). Implicit in this kind of study is the inference that these erythematous rashes would lead to the development or worsening of eczema if further doses of challenge material were given, but this is

319

Table 54.1 Classification of eczema[1]

Exogenous eczemas
Irritant dermatitis
Allergic contact dermatitis
Photoallergic contact dermatitis
Eczematous polymorphic light eruption
Infective dermatitis
Dermatophytide

Endogenous eczemas
Atopic eczema
Seborrhoeic dermatitis and pityrosporal folliculitis
Asteatotic eczema
Discoid eczema
Exudative discoid and lichenoid dermatitis
Chronic scaly superficial dermatitis
Pityriasis alba
Hand eczema
Gravitational eczema
Juvenile plantar dermatosis
Metabolic eczema or eczema associated with systemic disease
Eczematous drug eruptions

[1] Source: Burton (1992).

unproven. Challenges in these and related studies were given as little as 5 hours apart, precluding the observation of delayed onset reactions or worsening of eczema. The conventional dermatological view in the UK is that these immediate erythematous reactions are indeed common in children with atopic eczema but represent an entirely separate and unrelated problem (Allen 1988). A further problem with these kind of studies is that a single provocation with a small dose in the laboratory differs greatly from the real life situation of continuous or repeated exposure to larger doses of foods. For example, Hill found that whereas 8–10 g of cow's milk powder, corresponding to 60 to 70 ml of milk, was adequate to provoke a response in some patients with cow's milk protein intolerance, other patients with late onset symptoms and particularly eczema (Hill *et al.* 1984) required up to 10 times this volume of milk daily for more than 48 hours before symptoms developed (Hill *et al.* 1988).

delayed eczematous reactions   Challenge studies in children with cow's milk protein intolerance such as those of Goldman and Hill have repeatedly demonstrated that eczematous reactions tend to be delayed rather than immediate, and may not become apparent until a few days after ingestion (Goldman *et al.* 1963; Hill *et al.* 1984). A recent study of a particularly rigorous antigen avoidance regimen in children with atopic

Table 54.2 Diagnostic criteria for atopic eczema, according to Hanifin and Rajka.[1]

Must have three or more of the following basic features

Pruritus

Typical morphology and distribution
  Flexural lichenification or linearity in adults
  Facial and extensor involvement in infants and children

Chronic or chronically relapsing dermatitis

Personal or family history of atopy (asthma, allergic rhinitis, atopic eczema)

Plus three or more minor features

Xerosis

Ichthyosis/palmar hyperlinearity/keratosis pilaris

Immediate (type I) skin test reactivity

Elevated serum IgE

Early age of onset

Tendency toward cutaneous infections (especially *Staphylococcus aureus* and herpes simplex)/impaired cell-mediated immunity

Tendency toward non-specific hand or foot dermatitis

Nipple eczema

Cheilitis

Recurrent conjunctivitis

Dennie-Morgan infraorbital fold

Keratoconus

Anterior subcapsular cataracts

Orbital darkening

Facial pallor/facial erythema

Pityriasis alba

Anterior neck folds

Itch when sweating

Intolerance to wool and lipid solvents

Perifollicular accentuation

Food intolerance

Course influenced by environmental/emotional factors

White dermographism/delayed blanch

[1] Source: Hanifin & Rajka (1980).

eczema has highlighted the importance of these delayed reactions (Devlin *et al.* 1991b). A further example is the eczematous lesions which occur 1–8 days after eating incorrectly processed cashew nuts which had become contaminated with oil from the shell of the nut (Marks *et al.* 1984). The delayed nature of these reactions is important because it makes it far more difficult to identify food triggers from the history.

indirect evidence   There is good evidence that, in a proportion of children with atopic eczema, the elimination of certain foods from the diet is associated with improvement of the eczema (e.g. Devlin *et al.* 1991a, b), but without randomized controlled studies it is impossible to tell how

Table 54.3 Triggers which can exacerbate atopic eczema

Heat
Tiredness
Teething
Intercurrent viral infection
Woollen or nylon clothing
Enzyme-containing washing powder
Bacterial skin infection
Herpes simplex virus skin infection
Pet animals
House dust
Grass and pollen
Food intolerance

much of this improvement is due to a placebo effect. Some studies of dietary therapy have incorporated challenges of selected single foods, but the finding of positive challenges is no proof that the benefit of the diet was solely due to specific food avoidance (Juto *et al.* 1978; Veien *et al.* 1987a; Pike *et al.* 1989; Van Bever *et al.* 1989; Devlin *et al.* 1991a, b).

selected patients   These and other uncontrolled observational studies have been conducted on highly selected groups of patients. The problem is that such studies fail to provide information about what sort of success can be expected from the general clinical application of elimination diets in the treatment of atopic eczema in childhood.

effect of diet on long-term outcome   Even if an elimination diet is associated with improvement, an important area of uncertainty is whether such treatment has any long-term effect on the outcome. One study, in which the outcome at 12 months was the same regardless of whether the patient had initially responded to the diet or not, and regardless of whether the family were able to cope with the diet or whether they abandoned it, suggests that the benefit of diets may be in the short term rather than the long term (Devlin *et al.* 1991a).

Food additives   There is some evidence of occasional adverse reactions to challenges with food additives in children with atopic eczema, but no objective evidence of benefit from additive avoidance. Østergaard (1986) in a blinded and placebo-controlled study found that five out of 62 (8%) children with atopic eczema were intolerant to capsules which contained a combination of nine colouring agents. The reactions comprised either erythema and urticaria or increased itching, but data was not provided as to which additives were implicated in these five subjects. A study of placebo-controlled additive challenges in 101 patients (only five were under 10 years of age) who suspected that foods aggravated their eczema demonstrated reproducible reactions in only eight, but data was not provided as to which additives were implicated in these eight subjects (Veien *et al.* 1987b). Van Bever *et al.* (1989) reported positive blind challenges to tartrazine in two out of six children with atopic eczema, but no attempt was made to see if these reactions were reproducible, and the reactions comprised quick onset erythematous flares and not worsening of eczema. A recent study examined tartrazine intolerance in 12 children with atopic eczema whose parents reported worsening of eczema after tartrazine ingestion, and improvement after dietary avoidance (Devlin & David 1992). Multiple double-blind placebo-controlled challenges demonstrated a reproducible and consistent worsening of eczema in association with tartrazine ingestion in only one child, and the probability of this occurring by chance in one or more patients out of 12 was 0.46.

Role of dietary treatment

Two centres (Hospital for Sick Children, London, and Booth Hall Children's Hospital, Manchester) with a special interest in treating atopic eczema in childhood with elimination diets have independently come to the conclusion that the proportion of children with atopic eczema severe enough to warrant regular attendance at hospital who derive benefit from elimination diets is only of the order of 10% (Atherton 1988; David 1989). The difficulties of such diets (see chapters 70 to 75) means that on the whole they are best suited for the most severely affected cases (for selection of cases see next chapter). Even with the very best results from dietary treatment, complete disappearance of all skin lesions does not occur. Thus, the main role for a dietary approach is probably for the more severely affected patient who has failed to respond to simpler measures.

Pets and dust mites

It is likely that exposure to pet animals, house-dust mites and pollen are important triggers in atopic eczema, but trying to unravel the individual effect of these rather ubiquitous items, and separate their effect from that of, for example, food intolerance, has proved difficult. One line of evidence to indicate the importance of these antigens comes from a study where patients were treated with a particularly rigorous antigen avoidance regimen in hospital, and where the use of an elemental diet was combined with measures to reduce exposure to animal and dust-mite antigens upon return home (Devlin *et al.* 1991b). Once the skin lesions improved, it became much easier to recognize individual triggers. In 37 patients treated in this way, following discharge from hospital a clear history of a reaction to dust, pets or grass was noted in 19 out of 37 (51%) patients.

Table 54.4 Conventional treatment of atopic eczema in childhood

Treatment	Reference
Emollients (e.g. emulsifying ointment) for co-existing dry skin, which varies in severity with the weather (worse in the winter) and with the severity of the eczema	David & Ewing (1988)
Topical application of emulsifying ointment prior to a bath, rather than trying to dissolve it into the bath water. Possibly increased frequency of baths for those helped, but reduced frequency for the majority in whom bathing makes the skin worse	White *et al.* (1987)
Avoidance of soap (some cases)	White *et al.* (1987)
Coal tar and calamine ointment to relieve itching at night (helpful in some)	David *et al.* (1991)
Trimeprazine 10–50 mg 1 hour before bedtime, as a sedative	David & Ewing (1988)
Treatment of bacterial skin infection with an anti-staphylococcal and anti-streptococcal antibiotic (e.g. flucloxacillin)	David & Cambridge (1986)
Recognition of initial and recurrent herpes simplex skin infection, and prevention of secondary bacterial infection with topical antiseptic (e.g. povidone-iodine ointment) or oral antibiotic	David & Longson (1985)
Topical steroids	David (1987); David & Ewing (1988)
Avoidance of irritants, such as woollen clothing, heat, enzyme-containing washing powder	David & Ewing (1988)

Other treatment   Attention to detail of conventional treatment (Table 54.4) is the most important approach to the management of atopic eczema.

Key references   54.1   RAJKA G (1989) *Essential Aspects of Atopic Dermatitis*, Springer-Verlag, Berlin. *Major textbook covering all clinical and experimental aspects of atopic eczema.*

54.2   RUZICKA T, RING J & PRZYBILLA B (1991) (eds) *Handbook of Atopic Eczema*, Springer-Verlag, Berlin. *Multi-author textbook which reviews many aspects of atopic eczema.*

54.3   DEVLIN J, DAVID TJ & STANTON RHJ (1991) Six food diet for childhood atopic dermatitis. *Acta Derm Venereol* **71**:20–24. Sixty-three children with severe atopic dermatitis, aged 0.4 to 14.8 years, were treated with a diet eliminating all but six foods for a 6-week period. Nine (14%) abandoned the diet before 6 weeks had elapsed. Twenty-one (33%) completed the diet but did not benefit. Thirty-three (52%) patients obtained 20% or greater improvement in the disease severity score at 6 weeks, and in these patients foods were re-introduced singly at weekly intervals. The outcome at 12 months was the same for the group who responded to the diet, the group who failed to respond, and the group who failed to comply, because of the tendency for eczema to markedly improve in all three groups. *Although dietary elimination of this type may be associated with immediate improvement, the long term outcome appears to be unaffected by dietary success or failure.*

54.4   DEVLIN J, DAVID TJ & STANTON RHJ (1991) Elemental diet for refractory atopic eczema. *Arch Dis Child* **66**:93–99. Thirty-seven children with refractory widespread atopic eczema were treated with an antigen avoidance regimen comprising hospitalization, exclusive feeding with an elemental formula for a median duration of 30 days, and measures to reduce exposure to pet and dust-mite antigens at home. After the initial period of food exclusion, food challenges were performed at intervals of 7 days, and the patients followed up for at least 12 months. Ten of 37 (27%) either failed to respond to the regimen or relapsed within 12 months. Improvement in the eczema was seen in 27 of 37 (73%) patients, by discharge from hospital their disease severity score had fallen to a median of 27% of the pre-treatment figure, and only three of 27 required topical corticosteroids. Following discharge from hospital a clear history of a reaction to dust, pets or grass was noted in 19/37 (51%) patients; to cats in eight, dogs in 17, house dust in six, hamsters in three, horses in three, pet birds or feathers in three, guinea pigs in two, rabbits in two, cows in one, and skin contact with grass in 13. *A strict antigen avoidance regimen may be associated with improvement of atopic eczema where conventional treatments have failed; the degree to which the benefit was a placebo effect is unfortunately not identifiable from this study.*

54.5   JUTO P, ENGBERG S & WINBERG J (1978) Treatment of infantile atopic dermatitis with a strict elimination diet. *Clin Allergy* **8**:493–500. Of 20 infants with atopic eczema treated with an elemental diet for 2–6 weeks, 19 improved, and following this improvement an open challenge with cow's milk was performed. By this method, 12 out of the 19 were found to be intolerant to cow's milk. *Unfortunately the infants were not put back on to a normal diet, and there was no control group, so it is impossible to tell how many had grown out of their eczema or had a placebo response to the diet.*

54.6   SAMPSON HA & MCCASKILL CC (1985) Food hypersensitivity and atopic dermatitis. *J Pediat* **107**:669–675. One hundred and thirteen children with atopic eczema were put on an elimination diet. Three hundred and seventy double-blind placebo-controlled food challenges were then performed, and 101 were interpreted as positive in 63 (56%) patients. Erythematous rashes developed in 85 challenges, gastrointestinal symptoms in 53 and respiratory symptoms in 32. *The relationship between these erythematous rashes and atopic eczema is obscure. The assumption that continued administration of a food which triggers a rash will eventually lead to eczema is reasonable, but not proven by any sort of controlled or blind study.*

54.7   DAVID TJ & CAMBRIDGE GC (1986) Bacterial infection and atopic eczema. *Arch Dis Child* **61**:20–23. One hundred and ninety children with atopic eczema were studied prospectively for 2.5 years. Seventy-six children (40%) had between them 164 episodes of exacerbation of eczema due to bacterial infection, and in 52 (32%) infection recurred within 3 months of a previous infection. *Staphylococcus aureus* was recovered in 97% of episodes and beta-haemolytic streptococci in 62%. Physical signs suggesting infection were pustules, crusting and a weeping discharge. *It is worthwhile recognizing bacterial skin infection, as it is the most common and most easily treatable cause of flare-ups in atopic eczema.*

54.8   DAVID TJ & LONGSON M (1985) Herpes simplex infections in atopic eczema. *Arch Dis Child* **60**:338–343. One hundred and ninety-seven children with atopic eczema were studied prospectively for 2.75 years. Ten children had initial infection with herpes simplex virus (HSV), and there were 11 recurrent HSV infections among five patients. Four children with initial infections were very ill despite antipyretics and antibiotics, and required intravenous acyclovir. The signs of an initial infection are vesicles which become pustular, the lesions then developing an umbilicated appearance. Later the lesions may coalesce leading to superficial ulceration, and bacterial superinfection is common. Recurrent lesions consist of crops of adjacent thin walled vesicles which quickly burst leaving a raw patch of skin often indistinguishable from other patches of eczema. *Infection with HSV is common in children with atopic eczema. It is worthwhile identifying HSV infections for two reasons. Firstly, initial infections are occasionally life threatening, and secondly the identification of HSV as the cause of recurrences can help the family avoid the needless pursuit of alternative and incorrect explanations (e.g. food intolerance) for flare-ups.*

Summary 54   Eczema is a pattern of inflammatory response of the skin. Atopic eczema is the characteristic clinical type of eczema found in childhood. A precise agreed definition of atopic eczema is lacking. Elimination of food from the diet may benefit a small proportion (up to 10%) of children with atopic eczema. The successful treatment of eczema entails the close attention to details of conventional medical treatment, which includes use of emollients for the dryness of the skin, the recognition and treatment of bacterial and viral infections of the skin, the use of topical steroids, the use of sedating antihistamines at night, and where relevant the avoidance of triggers such as pets, house-dust mites, and certain types of washing powder and clothing.

55   Selection of patients for elimination diets
Choose the worst cases first

Patient selection   Some children with atopic eczema will be helped by an elimination diet, some will not be helped by a diet, and some can be harmed by a diet (David 1984; David *et al.* 1984). The hazards of elimination diets are dealt with elsewhere (see chapters 70 to 75).

Table 55.1 Relative indications for elimination diet in atopic eczema

History of food intolerance
Extensive area of skin affected (e.g. over 20%)
Under 5 years of age, particularly under 2 years of age, and especially under 6 months of age
Infants who are currently being exclusively breast-fed
Parents very enthusiastic to try a diet

Unfortunately there is no objective method to predict those who are likely to benefit from a diet. The guidelines described below and in Table 55.1 are entirely empirical and based on personal experience, a poor substitute for objective evidence.

History
look for triggers

It is sensible to seek a history of any items which the parents may have noted make the child's eczema worse, whether it is excessively frequent baths (e.g. a child who is having four baths a day), exposure to pets, or ingestion of a food. It is surprisingly common to find parents who have noted or suspected a food item as something that may worsen eczema, but who nevertheless have failed to act upon their observations or more commonly failed to pursue them with vigour. An example of the latter would be a parent who noted that ingestion of cow's milk made the eczema worse, but either failed to try and exclude cow's milk products from the diet or, more commonly, only partially excluded milk products, or tried exclusion for too short a period of time. Even in these days when parents are so aware of food intolerance, they often fail to volunteer their own observations, which need to be drawn out and evaluated.

document effect of each putative trigger

When taking a history, it is worth noting precisely what kind of adverse effects have been observed for each food item. It is common for different foods to have separate adverse effects in a child. These adverse effects may well include non-dermatological manifestations, such as wheezing or vomiting. In practice, in children with atopic eczema the most common types of adverse reaction observed by the parents are immediate reactions, usually urticaria, angioedema or vomiting. It is far less common to obtain a history that a food item only causes a deterioration of the eczema a day or two after the food has been eaten. This is either because delayed adverse effects are genuinely much less common, or because it is more difficult for parents to spot a link between a food and a deterioration a day or more later, or because of both reasons.

parental confusion

One reason for taking a careful history is that the parents may have discounted their own observations. This happens either when they are unable to see any logic in their observations or when they draw false conclusions. An example of the former would be that the eczema became worse after consumption of a cola drink, but only on certain occasions, a possible reason for this being the different composition of various cola drinks. An example of the latter is the parent who discounts cow's milk intolerance as a possibility because providing goat's milk (to which the child is also intolerant) fails to help the child.

history of food intolerance

A history of food intolerance is often considered to be an indication for trying an elimination diet, although it is a poor predictor of the outcome of an elimination diet (Devlin *et al.* 1991a, b). Perhaps more important, a history of food intolerance is one factor which may fuel parental enthusiasm for trying a diet.

Severity and extent

It is common sense to take the severity and extent of the eczema into account when deciding whether or not to embark on an elimination diet. Diets are not without their problems, and by imposing an elimination diet it is all too easy merely to add to the burden of the eczema itself. In most cases the skin lesions are confined to a small area, do not greatly disturb the child, and are most simply dealt with by topical treatment alone. As a general rule, the more extensive and the more severely inflamed the lesions, the greater the motivation for trying an elimination diet. In severe or extensive cases, where there has been a poor response to other treatment, it is entirely reasonable to engage in a trial of an elimination diet, for the alternative forms of treatment (e.g. systemic steroids, other immuno-suppressive drugs, PUVA therapy) are not without major drawbacks (David 1991).

Age of patient

As a general rule, the younger the child and the smaller the size of the family, the easier it is to employ an elimination diet. Trying to enforce a diet on a 2-year old while an older sibling is allowed a normal diet can be every bit as much a challenge for the parents as managing the eczema itself. Nevertheless, it is striking how well small children can cope with strict elimination diets, and it is not uncommon to see 2- or 3-year-old children refuse sweets or chocolate if they have been told that these may worsen their eczema. It is easy to underestimate how well children can cope with a restricted diet.

Age of onset

It is often suggested that the earlier the age of onset, the more likely is an elimination diet to be helpful, but there is no objective data to support this belief.

Breast-feeding Where extensive atopic eczema develops in a young infant who has been exclusively breast-fed, it is possible that the infant has become intolerant to traces of food protein in mother's milk (Cant *et al.* 1985), and placing the mother on an elimination diet may be helpful (Cant *et al.* 1986).

Site of eczema There is no evidence of a connection between the site which is predominantly affected and the likelihood of response to an elimination diet.

Parents' wishes A key matter is how enthusiastic the parents are to try an elimination diet. Parents who are not keen to try a diet, or who are unconvinced of the need for one, are less likely to succeed in adhering to a diet.

Doctor's attitude Most parents have heard of elimination diets and may wish to discuss the advantages and disadvantages. Dealing with this issue in a dismissive way is an important cause of parental dissatisfaction. In a child with troublesome eczema and parents who are insistent on trying a diet, it may be better to allow the family to try a diet under supervision than to leave them to initiate their own unsupervised and nutritionally unsafe diet. Parents seem happier to accept advice about diets if they know that they can try one if they so wish.

Underestimating parents' ability It is not always easy to predict which parents will be able to cope with an elimination diet. Occasionally apparently capable parents fail to cope. The most common problem is failing to ensure that specific food items are totally excluded from the diet. An inability to apply consistently other forms of treatment, or to cope with the child's illness or behaviour, make it less likely that parents will be able to cope with a diet. However, personal experience is that it is more common to underestimate than overestimate parents' ability to cope with elimination diets.

Key references 55.1 VAN ASPEREN PP, LEWIS M, ROGERS M, KEMP AS & THOMPSON S (1983) Experience with an elimination diet in children with atopic dermatitis. *Clin Allergy* **13**:479–485. Twenty-nine children with atopic eczema were placed on a diet consisting of 18 foods for a 2-week period, but 16 (55%) failed to complete the diet; eight felt it was too strict and eight failed to return for follow up. *The authors failed to indicate how the patients were selected for this study, making the results difficult to interpret. Failure to adhere to the diet suggests that either the patients or parents (or both) lacked enthusiasm for a diet. Failure to return for follow-up in patients who had been previously attending regularly for severe eczema is odd – maybe these patients spontaneously improved.*

55.2 HATHAWAY MJ & WARNER JO (1983) Compliance problems in the dietary management of eczema. *Arch Dis Child* **58**:463–464. Three of 14 children (21%)

under 3 years of age and 12 of 26 children (46%) over 3 years gave up their diets, with a subsequent relapse of their eczema. The authors give the emotional and financial burden of diets as the main reasons for this failure rate. *Non-adherence is partly related to the effectiveness of the diet and the parents' enthusiasm for a diet. Since diets do not result in complete disappearance of eczema, parents are faced with the constant problem of whether a diet is worthwhile. Furthermore it is common to find that certain foods cause much more severe adverse effects than other foods, and parents are usually best placed to decide how much relaxation of the diet is acceptable.*

55.3   DEVLIN J, DAVID TJ & STANTON RHJ (1991) Six food diet for childhood atopic dermatitis. *Acta Derm Venereol* **71**:20–24. Sixty-three children with severe atopic dermatitis, aged 0.4 to 14.8 years, were treated with a diet eliminating all but six foods for a 6-week period. Nine (14%) abandoned the diet before 6 weeks had elapsed. Twenty-one (33%) completed the diet but did not benefit. Thirty-three (52%) patients obtained 20% or greater improvement in the disease severity score at 6 weeks, and in these patients foods were re-introduced singly at weekly intervals. The outcome at 12 months was the same for the group who responded to the diet, the group who failed to respond, and the group who failed to comply, because of the tendency for eczema to markedly improve in all three groups. *Although dietary elimination of this type may be associated with immediate improvement, the long term outcome appears to be unaffected by dietary success or failure.*

55.4   DEVLIN J, DAVID TJ & STANTON RHJ (1991) Elemental diet for refractory atopic eczema. *Arch Dis Child* **66**:93–99. *The outcome of dietary treatment, whether a six food diet or an elemental diet, was unrelated to the age or sex of the patient, a previous history of food intolerance, pre-treatment disease severity, pre-treatment serum IgE concentration or the pre-treatment absolute eosinophil count.*

Summary 55   The advice for selecting patients with atopic eczema for elimination diets is entirely empirical. Factors favouring a trial of dietary treatment are extensive disease, a history of food intolerance, age (it is easier to impose diets on younger patients), severe disease in an infant who is being exclusively breast-fed, and parental enthusiasm for a diet. Not all parents can manage an elimination diet, but it is easy to under-estimate how well parents can cope.

56   Elimination diets for atopic eczema
The more restricted the better the result

Which type of diet to chose?   Having decided to try a diet for one or more of the above reasons, one has the no less empirical task of deciding which diet to try (Table 56.1). One also has to decide whether to combine a diet with

Table 56.1 Types of elimination diet

Have a go at cutting down intake of one or two foods
Eliminate food triggers identified from the history
Eliminate cow's milk protein and egg
Eliminate foods believed to be common triggers
Few food diet
Eliminate all foods and supply casein hydrolysate formula
Eliminate all foods and supply elemental diet

attempts to reduce exposure to pet and house-dust mite antigens, yet another area where there is a lack of objective data upon which to base recommendations. Unfortunately, the results of tests for specific IgE antibodies, whether in the skin or the circulation, are unhelpful in predicting the outcome of avoidance measures (see chapters 41 and 43).

Basic principles

The basic principles are:

1 choose which type of diet to try;

2 employ the help of a dietitian to ensure complete avoidance of individual foods, to ensure that the diet is nutritionally sound, and to give suggestions as to how to make the diet practical and palatable;

3 apply the diet for a fixed period of time; 6 weeks is long enough to ensure that any improvement will not have been missed, while also allowing for the inevitable day to day fluctuations in disease activity;

4 reassess the patient after this fixed period to see if the diet has helped; parents (and children) are sometimes so keen that a diet should succeed that they perceive improvement where none exists, and they need the help of an objective observer, otherwise there is a risk that a useless diet will be continued indefinitely;

5 help the parents to decide whether to continue or abandon the diet;

6 continue supervision if the diet is continued, and help the parents to distinguish between confounding variables (e.g. intercurrent infection, teething, holiday abroad, natural variation in disease severity) and adverse effects caused by re-introduction of specific foods.

Have a go at cutting down intake of one or two foods

Half-hearted attempts to cut down the intake of one or two foods (e.g. giving less chocolate) are often tried by parents. In the absence of any data supporting this approach, all one can say is that the very small quantity of food which can provoke an adverse reaction makes this type of tinkering with the diet unlikely to succeed. The advantage of a carefully conducted and supervised diet is that even if it fails at least the parents will be satisfied in the knowledge that it was tried properly.

Eliminate known triggers

Unless one believes that food intolerance and atopic eczema are unconnected events, as some do (Allen 1988), it makes sense to eliminate completely items from the diet which the parents have already noticed cause an adverse reaction. Many parents have already attempted this prior to being seen by a doctor, but the elimination may have been tried for too short a period of time (e.g. a day or two), it may have only been done incompletely or half-heartedly, or the parents may be unwittingly giving a food to which the child is known to be intolerant because they have not received advice (e.g. from a dietitian) as to how to exclude food items from the diet. It is common, for example, for parents to put a child on a cow's milk-free diet, but not realize that foods containing casein or whey contain cow's milk protein. Another common error is for parents to administer goat's milk without taking steps to eliminate cow's milk products from the diet. There are no data on the outcome of this simplest type of intervention. The author's impression is that although it makes sense, this approach is only rarely associated with benefit.

Cow's milk & egg avoidance

A relatively simple (compared with more complicated diets described below) diet is a trial of cow's milk protein and egg exclusion. Some published results support this approach (Atherton *et al.* 1978), but others do not (Neild *et al.* 1986). Personal experience is that the chances are poor (at best 10%) that this diet will cause useful improvement in atopic eczema. The major use for such a diet may be in an infant whose intake consists largely of a cow's milk formula, and therefore in whom replacement of cow's milk by a soya-based milk or a casein hydrolysate is most easily achieved.

Eliminate foods believed to be common triggers

The patient avoids foods for which there is a history of intolerance, plus approximately 10 common food triggers, such as cow's milk, egg, wheat, fish, legumes (pea, bean, soya, lentil), tomato, nuts, berries and currants, citrus fruit and food additives (azo dyes, benzoates and sulphites). Personal experience is that less than 20% of children with atopic eczema experience a useful clinical benefit.

Few food diet

This has in the past been called an oligo-antigenic diet. It consists of exclusion of all foods except for five or six items (Thomas 1988). Such diets comprise a meat (usually lamb or turkey), three vegetables (e.g. potato, rice, and carrot or a brassica – cauliflower, cabbage, broccoli or sprouts), a fruit (usually pear) and possibly a non-wheat or corn-based breakfast cereal (e.g. Rice Crispies). In the only carefully defined study of this diet in children with atopic eczema, nine out of 63 (14%) abandoned the diet before 6 weeks had elapsed, 21 out of 63 (33%) completed the diet but did not benefit, and 33 out of 63 (52%) patients obtained 20% or greater improvement in the disease severity score at 6 weeks (Devlin *et al.* 1991a). The outcome at 12 months was the same for the group who responded to the diet, the group who failed to respond, and the group who failed to comply, because of the tendency for eczema to markedly improve with time in all three groups.

Eliminate all foods and supply casein hydrolysate formula

Clearly, the larger the number of foods which are excluded, the greater are the chances that a trigger food will have been avoided. In practice this type of diet is most easily employed in infants, who are more likely than older children to be willing to drink poorly palatable formulae such as the casein hydrolysate formulae Pregestimil or Nutramigen. No data are available on the outcome of this type of diet.

Eliminate all foods and supply an elemental diet

The application of an in-patient regimen of 4–6 weeks of a so-called elemental diet (e.g. Vivonex) is the ultimate test of whether food intolerance is relevant or not. If one is going to go to such extremes, then it makes sense to also take steps to try to minimize exposure to pet and dust mite antigens. In one major study of this approach, 37 children with refractory widespread atopic eczema were treated with an antigen avoidance regimen comprising hospitalization, exclusive feeding with an elemental formula for a median duration of 30 days, and measures to reduce exposure to pet and dust mite antigens at home (Devlin *et al.* 1991b). After the initial period of food exclusion, food challenges were performed at intervals of 7 days, and the patients followed up for at least 12 months. Ten out of 37 (27%) either failed to respond to the regimen or relapsed within 12 months. Improvement in the eczema was seen in 27 out of 37 (73%) patients, by discharge from hospital their disease severity score had fallen to a median of 27% of the pre-treatment figure, and only three out of 27 required topical corticosteroids. The drawbacks comprise the lack of a guarantee of success, family disruption associated with 2–3 month's hospitalization, loose stools (due to hyperosmolarity of Vivonex), marked weight loss, and hypo-albuminaemia. The lack of a control group in this study means that it is impossible to tell how much of the benefit was simply due to a placebo effect of the regimen. Further information about Vivonex and other so-called elemental formulae is given in chapter 19.

Conclusions

Like many chronic diseases, there is a strong placebo effect of any new therapy applied with enthusiasm, particularly if the parents are convinced it will help. The lack of randomized studies of dietary treatment means that the role of elimination diets is uncertain. Since diets are difficult and potentially hazardous, and are possibly best employed in conjunction with pet and dust mite avoidance, it is logical to apply simpler conventional therapy first. Despite the somewhat disappointing overall results of diets, a number of patients with severe disease experience dramatic and lasting benefit associated with specific food avoidance, and the detection of these children by the application of empirically based diets is an important part of the management of atopic eczema.

Key references 56.1   WEBBER SA, GRAHAM-BROWN RAC, HUTCHINSON PE & BURNS DA (1989) Dietary manipulation in childhood dermatitis. *Br J Derm* **121**:91–98. The dietary habits of 73 children seen in a dermatology out-patient department were studied. Although most children had only 'mild flexural dermatitis', 52 (71%) had had alterations made to their diet before attendance at hospital. Over half had been started on diets before any professional advice had been sought. Despite a number of supposedly harmful or dangerous diets, there was no evidence of growth retardation, failure to thrive or specific deficiency symptoms. The authors condemned uncontrolled and unsupervised diets. *This paper reveals as much about professional attitudes as it does about the problem it supposedly addresses. If the eczema were so mild, why were these children referred to hospital? It would appear that the doctors' perceptions were out of keeping with those of the parents. Rightly or wrongly, parents are often concerned about the chronic nature of atopic eczema and about prolonged topical steroid use, and the idea of self-help ('let's try a diet') is understandable. The study rightly documented the lack of advice given to parents about when to expect benefit, how long to continue the diet, and when and if to re-introduce the excluded foods. However some control questions on knowledge of topical steroid use might well have revealed similar lacunae in knowledge. The disapproval voiced in this paper is evidence of a gulf between professional attitudes and parental desires.*

56.2   DEVLIN J, DAVID TJ & STANTON RHJ (1991) Six food diet for childhood atopic dermatitis. *Acta Derm Venereol* **71**:20–24. *The most clearly defined study of a few food diet in atopic eczema. At 1 year the group who responded to the diet fared no better than the groups who failed to respond or who could not cope with the diet at all; all three groups were much improved.*

56.3   DEVLIN J, DAVID TJ & STANTON RHJ (1991) Elemental diet for refractory atopic eczema. *Arch Dis Child* **66**:93–99. *The largest study of a stringent antigen avoidance regimen. Improvement (i.e. greater than 20% reduction in disease severity score) in the eczema was seen in 27 out of 37 (73%) patients, but the lack of a control group means that it is impossible to know how much of this benefit was a placebo effect.*

56.4   ATHERTON DJ (1988) Diet and atopic eczema. *Clin Allergy* **18**:215–228. *Useful detailed review.*

56.5   SAMPSON HA (1991) Eczema and food hypersensitivity. In Metcalfe DD, Sampson HA & Simon RA (eds) *Food Allergy: Adverse Reactions to Foods and Food Additives*, pp. 113–128, Blackwell Scientific Publications, Boston. *By employing large numbers of double-blind placebo-controlled food challenges in children with atopic eczema, Sampson has made an important contribution to our understanding of the importance of quick-onset reactions in eczema. This chapter reviews the authors' work.*

Summary 56 The role of elimination diets is uncertain. Since diets are difficult and possibly best employed in conjunction with pet and dust mite avoidance, it is logical to apply conventional therapy first. Despite the somewhat disappointing results of diets, a number of patients with severe disease experience lasting benefit associated with specific food avoidance, and the detection of these children by the application of empirically based diets is an important part of the management of atopic eczema. The main options are cow's milk and egg avoidance, elimination of commonly incriminated food triggers, a few food diet, or an elemental diet.

References to Chapters 54–56

ALLEN R (1988) Role of diet in treating atopic eczema: dietary manipulation has no value. *Br Med J* **297**:1459–1460.

ATHERTON DJ (1988) Diet and atopic eczema. *Clin Allergy* **18**:215–228.

ATHERTON DJ, SEWELL M, SOOTHILL JF, WELLS RS & CHILVERS CED (1978) A double-blind controlled crossover trial of an antigen-avoidance diet in atopic eczema. *Lancet* **1**:401–403.

BURKS AW, MALLORY SB, WILLIAMS LW & SHIRRELL MA (1988) Atopic dermatitis: clinical relevance of food hypersensitivity reactions. *J Pediat* **113**: 447–451.

BURTON JL (1992) Eczema, lichenification, prurigo and erythroderma. In Champion RH, Burton JL & Ebling FJG (eds) *Textbook of Dermatology*, vol. 1, 5th edn, pp. 537–588, Blackwell Scientific Publications, Oxford.

CANT AJ, BAILES JA, MARSDEN RA & HEWITT D (1986) Effect of maternal dietary exclusion on breast fed infants with eczema: two controlled studies. *Br Med J* **293**:231–233.

CANT A, MARSDEN RA & KILSHAW PJ (1985) Egg and cows' milk hypersensitivity in exclusively breast fed infants with eczema, and detection of egg protein in breast milk. *Br Med J* **291**:932–935.

CHAMPION RH & PARISH WE (1992) Atopic dermatitis. In Champion RH, Burton JL & Ebling FJG (eds) *Textbook of Dermatology*, vol. 1, 5th edn, pp. 589–610, Blackwell Scientific Publications, Oxford.

CHAPEL H & HAENEY M (1988) *Essentials of Clinical Immunology*, 2nd edn, Blackwell Scientific Publications, Oxford.

DAVID TJ (1984) Anaphylactic shock during elimination diets for severe atopic eczema. *Arch Dis Child* **59**:983–986.

DAVID TJ (1987) Steroid scare. *Arch Dis Child* **62**:876–878.

DAVID TJ (1989) Dietary treatment of atopic eczema. *Arch Dis Child* **64**: 1506–1509.

DAVID TJ (1991) Recent developments in the treatment of childhood atopic eczema. *J Roy Coll Phys Lond* **25**:95–101.

DAVID TJ & CAMBRIDGE GC (1986) Bacterial infection and atopic eczema. *Arch Dis Child* **61**:20–23.

DAVID TJ, DEVLIN J & EWING CI (1991) Atopic and seborrheic dermatitis. Practical management. *Pediatrician* **18**:211–217.

DAVID TJ & EWING CI (1988) Treatment of atopic eczema in childhood. *Comprehensive Therapy* **14**:21–26.

DAVID TJ & LONGSON M (1985) Herpes simplex infections in atopic eczema. *Arch Dis Child* **60**:338–343.

DAVID TJ, WADDINGTON E & STANTON RHJ (1984) Nutritional hazards of elimination diets in children with atopic eczema. *Arch Dis Child* **59**:323–325.

DEVLIN J & DAVID TJ (1992) Tartrazine in atopic eczema. *Arch Dis Child* **67**: 709–711.

DEVLIN J, DAVID TJ & STANTON RHJ (1991a) Six food diet for childhood atopic dermatitis. *Acta Derm Venereol* **71**:20–24.

DEVLIN J, DAVID TJ & STANTON RHJ (1991b) Elemental diet for refractory atopic eczema. *Arch Dis Child* **66**:93–99.

GOLDMAN AS, ANDERSON DW, SELLERS WA, SAPERSTEIN S, KNIKER WT & HALPERN SR (1963) Milk allergy. I. Oral challenge with milk and isolated milk proteins in allergic children. *Pediatrics* **32**:425–443.

HANIFIN JM & RAJKA G (1980) Diagnostic features of atopic dermatitis. *Acta Dermatovenereol* (suppl. 92):44–47.

HILL DJ, BALL G & HOSKING CS (1988) Clinical manifestations of cow's milk allergy in childhood. I. Associations with in-vitro cellular immune responses. *Clin Allergy* **18**:469–479.

HILL DJ, FORD RPK, SHELTON MJ & HOSKING CS (1984) A study of 100 infants and young children with cow's milk allergy. *Clin Rev Allergy* **2**:125–142.

JUTO P, ENGBERG S & WINBERG J (1978) Treatment of infantile atopic dermatitis with a strict elimination diet. *Clin Allergy* 8:493–500.

MARKS JG, DEMELFI T, MCCARTHY MA et al. (1984) Dermatitis from cashew nuts. *J Am Acad Dermatol* **10**:627–631.

NEILD VS, MARSDEN RA, BAILES JA & BLAND JM (1986) Egg and milk exclusion diets in atopic eczema. *Br J Dermatol* **114**:117–123.

ØSTERGAARD PA (1986) Incidensen af farvestofintolerans hos eksembørn. *Ugeskr Læger* **148**:711–714.

PIKE MG, CARTER CM, BOULTON P, TURNER MW, SOOTHILL JF & ATHERTON DJ (1989) Few food diets in the treatment of atopic eczema. *Arch Dis Child* **64**:1691–1698.

RAJKA G (1989) *Essential Aspects of Atopic Dermatitis*, Springer-Verlag, Berlin.

SAMPSON HA & JOLIE PA (1984) Increased plasma histamine concentration after food challenges in children with atopic dermatitis. *New Engl J Med* **311**: 372–376.

SAMPSON HA & MCCASKILL CC (1985) Food hypersensitivity and atopic dermatitis: evaluation of 113 patients. *J Pediat* **107**:669–675.

THOMAS B (1988) (ed) *Manual of Dietetic Practice*, pp. 527–531, Blackwell Scientific Publications, Oxford.

VAN BEVER HP, DOCX M & STEVENS WJ (1989) Food and food additives in severe atopic dermatitis. *Allergy* **44**:588–594.

VEIEN NK, HATTEL T, JUSTESEN O & NØRHOLM A (1987a) Dermatitis induced or aggravated by selected foodstuffs. *Acta Derm Venereol* **67**:133–138.

VEIEN NK, HATTEL T, JUSTESEN O & NØRHOLM A (1987b) Oral challenge with food additives. *Contact Derm* **17**:100–103.

WHITE MI, MCEWAN JENKINSON D & LLOYD DH (1987) The effect of washing on the thickness of the stratum corneum in normal and atopic individuals. *Br J Dermatol* **116**:525–530.

Part 13　Urticaria and Angioedema

57 Classification and mechanism of urticaria
Idiopathic is the largest category

Definition Urticaria (also known as nettle rash or hives) is a transient erythematous or oedematous swelling of the dermis. The characteristic lesion of urticaria is a weal. A weal is an area of dermal oedema, white, compressible and usually evanescent. Angioedema (formerly known as angioneurotic oedema) is a variant of urticaria in which the subcutaneous tissues, rather than the dermis, are mainly involved (Champion 1992).

Pathogenesis Urticaria is caused by the release of various pharmacological mediators which leads to a temporary local increase in the permeability of capillaries and small venules. These mediators are synthesized and released by mast cells, of which there are two types, connective tissue mast cells and mucosal mast cells (Seldin & Austen 1985), and also by circulating blood basophils.

Mediators Histamine is the best known mediator. Mast cells are the major source of histamine, but non-mast cell histamine has been found in the skin, the intestinal mucosa and submucosa, and the brain (Greaves 1985). Certain prostaglandins and leukotrienes, platelet-activation factor, eosinophilotactic factor, and a range of other substances whose pathophysiological role is at present unclear, have also been identified as mediators (Greaves 1985). Histamine is probably the most important mediator for acute allergic urticaria, but not in the majority of cases of chronic urticaria (Champion 1992).

Histamine receptors Histamine receptors are divided into two classes, H1 and H2. Using selective H1-receptor and H2-receptor agonists and antagonists, it has been shown that the vasodilatory and vascular permeability actions of histamine involve both H1 and H2 receptors (Greaves 1985). Induction of the axon reflex flare by histamine involves H1 receptors, and itching is also an H1 response (Champion 1992).

Angioedema Angioedema shares the same complex aetiology as urticaria, and the two conditions commonly co-exist. Almost any part of the body may be affected, but the most common sites are the lips, eyelids, tongue, larynx and genitalia. The lesions often develop within minutes, and the rapidity of swelling, particularly around the eyes, may cause alarm to the patient and parents.

Itching   Most, but not all, urticarial weals itch. Weals which have lasted more than 12 hours often have a burning or painful component, especially in urticarial vasculitis or the physical urticarias. Itching is likely to be more intense where the weals are superficial, and less intense where there is subcutaneous extension of the weal. Angioedema is not usually itchy (Warin & Champion 1974).

Duration of attacks   Urticarial weals usually last 3–4 hours, but some superficial lesions clear in 2 hours. Larger and deeper lesions persist longer and may last up to 2 or 3 days. The weals of the physical urticarias often clear in 30–60 min (Warin & Champion 1974).

Clearing of weals   As a weal fades its central whiteness tends to disappear, it becomes flatter and develops a more diffuse but paler red colour. Once the weal has cleared the skin appears completely normal, except in a few cases where there is residual purpura. Residual purpura suggests the presence of urticarial vasculitis (see below), but it may occur after ordinary idiopathic urticaria and is more often seen in children than adults (Warin & Champion 1974).

Classification
acute or chronic   Urticaria is sometimes classified into acute and chronic (i.e. recurrent episodes), with a time division at 2 months, but this subdivision is of little value in understanding the basic aetiology (Champion 1992).

allergic or non-allergic   Urticaria can be classified into allergic and non-allergic. This subdivision is difficult to apply as it is often not possible to prove whether there is a true allergic reaction, and in a large proportion of cases of urticaria no cause is ever found (Champion 1992).

main categories   The most useful categorization is to recognize the physical urticarias, hereditary angioedema, urticarial vasculitis, urticaria pigmentosa and papular urticaria as separate entities, and designate the remaining and largest groups of cases as ordinary or idiopathic urticaria and contact urticaria (Champion 1992). Food intolerance is only relevant to ordinary urticaria and exercise-induced anaphylaxis (one of the physical urticarias). An outline of all forms of urticaria is given in this book, as unravelling the cause of urticaria depends on the correct identification of the type of urticaria present.

Key references 57.1   CHAMPION RH (1992) Urticaria. In Champion RH, Burton JL & Ebling FJG (eds) *Textbook of Dermatology*, vol. 1, 5th edn, pp. 1865–1880, Blackwell Scientific Publications, Oxford. *Good general review of classification.*

57.2   CZARNETZKI BM (1986) *Urticaria*, Springer-Verlag, Berlin. *Detailed review.*

Summary 57   Urticaria is the result of the release of histamine and other chemical mediators, which cause increased capillary permeability and lead to the production of itchy weals in the skin. Angioedema is a closely related disorder which commonly co-exists with urticaria but affects the subcutaneous tissues rather than the dermis. It is simplest to classify urticaria by its aetiology, which leaves ordinary idiopathic urticaria as the most common category. Other forms of urticaria are the physical urticarias, hereditary angioedema, urticarial vasculitis, urticaria pigmentosa, papular urticaria and contact urticaria.

58 Physical urticarias, hereditary angioedema, papular urticaria, urticarial vasculitis, urticaria pigmentosa
Urticaria is an heterogenous entity

Physical urticarias   The physical urticarias are generally responses to physical stimuli. The main types of physical urticaria are shown in Table 58.1. It is not uncommon for different types to co-exist.

Triple response   The response of skin to firm stroking is called the triple response. This consists of an initial red line in 3–15 s (capillary dilatation), followed by an axon reflex flare accompanied by broadening erythema (arteriolar dilatation), and culminating in replacement of the red line with a weal (transudation of fluid through dilated capillaries). Itching is usually absent.

Dermographometer   It has been reported that a triple response can be elicited in 25–50% of normal persons (Champion 1992), but such estimates are of little value without some objective measurement of the intensity of the stimulus. The most commonly used testing device (Fig. 58.1) consists of a spring-loaded stylus, the pressure of which can be varied by a screw adjustment on the upper part of the instrument to produce graded pressures, which can be read off an arbitrary scale. The instrument is guided through a slot in a flat metal plate applied to the skin, to standardize scratching of the skin (James & Warin 1969). The instrument used at various pressures produces weals of fairly consistent size which can be readily measured. Warin and

Table 58.1 The main types of physical
urticaria and related disorders[1]

Dermographism
Delayed dermographism
Pressure urticaria
Solar urticaria
Cold urticaria
    Familial cold urticaria
    Idiopathic cold urticaria
    Cold urticaria caused by cryoglobulins or cold agglutinins
    Cold erythema
    Cold reflex urticaria
Heat urticaria
Cholinergic urticaria
Cholinergic pruritus
Aquagenic urticaria
Aquagenic pruritus
Vibratory angioedema

[1] Source: Champion RH (1992).

Champion (1974) reported that: 'the well manicured thumb nail of the average dermatologist produces a weal comparable with a pressure on the stylus in this instrument of 4900 g/cm^2'.

Dermographism

Dermographism (also called factitious urticaria) has been defined as wealing which is more than 2 mm across when the stylus of the instrument described above is loaded at 4900 g/cm^2. With the use of the dermographometer described above, when set at 4900 g/cm^2, 4.2% of 2813 normal adults produced a linear weal on the forearm of 2 mm width or more 10 min after scratching (Kirby *et al.* 1971). The site of testing is important. The effect of pressure is altered by the presence or absence of underlying bone, the looseness of the skin, the presence of hair and the degree of sweating. Skin normally exposed and weathered reacts much less than skin normally covered (Warin & Champion 1974). A difficulty in defining the nature of the trauma causing wealing is that it is more than a simple pressure effect, and is partly due to a stretching action on the skin (Warin & Champion 1974).

timing

The weals in dermographism reach a maximum size in 6–7 min, remain for 10–15 min before starting to fade (Warin & Champion 1974), and therefore disappear more quickly than the weals of idiopathic urticaria which tend to last several hours.

prick test sites

Skin which has been the site of a positive prick test or an insect bite weals on scratching for a period of 72–96 hours (James & Warin 1969).

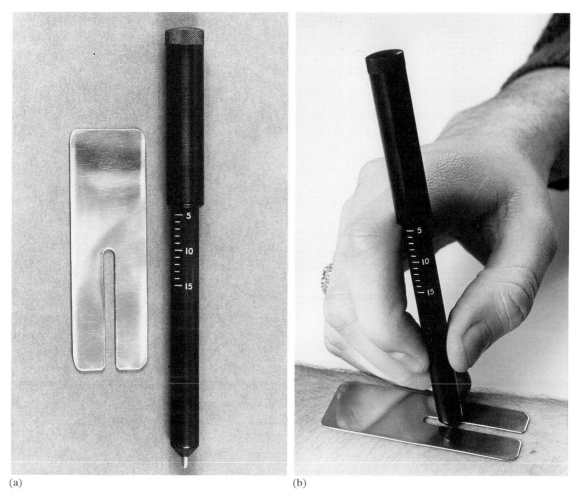

(a)   (b)

Fig. 58.1 (a) Instrument to produce a constant pressure effect on the skin. (b) The tension on the spring on the point of the instrument can be varied to produce known pressures. Because the shoulders run on the metal guide, rucking of the skin can be avoided.

Symptomatic dermographism

Dermographism commonly co-exists with other forms of urticaria, and is particularly pronounced in atopic eczema (Champion 1992). Dermographism has been sub-classified into simple dermographism, which is a constitutional wealing tendency, and symptomatic dermographism in which a different, possibly immunological, mechanism may be operative (Breathnach *et al.* 1983). Symptomatic dermographism is differentiated from simple dermographism by the presence of itching and the generally lower threshold required to induce wealing. Symptomatic dermographism may be passively transferred to unaffected human subjects in up to 50% of cases, although the serum factor responsible for passive transfer has yet to be identified with certainty (Murphy *et al.* 1987). Double-blind studies have shown that in the treatment of dermographism, a combination of an H1-receptor antagonist and an H2-receptor antagonist is more effective than either drug alone (Kaur *et al.* 1981).

White dermographism

White dermographism refers to a subsequent blanching of the initially produced erythematous line of the triple response. The term dermographism is a misnomer, as no wealing is found. The mechanism of white dermographism is unclear, but the condition is a common feature of atopic eczema (Wong *et al.* 1984) and other inflammatory dermatoses.

Pressure urticaria

In pressure urticaria, swelling develops some 2–6 hours after exposure to pressure, such as from the back or seat of a hard chair, pressure from tight clothes or standing on ladders (Champion 1992). The swellings last 24–48 hours, and give rise to burning and soreness rather than itching (Kobza-Black 1985). There is no standard objective test for pressure urticaria. The condition can sometimes be reproduced by hanging a weight (e.g. 15 lb for 10 min – Ryan *et al.* 1968) on the end of a crepe bandage over the shoulder, thigh or forearm, although it may not be easy to reproduce the continuous, greater, traction-like pressure which precipitates the condition. There are two potential sources of confusion. One is that about a third of patients with true pressure urticaria also have ordinary urticarial weals. The other is that in ordinary urticaria, weals may occur at sites of pressure against the skin. However, these develop at the height of the general urticarial eruption and have the same short duration as the general weals, which distinguishes them from true pressure urticaria (Kobza-Black 1985). In a variant, called delayed pressure urticaria, wealing occurs on average at 3.5 hours after the pressure stimulus, the weals come to a peak at about 10 hours, and the mean duration of the swellings is 40 hours (Dover *et al.* 1988; Lawlor *et al.* 1989). Systemic steroids are the only effective treatment (Dover *et al.* 1988).

Solar urticaria

Solar urticaria is an uncommon condition in which exposure to sunlight or artificial radiation results in an urticarial reaction within a few minutes of exposure (Kobza-Black 1985). Repeated exposure may lead to the development of tolerance, though the mechanism for this is not understood (Leenutaphong *et al.* 1990). Some patients with solar urticaria possess a circulating factor which is transferable, and plasmapheresis has been shown to be effective in one such patient (Duschet *et al.* 1987).

Cold urticaria   In cold urticaria, weals develop on skin sites exposed to cold, usually when the area is warmed again. Minor degrees of cold urticaria are quite common, and often occur suddenly after an intercurrent illness (Doeglas *et al.* 1986), and may last months or even years. The condition is probably the most common symptomatic form of physical urticaria seen in childhood. Out of 220 patients with cold urticaria reported from Finland, 25 (11%) were under 10 years of age and 88 (40%) were under 20 years old (Neittaanmaki 1985). Cold urticaria is often (30% in one large series) associated with other forms of urticaria (Neittaanmaki 1985). Common precipitating factors are exposure to cold windy weather with rain, immersion of hands in cold water, and handling cold objects. Systemic manifestations such as syncope and headache are common, and patients must be warned against pool and sea bathing because of a risk of loss of consciousness and drowning (Kobza-Black 1985). The diagnosis of cold urticaria can usually be confirmed by the application (without excess pressure which could cause dermographism) of an ice cube (wrapped in a plastic bag) to the skin for 5–10 min, or by the immersion of the patient's forearm in cold water at 5°C (Kobza-Black 1985). On rare occasions, the diagnosis can only be confirmed by total body exposure to cold (Kivity *et al.* 1990).

differential diagnosis   A large number of disorders can result from, or be exacerbated by, exposure to the cold (Table 58.2), and differentiation from other physical urticarias can be difficult. For example, a history of weals developing after sea bathing might be due to: (a) cholinergic urticaria from heat and exercise; (b) dermographism from trauma associated

Table 58.2 Skin disorders caused by or aggravated by cold[1]

Reaction to abnormal cold
Frostbite
Immersion or trench foot

Abnormal reaction to cold
Chilblains (perniosis)
Acrocyanosis
Erythrocyanosis
Livedo reticularis
Raynaud's phenomenon
Cryoglobulinaemia
Cold urticaria
Cold erythema
Cold panniculitis
Neonatal cold injury

[1] Source: Champion (1992).

with beach games; (c) solar urticaria; (d) aquagenic urticaria; or (e) cold urticaria.

treatment

The recommended treatment of cold urticaria consists of avoidance of the precipitating circumstances, and the administration of H1-receptor antagonists (Kobza-Black 1985). Induction of tolerance by repeated exposure to cold has been reported (Bentley-Phillips *et al.* 1976; Keahey *et al.* 1988).

Heat urticaria

Local urticarial reactions to direct contact with heat are rare (Kobza-Black 1985). Induction of tolerance has been reported after repeated and gradually increasing exposure to heat (Leigh & Ramsay 1975).

Cholinergic urticaria

Cholinergic urticaria consists of widespread tiny (1–3 mm) weals with variable erythema which last 30–60 min and occur in association with sweating (Champion 1992). In minor degrees the condition is common and merely a nuisance. The onset is most frequently in teenagers and young adults (Kobza-Black 1985). The cause of the sweating is not important, and heat, exercise, emotion or eating spicy food can all cause cholinergic urticaria. Itching may occur in the absence of wealing. The urticarial lesions in patients with cholinergic urticaria can be induced by the intradermal injection of acetyl choline and abolished by topical application of atropine, but the precise pathogenesis of the condition is obscure (Kobza-Black 1985). Attacks can sometimes be aborted by the prompt application of cold water to the skin at the first hint of an episode (Kobza-Black 1985). A refractory period of up to 24 hours may occur after an attack, and this effect can be used prior to a specific social event or as part of a programme to induce tolerance by the use of carefully graded increasing stimuli (Kobza-Black 1985). The androgenic steroid danazol has been used with benefit in some severe cases, although its mode of action is unclear (Wong *et al.* 1987).

Exercise-induced anaphylaxis

In what may (Champion 1992) or may not (Kaplan *et al.* 1981) be a separate entity from cholinergic urticaria, exercise may be followed by hypotension, accompanied by a varying combination of cholinergic urticaria, and angioedema of the face and pharynx (Kaplan *et al.* 1981; Lewis *et al.* 1981; Sheffer *et al.* 1983; Songsiridej & Busse 1983). The mechanism of exercise-induced anaphylaxis is unclear, although when attacks can be reproduced by exercise challenge an exercise-related rise in the serum histamine concentration has been documented (Sheffer *et al.* 1983).

role of food

In a curious but well described variant of exercise-induced anaphylaxis, attacks only occur when the exercise follows within a couple of hours of the ingestion of specific foods such as celery, shellfish (shrimps and oysters), squid, peaches or wheat (Maulitz *et al.* 1979; Buchbinder *et al.* 1983; Kidd *et al.* 1983; Kushimoto & Aoki 1985; Silverstein *et al.* 1986; Kivity *et al.* 1988; McNeil & Strauss 1988; Dohi *et al.* 1991). In a few cases specific food triggers cannot be identified, and it appears that the act of eating within 30 min of exercise is sufficient to provoke anaphylaxis (Novey *et al.* 1983; Dohi *et al.* 1991). This has been labelled postprandial exercise-induced anaphylaxis (Novey *et al.* 1983). The mechanisms which result in food-dependent exercise-induced anaphylaxis are obscure. This disorder, though rare, is important in the interpretation of dietary challenge studies of food intolerance, because in these patients a simple double-blind food challenge without exercise will fail to validate a history of food intolerance.

Aquagenic urticaria

Aquagenic urticaria is an urticaria resembling, but not identical with, cholinergic urticaria, which is precipitated by contact with water, irrespective of its temperature (Champion 1992). The weals are usually confined to the neck, the upper trunk and the arms. Treatment with H1- or H2-receptor antagonists is generally unhelpful (Steinman & Greaves 1985), but some benefit may be associated with the application of an inert oily substance prior to exposure to water (Sibbald *et al.* 1981), or with the addition of 25 to 200 g of sodium bicarbonate to the bath water (Bayoumi *et al.* 1986). Aquagenic pruritus is water-induced itching without any visible skin changes, and is therefore distinct from aquagenic urticaria. It sometimes responds well to H1-receptor antagonists (Greaves *et al.* 1981).

Hereditary angioedema

Hereditary angioedema is a rare disorder which is transmitted as an autosomal dominant trait, and is due to a total or partial reduction in the function of the C1-esterase inhibitor (Lachmann 1985). Because of this, usually following a trivial injury, unrestrained C1 esterase activates the complement cascade, with the formation of kinins and other vasoactive peptides. Usually the onset is in childhood, with recurrent deep swellings of the skin and mucous membranes. The swellings last approximately 24 hours and are usually not itchy. Attacks of colicky abdominal pain, attributed to oedema of the bowel, sometimes accompanied by vomiting, are common, and may or may not coincide with skin swellings (Lachmann 1985). As mentioned, the skin lesions may occur after trauma, dental trauma being one particularly hazardous factor. The disease may be relatively mild in some patients, but there is a major threat of oedema of the larynx, pharynx, trachea and bronchi in this condition, and in some families over 20% of affected members died of large airway obstruction before middle age (Champion 1992). As the oedema may extend as far down the airways as the upper bronchi, tracheostomy may be ineffective in restoring the airway (Lachmann 1985). The deficiency of C1-esterase inhibitor can be demonstrated easily in a laboratory in which complement investigations are performed. Emergency treatment is with transfusion of fresh frozen plasma or purified C1-esterase inhibitor. Prophylaxis with epsilon amino-caproic acid, tranexamic acid or anabolic steroids (stanazolol or danazol) may reduce the frequency and severity of attacks (Lachmann 1985; Champion 1992).

food intolerance

The evidence linking the rare acquired non-hereditary deficiency of C1-esterase inhibitor with food intolerance is flimsy, and comprises two patients who were said to be intolerant to multiple foods, but in whom no food challenges were performed (Morrison & Rabson 1987).

Papular urticaria

In papular urticaria, the lesions are itchy, and consist of weals, or firm papules, or weals surrounded by papules. There is often a central punctum. There may be bullae, especially on the legs. Each lesion persists for 2–10 days (Rook 1986). The lesions are caused by an allergic reaction to insect bites, and not by the bite itself (Croce 1980; Rook 1986). Whether the weal or the papule predominates depends on the type and degree of allergic sensitivity to the insect antigens. The species of insect responsible vary with the environment. Dog, cat and bird fleas are common offenders but the human flea, the bed bug, the mosquito and certain mites are sometimes incriminated (Rook 1986; Burns 1987). Treatment consists of removal or avoidance of the insect.

Urticarial vasculitis

Urticaria or angioedema are uncommon features of necrotizing vasculitis, secondary to disorders such as serum sickness, systemic lupus erythematosus or Sjögren's syndrome. Idiopathic urticarial vasculitis, which is almost exclusively confined to adults, is reviewed elsewhere (Soter 1985). In this disorder, the weals may or may not be itchy, but purpura is commonly seen during resolution of the lesions. Episodic arthralgia is the most common extra-cutaneous manifestation, but there may be fever, malaise, abdominal pain and occasionally enlargement of the spleen.

painful joints & urticaria in childhood

Although urticarial vasculitis is an adult disorder, a similar but poorly described and unnamed disorder is commonly seen in childhood. The patient presents with florid urticaria and transiently painful joints, usually in the limbs and most commonly the ankles or knees. Purpura may or may not be seen during resolution, but there is no abdominal pain or renal involvement, helping to distinguish this entity from Henoch–Schonlein purpura. There may be a mild degree of general malaise, and the disorder commonly follows a non-specific respiratory infection. The arthropathy and the urticaria quickly resolve, within a day or two, but often re-appear several times, over a period of 2–3 months. As the condition disappears the recurrences become less severe. Treatment with H1-receptor antagonists is unhelpful. In the patients seen by the author, obvious possible causes such as exposure to drugs or particular foods have not been identified. The condition is self-limiting and appears to be without long term consequences.

Henoch-Schönlein purpura

In the context of urticaria and vasculitis, Henoch–Schönlein purpura (also called anaphylactoid purpura) is mentioned because, in addition to the purpura, urticaria is a prominent feature. In a study of 85 attacks, 30% of patients had urticaria, and 45% had localized oedema, particularly involving the scalp, eyelids, hands, feet, back and perineum (Ansell 1970).

Urticaria pigmentosa

The lesions of urticaria pigmentosa, an uncommon disorder, usually appear within the first 2 years of life (Greaves 1992), and comprise pigmented maculopapular or nodular lesions, seen mainly on the trunk and limbs. The lesions consist of increased amounts of melanin, and a dense accumulation of mast cells. The diagnosis is established by rubbing the lesions, which causes local itching, redness and wealing, and Darier's sign (Greaves 1992). The main symptom is itching, which is aggravated by rubbing and scratching. Blistering may occur in this condition, but usually only in those under 3 years of age. Urticaria pigmentosa in childhood carries a good prognosis, with eventual spontaneous resolution in almost all cases (Greaves 1992). Treatment is usually not required, but where the symptoms are troublesome treatment with a combination of H1- and H2-receptor antagonists may be helpful (Greaves 1992).

Key references

58.1 WONG RC, FAIRLEY JA & ELLIS CN (1984) Dermographism: a review. *J Am Acad Derm* **11**:643–652. *Useful review of dermographism, including other forms such as delayed, follicular, cholinergic, red and black dermographism.*

58.2 WARIN RP & CHAMPION RH (1974) *Urticaria*, Saunders, London. *Detailed review of the clinical features of all types of urticaria. For more recent information about the pathogenesis of individual types of urticaria, see next reference.*

58.3 CHAMPION RH, GREAVES MW, KOBZA-BLACK A & PYE RJ. (1985) (eds) *The Urticarias*, Churchill Livingstone, Edinburgh. *Multi-author, 28 chapter textbook on urticaria. Excellent reviews of the basic mechanisms, clinical causes and clinical types of urticaria.*

58.4 ILLIG L (1973) Physical urticaria. Its diagnosis and treatment. *Curr Probl Derm* **5**:79–116. *General review.*

58.5 NEITTAANMAKI H (1985) Cold urticaria. Clinical findings in 220 patients. *J Am Acad Dermatol* **13**:636–644. *Useful clinical study of a large series of patients.*

58.6 HADJIYANNAKI K & LACHMANN PJ (1971) Hereditary angio-oedema: a review with particular reference to pathogenesis and treatment. *Clin Allergy* **1**:221–233. *General review.*

58.7 BURNS DA (1987) The investigation and management of arthropod bite reactions acquired in the home. *Clin Exper Dermatol* **12**:114–120. *Useful practical advice, showing how the distribution of insect bites gives a good clue as to which insect is responsible.*

58.8 DOHI M, SUKO M, SUGIYAMA H *et al.* (1991) Food-dependent, exercise-induced anaphylaxis: a study on 11 Japanese cases. *J Allergy Clin Immunol* **87**:34–40. *Report of 11 patients, aged 15–43 years. Seven experienced anaphylaxis only after eating certain foods (grape, crab, shrimp, abalone, squid, wheat) before exercise. In the remaining four, no specific food could be identified, but the act of eating itself predisposed to anaphylaxis — exercise without food intake within 30 min caused no adverse symptoms.*

Summary 58 Urticarias associated with rubbing the skin, pressure, sunlight, cold, heat, water, sweating or exercise are defined as physical urticarias. Hereditary angioedema is a rare autosomal dominantly inherited disorder where a reduction of C1-esterase inhibitor predisposes the patient to attacks of oedema of the skin, intestines and airway. Papular urticaria is the result of insect bites. Where vasculitis is a prominent feature of urticaria, the weals tend to cause purpura and are associated with an arthropathy. Urticaria and angioedema are common features of Henoch–Schönlein purpura. The lesions of urticaria pigmentosa contain melanin and mast cells, and rubbing the lesions in this rare condition causes wealing. Food intolerance is not a factor in any of the above forms of urticaria, except for food-dependent exercise-induced anaphylaxis. In this rare disorder, attacks of exercise-induced anaphylaxis occur only when exercise follows within a couple of hours of the ingestion of a specific food.

59 Contact urticaria
Irritant and allergic types

Contact urticaria

Contact urticaria is a weal and flare response provoked by the application of a wide range of compounds to the skin. The weal develops within minutes and is gone within hours (Cronin 1985). There are two types of contact urticaria, irritant contact urticaria, which is by far the more frequent, and allergic contact urticaria. Some agents are capable of producing both types of contact urticaria, for example certain insect bites. The bite may initially produce an irritant urticaria, but some individuals become sensitized, and subsequent exposure may produce an allergic urticaria (Fisher 1986).

Anatomical site

There is a range of skin permeability at different anatomical sites (Feldmann & Maibach 1967 and Table 59.1), and for this reason contact urticaria may only affect certain sites in individual subjects. For example, in one reported case urticarial reactions to 1% hydrocortisone cream which contained polysorbate 60 occurred when it was applied to the forehead but not when it was applied to the arm or back (Maibach & Conant 1977).

Irritant contact urticaria

Irritant contact urticaria affects most normal people and is elicited by a range of substances on their first (and subsequent) application to the skin. The reaction varies in severity from erythema to a weal (Cronin 1985). The reaction is localized, and, unlike allergic contact dermatitis, systemic effects do not occur (Cronin 1985).

Table 59.1 The skin penetration of hydrocortisone in humans at various sites[1]

Anatomical site	Penetration ratio
Forearm (ventral)	1.0
Forearm (dorsal)	1.1
Foot (sole)	0.14
Ankle (lateral)	0.42
Palm	0.83
Back	1.7
Scalp	3.5
Axilla	3.6
Forehead	6.0
Angle of jaw	13.0
Scrotum	42.0

[1] Source: Feldwann & Maibach (1967).

causes   Common causes of irritant contact urticaria are plants such as nettles (Emmelin & Feldberg 1947; Lahti 1986) or creatures such as jellyfish, moths and caterpillars (Cronin 1985). In all these cases the irritant substance is injected into the skin, but the result is nevertheless described as contact urticaria. This is not the contradiction it seems, for some kind of skin penetration is required for the contact urticaria to occur (see section above on skin permeability).

chemicals   Chemicals are a major cause of irritant contact urticaria, and this is important because the relevant chemicals are widely used in food, medicines and cosmetics (Cronin 1985). A good example of this condition occurred in a Danish nursery (Clemmensen & Hjorth 1982). Twenty children aged 1–4 years, after having 'a rather undisciplined lunch', decided to have fun and smeared a mayonnaise fruit salad around their mouths. Eighteen developed erythema around the mouth which lasted 30–60 min. The cause was identified by patch testing as 0.11% potassium sorbate and 0.11% sodium benzoate present as preservatives in the mayonnaise. The authors of this report posed the interesting question as to why the children did not complain of contact urticaria in the mouth. The answer was probably that, as the studies of allergic contact urticaria by Hannuksela and Lahti have shown, contact urticaria within the mouth often causes only minor itching and tingling, which may even be experienced as a pleasurable sensation by some people (Hannuksela & Lahti 1977).

common causes   Lahti in Finland tested a wide range of chemicals when applied to the skin of 110 adults. 5% benzoic acid produced a response in 88% of those tested, 5% cinnamic acid did so in 85% and 2.5% sorbic acid

Table 59.2 Chemicals which commonly cause irritant contact urticaria[1]

Trafuril (tetrahydrofurfuril ester of nicotinic acid)
Acetic acid
Ammonium persulphate
Balsam of Peru
Benzoic acid
Butyl alcohol
Butyric acid
Cinnamic acid
Cinnamic aldehyde
Dimethyl sulfoxide
Ethyl alcohol
Sodium benzoate
Sorbic acid

[1] Sources: Lahti (1980), Fisher (1986).

did so in 58% (Lahti 1980). Most of these reactions appeared within 45 min and disappeared within 2 hours. Atopic persons were no more liable to get irritant contact urticaria from these substances than non-atopic individuals. Other chemicals which commonly produced irritant contact urticaria are shown in Table 59.2. It is important to note that the incidence of contact dermatitis caused by chemicals depends on the concentration of the chemical, the base or solvent in which it is dissolved and applied to the skin, and the part of the body which is exposed to the agent. Thus in a study of irritant contact dermatitis from cinnamic aldehyde, it was found that this substance was more irritant in a base of 10% ethyl alcohol than in a base of petrolatum, and the number and strength of reactions was greater on the antecubital fossa than the forearm (Mathias *et al.* 1980).

specific causes   Dimethyl sulfoxide and Trafuril (the tetrahydrofurfuryl ester of nicotinic acid) are therapeutic agents that depend for their effect on producing erythema in most individuals. They do not produce allergic reactions. Benzoic acid, sorbic acid, cinnamic aldehyde and cinnamic acid can produce not only irritant contact urticaria, but also allergic contact urticaria and also contact dermatitis. Benzoic acid and sorbic acid are widely used antimicrobial agents. Their presence in dermatological preparations may cause stinging and worsening of eczema (Fisher 1986). Cinnamic aldehyde is a constituent of cinnamon and is one of the substances responsible for the typical odour and flavour of this spice. Its oxidation occurs readily on exposure to air, yielding cinnamic acid (Fisher 1986). Cinnamic aldehyde is used as a flavouring in soft drinks, chewing gum, ice cream, cakes, toothpaste and mouthwashes (Fisher 1986).

mechanism   The mechanism of irritant contact urticaria is uncertain, but it is thought to be partly due to a direct influence on vessel walls in the skin, and partly to the release of vasoactive mediators (Fisher 1986).

management   The usual test for irritant contact urticaria is the open application of a small amount of the test substance to the ventral aspect of the intact skin of the forearm. The result is recorded after 30–45 min (Fisher 1986). The management consists of identification and avoidance of the agent responsible.

Allergic contact urticaria   Allergic contact urticaria is generally thought to be attributable to a Gell and Coombs type I immediate hypersensitivity response (Cronin 1985; Chapel & Haeney 1988). It is important not to confuse this with contact dermatitis, which is a different disorder and which is thought to be due to a Gell and Coombs type IV delayed hypersensitivity response (Chapel & Haeney 1988). General features of allergic contact urticaria are:

1 a history of previous exposure to the cause without symptoms;

2 the degree of specific sensitization tends to increase with further exposure;

3 as a rule, a low proportion of exposed subjects are usually affected.

Allergic contact urticaria is potentially more serious than irritant contact urticaria, because the local urticarial weal may (rarely) be followed by generalized urticaria and anaphylaxis (Fisher 1986).

causes
Although it is known that certain *foods*, such as raw egg, cow's milk, raw potatoes, raw fish, apples and nuts are particularly common causes of allergic contact urticaria, it is probable that any food which contains protein can be a cause. Published reports mainly describe adults, particularly those with occupational allergic contact urticaria, occurring, or example, in food handlers (Fisher 1986). Occasionally sufficient protein is absorbed into the circulation to result in systemic symptoms; one such example is that of a 12-month old boy who developed severe bronchospasm and generalized urticaria after skin application to a napkin rash of an ointment which contained casein (Jarmoc & Primack 1987). The symptoms of food-induced allergic contact urticaria, in addition to erythema and urticarial weals, often include itching or tingling of the lips (Hannuksela & Lahti 1977). The tissues and secretions (especially saliva, dander, hair and urine) of hairy animals such as cats, dogs, horses, rabbits, guinea pigs, and mice are common causes of allergic contact urticaria in childhood. Chemicals can also cause allergic contact urticaria, and these include a number of drugs applied topically (see Tables 59.2 & 59.3), as well as a few vehicles contained in topical medicaments and miscellaneous other chemicals (Fisher 1986; Von Krogh *et al.* 1987). Finally, plants are a potential cause of allergic contact urticaria (Lahti 1986).

Table 59.3 Some topical medications which cause allergic contact urticaria[1]

Bacitracin
Benzocaine
Chloramphenicol
Chlorpromazine
Gentamycin
Menthol
Neomycin
Penicillin
Streptomycin
Vitamin E

[1] Source: Fisher (1986).

eczema

It is clear, though poorly documented (Von Krogh *et al.* 1987), that children with atopic eczema are unusually prone to allergic contact urticaria. This is one explanation for the high incidence of positive skin-prick tests to foods in children with eczema who are not sensitive to the foods when included in the diet. It is known that one of the factors influencing the incidence of positive diagnostic tests for allergic contact urticaria is whether the test is performed on normal unaffected skin, or on skin that is slightly involved or which has recently healed (Von Krogh *et al.* 1987). Although this may be irrelevant in some cases, there are others where tests on normal skin give a normal result, and a positive response can only be obtained by testing eczematous skin (Von Krogh *et al.* 1987). It is unclear whether the association between atopic eczema and allergic contact urticaria is due to the increased permeability of damaged epidermis or to immunological factors.

management

Testing for allergic contact urticaria requires either prick testing or the application of the raw food or test substance to the skin. If testing is negative on normal skin then it should be repeated on mildly affected skin. Skin testing on grossly eczematized skin is unhelpful, as a weal and flare response may be difficult to recognize or may not occur (Von Krogh *et al.* 1987). Patch testing seeks delayed responses and is therefore inappropriate. The management consists of identification and avoidance of the cause.

tolerance to food when ingested even though the same food causes allergic contact urticaria

The fact that a food causes allergic contact urticaria does not necessarily imply that it cannot be eaten safely by the same patient. There is no good systematic study of this, but the author's observations are consistent with published anecdotal reports. For example, there is a report of a woman who was able to consume kiwi fruit without adverse effects but who experienced urticaria on her hands, itching eyes, wheezing and shortness of breath when handling, peeling or slicing kiwi fruit (Fine 1981).

Contact dermatitis

Contact dermatitis and contact stomatitis are outside the scope of this book, and are well reviewed elsewhere (Cronin 1980; Fisher 1986, 1987).

Key references   59.1

FISHER AA (1986) *Contact Dermatitis*, 3rd edn, Lea & Febiger, Philadelphia. *Chapter 39, pp. 686–709 is a useful review of contact urticaria.*

59.2

LAHTI A (1980) Non-immunologic contact urticaria. *Acta Dermato-Venereol* **60**: 3–49 (suppl. 91). *A detailed, important and widely quoted investigation of a wide range of chemicals (see text above) when applied to the skin of 110 adults. Interpretation of the results is complicated by the heterogeneous nature of the subjects, who comprised 36 atopics (eczema 22, rhinitis 12, asthma two), 23* *with chronic idiopathic urticaria, 26 non-atopics (contact dermatitis, irritant or other forms of eczema) and 25 miscellaneous dermatological patients (mainly psoriasis).*

59.3   EMMELIN N & FELDBERG W (1947) The mechanism of the sting of the common nettle (*Urtica urens*). *J Physiol* **106**:440–455. The nettle hair consists of a fine capillary tube. The tube breaks when it comes into contact with the skin, and leaves exposed a fine needle-like end which penetrates the skin. Compression of the bladder-like base of the tube forces fluid down the tube and into the skin. The fluid contains histamine, which causes itching and urticaria, and acetylcholine, which, when accompanied by histamine, causes a burning sensation which precedes the itching.

Summary 59   Irritant contact urticaria affects most normal people, and is elicited by a range of substances on their first (and subsequent) application to the skin. Common causes are nettles, jellyfish or caterpillars, and a wide range of chemicals particularly some preservatives in foods, medicines and cosmetics. Unlike irritant contact urticaria, allergic contact urticaria affects only certain individuals and occurs only after prior exposure to the cause. Common causes are contact with foods, animals and a number of topical medications. Children with atopic eczema are especially prone to allergic contact urticaria.

60   Ordinary or idiopathic urticaria
Food or food additives can be triggers

Definition   The designation of ordinary or idiopathic urticaria includes all cases of acute and chronic urticaria that do not fall into any of the recognizable categories already described above. Ordinary urticaria is not a single entity, but represents the result of a variety of causes and mechanisms. In many cases no cause is found (e.g. 79% of 554 patients – see Champion *et al.* 1969), the proportion in published series (mainly in adults) depending upon the source of the patients and the interests and enthusiasm of the investigators.

'Recurrent urticaria is always a challenge to the dermatologist. Sometimes one can find a specific agent which causes the patient's urticaria but it is often time consuming and needs an observant patient and a doctor with a mind of Sherlock Holmes' (Juhlin 1981).

Chronic urticaria is less common in children than in adults, and in childhood, chronic urticaria is associated with atopy (Halpern 1965).

Bias in published studies

The provoking causes of urticaria will be considered below. It is important to note that figures given here for the incidence of specific items as a cause of urticaria are all based on patients who have attended hospital clinics, usually with severe urticaria that has lasted weeks or months, and the cause of which has been unclear. It is inappropriate and misleading to extrapolate these figures to the general population, as such studies inevitably exclude cases of shorter duration and those where a cause is easily identified without specialist help. This is particularly important in childhood, where a higher proportion of cases of acute urticaria are either caused by easily identified foods or are brief sequelae to acute infections.

Foods

acute urticaria in childhood

Foods are the most common cause of ordinary acute urticaria in childhood. Most cases never come to medical attention. A parent notices, for example, that whenever a child eats white fish his lips swell and he develops an urticarial rash. Fish is avoided, and the problem disappears. Occasional lapses of avoidance either demonstrate continued intolerance or, with time, loss of symptoms or enhanced symptoms. Cases which come to medical attention are mostly severe, atypical, or associated with other medical problems such as atopic eczema. The list of foods incriminated as possible causes is large (Champion & Muhlemann 1985). The common ones, egg, cow's milk, fish, nuts, tomatoes and fruit, are similar to those which cause allergic contact urticaria, the difference being that children are in general more likely to touch raw foods than to eat them, and raw foods are on the whole more likely to cause urticaria than cooked foods. As with allergic contact urticaria, it is probable that any food containing protein is capable of provoking urticaria. It is common (but not invariable – see chapter 59) for a food to cause in the same patient both ordinary urticaria when eaten and when touched allergic contact urticaria. Thus in one study of 52 mainly adult atopic subjects with urticaria caused by eating apples, 48 also reported itching and tingling of the lips and/or mouth with or without slight oedema of the lips or tongue (Hannuksela & Lahti 1977). Patients with urticaria caused by food may have other symptoms caused by food. In the study of 52 subjects with urticaria caused by apples referred to above, hoarseness or irritation of the throat (presumably due to oedema of the larynx and pharynx) was noted in five patients, abdominal pain was a feature in four patients, and rhinitis with conjunctivitis occurred in two patients.

chronic urticaria in childhood

Chronic urticaria in childhood is rarely caused by food intolerance, although there have been claims to the contrary. By taking a history and accepting parents reports about food reactions, Halpern claimed to identify one or more foods as a provoking cause in 25 of 75 (33%)

children with chronic urticaria (Halpern 1965). Harris and colleagues obtained a history of food-provoked attacks in 20 of 94 (21%) children with chronic urticaria, but were able to confirm this (it is unclear how this confirmation was sought) in only two of the 20 (Harris *et al.* 1983).

Yeast

Yeast or yeast-containing foods such as soft bread, cheese, vinegar and beer have been suggested as a potential cause of chronic urticaria in adults, mainly on the basis that a number of patients improve on a low-yeast diet (Holti 1967; James & Warin 1971; Juhlin 1985). The reasons why a low-yeast diet should be helpful are unclear, but such diets do involve the avoidance of a large number of foods which are potential causes for urticaria in their own right (Table 60.1). Nevertheless, challenges with brewer's yeast have been shown to provoke urticaria in 14% (Warin & Smith 1976) to 24% (James & Warin 1971) of adults with chronic urticaria. The ingestion of *Candida albicans* gives similar results (Warin & Smith 1976). It has been suggested that some adult patients with urticaria might benefit from oral nystatin (Holti 1967), but this is unconfirmed.

Food additives

Certain food additives, both synthetic and naturally occurring, can provoke urticaria and angioedema in both adults and children, although the supporting evidence is not as secure as many people believe. The incidence of food additive intolerance in chronic urticaria is far from clear, because most studies are seriously flawed. The major substances incriminated are azo dyes (tartrazine, new coccine, sunset yellow), benzoic acid and its derivatives, antioxidants (butylated hydroxyanisole (BHA), butylated hydroxytoluene

Table 60.1 Foods to be avoided in a low-yeast diet[1]

Bread – any kind except soda bread
Buns and tea-cakes
Bread puddings
Sausages
Bread sauce and stuffing
Breadcrumb coatings on fish or rissoles
Wines and beer
Grapes and sultanas
Cheese
Marmite
Bovril
Vinegar (including pickled food)
Tomato ketchup
Tinned foods containing yeast
Yeast tablets

[1] Source: Warin & Champion (1974).

(BHT)), sodium nitrite, annatto and canthaxanthine (Mikkelsen *et al.* 1978; Moneret-Vautrin *et al.* 1980; Juhlin 1985; Pollock 1992). Individual food additives are reviewed in greater detail in chapters 33 to 37.

Food additives: study design problems

The best known studies have been conducted by Juhlin and his colleagues in Sweden (Juhlin *et al.* 1972; Michaëlsson & Juhlin 1973; Michaëlsson *et al.* 1974; Ros *et al.* 1976; Juhlin 1981). In these studies, H1-receptor antagonists, salicylates and food colouring agents were withheld for 3–5 days. Then, in the studies which were placebo-controlled, the placebo was administered, followed by aspirin and then by an additive. Urticaria which occurred after withdrawal of H1-receptor antagonists tended to be ascribed to aspirin, the additive, or both. The reaction criteria were poorly defined – the challenge was said to be positive when the patient developed 'clear signs' (Juhlin 1981) within 24 hours. Juhlin noted that: 'judging whether a reaction is positive or negative is not always easy'.

If patients reacted to the lactose placebo they were re-tested with starch placebo, but 'several' patients had 'questionable' tests to both lactose and starch and further tests were then postponed until the patients was in a more 'stable phase' (Juhlin 1981). Questionable results to additive challenges led to re-testing. If the repeat test was positive, then the assumption was made that the original test was positive. Likewise, if the repeat test was negative, the first test was assumed to be negative. Despite this, in one series of 330 patients, one or more tests were 'uncertain' in 33% (Juhlin 1981).

importance of disease activity

A further problem with reported studies concerns the optimum time to perform challenges. Studies of aspirin intolerance in adults with chronic urticaria, employing objective measures for determining a positive reaction, indicated that while six of 10 patients with active urticaria were aspirin sensitive, only one of 15 patients with inactive urticaria were aspirin sensitive (Lumry *et al.* 1982), a phenomenon that was first described by Warin (Moore-Robinson & Warin 1967; James & Warin 1970). Similarly, Warin reported 12 adults with chronic urticaria who reacted to tartrazine only during an active phase or shortly afterwards, but not when the urticaria had been clear for 1–7 years (Warin & Smith 1982). Juhlin's studies were performed on patients with 'slight or no symptoms' (Juhlin 1981), so it is unclear whether they were in an active or inactive phase, both terms, incidentally, which lack any precise definition.

additive dose   The dose of additive employed for challenges is clearly important. In the studies of Juhlin described above (Michaëlsson & Juhlin 1973; Juhlin 1981), tartrazine was given in a dose of up to 10 mg, but in another multi-centre study only 0.22 mg was used, and a far smaller proportion of patients (three out of 38) were positive (Settipane *et al.* 1976).

need for blind challenges   The need for challenges to be blind is emphasized by a study comparing 'preservative 1' (500 mg benzoic acid) with 'preservative 2' (500 mg lactose) given double-blind in gelatin capsules to 29 adult patients with chronic urticaria (Lahti & Hannuksela 1981). Only two patients (7%) had 'objective' (i.e. visible) symptoms after benzoic acid, but four had objective symptoms after lactose.

Incidence of additive intolerance in adults with urticaria   Using the approach described above, Juhlin found that 31% of a series of 330 adults with chronic urticaria had a positive reaction to one or more food additives (Juhlin 1981). In another study, 52 patients (ages not stated but presumably mainly adults) with recurrent urticaria or angioedema were studied in hospital and compared with 33 healthy controls (Michaëlsson & Juhlin 1973). Thirty-nine out of the 52 patients tested had positive reactions to one or more additives. The additives which were reported to provoke urticaria were sodium benzoate (22 out of 37), benzoic acid (21 out of 37), tartrazine (19 out of 39), sunset yellow (10 out of 27), new coccine (nine out of 25), and amaranth (one out of seven). None of the patients reacted to patent blue V, which is a non-azo dye, or to sulphanilic acid, which is a metabolite of some azo dyes. Aspirin (see below) provoked urticaria in 35 out of the 39, and the placebo did not cause urticaria. None of the controls reacted to placebo or additives.

more recent data   In a more recent study of 49 adults with chronic urticaria, 24 had symptoms which appeared to remit on an additive-free diet (Murdoch *et al.* 1987). During double-blind challenges with capsules which contained various food additives, 15 of these 24 failed to react. Four reacted to aspirin (without having presented with a history of aspirin intolerance), two reacted to sodium benzoate, and only three reacted to challenge with a mixture of azo colours. Of these three, re-challenge with individual azo dyes confirmed reactions (to tartrazine, amaranth, sunset yellow and carmoisine) in two, but not in the third subject.

Incidence of additive intolerance in children with urticaria   A carefully performed double-blind placebo-controlled study of children with chronic urticaria, which avoided many of the pitfalls outlined above, was performed by Supramaniam and Warner (1986).

Twenty-four out of the 43 children with chronic urticaria of more than 2 months duration, and who were attending an allergy clinic (and who were therefore highly selected), developed urticarial lesions when challenged with artificial food additives. The highly selected nature of this sample explains the very high incidence of additive intolerance.

Dietary additive avoidance

One approach is to eliminate all additives from the diet and observe the effect. Although such studies have been performed, none were placebo-controlled or used blind challenges. In one study, which has been widely cited as evidence that food additives can provoke urticaria, 158 adults with chronic urticaria were allowed to eat only bread, rice, potato, cottage cheese and fresh meat for 5 days. If their condition improved they were allowed to eat normal food again, and if this was associated with a relapse they had a second period of restricted diet. No attempt was made to identify the food or additive responsible for the symptoms. Nevertheless, those 50 who improved on both periods of special diet and who relapsed on a normal diet were declared 'sensitive to food additives' (Rudzki *et al.* 1980). Gibson and Clancy placed patients (mainly adults) with chronic urticaria on a 2–4 week additive-free diet, but failed to study for comparison a control group of patients not treated with a diet (Gibson & Clancy 1980). They found that 54 of 76 patients came into 'remission' on the diet. These patients were then challenged with individual additives, though as with Juhlin's studies, the placebo was always given first.

Natural history of additive intolerance

The natural history of urticaria caused by artificial additives is unclear. In one small follow-up study, re-challenge with the relevant additive after 1 year failed to produce urticaria in one-quarter of the (mainly adult) patients (Gibson & Clancy 1980). In another small follow-up study, re-challenge 1–5 years after discovery of additive intolerance showed that three-quarters of the children were able to tolerate additives to which they had been previously intolerant (Pollock & Warner 1987). In the light of knowledge about aspirin as a trigger of urticaria (see below), it could be that such spontaneous loss of additive intolerance reflects a general improvement or disappearance of the urticarial state rather than the development of specific tolerance to additives in the presence of continued urticaria.

D-psicose

There is a single report in a 30-year old man of chronic urticaria induced by D-psicose (Nishioka *et al.* 1983). The mechanism was not identified, but both skin tests and oral challenge tests were positive in this patient. D-psicose is a constituent of high fructose syrup which is widely used to sweeten foods. D-psicose is easily generated by heating sugar, and is also found in caramel. It is also found in commercial mixtures of D-glucose and D-fructose obtained by hydrolysis of sucrose or isomerization of D-glucose (Nishioka *et al.* 1983).

Aspirin

Challenge studies have demonstrated aspirin as a trigger in between 20% (Moore-Robinson & Warin 1967) and 40% (Warin & Smith 1976) of adults with chronic urticaria. Patients with aspirin-sensitive urticaria have significantly higher resting plasma levels of histamine and prostaglandin F2α both of which fall after aspirin challenge (Asad *et al.* 1987). Dose dependence is apparent, and many patients do not respond to 300 mg but do so when the dose is increased to 600 mg or 1200 mg (Warin & Champion 1974). In one study of children with chronic urticaria, in which a small dose (100 mg) was used, aspirin provoked urticaria in only one out of 42 patients (Supramaniam & Warner 1986). It is not clear whether this is because a lower dose was used or because the incidence of aspirin as a provoking cause in childhood chronic urticaria is low. It has been stated that aspirin is more likely to provoke urticaria during minor febrile illnesses or during periods of stress or anxiety (Warin & Champion 1974). Urticarial reactions to aspirin usually begin 3–4 hours after ingestion, and although the weals may settle after a few hours, an increased tendency to wealing may last for up to 3 weeks (Warin & Champion 1974). Intolerance to salicylates is discussed in greater detail in chapter 38.

Penicillin

Urticaria is a common feature of penicillin allergy (Warin & Champion 1974). It is controversial whether minute quantities of penicillin present in food, for example in milk or meat, might cause or exacerbate urticaria (Warin & Champion 1974; Dewdney & Edwards 1984; Van Ketel & Boonk 1985).

Caffeine

There is a report of an adult with a history of acute urticaria following ingestion of coffee, tea, cola drinks and chocolate in whom double-blind placebo-controlled challenges with caffeine 25 mg demonstrated intolerance to caffeine (Gancedo *et al.* 1991). Pretreatment with terfenadine, an H1-receptor antagonist, prevented the reaction to caffeine.

Other drugs

A large number of drugs, particularly antibiotics, can cause urticaria (Warin & Champion 1974). The mechanism is often unknown. A number of drugs have a non-specific histamine-releasing effect, though often only in unusually high dosage (see Table 60.1 and Paton 1957).

Table 60.2 Some examples of drugs
with a histamine-releasing effect

Quinine
Codeine
Morphine
Pethidine
Curare derivatives
Atropine
Amphetamine

Inhalants

Pollens, mould spores, animal danders, house dust and other air-borne substances to which there is an allergy may provoke urticaria with or without associated asthma or rhinitis (Warin & Champion 1974). In one report from Detroit, of 26 cases of urticaria provoked by pollen, 12 only had urticaria during the pollen season; six being due to ragweed, four to grass pollens, one to both grass and ragweed pollen, and one to tree pollen (Waldbott & Merkle 1952). In the other 14, the urticaria started during each pollen season, but the symptoms continued after the pollen count had fallen.

osmylogenic urticaria

In some individuals minute quantities of allergens can provoke acute urticaria. Cases following inhalation of the fumes of food or cooking are well described, the phenomenon having been given the delightful name of osmylogenic urticaria (Rappaport & Hoffman 1941; Horesh 1943; Derbes & Krafchuk 1957). Osmyls are apparently minute particles given off by odoriferous substances (Derbes & Krafchuk 1957). Such events are not uncommon in children with food intolerance.

Viral infection

It is a general impression that in childhood it is common for acute urticaria to follow a brief pyrexial illness presumed to be due to a viral infection (Fineman & Ghory 1976; Voss et al. 1982; Kauppinen et al. 1984). Verification either of a cause and effect relationship, or indeed of a definite viral infection, is usually not sought. Hard evidence to support the impression of a viral cause for some cases of urticaria is not available, except for certain specific viral infections which are well recognized as causes of urticaria. Urticaria is recorded as one of several types of rash occasionally seen in hepatitis, mainly hepatitis B, occurring either in the prodromal or the icteric phase (Ljunggren & Moller 1971; Lockshaw & Hurley 1972). An uncontrolled study of 114 adults with chronic urticaria reported serological evidence of past infection with hepatitis B in 15 (17%) of patients, and a further two patients had hepatitis B antigenaemia (Vaida et al. 1983). The authors' claim of a causal association requires confirmation. Urticarial rashes and cold urticaria have been described in infectious mononucleosis (Africk & Halprin

1969; Cowdrey & Reynolds 1969; Tyson & Czarny 1981; Bonnetblanc *et al.* 1983; Wu *et al.* 1983), but maculopapular rashes are more typical.

Bacterial infection   In older reports, chronic urticaria was often considered to be due to foci of infection such as in the teeth, tonsils or sinuses, and improvement was reported to follow treatment of the infection or removal of the diseased part (Warin & Champion 1974). However, evidence for a causal relationship is lacking, and a study of the causes of chronic urticaria in 330 adults with chronic urticaria gave little support to the hypothesis (Juhlin 1981). In 10 of the 330 patients a 'possible dental focus' identified by 'poor dental status or a history of dental symptoms' was treated by dental extraction. The urticaria disappeared after a week in three. Recurrent infections of the urinary tract were found in six patients, and recurrent tonsillitis in three, and the effect of antibiotics was described as 'difficult to evaluate but not impressive'.

Fungal infection   Ringworm and other fungal infections have been mentioned as possible causes of urticaria, but evidence of a causal relationship is in general lacking (Weary & Guerrant 1967; Warin & Champion 1974; Champion & Muhlemann 1985). Of 100 adults with chronic urticaria in whom skin tests with a range of fungal organisms were carried out, 36 showed a positive response to *Candida albicans* and five patients had positive tests to other fungi (James & Warin 1971). As with other skin test results (see chapter 41), the significance of these positive results is unclear. The role of ingestion of yeasts is discussed above.

Sex hormones and stress   Exogenous or endogenous sex hormones can occasionally provoke urticaria (Warin *et al.* 1986; Basomba *et al.* 1987; Champion 1990), although this is unlikely to be a problem in childhood. In a study of 330 adults with chronic urticaria, 7% of patients felt that emotional stress provoked attacks of urticaria (Juhlin 1981). There are some interesting single case reports of stress-related urticaria in adults. One concerned a patient in whom urticaria occurred after he discovered he was the victim of a business fraud (Pistiner *et al.* 1979) and another occurred in a patient when he watched the English football team perform rather badly in the 1986 World Cup (Merry 1987)!

Management: principles   The management of idiopathic urticaria consists of attempting to identify an avoidable cause such as a food or a drug, and if this is not possible, treatment with an H1-receptor antagonist may be worth trying.

acute urticaria

The chances of finding a food trigger depend on the duration of the symptoms. Parents' histories are reliable in acute urticaria, where the first and all subsequent episodes may clearly (and often rather dramatically) follow the ingestion of a food such as egg or peanut. Such cases are often simple to deal with, so simple in fact that most parents avoid the food and the child never comes to medical attention. Occasional accidental ingestion demonstrates either continuing intolerance or the fact that the child has grown out of the problem.

chronic urticaria

It is much less easy to unravel chronic urticaria, of which a far smaller proportion of cases is provoked by a food or food additive. Such a link is usually not obvious to the observer, and parents come to consider the possibility of food intolerance in particular not through their own observations but rather through information or misinformation supplied by health professionals or the press. Some such parents (or adult sufferers) may come to believe so firmly in a link between the disease and food that the history they give about possible food triggers becomes unreliable.

investigations

If the history does not disclose a convincing precipitant in chronic urticaria, then skin-prick tests and RAST tests will not do so either. To perform a battery of skin-prick tests or RAST tests in the vague hope of finding an undetected positive result is unhelpful (Champion 1970), because of the low sensitivity and specificity of such tests in chronic urticaria. Individual tests are discussed further in chapters 41 and 43. In practice, if one wishes to look for a provoking food or food additive, then it is better to use an elimination diet (details below) for 14 days, followed by the re-introduction of single food items.

Management: additive avoidance

On the principal of trying the simplest approach first, an initial step is to employ a diet avoiding tartrazine and azo dyes, benzoic acid and benzoates, and the antioxidants BHA and BHT (for further details see chapter 75). The easiest approach is to use the diet to see if symptoms abate. If they do, then the diet is continued. The drawbacks to this simple approach are as follows.

1 Any improvement may have been spontaneous and nothing to do with the diet, or it may have been a placebo effect. In one series of 49 adults with chronic urticaria, 24 appeared to improve on an additive-free diet, but 15 of these 24 failed to react when challenged with a variety of food additives (Murdoch et al. 1987).

2 The patient may be on a needlessly restrictive diet, avoiding many more additives than necessary.

3 That failure of the diet may be misinterpreted as indicating that

Table 60.3 Additive challenge procedure in urticaria[1]

Day	Contents of capsule
First series of challenges	
1	Control (lactose)
2	Tartrazine 1 mg with lactose as filler
3	Control
4	Sodium benzoate 50 mg
5	Control
6	Benzoic acid 50 mg
7	Control
8	Brewer's yeast extract 600 mg
9	Control
10	Aspirin 100 mg
Second series of challenges	
1	Control
2	Tartrazine 50 mg
3	Control
4	Sodium benzoate 250 mg
5	Control
6	Benzoic acid 250 mg

[1] Adapted from: Warin & Smith (1976).

food additives are unimportant, when the diet has failed because other dietary causes have not been excluded.

To avoid these problems it is helpful, after the diet has been seen to be beneficial, to perform a battery of blind challenges, using opaque capsules which contain additives or lactose placebo (Warin & Smith 1976).

additive challenge   One procedure is outlined in Table 60.3. It is divided into two phases. The higher doses given in the second phase are only tried if the subjects did not react adversely to the lower doses used in the first phase. The parents need to keep a record of symptoms, and they need to be seen before proceeding to the second phase. If the child is too young to swallow capsules then one way to perform the challenges in a blind fashion is for the contents of the capsules to be dissolved in pure orange juice and administered by an independent observer such as a member of the nursing staff. The juice must be drunk through a straw, as drinks containing tartrazine leave a characteristic yellow stain around the mouth if taken from a cup (David 1986). Allowing parents to administer the capsules at home runs the small risk of interference, in that such capsules are easily taken apart and the contents inspected; certainly tartrazine would be easy to detect this way. In practice this does not seem to be a problem in children with urticaria, but it is a problem if the same procedure is used for children with behavioural symptoms, where a parent may be prepared to go to great lengths to convince others that the child has additive intolerance.

Management: food avoidance

If chronic urticaria persists despite elimination of additives, the condition remains sufficiently troublesome, and if a dietary cause cannot be identified from the history, it may be worthwhile as a last resort conducting a trial of an elimination diet. The choice of foods to be avoided and the duration of the therapeutic trial are empirical. The duration required partly depends upon the frequency of attacks. If the patient is having, for example, episodes of urticaria twice a week, then 2–3 weeks on a diet should be sufficient to establish whether the diet is going to be helpful or not. If the attacks are less frequent, then a longer period of diet will be required. Clearly if attacks are very infrequent it is likely to be easier to put up with the problem than try a prolonged elimination diet. An example of the type of elimination diet that can be used in this context is given in Table 60.3, but it must be said that dietary treatment of this type has never been validated by objective studies. If the urticaria disappears on the diet, then the next step is the re-introduction of single food items to see which, if any, cause exacerbation of the urticaria.

Management: antihistamines

H1-receptor antagonists may be of benefit in some cases of urticaria, but their failure to produce consistent suppression of urticaria is explained by the fact that histamine is only one of the mediators capable of producing the vascular changes seen in urticaria (Champion *et al.* 1985). Terfenadine, astemizole, cetirizine, loratadine and acrivastine are the preferred type of H1-receptor antagonists because of their low incidence of sedative side effects. (At the time of writing, only terfenadine and astemizole were licensed in the UK

Table 60.4 Example of food elimination diet which might be employed in the identification of foods causing urticaria, to be used in addition to the elimination of additives

Foods to be eliminated are
Cow's milk and cow's milk products (e.g. cheese)
Eggs
Pork
Fish and shellfish
Tomato
Celery
Carrot
Nuts
All fruit
All spices

for use in children under 12 years of age.) There is some evidence that the addition of an H2-receptor antagonist (e.g. ranitidine or cimetidine) may occasionally be helpful (Champion *et al.* 1985), and a trial of this combination is reasonable in a troublesome case. If antihistamines are thought to be helpful, it is sensible to discontinue treatment approximately every 6 months, to establish the need for continued therapy.

Management: nifedipine　A double-blind placebo-controlled crossover trial of nifedipine, a calcium channel antagonist, in 10 adults with chronic urticaria which was refractory to treatment, demonstrated significant therapeutic benefit when nifedipine was given in addition to existing antihistamine therapy (Bressler *et al.* 1989). Further data are needed before nifedipine can be recommended for use in urticaria.

Key references　60.1　CHAMPION RH & MUHLEMANN MF (1985) A list of the potential causes of urticaria. In Champion RH, Greaves MW, Kobza-Black A & Pye RJ (eds) *The Urticarias*, pp. 123–129, Churchill Livingstone, Edinburgh. *Provides a list of the potential causes of urticaria, and gives an approximate indication of those which are common and those which are rare.*

60.2　CHAMPION RH (1990) A practical approach to the urticarial syndromes – a dermatologist's view. *Clin Exper Allergy* **20**:221–224. *Lively, practical but adult-orientated review of the diagnosis and management of urticaria. The theme is that the aetiology of about 70% of cases which present to hospital is quite obscure.*

60.3　JUHLIN L (1985) Food additives in urticaria. In Champion RH, Greaves MW, Kobza-Black A & Pye RJ (eds) *The Urticarias*, pp. 105–112, Churchill Livingstone, Edinburgh. *Provides information on doses of additives to be used in challenge tests, a comparison of the results of challenge tests from a number of centres, and a comparison of the results of dietary treatment of urticaria from a number of centres.*

60.4　JAMES J & WARIN RP (1971) An assessment of the role of *Candida albicans* and food yeasts in chronic urticaria. *Br J Dermatol* **84**:227–237. Using an extract of *Candida albicans*, 100 consecutively seen patients with chronic urticaria were prick tested, and 36 were positive. This figure included 25 patients in whom the weal only appeared 4 hours after the test. Of the 36 patients with positive skin tests, 23 improved on a low-yeast diet and three improved on a combination of oral nystatin and amphotericin B. Of the 64 patients with negative prick tests, only two improved on a diet and one on anti-candida medication. Double-blind challenge tests using *Candida albicans* extract and yeast separately caused an exacerbation in 20 of 33 patients with a positive skin-prick test to *Candida* and four of 18 patients with a negative skin test. *Similar studies have not been performed in children with chronic urticaria.*

60.5　SIMON RA (1986) Adverse reactions to food additives. *New Engl Reg Allergy Proc* **7**:533–542. *Critical review of the evidence for adverse reactions to food additives.*

60.6   LEGRAIN V, TAÏEB A, SAGE T & MALEVILLE J (1990) Urticaria in infants: a study of forty patients. *Pediat Dermatol* **7**:101–107. Retrospective study of 40 infants aged 1–24 months with mainly acute urticaria. An underlying cause was identified or suspected in 65%; foods in 25% and drugs and infection in 37%. Under 6 months of age, 75% had cow's milk protein intolerance. Over 6 months, the main causes were drugs (mostly aspirin and antibiotics) and/or infections (presumed to be viral). 20% of patients were atopic.

60.7   FINEMAN S & GHORY JE (1976) The hospitalized child with urticaria. *J Asthma Res* **14**:27–32. Report of 40 children with urticaria (some were acute, others were chronic) who were admitted to hospital, sometimes because of fever or associated bronchospasm. Viral illness or upper respiratory infection was the most frequently incriminated cause, and was present in 18 cases (45%). *The highly selected nature of this sample is a drawback; children with urticaria are usually not admitted to hospital. For details of another hospitalized series of urticaria in childhood, see* Kauppinen K, Juntunen K & Lanki H (1984) Urticaria in children. Retrospective evaluation and follow-up. *Allergy* **39**:469–472.

60.8   MURDOCH RD, POLLOCK I, YOUNG E & LESSOF MH (1987) Food additive-induced urticaria: studies of mediator release during provocation tests. *J Roy Coll Phys Lond* **4**:262–266. Of 49 adults with chronic urticaria, 24 appeared to improve on an additive-free diet, but 15 of these 24 failed to react when challenged with a variety of food additives. Of the remaining nine, only three reacted to a mixture of azo colours. When re-challenged with individual azo colours, two subjects reacted to all four colours (tartrazine, sunset yellow, amaranth, carmoisine) and one failed to react to any. The reactions in the two subjects were accompanied by rises in the plasma and urinary histamine concentrations.

Summary 60   Ordinary or idiopathic urticaria includes all cases of acute and chronic urticaria which do not come into any of the other categories. In many cases no cause is found. Some known provoking causes are foods, food additives, aspirin, antibiotics and other drugs, inhalants, and viral, bacterial and fungal infections. The management consists of attempting to identify and then avoid the cause, or, if this is not possible, to try H1-receptor antagonists which are of uncertain efficacy.

References to Chapters 57–60

AFRICK JA & HALPRIN KM (1969) Infectious mononucleosis presenting as urticaria. *J Am Med Ass* **209**:1524–1525.

ANSELL BM (1970) Henoch–Schonlein purpura with particular reference to the prognosis of the renal lesion. *Br J Dermatol* **82**:211–215.

ASAD SI, MURDOCH R, YOULTEN LJF & LESSOF MH (1987) Plasma level of histamine in aspirin-sensitive urticaria. *Ann Allergy* **59**:219–222.

BASOMBA A, GUERRERO M, CAMPOS A, PELAZ A & VILLALMANZO IG (1987) Grave anaphylactic-like reaction in the course of menstruation. A case report. *Allergy* **42**:477–479.

BAYOUMI AHM & HIGHET AS (1986) Baking soda baths for aquagenic pruritus. *Lancet* **2**:464.

BENTLEY-PHILLIPS CB, KOBZA-BLACK A & GREAVES MW (1976) Induced tolerance in cold urticaria caused by cold-evoked histamine release. *Lancet* **2**:63–66.

BONNETBLANC JM, GUALDE N, GAILLARD J, BONNETBLANC F, PESTRE-ALEXANDRE M & MALINVAUD G (1983) Urticaire au froid révélatrice d'une mononucléose infectieuse. *Presse Méd* **12**:1174.

BREATHNACH SM, ALLEN R, MILFORD WARD A & GREAVES MW (1983) Symptomatic dermographism: natural history, clinical features, laboratory investigations and response to therapy. *Clin Exper Dermatol* **8**:463–476.

BRESSLER RB, SOWELL K & HUSTON DP (1989) Therapy of chronic idiopathic urticaria with nifedipine: demonstration of beneficial effect in a double-blinded, placebo-controlled, crossover trial. *J Allergy Clin Immunol* **83**:756–763.

BUCHBINDER EM, BLOCH KJ, MOSS J & GUINEY TE (1983) Food-dependent, exercise-induced anaphylaxis. *J Am Med Ass* **250**:2973–2974.

BURNS DA (1987) The investigation and management of arthropod bite reactions acquired in the home. *Clin Exper Dermatol* **12**:114–120.

CHAMPION RH (1970) Urticaria and angio-oedema. *Br J Hosp Med* **3**:233–238.

CHAMPION RH (1990) A practical approach to the urticarial syndromes – a dermatologist's view. *Clin Exper Allergy* **20**:221–224.

CHAMPION RH (1992) Urticaria. In Champion RH, Burton JL & Ebling FJG (eds) *Textbook of Dermatology*, vol. 3, 5th edn, pp. 1865–1880, Blackwell Scientific Publications, Oxford.

CHAMPION RH, GREAVES MW, KOBZA-BLACK A & PYE RJ (1985) (eds) *The Urticarias*, pp. 205–233, Churchill Livingstone, Edinburgh.

CHAMPION RH & MUHLEMANN MF (1985) A list of the potential causes of urticaria. In Champion RH, Greaves MW, Kobza-Black A & Pye RJ (eds) *The Urticarias*, pp. 123–129, Churchill Livingstone, Edinburgh.

CHAMPION RH, ROBERTS SOB, CARPENTER RG & ROGER JH (1969) Urticaria and angio-oedema. A review of 554 patients. *Br J Dermatol* **81**:588–597.

CHAPEL H & HAENEY M (1988) *Essentials of Clinical Immunology*, 2nd edn, Blackwell Scientific Publications, Oxford.

CLEMMENSEN O & HJORTH N (1982) Perioral contact urticaria from sorbic acid and benzoic acid in a salad dressing. *Contact Dermatitis* **8**:1–6.

COWDREY SC & REYNOLDS JS (1969) Acute urticaria in infectious mononucleosis. *Ann Allergy* **27**:182–187.

CROCE J (1980) Hypersensitivity to flea bites. In Oehling A, Mathov E, Glazer I & Arbesman C (eds) *Advances in Allergology and Clinical Immunology. Proceedings of the 10th International Congress of Allergology*, Jerusalem, November 1979, pp. 449–456, Pergamon Press, Oxford.

CRONIN E (1980) *Contact Dermatitis*, Churchill Livingstone, Edinburgh.

CRONIN E (1985) Contact urticaria. In Champion RH, Greaves MW, Korza-Black A & Pye RJ (eds) *The Urticarias*, pp. 118–122, Churchill Livingstone, Edinburgh.

DAVID TJ (1986) Reactions to dietary tartrazine. *Arch Dis Child* **62**:119–122.

DERBES VJ & KRAFCHUK JD (1957) Osmylogenic urticaria. *Arch Dermatol* **76**:103–104.

DEWDNEY JM & EDWARDS RG (1984) Penicillin hypersensitivity – is milk a significant hazard?: a review. *J Roy Soc Med* **77**:866–877.

DOEGLAS HMG, RIJNTEN WJ, SCHRODER FP & SCHIRM J (1986) Cold urticaria and virus infections: a clinical and serological study in 39 patients. *Br J Dermatol* **114**:311–318.

DOHI M, SUKO M, SUGIYAMA H *et al.* (1991) Food-dependent, exercise-induced anaphylaxis: a study on 11 Japanese cases. *J Allergy Clin Immunol* **87**:34–40.

DOVER JS, KOBZA-BLACK A, WARD AM & GREAVES MW (1988) Delayed pressure urticaria. Clinical features, laboratory investigations, and response to therapy of 44 patients. *J Am Acad Dermatol* **18**:1289–1298.

DUSCHET P, LEYEN P, SCHWARZ T, HOCKER P, GREITER J & GSCHNAIT F (1987) Solar urticaria – effective treatment by plasmapheresis. *Clin Exp Dermatol* **12**:185–188.

EMMELIN N & FELDBERG W (1947) The mechanism of the sting of the common nettle (*Urtica urens*). *J Physiol* **106**:440–455.

FELDMANN RJ & MAIBACH HI (1967) Regional variation in percutaneous penetration of ^{14}C cortisol in man. *J Investig Dermatol* **48**:181–183.

FINE AJ (1981) Hypersensitivity reaction to kiwi fruit (Chinese gooseberry, *Actinidia chinensis*). *J Allergy Clin Immunol* **68**:235–237.

FINEMAN S & GHORY JE (1976) The hospitalized child with urticaria. *J Asthma Res* **14**:27–32.

FISHER AA (1986) *Contact Dermatitis*, 3rd edn, Lea & Febiger, Philadelphia.

FISHER AA (1987) Contact stomatitis. *Dermatol Clin* **5**:709–717.

GANCEDO SQ, FREIRE P, FERNÁNDEZ RIVAS M, DÁVILA I & LOSADA E (1991) Urticaria from caffeine. *J Allergy Clin Immunol* **88**:680–681.

GIBSON A & CLANCY R (1980) Management of chronic idiopathic urticaria by the identification and exclusion of dietary factors. *Clin Allergy* **10**:699–704.

GREAVES MW (1985) Mast cells, histamine and histamine release. In Champion RH, Greaves MW, Kobza-Black A & Pye RJ (eds) *The Urticarias*, pp. 3–11, Churchill Livingstone, Edinburgh.

GREAVES MW (1992) Mastocytoses. In Champion RH, Burton JL & Ebling FJG (eds) *Textbook of Dermatology*, vol. 3, 5th edn, pp. 2065–2072, Blackwell Scientific Publications, Oxford.

GREAVES MW, BLACK AK, EADY RAJ & COUTTS A (1981) Aquagenic pruritus. *Br Med J* **282**:2008–2010.

HALPERN SR (1965) Chronic hives in children: an analysis of 75 cases. *Ann Allergy* **23**:589–599.

HANNUKSELA M & LAHTI A (1977) Immediate reactions to fruits and vegetables. *Contact Dermatitis* **3**:79–84.

HARRIS A, TWAROG FJ & GEHA RS (1983) Chronic urticaria in childhood: natural course and etiology. *Ann Allergy* **51**:161–165.

HOLTI G (1967) Management of pruritus and urticaria. *Br Med J* **1**:155–158.

HORESH AJ (1943) Allergy to food odors. Its relation to the management of infantile eczema. *J Allergy* **14**:335–339.

JAMES J & WARIN RP (1969) Factitious wealing at the site of previous cutaneous response. *Br J Dermatol* **81**:882–884.

JAMES J & WARIN RP (1970) Chronic urticaria: the effect of aspirin. *Br J Dermatol* **82**:204–205.

JAMES J & WARIN RP (1971) An assessment of the role of *Candida albicans* and food yeasts in chronic urticaria. *Br J Dermatol* **84**:227–237.

JARMAC LM & PRIMACK WA (1987) Anaphylaxis to cutaneous exposure to milk protein in a diaper rash ointment. *Clin Pediat* **26**:154–155.

JUHLIN L (1981) Recurrent urticaria: clinical investigation of 330 patients. *Br J Dermatol* **104**:369–381.

JUHLIN L (1985) Food additives in urticaria. In Champion RH, Greaves MW, Kobza-Black A & Pye RJ (eds), *The Urticarias*, pp. 105–112, Churchill

Livingstone, Edinburgh.

JUHLIN L, MICHAËLSSON G & ZETTERSTROM O (1972) Urticaria and asthma induced by food-and-drug additives in patients with aspirin hypersensitivity. *J Allergy Clin Immunol* **50**:92–98.

KAPLAN AP, NATBONY SF, TAWIL AP, FRUCHTER L & FOSTER M (1981) Exercise-induced anaphylaxis as a manifestation of cholinergic urticaria. *J Allergy Clin Immunol* **68**:319–324.

KAUPPINEN K, JUNTUNEN K & LANKI H (1984) Urticaria in children. Retrospective evaluation and follow-up. *Allergy* **39**:469–472.

KAUR S, GREAVES MW & EFTEKHARI N (1981) Factitious urticaria (dermographism): treatment by cimetidine and chlorpheniramine in a randomised double-blind study. *Br J Dermatol* **104**:185–189.

KEAHEY TM, INDRISANO J & KALINER MA (1988) A case study on the induction of clinical tolerance in cold urticaria. *J Allergy Clin Immunol* **82**:256–261.

KIDD JM, COHEN SH, SOSMAN AJ & FINK JN (1983) Food-dependent exercise-induced anaphylaxis. *J Allergy Clin Immunol* **71**:407–411.

KIRBY JD, MATTHEWS CNA, JAMES J, DUNCAN EHL & WARIN RP (1971) The incidence and other aspects of factitious wealing (dermographism). *Br J Dermatol* **85**:331–335.

KIVITY S, SCHWARTZ Y, WOLF R & TOPILSKY M (1990) Systemic cold-induced urticaria – clinical and laboratory characterization. *J Allergy Clin Immunol* **85**:52–54.

KIVITY S, SNEH E, GREIF J, TOPILSKY M & MEKORI YA (1988) The effect of food and exercise on the skin response to compound 48/80 in patients with food-associated exercise-induced urticaria-angioedema. *J Allergy Clin Immunol* **81**:1155–1158.

KOBZA-BLACK A (1985) The physical urticarias. In Champion RH, Greaves MW, Kobza-Black A & Pye RJ (eds) *The Urticarias*, pp. 168–190, Churchill Livingstone, Edinburgh.

KUSHIMOTO H & AOKI T (1985) Masked type 1 wheat allergy. Relation to exercise-induced anaphylaxis. *Arch Dermatol* **121**:355–360.

LACHMANN PJ (1985) Hereditary angio-oedema. In Champion RH, Greaves MW, Kobza-Black A & Pye RJ (eds) *The Urticarias*, pp. 194–201, Churchill Livingstone, Edinburgh.

LAHTI A (1980) Non-immunologic contact urticaria. *Acta Dermato-venerol* **60** (suppl. 91):3–49.

LAHTI A (1986) Contact urticaria to plants. *Clin Dermatol* **4**:127–136.

LAHTI A & HANNUKSELA M (1981) Is benzoic acid really harmful in cases of atopy and urticaria? *Lancet* **2**:1055.

LAWLOR F, KOBZA-BLACK A, WARD AM, MORRIS R & GREAVES MW (1989) Delayed pressure urticaria, objective evaluation of a variable disease using a dermographometer and assessment of treatment using colchicine. *Br J Dermatol* **120**:403–408.

LEENUTAPHONG V, HÖLZLE E & PLEWIG G (1990) Solar urticaria: studies on mechanisms of tolerance. *Br J Dermatol* **122**:601–606.

LEIGH IM & RAMSAY CA (1975) Localized heat urticaria treated by inducing tolerance to heat. *Br J Dermatol* **92**:191–194.

LEWIS J, LIEBERMAN P, TREADWELL G & ERFFMEYER J (1981) Exercise-induced urticaria, angioedema, and anaphylactoid episodes. *J Allergy Clin Immunol* **68**:432–437.

LJUNGGREN B & MOLLER H (1971) Hepatitis presenting as transient urticaria. *Acta Dermatovener* **51**:295–297.

LOCKSHIN NA & HURLEY H (1972) Urticaria as a sign of viral hepatitis. *Arch*

Dermatol **105**:570–571.

LUMRY WR, MATHISON DA, STEVENSON DD & CURD JC (1982) Aspirin in chronic urticaria and/or angioedema: studies of sensitivity and desensitisation. *J Allergy Clin Immunol* **69**(suppl.):135.

MAIBACH H & CONANT M (1977) Contact urticaria to a corticosteroid cream: polysorbate 60. *Contact Dermatitis* **3**:350–351.

MATHIAS CGT, CHAPPLER RR & MAIBACH HI (1980) Contact urticaria from cinnamic aldehyde. *Arch Dermatol* **116**:74–76.

MAULITZ RM, PRATT DS & SCHOCKET AL (1979) Exercise-induced anaphylactic reaction to shellfish. *J Allergy Clin Immunol* **63**:433–434.

MCNEIL D & STRAUSS RH (1988) Exercise-induced anaphylaxis related to food intake. *Ann Allergy* **61**:440–442.

MERRY P (1987) World Cup urticaria. *J Roy Soc Med* **80**:779.

MICHAËLSSON G & JUHLIN L (1973) Urticaria induced by preservatives and dye additives in food and drugs. *Br J Dermatol* **88**:525–532.

MICHAËLSSON G, PATTERSSON L & JUHLIN L (1974) Purpura caused by food and drug additives. *Arch Dermatol* **109**:49–52.

MIKKELSEN H, LARSEN JC & TARDING F (1978) Hypersensitivity reactions to food colours with special reference to the natural colour annatto extract (butter colour). *Arch Toxicol* **1**(suppl.):141–143.

MONERET-VAUTRIN DA, EINHORN C & TISSERAND J (1980) Le role du nitrite de sodium dans les urticaires histaminiques d'origine alimentaire. *Ann Nutr Alim* **34**:1125–1132.

MOORE-ROBINSON M & WARIN RP (1967) Effect of salicylates in urticaria. *Br Med J* **4**:262–264.

MORRISON RCA & RABSON AR (1987) The late onset form of C1 esterase-inhibitor deficiency presenting as food allergy. *J Allergy Clin Immunol* **79**:336–339.

MURDOCH RD, POLLOCK I, YOUNG E & LESSOF MH (1987) Food additive-induced urticaria: studies of mediator release during provocation tests. *J Roy Coll Phys Lond* **4**:262–266.

MURPHY GM, ZOLLMAN PE, GREAVES MW & WINKELMANN RK (1987) Symptomtic dermographism (factitious urticaria) – passive transfer experiments from human to monkey. *Br J Dermatol* **116**:801–804.

NEITTAANMAKI H (1985) Cold urticaria. Clinical findings in 220 patients. *J Am Acad Dermatol* **13**:636–644.

NISHIOKA K, KATAYAMA I & SANO S (1983) Urticaria induced by D-psicose. *Lancet* **2**:1417–1418.

NOVEY HS, FAIRSHTER RD, SALNESS K, SIMON RA & CURD JG (1983) Postprandial exercise-induced anaphylaxis. *J Allergy Clin Immunol* **71**:498–504.

PATON WDM (1957) Histamine release by compounds of simple chemical structure. *Pharmacol Rev* **9**:269–328.

PISTINER M, PITLIK S & ROSENFELD J (1979) Psychogenic urticaria. *Lancet* **2**:1383.

POLLOCK I (1992) Food additives. In David TJ (ed) *Recent Advances in Paediatrics*, No. 10, pp. 129–144, Churchill Livingstone, Edinburgh.

POLLOCK I & WARNER JO (1987) A follow-up study of childhood food additive intolerance. *J Roy Coll Phys Lond* **21**:248–250.

RAPPAPORT BZ & HOFFMAN MM (1941) Urticaria due to aliphatic aldehydes. *J Am Med Ass* **116**:2656–2659.

ROOK A (1986) Skin diseases caused by arthropods and other venomous or noxious animals. In Rook A, Wilkinson DS, Ebling FJG, Champion RH & Burton

JL (eds) *Textbook of Dermatology*, vol. 2, 4th edn, pp. 1031–1080, Blackwell Scientific Publications, Oxford.

ROS A-M, JUHLIN L & MICHAËLSSON G (1976) A follow-up study of patients with recurrent urticaria and hypersensitivity to aspirin, benzoates and azo dyes. *Br J Dermatol* **95**:19–24.

RUDZKI E, CZUBALSKI K & GRZYWA Z (1980) Detection of urticaria with food additives intolerance by means of diet. *Dermatologica* **161**:57–62.

RYAN TJ, SHIM-YOUNG N & TURK JL (1968) Delayed pressure urticaria. *Br J Dermatol* **80**:485–490.

SELDIN DC & AUSTEN KF (1985) Mast cell heterogeneity – the T-cell factor-dependent mast cell in vitro and in vivo. In Champion RH, Greaves MW, Kobza-Black A & Pye RJ (eds) *The Urticarias*, pp. 12–25, Churchill Livingstone, Edinburgh.

SETTIPANE GA, CHAFEE FH, POSTMAN IM *et al.* (1976) Significance of tartrazine sensitivity in chronic urticaria of unknown etiology. *J Allergy Clin Immunol* **57**:541–546.

SHEFFER AL, SOTER NA, McFADDEN ER & AUSTEN KF (1983) Exercise-induced anaphylaxis: a distinct form of physical allergy. *J Allergy Clin Immunol* **71**:311–316.

SIBBALD RG, KOBZA-BLACK A, EADY RAJ, JAMES M & GREAVES MW (1981) Aquagenic urticaria: evidence of cholinergic and histaminergic basis. *Br J Dermatol* **105**:297–302.

SILVERSTEIN SR, FROMMER DA, DOBOZIN B & ROSEN P (1986) Celery-dependent exercise-induced anaphylaxis. *J Emergency Med* **4**:195–199.

SONGSIRIDEJ V & BUSSE WW (1983) Exercise-induced anaphylaxis. *Clin Allergy* **13**:317–321.

SOTER NA (1985) Urticarial vasculitis. In Champion RH, Greaves MW, Kobza-Black A & Pye RJ (eds) *The Urticarias*, pp. 141–148, Churchill Livingstone, Edinburgh.

STEINMAN H & GREAVES MW (1985) Aquagenic pruritus: an analysis of 36 patients. *J Am Acad Dermatol* **13**:91–96.

SUPRAMANIAM G & WARNER JO (1986) Artificial food additive intolerance in patients with angio-oedema and urticaria. *Lancet* **2**:907–909.

TYSON CJ & CZARNY D (1981) Cold-induced urticaria in infectious mononucleosis. *Med J Aust* **1**:33–35.

VAIDA GA, GOLDMAN MA & BLOCH KJ (1983) Testing for hepatitis B virus in patients with chronic urticaria and angioedema. *J Allergy Clin Immunol* **72**:193–198.

VAN KETEL WG & BOONK WJ (1985) The role of penicillin in chronic urticaria. In Champion RH, Greaves MW, Kobza-Black A & Pye RJ (eds) *The Urticarias*, pp. 113–117, Churchill Livingstone, Edinburgh.

VON KROGH G & MAIBACH HI (1987) The contact urticaria syndrome. In Marzulli FN & Maibach HI (eds) *Dermatotoxicology*, 3rd edn, pp. 341–362, Hemisphere Publishing Corporation, Washington.

VOSS MJ, O'CONNELL EJ, HICK JF & SMITH TF (1982) Association of acute urticaria in children with respiratory tract infections (abstract). *J Allergy Clin Immunol* **69**:134.

WALDBOTT GL & MERKLE K (1952) Urticaria due to pollen. *Ann Allergy* **10**:30–35.

WARIN RP (1983) Urticarial vasculitis. *Br Med J* **286**:1919–1920.

WARIN RP & CHAMPION RH (1974) *Urticaria*, Saunders, London.

WARIN RP, CUNLIFFE WJ, GREAVES MW & WALLINGTON TB (1986) Recurrent angioedema: familial and oestrogen induced. *Br J Dermatol* **115**:731–734.

WARIN RP & SMITH RJ (1976) Challenge test battery in chronic urticaria. *Br J Dermatol* **94**:401–406.

WARIN RP & SMITH RJ (1982) Role of tartrazine in chronic urticaria. *Br Med J* **284**:1443–1444.

WEARY PE & GUERRANT JL (1967) Chronic urticaria in association with dermatophytosis. *Arch Dermatol* **95**:400–401.

WINKELMANN RK (1987) Food sensitivity and urticaria or vasculitis. In Brostoff J & Challacombe SJ (eds) *Food Allergy and Intolerance*, pp. 602–617, Baillière Tindall, London.

WONG E, EFTEKHARI N, GREAVES MW & WARD AM (1987) Beneficial effects of danazol on symptoms and laboratory changes in cholinergic urticaria. *Br J Dermatol* **116**:553–556.

WONG RC, FAIRLEY JA & ELLIS CN (1984) Dermographism: a review. *J Am Acad Derm* **11**:643–652.

WU LYF, MESKO JW & PETERSON BH (1983) Cold urticaria associated with infectious mononucleosis. *Ann Allergy* **50**:271–274.

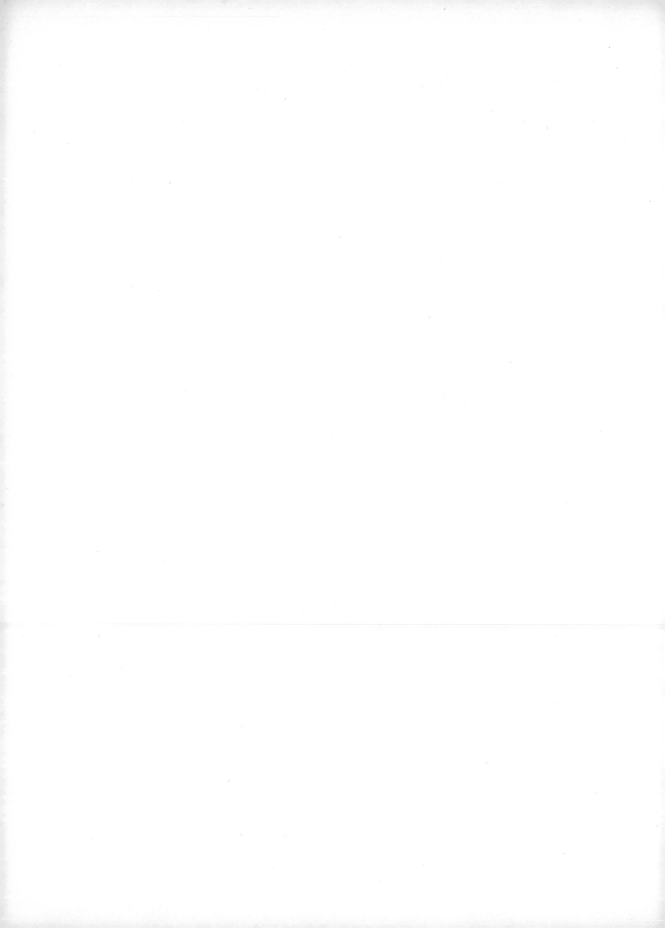

Part 14 Gastrointestinal Disorders

61 Mouth, oesophagus, stomach and small intestine
Common target organs for food intolerance

Aphthous ulcers
There are a number of uncontrolled reports suggesting that food intolerance may cause recurrent oral aphthous ulceration or stomatitis (Finn & Cohen 1978; Wray 1981; Wright *et al.* 1986). However, a single-blind controlled study of 105 dental students who suffered from recurrent aphthous ulceration, of whom a number had identified food triggers, and 113 control students, failed to confirm oral ulceration when food challenges were performed (Eversole *et al.* 1982). Jejunal biopsies were performed in 33 patients with recurrent oral aphthous ulcers who had been referred to either a dental (25 patients) or a gastroenterology department (eight patients), and eight (aged 12–25 years) had histological changes consistent with coeliac disease (Ferguson *et al.* 1975). The aphthous ulcers resolved in the eight patients when they were treated with a gluten-free diet, but unfortunately the group without coeliac disease were not followed up. The patients who were referred to the gastroenterology department presumably had symptoms pointing to an underlying gastrointestinal disorder; what the study does not tell us is what proportion of those who simply presented with oral ulcers had coeliac disease. Subsequent studies have suggested a much lower incidence of coeliac disease of 2–4% in adults with recurrent aphthous ulceration (Cooke *et al.* 1977; Lehner 1977; Ferguson *et al.* 1980). In reviewing the oral manifestations of food intolerance, Challacombe (1987) pointed out that the prevalence of recurrent oral ulceration (including herpetiform ulcers) is in the order of 10% of the population, and concluded that food intolerance is not the cause in most cases. It is worth remembering that recurrent oral ulceration is a mode of presentation in Crohn's disease.

management
Troublesome recurrent oral aphthous ulceration should raise a suspicion of coeliac disease (or possibly Crohn's disease). The presence of other features (e.g. chronic loose stools) would suggest the need for investigation. Apart from this, there is no objective evidence to support a causal association between food intolerance and recurrent oral aphthous ulceration, and there is therefore no basis for a therapeutic trial of an elimination diet.

379

Oral allergy syndrome

Some patients with food intolerance old enough to do so report oral symptoms, usually occurring immediately after ingestion of a trigger food. The symptoms are often poorly defined, such as irritation in the mouth or tightness in the lip or throat. Blebs may be present in the oral mucosa, and the above features may or may not be followed by others such as urticaria, conjunctivitis, asthma or anaphylaxis. The condition has been given the name oral allergy syndrome, and there is a strong association between positive skin-prick test results and the foods reported to provoke symptoms (Amlot *et al.* 1987; Ortolani *et al.* 1988). In practice, these oral symptoms may act as a useful warning of an impending severe reaction, and in those with a history of life-threatening anaphylactic reactions this warning may facilitate the prompt administration of adrenaline. The management is avoidance of the food trigger, although in cases where the reactions are mild treatment with astemizole may reduce the symptoms (Bindslev-Jensen *et al.* 1991).

sulphite intolerance

In a study of sulphite intolerance in children with asthma, it was noted that in all those who reacted the first symptom, which commenced within 1–2 min of sulphite ingestion, was a burning sensation in the throat (Towns & Mellis 1984).

Auriculotemporal syndrome

The auriculotemporal syndrome comprises gustatory flushing and sweating, and was originally classified (Weidman *et al.* 1969) as occurring:

1 after the ingestion of spicy foods;

2 in central nervous system disorders such as encephalitis;

3 secondary to disease of, or trauma to, the parotid gland (Glaister *et al.* 1958) e.g. forceps delivery;

4 secondary to sympathetic nerve section (Harper & Spielvogel 1986).

Subsequently it was appreciated that gustatory flushing and sweating probably occur in response to any stimulus which normally causes salivation in such individuals (Beck *et al.* 1989). Because it follows the consumption of food, it is understandable that parents should suspect food intolerance as a cause of the facial 'rash', but the symptom is non-specific and is not regarded as a form of food intolerance (Davis & Strunk 1981). Atropine is reported to be ineffective (Beck *et al.* 1989), in contrast to gustatory rhinitis (see chapter 61) in which facial flushing and sweating may also occur.

Gastro-oesophageal reflux

Sixty-six adults with gastro-oesophageal reflux were studied by Price *et al.* (1978). Those in whom acid infusion provoked symptoms were significantly more likely to also be sensitive to infusions of coffee, orange juice or a spicy drink (Tabasco Bloody Mary mix), even when these solutions were adjusted to a pH of 7. The mechanism of pain associated with ingestion of these foods was unrelated to temperature, acidity, or effect on the lower oesophageal sphincter.

Eosinophilic gastroenteritis Eosinophilic gastroenteritis is a disorder in which infiltration of the oesophagus, stomach and small intestine by eosinophils is accompanied by protein-losing enteropathy, peripheral eosinophilia, and iron-deficiency anaemia secondary to gastrointestinal blood loss (Katz *et al.* 1977; Min 1991). The condition is rare, especially in children, but has been documented in both infancy and childhood. The eosinophilic infiltration may be very patchy (Leinbach & Rubin 1970) and affect the mucosal layer, the muscularis layer, or the serosal layer (Klein *et al.* 1970; Trounce & Tanner 1985).

mucosal involvement Mucosal involvement is associated with vomiting, diarrhoea and blood loss, with resultant anaemia, malabsorption, protein-losing enteropathy and failure to thrive.

muscularis involvement Infiltration of the muscularis layer results in thickening of the gut wall and is associated with obstruction.

serosal involvement Infiltration of the serosa is associated with an exudative ascites, the ascitic fluid being rich in eosinophils and protein.

food intolerance The relationship of eosinophilic gastroenteritis to food intolerance is unclear. In some cases there is no response to an elimination diet, even though the patient may have been noted previously to have an anaphylactic reaction to certain foods (Caldwell *et al.* 1978; Katz *et al.* 1984; Keshavarzian *et al.* 1985). In others the disorder does respond to elimination of certain foods, most notably cow's milk protein (Waldmann *et al.* 1967; Trounce & Tanner 1985; El Mouzan *et al.* 1990; Vandenplas *et al.* 1990). Oral sodium cromoglycate was reported to be unhelpful in two siblings with eosinophilic gastroenteritis (Keshavarzian *et al.* 1985), but control can usually be achieved if necessary with systemic steroids.

Pyloric stenosis There is a quite well documented report of two infants, aged 6 and 35 days, in whom pyloric stenosis was attributed to cow's milk protein intolerance (Davanzo *et al.* 1987). The latter was suspected because of a circulating eosinophilia. In both cases the diagnosis was supported by contrast radiography, and in both the symptoms abated without the need for surgery when cow's milk protein was withdrawn from the diet. In addition, I am aware of a similar but unpublished anecdotal report (Miller, 1990). In the author's opinion, it is important not to over-value such reports, because of the most unappealing prospect of large numbers of infants with pyloric stenosis being detained unnecessarily in hospital with continued symptoms, simple and safe surgery having been deferred for what is likely to be a fruitless trial of cow's milk protein avoidance. The food intolerance enthusiast would doubtless reply, understandably enough, that needless surgery is an equally unattractive prospect. Whilst it is true that there are reports of patients with pyloric stenosis in whom symptoms failed to abate after surgery, and only improved after cow's milk protein avoidance (such cases have been reported, for example, by Clein 1954 and Minford *et al.* 1982), there is no evidence that the two conditions co-exist more commonly than one would expect by chance alone. The conclusion is that at present one cannot exclude the possibility that cow's milk protein intolerance may play a part in the aetiology of infantile pyloric stenosis in a small number of cases, but the supportive evidence of such an association is at best scanty.

Key references 61.1 CHALLACOMBE SJ (1987) Oral manifestations of food allergy and intolerance. In Brostoff J & Challacombe SJ (eds) *Food Allergy and Intolerance*, pp. 511–520, Baillière Tindall, London. *Review of possible relationship between oral ulceration and food intolerance.*

61.2 AMLOT PL, KEMENY DM, ZACHARY C, PARKES P & LESSOF MH (1987) Oral allergy syndrome (OAS): symptoms of IgE-mediated hypersensitivity to foods. *Clin Allergy* **17**:33–42. Of a highly selected group of 80 highly atopic patients, 31 reported immediate onset symptoms after ingesting a trigger food, at first confined to the mouth and throat. In a proportion of these patients, further symptoms such as urticaria, asthma or anaphylaxis developed. There was a strong association with positive skin-prick tests.

61.3 STEFFEN RM, WYLLIE R, PETRAS RE *et al.* (1991) The spectrum of eosinophilic gastroenteritis. Report of six pediatric cases and review of the literature. *Clin Pediat* **30**:404–411. *Detailed case reports (all six patients required treatment with prednisolone) and review of literature.*

Summary 61 There is no objective evidence to support claims that food intolerance causes recurrent oral aphthous ulceration, with the exception of the observation that a very small proportion of patients (*circa* 2%) with severe recurrent oral aphthous ulceration have coeliac disease. In these patients, the ulceration responds to a gluten-free diet. Irritation in the mouth, tightness in the lip or throat, and blebs in the oral mucosa, sometimes called the oral allergy syndrome, are recognized features of food intolerance and occur immediately after ingestion of a trigger food, sometimes to be followed by other symptoms. The auriculotemporal syndrome comprises gustatory flushing and sweating, which probably occur in response to any stimulus which normally causes salivation. Eosinophilic gastroenteritis is a rare disorder in which infiltration of the oesophagus, stomach and small intestine by eosinophils is accompanied by protein-losing enteropathy, peripheral eosinophilia, and gastrointestinal blood loss; some cases in childhood may be related to food intolerance, but others are not.

62   Colon and rectum
Less commonly affected in food intolerance

Enteropathy   Abnormalities of the small intestinal mucosa can occur in children with gastrointestinal features (e.g. loose stools, failure to thrive) of food intolerance. The histological changes are usually not as severe as that seen in coeliac disease, although a flat mucosa may occasionally be seen (Walker-Smith 1988). The most common food trigger is cow's milk protein, and enteropathy as a feature of cow's milk protein intolerance is discussed in chapter 8. Other recognized triggers are cow's milk protein hydrolysates, soya, egg, chicken, rice and fish (Ament & Rubin 1972; Iyngkaran et al. 1982; Vitoria et al. 1982; Iyngkaran et al. 1989a; Rosenthal et al. 1991). Most affected children develop symptoms in the first 9 months of life.

relationship to gastroenteritis   In many infants, the symptoms mimic those of acute gastroenteritis, with vomiting and loose stools. It has been suggested that the acute small bowel injury of viral gastroenteritis predisposes to the development of a food-induced enteropathy (Iyngkaran et al. 1978, 1988; Walker-Smith 1982, 1988; Firer et al. 1988).

does damage from one food lead to trouble with others?   It has been suggested that acute injury from cow's milk protein may predispose to subsequent intolerance to soya or gluten (Gryboski et al. 1968; Whitington & Gibson 1977). Evidence of challenge studies in infants with cow's milk protein-sensitive enteropathy showed that during cow's milk protein avoidance the intestinal mucosa had normal levels of peptidases, but these decreased 24 hours after challenge (Iyngkaran et al. 1991). The suggestion is that the observed decrease in peptidases may lead to abnormal protein digestion and facilitate the movement of antigenic macromolecules across the intestine, leading to intolerance to other proteins.

clinical features

The main symptoms are vomiting, loose stools and failure to thrive. There may be some degree of gastrointestinal protein loss. Anaemia is common, although there is debate as to whether this is due to malabsorption of iron or to gastrointestinal loss (Walker-Smith 1988; Lake 1991). The condition is usually transient, and in most cases tolerance to the food trigger has developed by the ages of 2–3 years (Walker-Smith 1988; Lake 1991).

diagnosis

The way the diagnosis is made, and the need for one or more small intestinal biopsies depends upon the circumstances. The child who presents with features of malabsorption, and who is referred to a gastroenterologist, is likely to receive a biopsy as a key investigation to establish a diagnosis. The majority of biopsy specimens reveal a patchy, partial villous atrophy, with an increased intraepithelial lymphocyte count (not usually to the level found in untreated coeliac disease) and a variable degree of eosinophil infiltration. Reduced mucosal thickness is a consistent feature, but, unlike coeliac disease, the mucosa remains thin even after withdrawal of the offending food (Walker-Smith 1988; Lake 1991). In theory the diagnosis of intolerance to the individual food is based on the response to withdrawal and subsequent re-introduction of the offending food. In practice, if the child has had severe and protracted symptoms which have been completely abolished by specific food avoidance, there may be reluctance to perform a diagnostic food challenge (Walker-Smith 1988) for several reasons:

1 reluctance to cause recurrence of severe and possibly protracted symptoms;

2 risk of anaphylactic shock (Walker-Smith 1988);

3 probable temporary nature of the food intolerance.

Thus, in practice, challenge is often deferred until the age of say 12 months, by which time a large proportion of infants will have developed tolerance.

less severe cases

There is no need to perform a small intestinal biopsy in less severe cases, which have not required referral to a gastroenterologist, and in which symptoms and signs were abolished after food withdrawal, returned after re-introduction and were abolished again after continued withdrawal.

Coeliac disease

Coeliac disease is discussed in a separate chapter (27).

Colic
a much abused term

Colic means the intermittent painful contraction of any hollow viscus whose wall contains smooth muscle. Thus there can be ureteric colic, biliary colic, and intestinal colic. It is common, but erroneous and unsafe, to equate all crying in infants with intestinal colic. Crying or screaming are non-specific symptoms in infants, are often accompanied by drawing-up of the legs, have a number of physiological and pathological causes including hunger, tiredness, infection or pain, and may well indicate a serious pathological disorder (Poole 1991). Most studies of so-called colic as a possible symptom of cow's milk protein or other food intolerance are diminished in value by failure to define the term colic, by failure to record associated symptoms that might suggest cow's milk protein intolerance, by omitting to record any temporal relationship between symptoms and milk ingestion, and by being uncontrolled (Jakobsson & Lindberg 1978; Evans *et al.* 1981; Lothe *et al.* 1982; Jakobsson & Lindberg 1983; Ståhlberg & Savilahti 1986; Lothe & Lindberg 1989; Sampson 1989).

cow's milk protein intolerance

In one study designed to overcome the pitfalls described above, and to overcome the very marked placebo effect of changing an infant formula (Taitz & Scholey 1989), 17 formula-fed infants aged 8 weeks or less with crying at least 3 hours per day were studied (Forsyth 1989). The infants were alternately fed a casein hydrolysate formula (Nutramigen) or a casein hydrolysate formula plus cow's milk formula for four periods of 4 days each. Significant decreases in overall crying and crying attributed to colic by mothers were seen with the initial formula change, and a significant decrease in crying attributed to colic but not in overall crying was seen with the second formula change. No significant change was seen with the third formula change. Only two (12%) of the 17 infants had changes in crying behaviour that were consistent with cow's milk protein intolerance. If the findings of this small but careful study can be extrapolated, then the implication is that cow's milk protein intolerance may cause increased crying in approximately 10% of infants reported by their mothers to have colic.

poor sleeping

Some babies with disturbed sleep patterns may have cow's milk protein intolerance. The basis for this is the observation that 17 of 146 children (12%) referred to a sleep clinic for repeated waking and crying during sleep hours responded to a cow's milk protein free diet and relapsed during double-blind crossover challenge (Kahn *et al.* 1987, 1989).

altered motility

Why can cow's milk protein intolerance cause crying? Experiments in rats sensitized to egg albumen showed that installation of egg albumen into the jejunum caused disruption of myoelectric complexes in the small intestine, increased gastrointestinal motility, and diarrhoea (Maric *et al.* 1989). Thus it is possible that this hyperperistalsis, if it also occurs in human infants with food intolerance, could cause intestinal colic and pain.

feeding mismanagement

It has been suggested, but not proven, that a rigidly applied breast-feeding regimen, which curtails nursing at the first breast in order to encourage intake from the second breast, may result in a diminished calorie intake as the baby consumes foremilk from both breasts but no hindmilk, leading in turn to symptoms of hunger such as crying and fretfulness (Woolridge & Fisher 1988). The solution to this problem is to allow the infant to finish sucking from one breast before being offered the second breast.

Crohn's disease

The hallmark of Crohn's disease is chronic transmural inflammation that may affect any segment of the gastrointestinal tract. Its clinical course is characterized by unpredictable exacerbations (Griffiths 1992). The mainstays of treatment are steroids, sulphasalazine and 5-aminosalicylic acid analogues. Controlled trials have shown that, except for those with isolated colonic disease, the use of 'bowel rest' plus an elemental diet induces clinical remission with a frequency comparable to steroids (Ó'Moráin *et al.* 1983, 1984; Sanderson *et al.* 1987; Malchow *et al.* 1990). It should be pointed out that these diets were not always elemental diets in the usually accepted sense of the word (see chapter 19). Although Ó'Moráin *et al.* did use a so-called elemental formula (Vivonex), Sanderson *et al.* employed a formula (Flexical) which was based on hydrolysed casein, glucose syrup and modified tapioca starch. The mechanism of action of diet therapy is unknown. Hunter and his colleagues reported provocative but uncontrolled data suggesting that adult patients with Crohn's disease had intolerance to individual foods, and that continued avoidance of the trigger foods was associated with prolonged remission from disease (Alun Jones *et al.* 1985). However, subsequent double-blind challenge studies performed at the same centre failed to confirm food intolerance in patients with Crohn's disease (Fotherby 1989). There is no objective evidence to support an aetiological association between food intolerance and Crohn's disease.

Oedema of the ileum

There is an anecdotal report of a 39-year old woman with recurrent episodes of urticaria, accompanied by abdominal pain, in whom mucosal oedema of the terminal ileum was found in a barium follow-through examination (Robertson & Wright 1987). The symptoms persisted despite treatment with a few food diet and avoidance of food additives, but the abdominal pain responded to treatment with the H1-receptor antagonist terfenadine, and the urticaria improved when this was accompanied by an H2-receptor antagonist cimetidine. A normal diet was restarted without recurrence of symptoms. It is not clear why these symptoms were attributed to food intolerance, given the absence of response to dietary elimination and the lack of relapse upon resumption of a normal diet.

Pneumatosis intestinalis   Neonatal pneumatosis intestinalis has been reported in a pre-term infant with bloody diarrhoea. The condition improved on a cow's milk-free diet, and relapsed when cow's milk was re-introduced (Aziz 1973).

Pancreatitis   There are anecdotal reports of three adults in whom recurrent attacks of pancreatitis were attributed to food intolerance (Matteo & Sarles 1990), but confirmation by double-blind placebo-controlled challenge was not attempted.

Infantile colitis   Infancy is one of the two periods of childhood in which colitis may present, the second being late childhood and early adolescence. The main symptom in affected infants is chronic bloody loose stools or simply rectal bleeding in the first few weeks or months of life. The most common cause is infection (Hill & Milla 1991). When no infectious agent is detectable, it has been claimed by some that the most common cause is food intolerance, and in one study of non-infectious colitis in infancy, the cause was found to be food intolerance in all eight patients (Jenkins *et al.* 1984). In contrast, in another report of 11 children under 1 year of age with non-infective colitis, only four had food intolerance (Chong *et al.* 1984). At colonoscopy there is a characteristic patchy appearance with areas of inflammation but without ulceration, in contrast to Crohn's disease where there is usually aphthous or 'snail-track' ulceration (Hill & Milla 1991). The key histological feature is an infiltrate of the lamina propria with eosinophils and plasma cells (Hill & Milla 1991), sometimes accompanied by granulomatous-like lesions with giant cells (Raafat *et al.* 1990). In a study in which both jejunal and rectal biopsies were performed in six infants with an enteropathy due to cow's milk protein intolerance, two infants had severe proctitis without evidence of injury to the jejunum (Iyngkaran *et al.* 1989b).

foods implicated   Cow's milk protein, goat's milk protein, soya, beef, wheat, fish, soya and pork have all been implicated (Rubin 1940; Gryboski 1967; Powell 1978; Perisic *et al.* 1988; Hill & Milla 1990; Harrison *et al.* 1991).

breast-feeding   There have been a number of reports of infantile colitis as a result of intolerance to foods consumed by an infant's mother, the food having passed to the infant via the mother's breast milk (Lake *et al.* 1982; Harmatz & Bloch 1988; Perisic *et al.* 1988; Wilson *et al.* 1990). The passage of drugs, chemicals, toxins and foods into breast milk is a well recognized phenomenon. (In one bizarre report, a breast-fed infant died of turtle-flesh poisoning after his mother alone consumed turtle – Chandrasiri *et al.* 1988.) The passage of foods into breast milk, the possible factors which might influence this process, and resulting food intolerance are well reviewed in detail elsewhere and are not dealt with further in this book. For further information see Donnally 1930; Kuroume *et al.* 1976; Warner 1980; Shacks & Heiner 1982; Gerrard 1984; Kilshaw & Cant 1984; Cant *et al.* 1986; Machtinger & Moss 1986; Van Asperen *et al.* 1987; Fälth-Magnusson 1989; Høst *et al.* 1990.

management   The management of food-provoked infantile colitis comprises exclusion of other causes of rectal bleeding or bloody loose stools in infancy (e.g. stool microscopy and culture to exclude infection and investigations to exclude coagulation disorders), the demonstration of loss of symptoms with specific food avoidance and relapse on challenge, followed by a further period of specific food avoidance (Powell 1986). The food intolerance is usually transient, and by the age of 5 years most trigger foods are likely to be tolerated (Hill & Milla 1990).

Ulcerative colitis   Unlike colitis in infancy, ulcerative colitis occurring in later childhood and adolescence does not appear to be associated with food intolerance, although there have been no objective studies of food intolerance in colitis in this age group. In adults with ulcerative colitis the data are scanty. In one study, 77 adults with ulcerative colitis were allocated at random to receive for 1 year either a cow's milk-free diet, a gluten-free plus cow's milk-free diet, or a diet in which the patient was advised to avoid fried foods, condiments and ice cream, but to consume milk and milk products liberally (Wright & Truelove 1965). The results were not easy to interpret. It appears that some of the milk-free diets included butter and margarine which contained powdered milk, and in addition a number of patients on the gluten- and milk-free diets were unable to adhere to the diet so the results for this group were excluded. Of the 26 who received a milk-free diet, 10 had no relapses during the study period, compared to five out of 24 who received the 'dummy' diet, a difference which did not reach statistical significance.

Constipation   The only evidence that food intolerance can cause constipation consists of:

1 Two poorly documented anecdotal case reports of constipation associated with cow's milk protein intolerance (Chin *et al.* 1983; McGrath 1984).

2 The uncontrolled observation that of 206 infants with suspected cow's milk protein intolerance, 10 (6%) had constipation (Clein 1954).

3 The comment in a brief report of an atypical series of 79 patients with cow's milk protein intolerance that 'constipation was more common than diarrhoea', a conclusion that was entirely predictable in view of the exclusion from study of those in whom the sole presenting symptom was diarrhoea (Buisseret 1978).

4 The report of an 8-year-old boy in whom constipation followed cessation of breast-feeding at 2 months of age (Frithz *et al.* 1991). Withdrawal of cow's milk and its products was associated with improvement, and re-introduction with relapse. The authors suggested that this was not cow's milk protein intolerance because cow's milk antibodies could not be demonstrated, and on the basis of challenge studies with calcium carbonate and trials of a low calcium diet it was concluded that the constipation was caused by a local effect on the intestine of dietary calcium!

5 Hill *et al.* stated that 'a small number of infants have constipation in association with their disease' (cow's milk protein intolerance) but no data were provided and no control population was studied (Hill *et al.* 1984).

Key references   **62.1**   WALKER-SMITH J (1988) *Diseases of the Small Intestine in Childhood*, 3rd edn, Butterworths, London. *Detailed review of cow's milk protein-induced enteropathy, including pathogenesis, clinical features and histological changes. It is suggested that there are two syndromes, one a primary disorder of immunological origin and a secondary disorder, a sequel of mucosal damage (e.g. caused by gastroenteritis).*

62.2   LAKE AM (1991) Food protein-induced gastroenteropathy in infants and children. In Metcalfe DD, Sampson HA & Simon RA (eds) *Food Allergy: Adverse Reactions to Foods and Food Additives*, pp. 173–185, Blackwell Scientific Publications, Boston. *Review.*

62.3   FORSYTH BWC (1989) Colic and the effect of changing formulas: a double-blind, multiple-crossover study. *J Pediat* **115**:521–526. *The best study to date, indicating that cow's milk protein intolerance may cause increased crying in approximately 10% of infants reported by their mothers to have colic.*

62.4   CLYNE PS & KULCZYCKI A (1991) Human breast milk contains bovine IgG. Relationship to infant colic? *Pediatrics* **87**:439–444. In a study of the breast milk from 97 healthy mothers, the milk was found to contain greater than 0.1 µg/ml of bovine IgG. The breast milk concentration of bovine IgG was statistically significantly greater in mothers of colicky infants (median 0.42 µg/ml) than in mothers of non-colicky infants (median 0.32 µg/ml). The authors concluded that appreciable quantities of bovine IgG are commonly present in human milk, that significantly higher levels are present in milk from mothers of colicky infants, and that bovine IgG might be involved in the pathogenesis of infant colic.

62.5   SANDERSON IR, UDEEN S, DAVIES PSW, SAVAGE MO & WALKER-SMITH JA (1987) Remission induced by an elemental diet in small bowel Crohn's disease. *Arch Dis Child* **61**:123–127. Seventeen children with active Crohn's disease of the small intestine were entered into a randomized trial which compared the efficacy of a so-called elemental diet (Flexical given for 6 weeks via a nasogastric tube) with a high dose steroid regimen. The diet was as effective as steroids in inducing improvement in indices of disease activity, but had the advantage over steroid therapy of improved linear growth as assessed by height velocity. *Because of the long-term effect of steroid therapy on growth, and the well recognized association between permanent growth stunting and Crohn's disease, the authors concluded that diet is the treatment of choice in the treatment of small intestinal Crohn's disease. Note that the diet was not an elemental diet in the usually accepted sense of the word (see chapter 19) and was in fact a formula based on hydrolysed casein, glucose syrup and modified tapioca starch.*

62.6   POWELL GK (1986) Food protein-induced enterocolitis of infancy: differential diagnosis and management. *Comprehens Therapy* **12**:28–37. *Useful review.*

62.7   HILL SM & MILLA PJ (1990) Colitis caused by food allergy in infants. *Arch Dis Child* **65**:132–133. Report of 13 infants; 54% and 92% had a personal or first-degree family history of atopy respectively, but there was no family history of inflammatory bowel disease.

Summary 62   Gastrointestinal symptoms of intolerance to cow's milk protein, or occasionally other foods such as soya, egg, rice, chicken or fish, may be associated with histological changes in the small intestinal mucosa. The typical features are a partial villous atrophy, an increased intra-epithelial lymphocyte count, and thinning of the mucosa which persists even after withdrawal of the offending food. The term colic is much misused, and the evidence that persistent or excessive crying is caused by painful hyperperistalsis is largely lacking. Cow's milk protein intolerance is a proven cause of excessive crying in infancy, and may be found in up to 10% of infants reported to have 'colic'. Crohn's disease of the small intestine responds to treatment with elemental diets, but there is no evidence that these patients have intolerance to individual foods and the reason for benefit is not known. Food intolerance is an important cause of colitis in infancy, but not of ulcerative colitis in older children.

References to Chapters 61 and 62

ALUN JONES V, DICKINSON RJ, WORKMAN E, WILSON AJ, FREEMAN AH & HUNTER JO (1985) Crohn's disease: maintenance of remission by diet. *Lancet* **2**:177–180.

AMENT ME & RUBIN CE (1972) Soy protein – another cause of the flat intestinal lesion. *Gastroenterol* **62**:227–234.

AMLOT PL, KEMENY DM, ZACHARY C, PARKES P & LESSOF MH (1987) Oral allergy syndrome (OAS): symptoms of IgE-mediated hypersensitivity to foods. *Clin Allergy* **17**:33–42.

AZIZ EM (1973) Neonatal pneumatosis intestinalis associated with milk intolerance. *Am J Dis Child* **125**:560–562.

BECK SA, BURKS AW & WOODY RC (1989) Auriculotemporal syndrome seen clinically as food allergy. *Pediatrics* **83**:601–603.

BUISSERET PD (1978) Common manifestations of cow's milk allergy in children. *Lancet* **1**:304–305.

CALDWELL JH, MEKHJIAN HS, HURTUBISE PE & BEMAN FM (1978) Eosinophilic gastroenteritis with obstruction. Immunological studies of seven patients. *Gastroenterol* **74**:825–829.

CANT AJ, BAILES JA, MARSDEN RA & HEWITT D (1986) Effect of maternal dietary exclusion on breast fed infants with eczema: two controlled studies. *Br Med J* **293**:231–233.

CHALLACOMBE SJ (1987) Oral manifestations of food allergy and intolerance. In Brostoff J & Challacombe SJ (eds) *Food Allergy and Intolerance*, pp. 511–520, Bailliére Tindall, London.

CHANDRASIRI N, ARIYANANDA PL & FERNANDO SSD (1988) Autopsy findings in turtle flesh poisoning. *Med Sci Law* **28**:142–144.

CHIN KC, TARLOW MJ & ALLFREE AJ (1983) Allergy to cows' milk presenting as chronic constipation. *Br Med J* **287**:1593.

CHONG SKF, SANDERSON IR, WRIGHT V & WALKER-SMITH JA (1984) Food allergy and infantile colitis. *Arch Dis Child* 1984 **59**:690–691.

CLEIN NW (1954) Cow's milk allergy in infants. *Pediat Clin North Am* **4**:949–962.

COOKE BED, CHALLACOMBE S, ROSE MS, RITCHKEN S & LEHNER T (1977) Recurrent oral ulceration. *Proc Roy Soc Med* **70**:354–357.

DAVANZO R, PERINI R, VENTURA A & GUASTALLA P (1987) Infantile hypertrophic pyloric stenosis and cow's milk intolerance. *Ped Med Chir* **9**:77–80.

DAVIS RS & STRUNK RC (1981) Auriculotemporal syndrome in childhood. *Am J Dis Child* **135**:832–833.

DONNALLY HH (1930) The question of the elimination of foreign protein (egg-white) in woman's milk. *J Immunol* **19**:15–40.

EL MOUZAN MI, AL QUORAIN AA & ANIM JT (1990) Cow's-milk-induced erosive gastritis in an infant. *J Pediat Gastroenterol Nutr* **10**:111–113.

EVANS RW, FERGUSON DM, ALLARDYCE RA & TAYLOR B (1981) Maternal diet and infantile colic in breast-fed infants. *Lancet* **1**:1340–1342.

EVERSOLE LR, SHOPPER TP & CHAMBERS DW (1982) Effects of suspected foodstuff challenging agents in the etiology of recurrent apthous stomatitis. *Oral Surg* **54**:33–38.

FÄLTH-MAGNUSSON K (1989) Breast milk antibodies to foods in relation to maternal diet, maternal atopy and the development of atopic disease in the baby. *Int Arch Allergy Appl Immunol* **90**:297–300.

FERGUSON MM, WRAY D, CARMICHAEL HA, RUSSELL RI & LEE FD (1980) Coeliac disease associated with recurrent aphthae. *Gut* **21**:223–236.

FERGUSON R, BASU MK, ASQUITH P & COOKE WT (1975) Jejunal mucosal abnormalities in patients with recurrent aphthous ulceration. *Br Med J* **1**:11–13.

FINN R & COHEN HN (1978) 'Food allergy': fact or fiction? *Lancet* **1**:426–428.

FIRER MA, HOSKING CS & HILL DJ (1988) Possible role for rotavirus in the development of cows' milk enteropathy in infants. *Clin Allergy* **18**:53–61.

FORSYTH BWC (1989) Colic and the effect of changing formulas: a double-blind, multiple-crossover study. *J Pediat* **115**:521–526.

FOTHERBY KJ (1989) Crohn's disease: an assessment of dietary therapy, MD thesis, University of Cambridge.

FRITHZ G, WICTORIN B & RONQUIST G (1991) Calcium-induced constipation in a prepubescent boy. *Acta Paediat Scand* **80**:964–965.

GERRARD JW (1984) Allergies in breast-fed babies to foods ingested by the mother. *Clin Rev Allergy* **2**:143–149.

GLAISTER DH, HEARNSHAW JR, HEFFRON PF, PECK AW & PATEY DH (1958) The mechanism of post-parotidectomy gustatory sweating (the auriculotemporal syndrome). *Br Med J* **2**:942–946.

GRIFFITHS AM (1992) Crohn's disease. In David TJ (ed) *Recent Advances in Paediatrics*, vol. 10, pp. 145–160, London, Churchill Livingstone.

GRYBOSKI JD (1967) Gastrointestinal milk allergy in infants. *Pediatrics* **40**:354–362.

HARMATZ PR & BLOCH KJ (1988) Transfer of dietary protein in breast milk. *Ann Allergy* **61**:21–24.

HARPER KE & SPIELVOGEL RL (1986) Frey's syndrome. *Int J Dermatol* **25**:524–526.

HARRISON CJ, PUNTIS JWL, DURBIN GM, GORNALL P & BOOTH IW (1991) Atypical allergic colitis in preterm infants. *Acta Paediat Scand* **80**:1113–1116.

HILL DJ, FORD RPK, SHELTON MJ & HOSKING CS (1984) A study of 100 infants and young children with cow's milk allergy. *Clin Rev Allergy* **2**:125–142.

HILL SM & MILLA PJ (1990) Colitis caused by food allergy in infants. *Arch Dis Child* **65**:132–133.

HILL SM & MILLA PJ (1991) Infantile colitis. Allergy to food is the main non-infective cause and is easily treatable. *Br Med J* **302**:545–546.

HØST A, HUSBY S, HANSEN LG & ØSTERBALLE O (1990) Bovine β-lactoglobulin in human milk from atopic and non-atopic mothers. Relationship to maternal intake of homogenized and unhomogenized milk. *Clin Exper Allergy* **20**:383–387.

IYNGKARAN N, ABIDAIN Z, MENG LL & YADAV M (1982) Egg-protein-induced villous atrophy. *J Pediat Gastroenterol Nutr* **1**:29–35.

IYNGKARAN N, ROBINSON MJ, PRATHAP K, SUMITHRAN E & YADAV M (1978) Cow's milk protein-sensitive enteropathy. *Arch Dis Child* **53**:20–26.

IYNGKARAN N, YADAV M & BOEY CG (1989b) Rectal mucosa in cow's milk allergy. *Arch Dis Child* **64**:1256–1260.

IYNGKARAN N, YADAV M & BOEY CG (1991) Intestinal brush border peptidases in cow's milk protein-sensitive enteropathy. *Acta Paediat Scand* **80**:549–550.

IYNGKARAN N, YADAV M, BOEY CG, KAMATH KR & LAM KL (1989a) Causative effect of cow's milk protein and soy protein on progressive small bowel mucosal damage. *J Gastroenterol Hepatol* **4**:127–136.

IYNGKARAN N, YADAV M, LOOI LM et al. (1988) Effect of soy protein on the small bowel mucosa of young infants recovering from acute gastroenteritis. *J Pediatr Gastroenterol Nutr* **7**:68–75.

JAKOBSSON I & LINDBERG T (1978) Cow's milk as a cause of infantile colic in breast-fed infants. *Lancet* **2**:437–439.

JAKOBSSON I & LINDBERG T (1983) Cow's milk proteins cause infantile colic in breast-fed infants: a double-blind crossover study. *Pediatrics* **71**:268–271.

JENKINS HR, PINCOTT JR, SOOTHILL JF, MILLA PJ & HARRIES JT (1984) Food allergy: the major cause of infantile colitis. *Arch Dis Child* **59**:326–329.

KAHN A, MOZIN MJ, REBUFFAT E, SOTTIAUX M & MULLER MF (1989) Milk intolerance in children with persistent sleeplessness: a prospective double-blind crossover evaluation. *Pediatrics* **84**:595–603.

KAHN A, REBUFFAT E, BLUM D *et al.* (1987) Difficulty in initiating and maintaining sleep associated with cow's milk allergy in infants. *Sleep* **10**:116–121.

KATZ AJ, GOLDMAN H & GRAND RJ (1977) Gastric mucosal biopsy in eosinophilic (allergic) gastroenteritis. *Gastroenterol* **73**:705–709.

KATZ AJ, TWAROG FJ, ZEIGER RS & FALCHUK ZM (1984) Milk-sensitive and eosinophilic gastroenteropathy: similar clinical features with contrasting mechanisms and clinical course. *J Allergy Clin Allergy* **74**:72–78.

KESHAVARZIAN A, SAVERYMUTTU SH, TAI PC *et al.* (1985) Activated eosinophils in familial eosinophilic gastroenteritis. *Gastroenterol* **88**:1041–1049.

KILSHAW PJ & CANT AJ (1984) The passage of maternal dietary proteins into human breast milk. *Int Arch Allergy Appl Immunol* **75**:8–15.

KLEIN NC, HARGROVE RL, SLEISENGER MH & JEFFRIES GH (1970) Eosinophilic gastroenteritis. *Medicine* **49**:299–319.

KUROUME T, OGURI M, MATSUMURA T *et al.* (1976) Milk sensitivity and soybean sensitivity in the production of eczematous manifestations in breast-fed infants with particular reference to intra-uterine sensitization. *Ann Allergy* **37**:41–46.

LAKE AM (1991) Food protein-induced gastroenteropathy in infants and children. In Metcalfe DD, Sampson HA & Simon RA (eds) *Food Allergy: Adverse Reactions to Foods and Food Additives*, pp. 173–185, Blackwell Scientific Publications, Boston.

LAKE AM, WHITINGTON PF & HAMILTON SR (1982) Dietary protein-induced colitis in breast-fed infants. *J Pediat* **101**:906–910.

LEHNER T (1977) Oral ulceration and Behçet's syndrome. *Gut* **8**:491–511.

LEINBACH GE & RUBIN CE (1970) Eosinophilic gastroenteritis: a simple reaction to food allergens? *Gastroenterol* **59**:874–889.

LOTHE L & LINDBERG T (1989) Cow's milk whey protein elicits symptoms of infantile colic in colicky formula-fed infants: a double-blind crossover study. *Pediatrics* **83**:262–266.

LOTHE L, LINDBERG T & JAKOBSSON I (1982) Cow's milk formula as a cause of infantile colic: a double-blind study. *Pediatrics* **70**:7–10.

MACHTINGER S & MOSS R (1986) Cow's milk allergy in breast-fed infants: the role of allergen and maternal secretory IgA antibody. *J Allergy Clin Immunol* **77**:341–347.

MALCHOW H, STEINHARDT HJ, LORENZ-MEYER H *et al.* (1990) Feasibility and effectiveness of a defined-formula diet regimen in treating active Crohn's disease. European Cooperative Crohn's Disease Study III. *Scand J Gastroenterol* **25**:235–244.

MARIC M, GALL DG & SCOTT RB (1989) The effect of food protein-induced intestinal anaphylaxis on rate of transit. *Can J Physiol Pharmacol* **67**:1437–1441.

MATTEO A & SARLES H (1990) Is food allergy a cause of acute pancreatitis? *Pancreas* **5**:234–237.

MCGRATH J (1984) Allergy to cows' milk presenting as chronic constipation. *Br*

Med J **288**:236.

MIN KU (1991) Eosinophilic gastroenteritis. In Metcalfe DD, Sampson HA & Simon RA (eds) *Food Allergy: Adverse Reactions to Foods and Food Additives*, pp. 164–172, Blackwell Scientific Publications, Boston.

MINFORD AMB, MACDONALD A & LITTLEWOOD JM (1982) Food intolerance and food allergy in children: a review of 68 cases. *Arch Dis Child* **57**:742–747.

Ó'MORÁIN C, SEGAL AW & LEVI AJ (1984) Elemental diet as primary treatment of acute Crohn's disease: a controlled trial. *Br Med J* **288**:1859–1862.

Ó'MORÁIN C, SEGAL AW, LEVI AJ & VALMAN HB (1983) Elemental diet in acute Crohn's disease. *Arch Dis Child* **58**:44–47.

ORTOLANI C, ISPANO M, PASTORELLO E, BIGI A & ANSALONI R (1988) The oral allergy syndrome. *Ann Allergy* **61**:47–52.

PERISIC VN, FILIPOVIC D & KOKAI G (1988) Allergic colitis with rectal bleeding in an exclusively breast-fed neonate. *Acta Paediat Scand* **77**:163–164.

POOLE SR (1991) The infant with acute, unexplained, excessive crying. *Pediatrics* **88**:450–455.

POWELL GK (1978) Milk- and soy-induced enterocolitis of infancy. *J Pediat* **93**:553–560.

PRICE SF, SMITHSON KW & CASTELL DO (1978) Food sensitivity in reflux esophagitis. *Gastroenterology* **75**:240–243.

POWELL GK (1986) Food protein-induced enterocolitis of infancy: differential diagnosis and management. *Comprehens Therapy* **12**:28–37.

RAAFAT F, CASTRO R & BOOTH IW (1990) Eosinophilic proctitis with giant cells: a manifestation of cow's milk protein intolerance. *J Pediat Gastroenterol Nutr* **11**:128–132.

ROBERTSON D & WRIGHT R (1987) Oedema of the ileum: a possible manifestation of food allergy. *Br Med J* **294**:350.

RUBIN MI (1940) Allergic intestinal bleeding in the newborn; a clinical syndrome. *Am J Med Sci* **200**:385–390.

SAMPSON HA (1989) Infantile colic and food allergy: fact or fiction? *J Pediat* **115**:583–584.

SANDERSON IR, UDEEN S, DAVIES PSW, SAVAGE MO & WALKER-SMITH JA (1987) Remission induced by an elemental diet in small bowel Crohn's disease. *Arch Dis Child* **61**:123–127.

SHACKS SJ & HEINER DC (1982) Allergy to breast milk. *Clin Immunol Allergy* **2**:121–136.

STÅHLBERG MR & SAVILAHTI E (1986) Infantile colic and feeding. *Arch Dis Child* **61**:1232–1233.

TAITZ LS & SCHOLEY E (1989) Are babies more satisfied by casein based formulas? Arch Dis Child **64**:619–621.

TOWNS SJ & MELLIS CM (1984) Role of acetyl salicylic acid and sodium metabisulphite in chronic childhood asthma. *Pediatrics* **73**:631–637.

TROUNCE JQ & TANNER MS (1985) Eosinophilic gastroenteritis. *Arch Dis Child* **60**:1186–1188.

VAN ASPEREN PP, KEMP AS & MELLIS CM (1987) Immediate food hypersensitivity reactions on first known exposure — the role of breast feeding in sensitisation. In Chandra RK (ed) *Food Allergy*, pp. 217–223, Nutrition Research Education Foundation, St. John's, Newfoundland.

VANDENPLAS Y, QUENON M, RENDERS F, DAB I & LOEB H (1990) Milk-sensitive eosinophilic gastroenteritis in a 10-day old boy. *Eur J Pediatr* **149**:244–245.

VITORIA JC, CAMARERO C, SOJO A, RUIZ A & RODRIGUEZ-SORIANO J (1982) Enteropathy related to fish, rice and chicken. *Arch Dis Child* **57**:44–48.

WALDMAN TA, WOCHNER RD, LASTER L & GORDON RS (1967) Allergic gastroenteropathy. A cause of excessive gastrointestinal protein loss. *New Engl J Med* **276**:761–769.

WALKER-SMITH JA (1982) Cow's milk intolerance as a cause of post-enteritis diarrhea. *J Pediatr Gastroenterol Nutr* **1**:163–166.

WALKER-SMITH JA (1988) *Diseases of the Small Intestine in Childhood*, 3rd edn, Butterworths, London.

WARNER JO (1980) Food allergy in fully breast-fed infants. *Clin Allergy* **10**:133–136.

WEIDMAN AI, NATHAN D & FRANKS AG (1969) Gustatory sweating associated with unilateral hyperpigmentation. *Arch Dermatol* **99**:734–738.

WILSON NW, SELF TW & HAMBURGER RN (1990) Severe cow's milk induced colitis. In an exclusively breast-fed neonate. Case report and clinical review of cow's milk allergy. *Clin Pediat* **29**:77–80.

WOOLRIDGE MW & FISHER C (1988) Colic, 'overfeeding', and symptoms of lactose malabsorption in the breast-fed baby: a possible artifact of feed management? *Lancet* **2**:382–384.

WRAY D (1981) Gluten-sensitive recurrent aphthous stomatitis. *Dig Dis Sci* **26**:737–740.

WRIGHT A, RYAN FP, WILLINGHAM SE, HOLT S & PAGE AC (1986) Food allergy or intolerance in severe recurrent aphthous ulceration of the mouth. *Br Med J* **292**:1237–1238.

WRIGHT R & TRUELOVE SC (1965) A controlled therapeutic trial of various diets in ulcerative colitis. *Br Med J* **2**:138–141.

Part 15 Other Disorders

63 Anaphylactic shock
An occasional complication of food intolerance

Definition   The terms anaphylaxis or anaphylactic shock are used in this book to mean a severe reaction of rapid onset, with circulatory collapse and hypotension. Some have used the term anaphylaxis to describe any immediate allergic reaction mediated by IgE antibodies, however mild, but such usage fails to distinguish between a trivial event (e.g. skin test reaction) and a life-threatening one.

Timing   Although delayed (12 hours or more) anaphylactic reactions to foods can occur (David 1984), most cases of anaphylaxis produce symptoms within minutes after ingestion of the causative agent. In general, the sooner the symptoms occur, the more severe is the reaction.

Features   The first symptoms are often first noted in the mouth, with a sensation of burning, irritation or itching in the lips, mouth or throat, and this can provide a patient with immediate warning of a reaction to a food. These may be followed by feeling unwell, feeling warm, fear, generalized pruritus, faintness and sneezing. In severe cases these early symptoms are quickly (in seconds or minutes) followed by loss of consciousness, and death from suffocation (oedema of the larynx, epiglottis and pharynx) or from shock and cardiac arrhythmia (Booth & Patterson 1970; Criep & Woehler 1971; Delage & Irey 1972). Generalized erythema progressing to urticaria, angioedema, severe bronchospasm, and conjunctivitis are common features, but in severe cases may not occur at all.

Death   The major causes of death in anaphylaxis are obstruction to the upper airway or shock and cardiac arrhythmia (Barnard 1967, 1973). Death may occur within minutes of ingestion of a food (see Fig. 15.1).

Mechanisms   The mechanisms are believed to be either:
1 IgE mediated (e.g. certain cases of food-provoked anaphylaxis, and penicillin or insulin allergy);
2 the generation of immune complexes (e.g. reactions to blood products);
3 a direct (i.e. not involving antigens or antibodies) effect on mast

399

cells or basophils causing inflammatory mediator release (e.g. reactions to radiocontrast media);

4 presumed abnormalities of arachidonic acid metabolism (e.g. anaphylactic reactions to aspirin).

Anaphylactoid reactions

In theory one can differentiate between immunologically mediated reactions and non-immunologically mediated (so-called anaphylactoid) reactions. Previous sensitization is required for the former but not the latter. In practice it is not always obvious whether a reaction is or is not immunologically mediated.

Potentiation by beta blockers

Mild allergic reactions may be greatly enhanced in patients receiving beta blockers (e.g. propranolol). Beta-adrenergic blocking agents may potentiate anaphylactic shock and decrease the response to inhaled or injected β-2 agonists (Jacobs *et al.* 1981; Togood, 1988).

Food triggers

Almost any food can cause anaphylaxis (for some examples see Table 63.1), but the foods most commonly responsible are nuts, fish, shellfish, cow's milk and eggs. It is unclear why some foods should be more likely than others to provoke anaphylaxis. Fatal reactions can occur, and are particularly associated with peanuts (Evans *et al.* 1988; Yunginger *et al.* 1988; Assem *et al.* 1990). In some cases

Table 63.1 Miscellaneous examples of food-provoked anaphylaxis

Food	Age	Fatal	Reference
Nuts/seeds			
Peanut	15–23 years	*	Assem *et al.* (1990)
	28 years		Donovan & Peters (1990)
	24 years	*	Evans *et al.* (1988)
	11–19 years	*	Yunginger *et al.* (1988)
Pecan	16 years	*	Yunginger *et al.* (1988)
Pistachio	28 years		Golbert *et al.* (1969)
Cashew	28 years		Golbert *et al.* (1969)
Brazil	28 years		Golbert *et al.* (1969)
Millet seed	25 years		Parker *et al.* (1981)
Sunflower seed	11–58 years		Noyes *et al.* (1979)
Sesame seed	31–72 years		Malish *et al.* (1981)
	31 years		Rubenstein (1950)
	40 years		Uvitsky (1956)
	6–64 years		Torsney (1964)
Fish and shellfish			
Cod	31 years	*	Yunginger *et al.* (1988)
Crab	40 years	*	Yunginger *et al.* (1988)
	17 years		Coleman & Derbes (1964)
Halibut	27 years		Golbert *et al.* (1969)

continued on p. 401

Table 63.1 *Continued*

Food	Age	Fatal	Reference
Shrimp	24 years		Golbert *et al.* (1969)
	42 years		Coleman & Derbes (1964)
Lobster	24 years		Golbert *et al.* (1969)
Grand keyhole limpet	3–27 years		Morikawa *et al.* (1988)
Cereals			
Wheat	10 weeks		Rudd *et al.* (1981)
Fruit			
Orange	49 years		Williamson (1961)
	48 years		Bendersky & Lupas (1960)
Tangerine	33 years		Golbert *et al.* (1969)
Mango	22 years		Rubin *et al.* (1965)
	24 years		Dang & Bell (1967)
Banana	15 years		Linaweaver *et al.* (1976)
Vegetables			
Potato	5 months		Castells *et al.* (1986)
	17 years		Golbert *et al.* (1969)
Celery	55 years		Forsbeck & Ros (1979)
Pinto bean	37 years		Golbert *et al.* (1969)
Rice	21 years		Golbert *et al.* (1969)
Pea	2 years		David (1989)
Corn	5 months		David (1984)
Soya	4 years		David (1984)
Chick pea	39 years		Golbert *et al.* (1969)
Dairy products			
Cow's milk	6 months	*	Finkelstein (1905)
	'Nursling'	*	Richet (1931)
	10 months	*	Kerley (1936)
	Early childhood		Goldman *et al.* (1963)
	5 month		Golbert *et al.* (1969)
	12 months		David (1984)
	1–6 months		Bock (1985)
	5 years		David (1989)
Meat			
Chicken	2 years		David (1984)
Egg			
Hen's egg	8 years		Richet (1931)
	12 months		Bock (1985)
	2–3 years		Kemp *et al.* (1988)
Miscellaneous			
Chamomile tea	35 years		Benner & Lee (1973)
	54 years		Casterline (1980)
Wine	31 years		Clayton & Busse (1980)

anaphylaxis only occurs when a food is taken in conjunction with exercise – see chapter 58. For obvious reasons there are no studies which have prospectively studied the quantity of food required to provoke anaphylaxis, but anecdotal reports indicate that milligram quantities may be sufficient.

Concealed food ingredients

Most patients with a history of anaphylactic reactions to a food take great care to avoid accidental exposure. A major problem for such patients is the use of food items, most notably peanut, as a concealed or undeclared ingredient in manufactured foods or restaurant meals. Examples which have led to anaphylaxis are the inclusion of peanut in almond icing (Evans *et al.* 1988), dried food dressing (Assem *et al.* 1990), Chinese food (Assem *et al.* 1990) and vegetable burgers (Donovan & Peters 1990).

Misinformation at health food shops

Normally vigilant parents of children with food intolerance may be caught off guard when reassured in a health food shop that a particular food is, for example, dairy-free (i.e. free from cow's milk protein). The author has seen two instances of anaphylactic shock to cow's milk protein arise in this way. In one, the parent was assured that 'vegetarian cheese' was dairy-free, whereas vegetarian cheese is derived from cow's milk and is called vegetarian because animal-derived rennet is not used in the production. In another instance, the parent of another child with cow's milk protein intolerance was incorrectly assured that a soya cheese was dairy-free, and the child died of an anaphylactic reaction.

Natural history

The severity of an adverse reaction to a food gives no indication as to the chances of the child growing out of the food intolerance. With the exception of peanut intolerance, which is usually life-long (Bock & Atkins 1989), children with very severe reactions to a food during the first 2 years of life are likely to grow out of their intolerance or at least become tolerant to small amounts of the food (Bock 1985).

Effect of food avoidance

A definite sequence of events can occasionally be recognized in which specific food avoidance in a child with relatively mild symptoms of food intolerance is followed by anaphylactic shock when the food is re-introduced. The best known example is cow's milk protein intolerance in infancy, when it is well established that there is a clear risk of anaphylaxis during a milk challenge performed after a period of cow's milk protein avoidance (Goldman *et al.* 1963). It is for this reason that milk challenges are often performed in hospital (see chapter 14). It has been suggested that enhanced sensitivity is a small risk of food avoidance in a case of food intolerance (Esteban *et al.* 1988), and this may apply particularly to children with atopic eczema who are treated with elemental diets (David 1984, 1989).

Precautions during food challenges

Given that anaphylaxis is a hazard of food challenges or food re-introductions, what precautions can be taken? The conduct of cow's milk challenges is discussed elsewhere in this book (see chapter 14). For other items, the possible strategies when re-introducing a food are:

1 Do not re-introduce food and continue life-long avoidance. This may be appropriate for peanut intolerance, but is otherwise likely to be needlessly restrictive.

2 Perform all food re-introductions in hospital. This is clearly impractical.

3 If there is a history of a recent (e.g. in last 6 to 12 months) severe reaction, defer the re-introduction.

4 Warn parents of the possible danger of severe reactions if a food is re-introduced at home. This is very important. Parents are more likely to appreciate the potential seriousness of an unexpected adverse reaction if they have received advance warning.

5 Prior to food re-introduction, rub a small quantity of the food onto the skin, and defer re-introduction if there is an obvious urticarial reaction (see chapter 42). Problems with this approach are:

(a) reaction may be suppressed in those receiving H1-histamine antagonists, leading to a false sense of security;

(b) patients with a positive reaction to skin contact with a food are commonly able to tolerate the food when it is taken by mouth, so applying this test may result in needless dietary restriction;

(c) the test is only likely to be positive in IgE-mediated adverse reactions. If another mechanism is operating, or if the test is false negative for other reasons (e.g. infancy) then a negative test may give a false sense of security.

6 When re-introducing a food, start with a minute quantity (e.g. the size of a quarter of a grain of rice). The problem here is that there is no guarantee that a tiny quantity will prevent a severe reaction, but it seems a reasonable precaution.

7 There is no need to employ special precautions for food re-introductions where there is a clear history that accidental ingestion of the food is without untoward effect.

Precautions at other times

1 Make sure that the child's carers and the older child are all aware of the situation.

2 Where there is a history of food-provoked anaphylactic shock, beware of eating in restaurants, when it may be difficult to be sure about food ingredients.

3 Be especially careful of manufactured foods, particularly chocolate or cocoa products (in the UK exempt from the usual regulations for listing ingredients) and food which has not been wrapped (e.g. bread or cake), in which case there will be no label to indicate the ingredients.

4 Consider carrying syringes pre-loaded with adrenaline (see below).

5 Wear a Medic-Alert bracelet or neck pendant, to warn others of intolerance in the event of an accident. These bracelets are obtainable from Medic-Alert Foundation, 12 Bridge Wharf, 156 Caledonian Road, London N1 9UU.

Treatment — secure the airway

As a major cause of death in anaphylaxis is obstruction to the upper airway, protection of the airway is vital, with endotracheal intubation if necessary, or if this is impossible, cricothyroid puncture or tracheostomy (Yunginger *et al.* 1988).

Treatment — oxygen

Oxygen should be given early to prevent myocardial hypoxia.

Treatment – adrenaline

anaphylaxis without cardiac arrest

Adrenaline, 0.1 ml/kg of a 1:10 000 solution ($=10\,\mu g/kg$), is the most important drug. It should be given subcutaneously or intramuscularly. Adrenaline has a short half-life, and the injection can be repeated. The standard advice has been to repeat at intervals of 15–20 min (Smith 1990), but this may be insufficient. Therefore if a patient responds to adrenaline and then appears to be deteriorating a further injection of the same quantity of adrenaline should be given without delay (Ackroyd 1990). If there is then no improvement after 5 min, a further injection should be given (Ackroyd 1990).

anaphylaxis with cardiac arrest

Once basic life support (e.g. external cardiac massage) has been established, adrenaline should be diluted in 10 ml saline and given intravenously (via a central vein if possible) slowly over 3–5 min, remembering that this route carries the risk of ventricular tachycardia and fibrillation. If the child is intubated, and there is no cardiac response, then 1 mmol/kg ($=1\,ml/kg$) of 8.4% sodium bicarbonate should be given, and a double dose ($20\,\mu g/kg$) of adrenaline given.

via endotracheal tube

It is also possible to give adrenaline via an endotracheal tube, which may be useful in the event of a cardiac arrest if an intravenous line has not been established. In this case, the dose is twice the intravenous dose (i.e. the dose is $20\,\mu g/kg$). The drug is squirted rapidly via a fine suction catheter which has been passed through the endotracheal tube so that the tip of the catheter lies just beyond the end of the endotracheal tube. This is immediately followed by 2 ml

0.9% sodium chloride solution, and then the patient is 'bagged' vigorously.

home treatment For home treatment with adrenaline, see below.

Treatment — intravenous fluids Once adrenaline has been given, persisting hypotension can be treated further with intravenous fluids as a 20 ml/kg bolus, with inotropic support (e.g. dopamine) if there is no response.

Treatment — bronchodilators Bronchoconstriction is treated with a nebulized or intravenous β-2 agonist (e.g. salbutamol or terbutaline).

Treatment — histamine antagonists After injection of adrenaline, an H1-histamine antagonist (e.g. chlorpheniramine) is administered by intramuscular or intravenous injection, and continued for 48 hours to prevent recurrence of urticaria.

Treatment — steroids Steroids take some hours to be effective and are unhelpful in the immediate treatment of anaphylaxis. The important exception to this is where anaphylaxis occurs in an asthmatic who has received oral or inhaled steroids in the previous 12 months. Such patients may have some degree of adrenal atrophy (Kravis & Kolski 1986) and adrenal-pituitary axis suppression, and if this exists then additional steroid therapy (e.g. intravenous hydrocortisone succinate 4 mg/kg) may be life-saving. Adrenal atrophy and adrenal-pituitary axis suppression is one possible explanation for the undocumented general impression that asthmatics are at increased risk for severe or fatal anaphylaxis (Settipane & Settipane 1991).

Treatment after recovery The further management consists of avoidance of the cause.

Home treatment of anaphylaxis There have been no controlled studies, so the recommendations made here are based on theoretical considerations, on the results of studies performed in healthy individuals, and on experience obtained from clinics which have employed hyposensitization injections for adults with bee or wasp venom allergy.

induced vomiting It would be extremely hazardous to attempt to induce vomiting in a child who was in the midst of an anaphylactic reaction. This would carry a major risk of inhalation of vomit. However, there are a few parents of children with food-provoked anaphylaxis who have developed the trick, by stimulating the child's throat, of inducing vomiting immediately after ingestion of a trigger food. This is only possible where the child has immediate oral symptoms. It may enable vomiting to be stimulated within seconds of ingestion, possibly preventing the systemic absorption of most of the food.

H1-receptor antagonist

Although there is no proof that it is beneficial, it is reasonable to recommend giving an H1-receptor antagonist at the first sign of a severe reaction. It makes sense to use a non-sedating and quick-acting agent, so the drug of choice is terfenadine, a suggested approximate dose being 15 mg for those under 2 years, 30 mg for those aged 2–5 years, 60 mg for those aged 6–10 years, and 120 mg for those of 11 years or over.

pre-loaded syringes with adrenaline

Where the cause is difficult to avoid (e.g. peanut in manufactured or restaurant food), or where accidental ingestion is a possibility, then it may be helpful to supply syringes pre-filled with adrenaline for the parents to use. When should one issue parents with adrenaline pre-filled syringes? There have been no controlled trials of adrenaline in this situation. Our practice is to issue adrenaline to parents only if the child has had a life-threatening episode of anaphylaxis.

two types of syringe

In Britain, there are two types of adrenaline pre-filled syringes, distributed by International Medical Systems, Daventry, North-amptonshire NN11 5PJ, England & So.El Monte, CA 91733, USA, and Commonwealth Serum Laboratories, 45 Poplar Road, Parkville, Victoria, Australia. Both contain adrenaline at a concentration of 1:1000, and sodium bisulphite as a preservative. The choice of syringe will depend on the dose which is intended, and whether the drug is to be given subcutaneously or by intramuscular injection.
1 500 μg in a 0.5 ml syringe, with a 25 gauge, one-quarter inch, (6.4 mm) long needle, for subcutaneous injection. The gradations on the syringe mean that in theory increments of 100 μg can be given (in practice it is not easy to be very accurate), so at a dose of 10 μg/kg the syringe could not be used for children less than 10 kg body weight.
2 1 mg in a 1 ml syringe, with a 21 gauge, 1.5 inch (38 mm) long needle, for intramuscular injection. The distributors do not recommend this syringe for use outside hospital.

adrenaline inhalers

Adrenaline acid tartrate (adrenaline base 160 μg/puff) is available as a metered dose aerosol (Medihaler-Epi). About 10% of the drug reaches the lungs and is absorbed, the remainder being exhaled or deposited in the mouth and pharynx and swallowed (Warren *et al.* 1986). In healthy individuals, large doses (15–30 puffs) have to be given to achieve the same plasma levels as a 300 μg subcutaneous injection (Warren *et al.* 1986) and the recommended dose for children is 10–15 puffs. In theory, the advantages of adrenaline aerosol over subcutaneous injection (Müller 1991) are:
1 quick absorption into the circulation;
2 possible direct effect on mucosal oedema.

The disadvantages (Warren *et al.* 1986; Ewan 1991) are:

1 more reliable, rapid and prolonged rise of plasma adrenaline after subcutaneous injection;

2 absorption of adrenaline in the lungs may be impaired in patients with laryngeal oedema, bronchoconstriction or bronchial mucosal oedema;

3 studies of absorption after inhalation were performed in normal subjects who were able to perform the correct inhalation technique. It is unlikely that acutely ill children with respiratory distress could obtain as good results.

Key references 63.1 YUNGINGER JW, SWEENEY KG, STURNER WQ *et al.* (1988) Fatal food-induced anaphylaxis. *J Am Med Ass* **260**:1450–1452. Report of seven cases, six of whom ingested the food while away from home. The patients were aged 11, 16, 18, 19, 31, 40 and 43 years. Factors contributing to the severity of individual reactions were denial of symptoms, reliance on oral antihistamines alone to treat symptoms, adrenal suppression by chronic glucocorticoid therapy for co-existing asthma, and concomitant intake of alcohol. In no case was adrenaline given immediately after the onset of symptoms. *Laryngeal oedema was a feature in four out of seven, indicating the importance of tracheostomy as a potentially life-saving manoeuvre in some cases of anaphylactic shock. Only one patient was a child; fatal food-induced anaphylaxis has been most commonly reported in young adults.*

63.2 DAVID TJ (1984) Anaphylactic shock during elimination diets for severe atopic eczema. *Arch Dis Child* **59**:983–986. Anaphylactic shock occurred when single foods (soya, chicken, corn, cow's milk) were re-introduced into the diet of four of 80 children with atopic eczema who had been treated with dietary elimination. Spontaneous recovery occurred in two patients, but two required resuscitation and intensive care and one of these narrowly escaped death. *In none of these children was there a prior history of severe reaction to the food which triggered anaphylaxis. Anaphylaxis is a hazard of an elimination diet for atopic eczema.*

63.3 SETTIPANE R & SETTIPANE GA (1991) Anaphylaxis and food allergy. In Metcalfe DD, Sampson HA & Simon RA (eds) *Food Allergy: Adverse Reactions to Foods and Food Additives*, pp. 150–163, Blackwell Scientific Publications, Boston, *Review.*

63.4 FINKELSTEIN H (1905) Kuhmilch als Ursache akuter Ernährungsstörungen bei Säuglingen. *Monatschr Kinderheilk* **4**:65–72. A 10-day-old infant developed 'dyspepsia', which was made worse when he was given buttermilk. Breast-feeding was recommenced at 5 weeks of age, and he thrived. At 11 weeks he was given 60 ml of one-third strength cow's milk, which resulted in an immediate reaction comprising pallor, collapse, profuse vomiting and loose stools and pyrexia. At 14 weeks he was given 50 ml of one-third strength cow's milk, with a similar but more severe immediate reaction, with the additional features of blood in the stools and spasms in the arms and legs. At 18 weeks he was given 60 ml of one-third strength cow's milk, with an even more severe immediate reaction. At 26 weeks of age, he was again tried on one-third strength diluted cow's milk. He received 10 ml, but suffered a more severe immediate reaction, but instead of recovering he deteriorated with increased fever, seizures, coma and death on the

9th day. Enterocolitis was found at necropsy. *This case is usually quoted as the first published example of death due to anaphylaxis to cow's milk protein. Such details as are available do suggest that anaphylaxis did occur, but it is not entirely clear why the child died 9 days later.*

Summary 63

The term anaphylaxis means a severe reaction of rapid onset, with circulatory collapse. Symptoms usually occur seconds or minutes after ingestion of the causative food. The major causes of death in anaphylaxis are obstruction to the upper airway or hypotension, circulatory failure and cardiac arrhythmia. Almost any food can cause anaphylaxis, but the foods most commonly reported to be responsible are nuts, fish, shellfish, cow's milk and eggs. With a history of anaphylaxis, avoidance of the relevant food trigger is imperative, but where there is a risk of accidental exposure then it may be appropriate to carry a pre-loaded syringe with adrenaline. The treatment of anaphylactic shock comprises:

1 maintenance of a patent airway, with cricothyrotomy or tracheostomy if necessary;

2 oxygen;

3 adrenaline given subcutaneously, intramuscularly, intravenously or via an endotracheal tube, and repeated if there is no effect or the effect wears off;

4 circulatory support with intravenous fluids;

5 inhaled or intravenous bronchodilators for bronchoconstriction;

6 intravenous H1-receptor antagonist.

64 Headache and migraine
Can be provoked by food but mechanism uncertain

What is migraine?

Although there is no universal agreement on a precise definition, migraine can be defined (modified from Blau 1984) as:

1 recurrent headaches, which last 2–72 hours, and with total freedom between attacks;

2 commonly unilateral in onset;

3 associated with visual or gastrointestinal disturbances or both;

4 the visual symptoms occurring as an aura before, and/or photophobia during, the headache phase;

5 often familial.

Abdominal migraine

Abdominal migraine is an unsatisfactory term, now out of fashion, which was formerly used to describe a common and rather striking childhood disorder, the periodic syndrome. This comprises recurrent attacks of abdominal pain, facial pallor, vomiting and pyrexia. The pathogenesis is unknown, and the relationship to migraine is unclear, although there is commonly a family history of migraine or travel sickness. The periodic syndrome is poorly defined and has not been systematically studied in recent years. However it appears to be unrelated to food ingestion or food intolerance, although it is worth pointing out that an immediate gastrointestinal reaction to a food trigger in a child with food intolerance could produce similar symptoms.

Triggers

A variety of triggers have been reported to provoke attacks of migraine in childhood (Table 64.1). Most are unrelated to food intake (Hockaday 1988).

Poor data on food and migraine

No aspect of food intolerance is more confusing than the relationship with migraine, a legacy of poor data. Although it is often asserted (e.g. see Dalton 1975 or Pryse-Phillips 1987) that certain foods, most notably chocolate, cheese, red wine, citrus fruit and coffee can provoke attacks in certain individuals with migraine, there is a singular lack of objective information about the frequency with which this occurs either in children or adults with migraine. Such data as there is suggests that food may have been over-rated as a trigger of migraine. For example, Moffett *et al.* (1974) administered double-blind placebo-controlled challenges with chocolate to 25 adults who reported that they were unable to eat even small quantities of chocolate or other cocoa products without suffering headache. Only two subjects responded consistently to chocolate. The

Table 64.1 Trigger factors reported to provoke attacks of migraine in childhood

Anxiety
Examinations
Family tension
Late nights
Minor head trauma
Fasting
Dietary constituents
Sex hormone variations
Bright light
Sunlight
Television
Discotheques
Loud noise
Cold weather

[1] Source: Hockaday (1988).

possible mechanisms of food-provoked migraine will be discussed below.

Tyramine and headache

Dietary tyramine is known to induce hypertension and headache in non-migrainous patients taking monoamine oxidase inhibitor drugs. This effect has been shown to be due to inhibition, by these drugs, of intestinal and hepatic metabolism of tyramine so that the amine accumulates. An hypothesis is that about 5–10% of patients with migraine have defective metabolism of ingested tyramine in the intestinal wall, which leads to increased absorption, apparently explaining why foods which contain tyramine can provoke attacks in susceptible individuals. However, there is no evidence that the activity of monoamine oxidase, the main tyramine metabolizing enzyme, is lower in patients with food-induced migraine than in other individuals prone to migraine, although levels of monoamine oxidase in platelets are generally lower in patients with migraine (Sandler *et al*. 1974).

tyramine challenge & exclusion

In spite of an early claim (Hanington 1967), most attempts to induce migraine by tyramine challenge in children and adults have been unsuccessful (Moffett *et al*. 1972; Forsythe & Redmond 1974), and a controlled study of exclusion of dietary vasoactive amines in children with migraine failed to demonstrate benefit (Salfield *et al*. 1987). In the latter study, patients were randomly allocated to either a high-fibre diet low in dietary amines or a high fibre diet alone. Although there was no significant difference in the results for the two groups, both groups showed a highly significant decrease in the number of headaches, emphasizing the need for a control diet in studies designed to show that dietary manipulation improves disease.

tyramine in foods

Of the foods commonly believed to trigger migraine, only cheese is rich in tyramine. Chocolate is low in this and other vasoactive amines including phenylethylamine (Schweitzer *et al*. 1975; Hurst & Toomey 1981), and red wine usually contains no more tyramine than white wine (Littlewood *et al*. 1988).

Red wine

Alcoholic drinks, particularly red wine, are commonly reported to provoke attacks of migraine in adults (Masyczek & Ough, 1983; Kaufman 1986). Whether these attacks are due to alcohol itself or some other compound has been disputed. The major chemical difference between red and white wines is the former's high concentration of phenolic flavanoids such as anthocyanins and catechins (Coultate 1984), which as well as having direct effects on blood vessels may also inhibit the enzyme phenolsulphotransferase (PST)

(Littewood *et al.* 1988). Patients with food-induced migraine were shown to have significantly lower levels of platelet PST activity, and it was hypothesized that low activity of PST could lead to an accumulation of phenolic or monoamine substrates which in turn might directly or indirectly provoke attacks of migraine (Sandler *et al.* 1974; Littlewood *et al.* 1982).

Migraine after transplantation Two cases have been reported in whom migraine developed after bone marrow transplantation (Williams & Franklin 1989; Lonnqvist & Ringden 1990). In the first report, the attacks were unrelated to food. In the second case, the attacks were provoked by red wine in both donor and recipient, and it was hypothesized that intolerance to red wine after transplantation could be due to low platelet PST activity, the enzyme defect having been transferred by bone marrow transplantation (Lonnqvist & Ringden 1990).

Aspartame and headache in childhood There is no data linking aspartame with headache or migraine in childhood.

in adults Observational reports of aspartame having provoked attacks of migraine led to a double-blind cross over study, which compared the effect of aspartame and placebo ingestion in 40 adults who reported headaches repeatedly after consuming aspartame (Schiffman *et al.* 1987). The incidence of headache after aspartame (35%) was not significantly different from that after placebo (45%). In a further cross over study of 25 adults with migraine, data on 14 was excluded, but analysis of the remaining results suggested a statistically significant increase in the number of attacks of migraine while taking aspartame (Koehler & Glaros 1988). When questioned, 8% of 171 patients with migraine reported that ingestion of aspartame provoked attacks (Lipton *et al.* 1989). However, self-reported headaches (and a number of other symptoms such as dizziness, urticaria, dysphagia, diarrhoea and rhinitis) as a result of aspartame ingestion could not be confirmed in a challenge study of 12 adults (Garriga *et al.* 1991).

Food intolerance in migraine The studies hitherto performed in this area are a model of confusion. In short, there is as yet no convincing clinical or laboratory evidence to incriminate immunologically mediated reactions as a cause of symptoms in adults or children with migraine. Grant (1979) treated 80 migrainous adults with a diet: lamb, pears and bottled 'spring water' were given for 5 days, and then other foods were re-introduced singly, and records made of the pulse rate and symptoms for 90 min. 85% of patients became headache-free. The patients were reported to be 'allergic' to a wide range of foods as well as gas and tobacco smoke. The study was seriously undermined by the lack of evidence that any of the 'reactions' were objectively reproducible or immunologically mediated, the absence of a control group and the use of pulse testing, an unvalidated method of allergy diagnosis (see chapter 77). Other studies have made similar claims for the benefit of dietary treatment in adults (Monro *et al.* 1980, 1984 – problem: uncontrolled data, see key reference 64.3 below) and children with migraine (Egger *et al.* 1983 – problem: very atypical patients, see key reference 64.4 below). Atkins and colleagues studied 36 children, aged 6–16 years, with migraine (Atkins *et al.* 1988). A history suggested a specific food or food additive as a provoking factor in 16 children. In two of these the skin test result was positive for the suspect food. The food triggers identified by the history were studied by double-blind placebo-controlled challenge, but in no case was migraine precipitated.

Management

Any role for elimination diets in the management of migraine remains to be established. If the history has pinpointed an obvious trigger then avoidance should be straightforward and effective, and lapses should result in attacks. A history is not, however, entirely reliable in excluding a food trigger, especially for a food or drink, such as for example coffee, which is taken daily or more. Given that laboratory and skin-prick tests are unhelpful, the only logical approach, if the possibility of food intolerance is to be explored, is to try an empirical regimen avoiding the commonly recognized food triggers such as chocolate, cheese, red wine, fish and coffee for a defined period which is long enough for a reduction in attacks to be detected. In other words, if the attacks occur every 2 weeks, then it is no use trying a diet for only a week. The likelihood of a placebo response means that a successful outcome is best followed by challenges, to avoid unnecessary life-long food avoidance.

Key references 64.1

LITTLEWOOD JT, GIBB C, GLOVER V, SANDLER M, DAVIES PTG & ROSE FC (1988) Red wine as a cause of migraine. *Lancet* **1**:558–559. In a double-blind study of patients with migraine who reported that attacks were provoked by red wine, 300 ml of a Spanish red wine or 300 ml of vodka-lemonade mixture of equivalent total alcohol content were administered chilled and drunk from a brown glass bottle through a dark straw to conceal the colour and flavour. The red wine induced a migraine in nine out of 11 patients, the headache starting within 3 hours of the challenge in all but one. Vodka failed to provoke migraine in all eight patients. Five patients with migraine who did not regard themselves as intolerant to red wine, and eight healthy subjects, were used as controls, and neither red wine or vodka provoked a headache in any of the subjects. *The blind nature of the study was insecure; it was claimed that the subjects seemed to be unsure of what they were drinking, but this claim was not validated. Nevertheless, the data do not support the view that alcohol in red wine is its sole noxious component.*

64.2   MOFFETT AM, SWASH M & SCOTT DF (1974) Effect of chocolate in migraine: a double blind study. *J Neurol Neurosurg Psychiat* **37**:445–448. The effect of chocolate was studied in 25 volunteer adult migrainous subjects who had reported that headache regularly occurred after the ingestion of cocoa products. In two separate double-blind placebo-controlled studies, only 13 headaches occurred after chocolate in 80 challenges, and only two subjects responded consistently to chocolate. *Contrary to popular belief, chocolate is only rarely a precipitant of migraine.*

64.3   MONRO J, BROSTOFF J, CARINI C & ZILKHA K (1980) Food allergy in migraine. Study of dietary exclusion and RAST. *Lancet* **2**:1–4. Forty-seven adult patients with migraine were given undefined 'rotation and elimination diets'. Fourteen withdrew from the study, leaving 33 patients. The 'diet' resulted in relief ('complete in most cases') in 23. *However*

1 *The absence of a control group made it impossible to exclude the striking placebo effect associated with dietary regimens.*

2 *It was claimed that there was a 'good correlation' between the positive tests for specific IgE antibodies (RAST tests) and the clinically relevant foods, but food challenges were uncontrolled and open, and other workers (e.g. key reference 64.5 – see below) have been unable to confirm positive RAST tests in patients with migraine.*

3 *The authors reported complete or 'partial' protection by giving oral sodium cromoglycate, but these observations were undermined by the varying doses used, the open nature of the food challenges and the lack of a control group. A subsequent study from the same team claimed to confirm that migraine is a food-allergic disease (Monro et al. (1984) Lancet **2**:719–721). The methodology was similar to the previous study, but with the addition of skin-prick and intradermal tests and blinding of the cromoglycate challenges. Only nine patients were studied, the patients were challenged on three occasions but only one response was reported, and most of the symptoms provoked (e.g. flatulence, nausea, diarrhoea) were unrelated to migraine; only one had teichopsia.*

64.4   EGGER J, CARTER CM, WILSON J, TURNER MW & SOOTHILL JF (1983) Is migraine food allergy? A double-blind controlled trial of oligoantigenic diet treatment. *Lancet* **2**:865–869. Of 88 children with migraine (defined as headaches occurring at least once a week for 6 months) who were treated with a so-called oligoantigenic diet, 78 'recovered completely', and 40 were entered into a double-blind placebo-controlled trial which tested the response to one of the foods that provoked symptoms. *Despite the authors claim that 'most children with severe frequent migraine recover on an appropriate diet', there are a number of major problems with this study.*

1 *The patients were highly selected and very atypical; indeed it is questionable as to whether they had migraine at all.*

2 *A high proportion had features not usually associated with migraine. Thus, 72% were atopic, 69% had diarrhoea or flatulence, 47% had a behaviour disorder, 47% had 'aches in limbs', 16% had seizures and 26% of the girls had a vaginal discharge.*

3 *The co-existence of atopic disease in a high proportion was a major source of confusion, and many of the food triggers supposedly identified are notable as triggers of atopic disease rather than migraine.*

4 *The need to administer trigger foods for at least 2 and often up to 7 days before any response occurred, which first took the form of abdominal symptoms* *(and was not always followed by headache), is inconsistent with parents' reports of migrainous responses to foods within at most a few hours of ingestion.*

64.5   MERRETT J, PEATFIELD RC, ROSE FC & MERRETT TG (1983) Food related antibodies in headache patients. *J Neurol Neurosurg Psychiat* **46**:738–742. IgE serum antibodies were assayed in 74 adults with migraine, in whom attacks were reported to be precipitated by ingestion of cheese, chocolate or citrus fruit. Also studied were 45 adults with migraine but no history of food triggers, 29 with cluster headache and 60 normal control subjects. There was no difference in the total or food-specific IgE levels between the dietary and non-dietary subjects. There was no evidence that food intolerance, reported by adults with migraine, was associated with an IgE-mediated immunological mechanism.

64.6   PERKIN JE & HARTJE J (1983) Diet and migraine: a review of the literature. *J Am Diet Assoc* **83**:459–463. Review of food intolerance, chemical triggers, hypoglycaemia and taste aversion.

Summary 64   Although the strands may be weak, and some are almost threadbare, the net of evidence is strong that certain foods can provoke attacks in some patients with migraine. The available data point away from an immunological mechanism, although the precise mechanism remains to be elucidated. There is a dearth of reliable information about the incidence of food as a trigger of attacks of migraine. The role of elimination diets in the identification of food intolerance in migraine in childhood remains to be established.

65 Arthritis
Probably not a symptom of food intolerance

Unlikely association   There is only scanty evidence to support an occasional causal association between food intolerance and arthritis. There are, however, sufficiently interesting case reports and animal studies to merit a brief discussion here.

Childhood arthritis   There is a report of a 14-year-old girl with a 6-year history of polyarticular, seronegative juvenile rheumatoid arthritis with a systemic onset, in whom relapse followed consumption of cow's milk (Ratner *et al.* 1985). The institution of a cow's milk protein-free diet was followed by remission within 10 days, and on four separate occasions consumption of cow's milk was followed by fever, joint pains and joint swelling within 2–4 weeks. The child had co-existing lactase deficiency. Unfortunately, double-blind challenges were not performed.

Arthritis in adults   A most striking report is that of a 38-year old woman with an 11-year history of progressive, erosive, seronegative rheumatoid arthritis, which was poorly responsive to conventional treatment which included systemic steroids (Parke & Hughes 1981). She ate 1 lb (0.4 kg) of cheese a day. Within 3 weeks of avoidance of cow's milk and cheese improvement was first noted, and this was followed by almost complete resolution of synovitis and stiffness after a few months. Consumption of cow's milk was followed by recurrence of symptoms within 12 hours. Open challenge in hospital with 3 lb (1.4 kg) of cheese and 7 pints (4095 ml) of cow's milk over 3 days was associated with objective changes in stiffness, grip strength and size of digits within 24 hours.

other reports   There are a number of other unconfirmed observations or uncontrolled studies which have claimed a causal association between food intolerance (mainly cow's milk) and synovitis or arthritis in adults (Vaughan & Hawke 1931; Hicklin *et al.* 1980; Denman *et al.* 1983; Breneman 1984; Darlington *et al.* 1986; Carini *et al.* 1987; Wojtulewski 1987; Prier 1988; Golding 1990; Darlington 1991; Panush 1991). Attempts to confirm such an association with double-blind challenges have been largely unsuccessful (Felder *et al.* 1987; Panush 1990).

Fasting   There is some evidence that rheumatoid arthritis in adults improves during a 1-week fast, but the reasons for improvement have not been clearly identified (Palmblad *et al.* 1991; Sköldstam & Magnusson 1991).

Reports in animals   Numerous studies have demonstrated an inflammatory synovitis in certain strains of rabbit given cow's milk to drink (Welsh *et al.* 1986; Coombs *et al.* 1988; Panush *et al.* 1990). This synovitis was first evident after 5 weeks of milk consumption, it peaked at approximately 12 weeks, but it was transient and resolved by 32 weeks. It was suggested that the transient nature of the synovitis was due to the development of specific secretory IgA antibodies which blocked continued antigen absorption (Welsh *et al.* 1986). Egg albumin had a similar but less marked arthritogenic effect. Similar administration of cow's milk to rats and mice did not result in synovitis (Welsh *et al.* 1986). It is not known whether there is any relationship between transient milk-induced synovitis in rabbits and arthritis in humans.

Summary 65   The evidence of a causal relationship between food intolerance (mainly cow's milk) and synovitis or arthritis in humans is anecdotal and scanty. Nevertheless, the possibility that such an association might exist on very rare occasions is possibly supported by the occurrence of transient synovitis in rabbits who are fed cow's milk.

66   Renal tract disorders
No proven link with food intolerance

Unlikely association   There is no convincing evidence to support an association between food intolerance and urinary tract disorders. However, the subject is dealt with briefly here because of the large number of published claims.

Nocturnal enuresis   The suggestions that nocturnal enuresis may be attributable to food intolerance, and that it can be abolished by dietary elimination are anecdotal and have never been validated objectively (Bray 1931; Burkland 1951; Breneman 1965, 1984; Esperanca & Gerrard 1969; Crook 1973; Bahna & Ghandi 1987; Sandberg 1987). Were enuresis to be a genuine feature of food intolerance, then one might have expected it to have been observed in the large number of studies of food intolerance which have examined the response to double-blind placebo-controlled challenges.

Nephrotic syndrome
antigen exposure   Anecdotal reports of the nephrotic syndrome occurring after exposure to grass pollen (Editorial 1969) led to a large study which appeared to support the subsequent suggestion (Zaleski *et al.* 1972) of an association between the nephrotic syndrome and atopic disease (Meadow & Sarsfield 1981). However, there was no confirmation of any temporal relationship between antigen exposure and exacerbation of the nephrotic syndrome.

food intolerance   There have been a number of anecdotal reports, unsupported by double-blind placebo-controlled challenge, which have suggested a temporal association between ingestion of certain foods and the nephrotic syndrome (Sandberg *et al.* 1977; Howanietz & Lubec 1985; McCrory *et al.* 1986; Genova *et al.* 1987; Lagrue *et al.* 1987; Laurent *et al.* 1987, 1988; Laurent & Lagrue 1989). The claims for a causal relationship between food intolerance and the nephrotic syndrome are not likely to be accepted without further supporting data.

Cystitis/urinary infection   It is has been suggested that over 80% of 900 children with recurrent urinary tract symptoms responded to elimination diets (details not specified), control of environmental factors (no details provided) and unspecified hyposensitization injections (Powell *et al.* 1972). There is no objective data to support a causal association between food intolerance and cystitis or urinary tract infection, despite the large number of anecdotal claims (Eisenstaedt 1951; Powell & Powell 1954; Pastinszky 1959; Unger *et al.* 1959; Horesh 1976; Littleton *et al.* 1982; Palacios *et al.* 1984).

Other renal disorders   Claims for a causal relationship between food intolerance and haematuria, IgA nephropathy, orthostatic proteinuria, renal colic, retention of urine due to angioedema of the urethra, or non-specific symptoms such as dysuria or frequency of micturition are based either on anecdotal evidence or studies of circulating antibodies to dietary antigens (Duke 1922; Vaughan & Hawke 1931; Thomas & Wickstein 1944; Burkland 1951; Dees & Simmons 1951; Powell 1961; Matsumura *et al.* 1966; Powell *et al.* 1970; Lelong & Pigeon 1989; Kolacek *et al.* 1990).

Summary 66   Despite a huge amount of anecdotal literature on the subject, there is as yet no systematic objective evidence of a causal relationship between food intolerance and disorders of the renal tract.

67 Epilepsy
Links with food intolerance very doubtful

Fasting   Diets have been used extensively in attempts to control epilepsy. The first assessments were reported early this century, when it was found that seizures ceased during absolute fasting in some patients (Geyelin 1921). Impracticability limited this approach.

Ketogenic diets   It was suggested that a high fat, low protein and low carbohydrate diet would be ketogenic, would mimic the effects of fasting, and would thereby help some patients with epilepsy. Such diets were helpful, but were overshadowed by the advent of more effective anti-epileptic drugs. More recently there has been a resurgence of interest in ketogenic diets, particularly for those poorly controlled by drug therapy.

Medium-chain triglyceride ketogenic diets

The unpalatability of ketogenic diets based on an intake high in long-chain saturated fats was associated with non-adherence to the diet. This led to the development of various modified ketogenic diets which used medium-chain triglycerides (MCT), which have also been shown to induce ketosis. A recent study of the original and the modified ketogenic diets (Table 67.1) showed no difference in the effectiveness of the two diets. During a 3-month treatment period, 51 of 63 treatment episodes showed a greater than 50% reduction in seizure frequency (Schwartz et al. 1989a). The mechanism by which ketogenic diets operate is obscure (Schwartz et al. 1989b), and the uncontrolled nature of the studies to date means that a placebo effect cannot be excluded.

Epilepsy

early unsatisfactory reports

The suggestion that food intolerance can provoke epilepsy has been the subject of numerous anecdotal and uncontrolled reports in the medical literature this century. Dees & Lowenbach reported in 1948 that the electroencephalogram was abnormal in a high proportion of children with 'allergy'. The clinical conditions encountered under this umbrella were, however, diverse, and included, as well as atopic disease, miscellaneous items such as nausea, vomiting or diarrhoea ('gastro-intestinal allergy'), behaviour problems, and 'superior intelligence'. By 1968, Fein and Kamin were able to review no fewer than 26 studies which examined a possible relationship between allergy and epilepsy, and concluded that pollen, dust and moulds were the principal allergens involved.

recent unsatisfactory reports

An open study of the effects of a non-standardized elimination diet on 76 selected children with hyperkinesis included 14 children who also had epilepsy (Egger et al. 1985). Seizures ceased while on the diet in 13 of the 14. Similar observations had been made at the same

Table 67.1 Composition of ketogenic diets[1]

Type of diet	Calculation based on	MCT[2] oil	Long-chain saturated fats	Protein	Carbohydrate
Original	75 kcal/kg bodyweight; 1 g protein/kg bodyweight	36 kcal from fat to 4 kcal from protein and carbohydrate			
MCT	RDA[3]	60%	11%	10%	19%
Modified MCT	RDA	30%	41%	10%	19%

[1] Source: Schwartz et al. (1989).
[2] MCT, medium chain triglyceride.
[3] RDA, recommended daily amounts.

centre during a previous study of dietary treatment of migraine (Egger *et al.* 1983). A few further patients were studied, and it was reported that dietary treatment was associated with improvement in seizures in 37 of 45 children with epilepsy, recurrent headaches, abdominal symptoms or hyperkinetic behaviour, but not in 18 children who had epilepsy alone (Egger *et al.* 1989). A further study of the same elimination diet failed to demonstrate benefit in nine children with idiopathic epilepsy (Van Someren *et al.* 1990). Until benefit from dietary treatment can be confirmed by controlled studies, most observers will continue to doubt whether improvement on diets is anything other than a placebo effect.

Seizures and anaphylaxis It appears that anaphylaxis can on rare occasions provoke a seizure. Goldman's classic report of oral cow's milk challenges in 89 children with cow's milk protein intolerance included one infant who was reported to develop anaphylactic shock, tonic-clonic seizures and loose stools after open challenge with cow's milk (Goldman *et al.* 1963). In this patient the seizures occurred within a few minutes to 8 hours after cow's milk ingestion, but seizures were only associated with anaphylaxis on one occasion. Wilken-Jensen & Melchior (1970) reported two children in whom paroxysmal activity in the electro-encephalogram was associated with ingestion of foods to which the child was thought to be intolerant. One of these children exhibited myoclonic jerks during an episode of egg-provoked anaphylactic shock, but since he also experienced episodes of focal myoclonic jerks on other occasions when trigger foods had not been ingested, a causal relationship between food ingestion and seizures was uncertain.

Key references 67.1 SCHWARTZ RH, EATON J, BOWER BD & AYNSLEY-GREEN A (1989) Ketogenic diets in the treatment of epilepsy: short-term clinical effects. *Dev Med Child Neurol* **31**:145–151. The original long-chain triglyceride ketogenic diet, the MCT ketogenic diet, and a modified MCT diet were used in the treatment of 55 children and four adults with intractable epilepsy. During a 3-month treatment period, 51 of 63 studies (81%) showed a >50% reduction in seizure frequency. There was no correlation between EEG changes and clinical response. *All three ketogenic diets were effective in the short-term management of children whose epilepsy was poorly controlled with anticonvulsant drugs.*

67.2 SCHWARTZ RM, BOYES S & AYNSLEY-GREEN A (1989) Metabolic effects of three ketogenic diets in the treatment of severe epilepsy. *Dev Med Child Neurol* **31**:152–160. *All three ketogenic diets induced ketosis, but the mechanism whereby the diets were associated with reduction in seizures was obscure.*

67.3 GOLDMAN AS, ANDERSON DW, SELLERS WA, SAPERSTEIN S, KNIKER WT & HALPERN SR (1963) Milk allergy. I. Oral challenge with milk and isolated milk proteins in allergic children. *Pediatrics* **32**:425–443. In a study of 89 children with cow's milk protein intolerance, anaphylactic shock occurred during milk challenge reactions in eight patients. One of these was a breast-fed boy who exhibited a tonic-clonic seizure of 30 min duration 3 hours after ingestion of homogenized cow's milk; watery loose stools were passed 10 hours later. Exclusive breast feeding continued until 2 months, when ingestion of homogenized milk was immediately followed by the frequent passage of loose watery stools. The onset of status epilepticus, lasting 24 hours and associated with a left facial paralysis, began 8 hours after milk ingestion. At 3 months, when homogenized milk was given accidentally, tonic-clonic seizures lasting 1 hour began within 10 min of milk ingestion. *Note an inconsistent time interval between milk ingestion and onset of seizures, which makes a causal relationship less likely.*

Summary 67   Ketogenic diets are occasionally used in the management of refractory epilepsy, where seizures are uncontrolled on anti-convulsant medication. Although there are a number of reports describing improvement on such diets, objective controlled data to support the use of such diets is lacking. The data to suggest that epileptic seizures may occur as part of an adverse reaction to foods is at best exceedingly scanty. Controlled studies are required before elimination diets can be recommended as treatment for epilepsy in childhood.

68 Behaviour problems
Not usually caused by food

Long history
Randolph 1947

It has long been recognized that acute or chronic illness can make a child irritable, restless and difficult to manage. Thus it is no surprise that food-provoked exacerbations of, for example, atopic eczema, may be associated with behavioural changes such as poor concentration, poor sleeping and irritability. The conceptual leap from 'food intolerance makes children miserable' to 'therefore miserable children have food intolerance' was first made in the 1920s and 1930s. In 1947, Randolph presented the idea that 'allergy' caused fatigue, irritability and behaviour problems in children. On the basis of purely anecdotal evidence, he divided affected children into two groups. One comprised those who were 'chronically tired, sluggish and depressed' and the other consisted of those who were 'hyperkinetic and hyperexcited'. Irritability, fretfulness, maladjusted behaviour, poor concentration, and memory impairment were common to both groups. Randolph claimed that any food could cause these symptoms, but alleged that the major foods responsible were wheat and corn.

Crook 1975   Crook attributed an even wider range of behavioural symptoms to food intolerance, and coined the term 'allergic tension-fatigue syndrome' (Crook 1975).

Feingold 1975a, b   Feingold claimed that hyperactivity and learning disorders were commonly caused by intolerance to food additives and foods rich in naturally occurring salicylates. This gave rise to the 'Feingold diet', which aimed to exclude all artificial food additives and foods rich in naturally occurring salicylates (Feingold 1975a, b).

Current situation   Despite the lack of objective data to support the beliefs described above, and the wealth of objective data to the contrary, it is currently widely believed by parents, professionals (e.g. teachers – see McLoughlin & Nall 1988) and others that food intolerance is an important and common cause of a wide range of childhood behaviour problems (Smith 1976; Rapp 1979; Stevens & Stoner 1979; Barnes & Colquhoun 1984; Mansfield & Monro 1987). The persistence of belief in a dietary basis for behavioural disturbance in the face of all scientifically valid studies failing to confirm any link sounds a cautionary note for those who believe that medicine based on rationality should be the basis of our practice. It also emphasizes the pressure society, from teachers to mothers-in-law, exerts on mothers whose children are labelled as misbehaving and the paradoxical thirst for a 'rational' biological non-judgemental explanation for this.

Hyperactivity/hyperkinesis
definition   The term hyperactivity has been devalued by its widespread use to describe such differing phenomena as poor sleeping, disobedience, aggression, temper tantrums and restlessness, as well as true hyperkinesis. The term has been most clearly defined in the *Diagnostic and Statistical Manual of Mental Disorders* published by the American Psychiatric Association (1980) – see Table 68.1. Several age-related scales have been devised for scoring the features of hyperkinesis, thus enabling objective studies to be undertaken (Conners 1980; Barkley 1982).

food intolerance   Numerous anecdotal or methodologically unsound studies have claimed to support the use of Feingold or other diets in the management of hyperkinesis, but the results of sound controlled studies which have incorporated double-blind placebo-controlled challenges have all failed to support a causal link between food intolerance and hyperkinesis (Goyette *et al.* 1978; Harley *et al.* 1978; Levy *et al.* 1978; Mattes & Gittelman 1981; Thorley 1984). It is clear that the behaviour of some children improved temporarily after the introduction

Table 68.1 Diagnostic criteria for attention deficit disorder with hyperactivity[1]

A   *Inattention*: at least three of the following
1 often fails to finish things he or she starts
2 often doesn't seem to listen
3 easily distracted
4 has difficulty concentrating on schoolwork or other tasks requiring sustained attention
5 has difficulty sticking to a play activity

B   *Impulsivity*: at least three of the following
1 often acts before thinking
2 shifts excessively from one activity to another
3 has difficulty organizing work (this not being due to cognitive impairment)
4 needs a lot of supervision
5 frequently calls out in class
6 has difficulty awaiting turns in games or group situations

C   *Hyperactivity*: at least two of the following
1 runs about or climbs on things excessively
2 has difficulty sitting still or fidgets excessively
3 has difficulty staying seated
4 moves about excessively during sleep
5 is always 'on the go' or acts as if 'driven by a motor'

D   *Onset before the age of 7 years*

E   *Duration of at least 6 months*

F   *Not due to schizophrenia, affective disorder, or severe or profound mental retardation*

---

[1] Source: American Psychiatric Association (1980).

of additive-free diets, but those who responded to the diet failed to deteriorate when food additives were re-introduced under double-blind conditions, suggesting that improvement on such diets was a placebo response.

Food additives   There is a notable lack of objective evidence to support the hypothesis that food additives can have adverse behavioural effects. A major source of confusion has been the presence of atopic disease. Thus, in one study of 76 patients where intolerance to food and food additives was said to contribute to behaviour disorders, a large proportion of patients had atopic disease (Egger *et al.* 1985). If a food additive makes urticaria, asthma or atopic eczema worse, the concentration and behaviour may also be expected to suffer, but there is no evidence that this is anything other than an indirect effect (David 1987).

parents' reports unreliable   Parents' reports of behaviour changes as a result of food or food additives are especially unreliable. Double-blind challenges with tartrazine and benzoic acid were performed in hospital in 24 children whose parents gave a definite history of a purely behavioural immediate adverse reaction to tartrazine (David 1987). In no patient was any change in behaviour noted. In another study of 39 children whose parents also reported adverse behavioural effects of food additives, the parents were unable to detect any changes in behaviour when the additives were introduced under double-blind conditions (Pollock & Warner 1990).

Sucrose

Objective studies have failed to confirm adverse effects after the ingestion of sucrose in both normal children and those with hyperkinesis or aggressive behaviour (Behar *et al.* 1984; Gross 1984; Wolraich *et al.* 1985; Ferguson *et al.* 1986; Mahan *et al.* 1988; Wender & Solanto 1991). The suggestion that sucrose ingestion causes reactive hypoglycaemia and adversely affects behaviour of juvenile delinquents has not been confirmed by objective studies (Bachorowski *et al.* 1990; Gans *et al.* 1990). Indeed a recent study has suggested that sucrose may have an analgesic effect in infants; those who drank 2 ml of a 12% sucrose solution prior to blood collection cried 50% less than control infants who received sterile water (Blass & Hoffmeyer 1991).

Caffeine

Studies of the behavioural effects of caffeine, which is found in tea, coffee, cola and certain other soft drinks, and chocolate, are complicated by the different responses of 'high consumers' (intake greater than 500 mg/day) and 'low consumers' and by the possibility that a high level of caffeine intake may to some extent be self-selected by children who tolerate or benefit from it (Rapoport *et al.* 1984). Children who select high-caffeine diets demonstrate greater impulsiveness and lower autonomic arousal (as assessed by skin conductance) when not consuming caffeine. Children who select low-caffeine diets are perceived to be more emotional, inattentive and restless while receiving caffeine 10 mg/day (Rapoport *et al.* 1984).

Theophylline

There have been a number of suggestions that theophylline, a theobromine which is closely related to caffeine, and which is used in the treatment of asthma, may have adverse cognitive or behavioural effects, but there has been no sound objective data to support this belief, and there has been little attempt to unravel the effects of theophylline from those of the co-existing caffeine intake (Creer *et al.* 1988; Creer & McLoughlin 1989).

Management
diagnosis and explanation

It is helpful to correctly delineate the behaviour problem. Is the child abnormal, or is the difficulty within the range of normal childhood behaviour? It is useful to make the distinction between cases where the main problem is anxiety about normal behaviour and cases where the notion of food intolerance is a family's current solution to what is, in fact, a very real problem. The latter group are more difficult to reassure, and show evidence of more widespread difficulty.

the label 'hyperactive'

Many children are unhelpfully and incorrectly labelled as hyperactive, and often the perceived behaviour problem is less serious than the parents fear. One needs to be alert here to parents who have become so over alert and anxious that ordinary behaviour is dramatized and exaggerated as an 'allergic' response. Parents often believe that foods or food additives are the cause of their child's behaviour problem. Parents' anxieties are best dealt with without being dismissive or confrontational (Varley 1984). Most parents are happy to accept an explanation as to why diets are not the solution for behaviour problems.

go easy on parents

Some parents are firmly wedded to their beliefs in food or additive intolerance. It is not necessarily helpful to strive to alter these beliefs, particularly if the resulting dietary restriction is associated with behavioural improvement and is nutritionally safe. Excessive confrontation may be counterproductive and lead to alienation, parental isolation, and escalation of dietary measures. Most important of all it may undermine parental confidence in any discussion of other approaches to the perceived problem. For a useful and practically based book written specially for parents, see Taylor 1985. To some extent the current fears about food additives arise from a background of general ecological anxiety, the validity or otherwise of which is outside the scope of this book; when talking to parents it is all too easy to find oneself taking part in a wider debate.

the focus on food

Parental beliefs in the importance of food or additive intolerance are often fuelled by an initial response to a dietary change. Food or additive challenges may be the only way to help parents understand the placebo nature of such improvements, although even after negative challenges a few parents still insist on continuing with dietary measures (David 1987). The focus on food is an attribution which places the causal agent for the behaviour problem outside both the child and the family. It is also a simple linear causal link. What is not considered is the possibility of a cause within the child or family, or of a more circular causality, i.e. where the child has effects on the parent who then has effects on the child. One of the least confrontational ways of introducing these other possibilities is simply to consider the effect of the child's difficult behaviour (however caused) on the parents. What is their experience of the child when he or she is like this and what is their behaviour at the time? Then one is talking about the parent/child relationship without challenging the initial cause of the problem, and the idea of a 'vicious circle' can be used to work on the parental behaviour. Parents' use of dietary control is possibly successful in addition to any placebo effect because it structures parental reactions in a helpful way, and gets parents and child 'on the same side' in fighting the 'external' problem.

difficult problems

The most difficult cases are those where a parental quest for other dietary 'causes' leads to escalating dietary restriction and unacceptable interference in the child's activities or nutrition. Helping such families to reach a more realistic approach may take many months and much discussion, often with the help of the child psychiatry service.

outlandish factitious illness

There remains a small hard core of cases where inappropriate parental belief in food or additive intolerance, often accompanied by overvalued beliefs in other forms of 'allergy', leads to grossly unreasonable restrictions on the child's eating and other activities. Such cases come in to the category of Meadow's syndrome (parental fabrication of symptoms), most recently also described as outlandish factitious illness (Taylor 1992). These beliefs are often shared and supported by an unorthodox medical practitioner, and this makes it much more difficult for social workers or local authorities to deal with such cases within the context of child protection (Taylor 1992).

Key references 68.1

HARLEY JP, RAY RS, TOMASI L et al. (1978) Hyperkinesis and food additives: testing the Feingold hypothesis. *Pediatrics* **61**:818–828. Teacher ratings, objective classroom and laboratory observational data, attention-concentration and other psychological measures obtained on 36 school-age hyperactive boys under experimental and control diet conditions yielded no support for the Feingold hypothesis.

68.2

LEVY F, DUMBRELL S, HOBBES G, RYAN M, WILTON N & WOODHILL JM (1978) Hyperkinesis and diet. A double-blind crossover trial with a tartrazine challenge. *Med J Aust* **1**:61–64. Twenty-two children with hyperactivity were treated with a Feingold diet for 4 weeks. There was a significant improvement in the mothers' ratings of the childrens' behaviour after on the diet, but teacher ratings of behaviour and objective tests of attention and motor performance failed to substantiate any improvement, and blind challenges with tartrazine failed to provoke symptoms. *This study: (a) failed to support the Feingold hypothesis;*

(b) suggested that any benefit of the Feingold diet as perceived by parents is probably a placebo effect; (c) showed that there was a 25% increase in symptoms as assessed by mothers during food challenges, whether with tartrazine or placebo; and (d) showed that even where parents claim to be convinced of the benefits of a Feingold diet, lapses in the diet are common.

68.3 EGGER J, CARTER CM, GRAHAM PJ, GUMLEY D & SOOTHILL JF (1985) Controlled trial of oligoantigenic treatment in the hyperkinetic syndrome. *Lancet* **1**:540–545. Seventy-six children with hyperkinesis, accompanied by an assortment of other disorders such as developmental delay, headaches, epilepsy, abdominal pain, chronic rhinitis, chronic limb pains, skin rashes, mouth ulcers and atopic disease, were openly treated with a non-standardized diet which basically comprised a variable combination of two meats, two sources of carbohydrate, vegetables, two fruits, calcium and vitamins. Symptoms improved in 21. Blind challenges with selected food items reproduced certain symptoms in 31 selected cases. *The major problems with this study are: (a) the highly atypical nature of the sample; (b) the high proportion of cases with atopic disease; (c) treatment order effect suggesting placebo response to diet; (d) failure to standardize the diet, so that different foods were avoided in each case; (e) positive food challenges do not prove that the cause of improvement on a diet is food avoidance.*

68.4 DAVID TJ (1987) Reactions to dietary tartrazine. *Arch Dis Child* **62**:119–122. Double-blind placebo-controlled challenges with tartrazine and benzoic acid were performed in hospital in 24 children whose parents gave a definite history of a purely behavioural immediate adverse reaction to one of these substances. The patients, aged 1.6–12.4 years, were all on a diet that avoided these items, and in all there was a clear history that any lapse of the diet caused an obvious adverse behavioural reaction within 2 hours. In no patient was any change in behaviour noted either by the parents or the nursing staff after the administration of placebo or active substances. Twenty-two returned to a normal diet without problems, but the parents of two insisted on continuing the diet. Parents' beliefs in the purely behavioural effects of tartrazine and benzoic acid are often unreliable.

68.5 SARAVIS S, SCHACHAR R, ZLOTKIN S, LEITER LA & ANDERSON GH (1990) Aspartame: effects on learning, behavior, and mood. *Pediatrics* **86**:75–83. When 20 healthy 9–10 year olds were given a drink containing either aspartame or sodium cyclamate, there was no difference in measures of associative learning, arithmetic calculation, activity level, social interaction and mood. *The consumption of aspartame by normal 9–10 year olds did not have identifiable detrimental effects on learning, behaviour or mood.*

68.6 KRUESI MJP & RAPOPORT JL (1986) Diet and human behavior: how much do they affect each other? *Ann Rev Nutr* **6**:113–130. *Very little, is the conclusion of this useful review.*

68.7 GLINSMANN WH, IRAUSQUIN H & PARK YK (1986) Evaluation of health aspects of sugars contained in carbohydrate sweeteners. Report of Sugars Task Force, 1986. *J Nutrition* **116** (suppl.):S1–S216. *Detailed review of all aspects, such as diabetes and atherosclerosis. Part VII (pp. S101–S117) examines behaviour, and concludes that sugar consumption does not cause significant changes in behaviour.*

68.8   VARLEY CK (1984) Diet and behavior of children with attention deficit disorder. *J Am Acad Child Psychiat* **23**:182–185. *Particularly lucid discussion of the reasons why belief in dietary strategies persists in the face of clear evidence that they are unhelpful, and the reasons why tacit endorsement of placebo therapy (diets) is undesirable.*

Summary 68   It is popularly believed that food additives are a common cause of a wide range of behaviour problems in childhood. Objective studies have failed to confirm this belief. Children with behaviour disorders often temporarily improve for a few weeks when given a diet which avoids food additives, but this appears to be a placebo effect.

69 Rhinitis and otitis media
Dietary treatment unlikely to help

Gustatory rhinitis   Watery rhinorrhoea, lacrimation, sweating of the forehead and scalp, facial flushing following the consumption of spicy food are well recognized symptoms which probably affect all people to some degree provided a sufficient quantity of spice is ingested. The nasal component has recently been described under the label of gustatory rhinitis (Raphael *et al.* 1989). Foods shown under controlled conditions to provoke these symptoms are listed in Table 69.1. The mechanisms whereby certain foods such as onions (which when cut produce a lachrymatory substance allicin – Brouk 1975), peppers and spices provoke irritant reactions are not fully understood. However, chilli powder, which can also provoke gustatory rhinitis, contains capsaicin, which is known to induce inflammation by the release of bioactive peptides. In one challenge study nasal

Table 69.1 Examples of foods that have been shown to provoke gustatory rhinitis[1]

Hot chilli peppers
Spicy foods
Horseradish
Hot and sour soup
Red cayenne pepper
Tabasco sauce
Black pepper
Onion
Vinegar
Mustard

[1] Source: Raphael *et al.* (1989).

pretreatment with nebulized atropine suppressed rhinorrhoea after ingestion of spicy foods (Raphael *et al.* 1989).

Rhinitis & food intolerance

A wide variety of stimuli can provoke rhinitis (Table 69.2). The literature on the relationship between rhinitis and intolerance to non-spicy foods is generally anecdotal, uncontrolled, and unsupported by double-blind placebo-controlled challenges (Gerrard 1966; Ogle & Bullock 1980; Wraith 1982; Heiner 1984; Pastorello *et al.* 1985; Pelikan 1987; Pelikan 1988; Pelikan & Pelikan-Filipek 1989; Sabbah *et al.* 1990). However, sneezing, nasal congestion, and a mucoid nasal discharge are features of cow's milk protein intolerance that have been confirmed by double-blind challenge studies (see chapter 9). In addition, a nasal discharge was confirmed by blind food challenge in seven out of 100 assorted patients with food intolerance reported by Lessof *et al.* (1980). Nasal symptoms are usually only one of several clinical features, and there are no reports supported by double-blind placebo-controlled challenges where rhinitis was the sole feature of food intolerance. There has been no systematic study comparing the incidence of food intolerance in children with rhinitis with and without other symptoms. Given the fact that solitary symptoms of food intolerance are uncommon, and considering that recurrent or chronic rhinitis in childhood are common, the chance that rhinitis is due to food intolerance in an individual child appears slight.

Serous otitis media

Since it is clearly possible (see above) for food intolerance adversely to affect the nasal mucosa, it would not be surprising to find secondary Eustachian tube obstruction contributing to serous otitis media. Regrettably, given the high incidence of serous otitis media and associated hearing loss (e.g. 20% of 5-year-old children – Brooks 1969), there is a lack of objective studies which bear on this issue. There are a number of anecdotal claims of benefit from elimination diets in children with serous otitis media and hearing loss (Viscomi 1975; Clemis 1976; Ruokonen *et al.* 1982; Rapp 1984; Pelikan 1987; Hurst 1990), but no proper controlled studies.

Table 69.2 Examples of stimuli that can provoke rhinitis

Viral respiratory infections
Inhalant allergens
Cold air
Recumbent position
Exercise
Irritant gases, dusts or fumes
Food intolerance

Hay fever & food intolerance   It is claimed that there is an association between allergy to pollen, such as mugwort or birch tree pollen, and intolerance to certain foods. This is discussed briefly in chapter 71. Pollen hyposensitization, despite being associated with improvement in hay-fever symptoms, does not appear to lead to loss of co-existing food intolerance (Möller 1989).

Management   The chances that solitary rhinitis or serous otitis media are due to food intolerance are highly remote. Even if these symptoms are predominant, but accompanied by other atopic disorders, there is little evidence that an elimination diet will be beneficial.

Key reference 69.1   RAPHAEL G, RAPHAEL MH & KALINER M (1989) Gustatory rhinitis: a syndrome of food-induced rhinorrhea. *J Allergy Clin Immunol* **83**:110–115. Twelve adult subjects ingested foods well known to produce rhinorrhoea, and control foods not associated with rhinorrhoea, such as potato crisps, hot tea and gefilte fish balls. Spicy foods, but not control foods, induced rhinorrhoea in all subjects, and increased the albumin and total protein content of nasal secretions. Nasal pretreatment with atropine blocked the food-induced rhinorrhoea.

Summary 69   Ingestion of spicy or irritant foods can produce watery rhinorrhoea, lacrimation, sweating of the forehead and scalp and facial flushing in most if not all normal people. Although logic dictates that chronic rhinitis or serous otitis media could in theory be caused by food intolerance, there is at present no good data to support the use of dietary manipulation in the management of either disorder.

References to Chapters 63–69

ACKROYD JF (1990) Allergy to peanuts. *Br Med J* **301**:120.

AMERICAN PSYCHIATRIC ASSOCIATION (1980) *Diagnostic and Statistical Manual of Mental Disorders*, 3rd edn, pp. 43–44, American Psychiatric Association, Washington DC.

ASSEM ESK, GELDER CM, SPIRO SG, BADERMAN H & ARMSTRONG RF (1990) Anaphylaxis induced by peanuts. *Br Med J* **300**:1377–1378.

ATKINS FM, BALL BD & BOCK A (1988) The relationship between the ingestion of specific foods and the development of migraine headaches in children (abstract). *J Allergy Clin Immunol* **81**:185.

BACHOROWSKI JA, NEWMAN JP, NICHOLS SL, GANS DA, HARPER AE & TAYLOR SL (1990) Sucrose and delinquency: behavioral assessment. *Pediatrics* **86**:244–253.

BAHNA SL & GANDHI MD (1987) Pediatric food allergy. In Breneman JC (ed) *Handbook of Food Allergies*, pp. 55–69, Dekker, New York.

BARKLEY RA (1982) *Hyperactive Children. A Handbook for Diagnosis and Treatment*, John Wiley, Chichester.

BARNARD JH (1967) Allergic and pathologic findings in fifty insect-sting fatalities. *J Allergy* **40**:107–114.

BARNARD JH (1973) Studies of 400 Hymenoptera sting deaths in the United States. *J Allergy* **52**:259–264.

BARNES B & COLQUHOUN I (1984) *The Hyperactive Child*, Thorsons, Wellingborough.

BEHAR D, RAPOPORT JL, ADAMS AJ, BERG CJ & CORNBLATH M (1984) Sugar challenge testing with children considered behaviourally 'sugar reactive'. *Nutr Behavior* **1**:277–288.

BENDERSKY G & LUPAS JA (1960) Anaphylactoid reaction to ingestion of orange. *J Am Med Ass* **173**:255–256.

BENNER MH & LEE HJ (1973) Anaphylactic reaction to chamomile tea. *J Allergy Clin Immunol* **52**:307–308.

BLASS EM & HOFFMEYER LB (1991) Sucrose as an analgesic for newborn infants. *Pediatrics* **87**:215–218.

BLAU JN (1984) Towards a definition of migraine headache. *Lancet* **1**:444–445.

BOCK SA (1985) Natural history of severe reactions to foods in young children. *J Pediat* **107**:676–680.

BOCK SA & ATKINS FM (1989) The natural history of peanut allergy. *J Allergy Clin Immunol* **83**:900–904.

BOOTH BH & PATTERSON R (1970) Electrocardiographic changes during human anaphylaxis. *J Am Med Ass* **211**:627–631.

BRAY GW (1931) Enuresis of allergic origin. *Arch Dis Child* **6**:251–253.

BRENEMAN JC (1965) Nocturnal enuresis, a treatment regimen for general use. *Ann Allergy* **23**:185–191.

BRENEMAN JC (1984) *Basics of Food Allergy*, 2nd edn, Charles C Thomas, Springfield.

BROOKS DN (1969) The use of the electro-acoustic impedance bridge in the assessment of middle ear function. *Internat Audiol* **8**:563–569.

BROUK B (1975) *Foods Consumed by Man*, Academic Press, London.

BURKLAND CE (1951) Manifestations of hypersensitivity in the genito-urinary system. *Urol Cutan Rev* **55**:290–295.

CARINI C, FRATAZZI C & AIUTI F (1987) Immune complexes in food-induced arthralgia. *Ann Allergy* **59**:422–428.

CASTELLS MC, PASCUAL C, ESTEBAN MM & OJEDA JA (1986) Allergy to white potato. *J Allergy Clin Immunol* **78**:1110–1114.

CASTERLINE CL (1980) Allergy to chamomile tea. *J Am Med Ass* **244**:330–331.

CLAYTON DE & BUSSE W (1980) Anaphylaxis to wine. *Clin Allergy* **10**:341–343.

CLEMIS JD (1976) Allergic factors in management of middle ear effusions. *Ann Otol Rhinol Laryngol* **85** (suppl.):259–262.

COLEMAN WP & DERBES VJ (1964) Anaphylactic reactions from shellfish. *Dermatol Tropica* **3**:91–94.

CONNERS CK (1980) *Food Additives and Hyperactive Children*, Plenum, New York.

COULTATE TP (1984) *Food – the Chemistry of its Components*, pp. 112–116 and 136, Royal Society of Chemistry, London.

CREER TL, KOTSES H, GUSTAFSON KE et al. (1988) A critique of studies investigating the association of theophylline to psychologic or behavioral performance. *Pediat Asthma Allergy Immunol* **2**:169–184.

CREER TL & McLOUGHLIN JA (1989) The effects of theophylline on cognitive and behavioral performance. *J Allergy Clin Immunol* **83**:1027–1029.

CRIEP LH & WOEHLER TR (1971) The heart in human anaphylaxis. *Ann Allergy* **29**:399–409.

CROOK WG (1973) Genitourinary allergy. In Speer F & Dockhorn RJ (eds) *Allergy and Immunology in Children*, pp. 690–694, Charles C Thomas, Springfield.

CROOK WG (1975) Food allergy – the great masquerader. *Pediat Clin N Am* **22**:227–238.

DALTON K (1975) Food intake prior to a migraine attack – study of 2,313 spontaneous attacks. *Headache* **15**:188–193.

DANG RWM & BELL DB (1967) Anaphylactic reaction to the ingestion of mango. Case report. *Hawaii Med J* **27**:149–150.

DARLINGTON LG (1991) Dietary therapy for arthritis. *Rheum Dis Clin N Am* **17**:273–285.

DARLINGTON LG, RAMSEY NW & MANSFIELD JR (1986) Placebo-controlled, blind study of dietary manipulation therapy in rheumatoid arthritis. *Lancet* **1**:236–238.

DAVID TJ (1984) Anaphylactic shock during elimination diets for severe atopic eczema. *Arch Dis Child* **59**:983–986.

DAVID TJ (1987) Reactions to dietary tartrazine. *Arch Dis Child* **62**:119–122.

DAVID TJ (1989) Hazards of challenge tests in atopic dermatitis. *Allergy* (suppl. 9):101–107.

DEES SC & LOWENBACH H (1948) The electroencephalograms of allergic children. *Ann Allergy* **6**:99–108.

DEES SC & SIMMONS EC (1951) Allergy of the urinary tract. A critical review of the literature with an analysis of 613 cases of urologic disease in relation to allergy. *Ann Allergy* **9**:714–725.

DELAGE C & IREY NS (1972) Anaphylactic deaths: a clinicopathologic study of 43 cases. *J Forensic Sci* **17**:525–539.

DENMAN AM, MITCHELL B & ANSELL BM (1983) Joint complaints and food allergic disorders. *Ann Allergy* **51**:260–263.

DONOVAN KL & PETERS J (1990) Vegetable burger allergy: all was nut as it appeared. *Br Med J* **300**:1378.

DUKE WW (1922) Food allergy as a cause of bladder pain. *Ann Clin Med* **1**:117–126.

EDITORIAL (1969) Pollen, mold allergies linked to nephrosis. *J Am Med Ass* **210**:1851.

EGGER J, CARTER CM, GRAHAM PJ, GUMLEY D & SOOTHILL JF (1985) Controlled trial of oligoantigenic treatment in the hyperkinetic syndrome. *Lancet* **1**:540–545.

EGGER J, CARTER CM, SOOTHILL JF & WILSON J (1989) Oligoantigenic diet treatment of children with epilepsy and migraine. *J Pediatr* **114**:51–58.

EGGER J, CARTER CM, WILSON J, TURNER MW & SOOTHILL JF (1983) Is migraine food allergy? A double-blind controlled trial of oligoantigenic diet treatment. *Lancet* **2**:865–869.

EISENSTAEDT JS (1951) Allergy and drug hypersensitivity of the urinary tract. *J Urol* **65**:154–159.

ESPERANCA M & GERRARD JW (1969) Nocturnal enuresis. Comparison of the effect of imipramine and dietary restriction on bladder capacity. *Can Med Ass J* **101**:65–70.

ESTEBAN MM, PASCUAL C FIANDOR A & OJEDA JA (1988) A possible consequence of long-term elimination diet in IgE mediated subclinical food hypersensitivity. *Allergie Immunol* **20**:55–56.

EVANS S, SKEA D & DOLOVICH J (1988) Fatal reaction to peanut antigen in almond icing. *Can Med Ass J* **139**:231–232.

EWAN PW (1991) Route of administration of adrenaline for the treatment of anaphylactic reactions to bee or wasp stings. *Clin Exper Allergy* **21**:753–755.

FEIN BT & KAMIN PB (1968) Allergy, convulsive disorders and epilepsy. *Ann Allergy* **26**:241–247.

FEINGOLD BF (1975a) *Why Your Child Is Hyperactive*, Random House, New York.

FEINGOLD BF (1975b) Hyperkinesis and learning disabilities linked to artificial food flavors and colours. *Am J Nurs* **75**:797–803.

FELDER M, DE BLECOURT ACE & WÜTHRICH B (1987) Food allergy in patients with rheumatoid arthritis. *Clin Rheumatol* **6**:181–184.

FINKELSTEIN H (1905) Kuhmilch als Ursache akuter Ernährungsstörungen bei Säuglingen. *Monatschr Kinderheilk* **4**:65–72.

FORSBECK M & ROS AM (1979) Anaphylactoid reaction to celery. *Contact Derm* **5**:191.

FORSYTHE WI & REDMOND A (1974) Two controlled trials of tyramine in children with migraine. *Dev Med Child Neurol* **16**:794–799.

GANS DA, HARPER AE, BACHOROWSKI JA, NEWMAN JP, SHRAGO ES & TAYLOR SL (1990) Sucrose and delinquency: oral sucrose tolerance test and nutritional assessment. *Pediatrics* **86**:254–262.

GARRIGA MM, BERKEBILE C & METCALFE DD (1991) A combined single-blind, double-blind, placebo-controlled study to determine the reproducibility of hypersensitivity reactions to aspartame. *J Allergy Clin Immunol* **87**:821–827.

GENOVA R, SANFILIPPO M, ROSSI ME & VIERUCCI A (1987) Food allergy in steroid-resistant nephrotic syndrome. *Lancet* **1**:1315–1316.

GERRARD JW (1966) Familial recurrent rhinorrhea and bronchitis due to cow's milk. *J Am Med Ass* **198**:137–139.

GEYELIN HR (1921) Fasting as a method for treating epilepsy. *Medical Record* **99**:1038–1039.

GIAFFER MH, NORTH G & HOLDSWORTH CD (1990) Controlled trial of polymeric versus elemental diet in treatment of active Crohn's disease. *Lancet* **335**:816–819.

GOLBERT TM, PATTERSON R & PRUZANSKY JJ (1969) Systemic allergic reactions to ingested antigens. *J Allergy* **32**:96–107.

GOLDING DN (1990) Is there an allergic synovitis? *J Roy Soc Med* **83**:312–314.

GOLDMAN AS, ANDERSON DW, SELLERS WA, SAPERSTEIN S, KNIKER WT & HALPERN SR (1963) Milk allergy. I. Oral challenge with milk and isolated milk proteins in allergic children. *Pediatrics* **32**:425–443.

GOYETTE CH, CONNORS CK, PETTI TA & CURTIS LE (1978) Effects of artificial colors on hyperkinetic children: a double-blind challenge study. *Psychopharmacol Bull* **14**:39–40.

GRANT ECG (1979) Food allergies and migraine. *Lancet* **1**:966–969.

HAND JR (1949) Interstitial cystitis: report of 233 cases (204 women and 19 men). *J Urol* **61**:291–310.

HANINGTON E (1967) Preliminary report on tyramine headache. *Br Med J* **2**:550–551.

HARLEY JP, RAY RS, TOMASI L *et al.* (1978) Hyperkinesis and food additives: testing the Feingold hypothesis. *Pediatrics* **61**:818–828.

HEINER DC (1984) Respiratory diseases and food allergy. *Ann Allergy* **53**:657–664.

HICKLIN JA, MCEWEN LM & MORGAN JM (1980) The effect of diet in rheumatoid arthritis (abstract). *Clin Allergy* **10**:463.

HOCKADAY JM (1988) (ed) *Migraine in Childhood and Other Non-Epileptic Paroxysmal Disorders*, pp. 102–104, Butterworths, London.

HORESH AJ (1976) Allergy and recurrent urinary tract infections in childhood. I. *Ann Allergy* **36**:16–22.

HOWANIETZ H & LUBEC G (1985) Idiopathic nephrotic syndrome, treated with steroids for five years, found to be allergic reaction to pork. *Lancet* **2**:450.

HURST DS (1990) Allergy management of refractory serous otitis media. *Otolaryngol Head Neck Surg* **102**:664–669.

HURST WJ & TOOMEY PB (1981) High-performance liquid chromatographic determination of four biogenic amines in chocolate. *Analyst* **106**:394–402.

JACOBS RL, RAKE GW, FOURNIER DC, CHILTON RJ, CULVER WG & BECKMANN CH (1981) Potentiated anaphylaxis in patients with drug-induced beta-adrenergic blockade. *J Allergy Clin Immunol* **68**:125–127.

KAUFMAN HS (1986) The red wine headache: a pilot study of a specific syndrome. *Immunol Allergy Practice* **8**:279–284.

KEMP AS, VAN ASPEREN PP & DOUGLAS J (1988) Anaphylaxis caused by inhaled pavlova mix in egg-sensitive children. *Med J Aust* **149**:712–713.

KERLEY CG (1936) Allergic manifestations to cows' milk. *New York J Med* **36**:1320–1322.

KOEHLER SM & GLAROS A (1988) The effect of aspartame on migraine headache. *Headache* **28**:10–13.

KOLACEK S, BOOTH IW & TAYLOR CM (1990) Food, mucosal immunity, and IgA nephropathy. *J Pediatr Gastroenterol* **11**:175–178.

KRAVIS LP & KOLSKI GB (1986) Asthma mortality in children: a 16-year experience at Children's Hospital of Philadelphia. *New Engl Reg Allergy Proc* **7**:442–447.

LAGRUE G, LAURENT J, ROSTOKER G & LANG P (1987) Food allergy in idiopathic nephrotic syndrome. *Lancet* **2**:277.

LAURENT J & LAGRUE G (1989) Dietary manipulation for idiopathic nephrotic syndrome. A new approach to therapy. *Allergy* **44**:599–603.

LAURENT J, ROSTOKER G, ROBEVA R, BRUNEAU C & LAGRUE G (1987) Is adult idiopathic nephrotic syndrome food allergy? Value of oligoantigenic diets. *Nephron* **47**:7–11.

LAURENT J, WIERZBICKI N, ROSTOKER G, LANG P & LAGRUE G (1988) Syndrome néphrotique idiopathique et hypersensibilité alimentaire. Valeur des régimes d'éviction. *Arch Fr Pediatr* **45**:815–819.

LELONG M & PIGEON B (1989) L'allergie immédiate peut-elle être à l'origine d'hématuries chez i'enfant? *Arch Fr Pediatr* **46**:447–448.

LESSOF MH, WRAITH DG, MERRETT TG, MERRETT J & BUISSERET PD (1980) Food allergy and intolerance in 100 patients – local and systemic effects. *Quart J Med* **49**:259–271.

LEVY F, DUMBRELL S, HOBBES G, RYAN M, WILTON N & WOODHILL JM (1978) Hyperkinesis and diet. A double-blind crossover trial with a tartrazine challenge. *Med J Aust* **1**:61–64.

LINAWEAVER WE, SAKS GL & HEINER DC (1976) Anaphylactic shock following banana ingestion. *Am J Dis Child* **130**:207–209.

LIPTON RB, NEWMAN LC, COHEN JS & SOLOMON S (1989) Aspartame as a dietary trigger of headache. *Headache* **29**:90–92.

LITTLETON RH, FARAH RN & CERNY JC (1982) Eosinophilic cystitis: an uncommon form of cystitis. *J Urol* **127**:132–133.

LITTLEWOOD JT, GIBB C, GLOVER V, SANDLER M, DAVIES PTG & ROSE FC (1988) Red wine as a cause of migraine. *Lancet* **1**:558–559.

LITTLEWOOD J, GLOVER V, SANDLER M, PETTY R, PEATFIELD R & ROSE FC

(1982) Platelet phenolsulphotransferase deficiency in dietary migraine. *Lancet* **1**:983–986.

LONNQVIST B & RINGDEN O (1990) Migraine precipitated by red wine after bone-marrow transplantation. *Lancet* **1**:364.

MAHAN LK, CHASE M, FURUKAWA CT *et al.* (1988) Sugar 'allergy' and children's behavior. *Ann Allergy* **61**:453–458.

MALISH D, GLOVSKY MM, HOFFMAN DR, GHEKIERE L & HAWKINS JM (1981) Anaphylaxis after sesame seed ingestion. *J Allergy Clin Immunol* **67**:35–38.

MANSFIELD P & MONRO J (1987) *Chemical Children. How to Protect Your Family from Harmful Pollutants*, Century, London.

MASYCZEK R & OUGH CS (1983) The 'red wine reaction' syndrome. *Am J Enol Vitic* **34**:260–264.

MATSUMURA T, KUROUME T & FUKUSHIMA I (1966) Significance of food allergy in the etiology of orthostatic albuminuria. *J Asthma Res* **3**:325–329.

MATTES JA & GITTELMAN R (1981) Effects of artificial food colorings in children with hyperactive symptoms. *Arch Gen Psychiat* **38**:714–718.

MCCRORY WW, BECKER CG, CUNNINGHAM-RUNDLES C, KLEIN RF, MOURADIAN J & REISMAN L (1986) Immune complex glomerulopathy in a child with food hypersensitivity. *Kidney International* **30**:592–598.

MCLOUGHLIN JA & NALL M (1988) Teacher opinion of the role of food allergy on school behavior and achievement. *Ann Allergy* **61**:89–91.

MOFFETT AM, SWASH M & SCOTT DF (1972) Effect of tyramine in migraine: a double-blind study. *J Neurol Neurosurg Psychiat* **35**:496–499.

MOFFETT AM, SWASH M & SCOTT DF (1974) Effect of chocolate in migraine: a double blind study. *J Neurol Neurosurg Psychiat* **37**:445–448.

MÖLLER C (1989) Effect of pollen immunotherapy on food hypersensitivity in children with birch pollinosis. *Ann Allergy* **62**:343–345.

MONRO J, BROSTOFF J, CARINI C & ZILKHA K (1980) Food allergy in migraine. Study of dietary exclusion and RAST. *Lancet* **2**:1–4.

MONRO J, CARINI C & BROSTOFF J (1984) Migraine is a food-allergic disease. *Lancet* **2**:719–721.

MORIKAWA A, KATO M, TOKUYAMA K, TAJIMA K & KUROUME T (1988) Anaphylaxis due to grand keyhole limpet (baby abalone like shellfish). *New Engl Reg Allergy Proc* **9**:406.

MÜLLER UR (1991) Route of administration of adrenaline for the treatment of anaphylactic reactions to bee or wasp stings. *Clin Exper Allergy* **21**:755–756.

NOYES JH, BOYD GK & SETTIPANE GA (1979) Anaphylaxis to sunflower seed. *J Allergy Clin Immunol* **63**:242–244.

OGLE KA & BULLOCK JD (1980) Children with allergic rhinitis and/or bronchial asthma treated with elimination diet: a five-year follow-up. *Ann Allergy* **44**: 273–278.

PALACIOS AS, DE JUANA AQ, SAGARRA JM & DUQUE RA (1984) Eosinophilic food-induced cystitis. *Allergol Immunopathol* **12**:463–469

PALMBLAD J, HAFSTRÖM I & RINGERTZ B (1991) Antirheumatic effects of fasting. *Rheum Dis Clin N Am* **17**:351–362.

PANUSH RS (1990) Food induced ('allergic') arthritis: clinical and serologic studies. *J Rheumatol* **17**:291–294.

PANUSH RS (1991) Does food cause or cure arthritis? *Rheum Dis Clin N Am* **17**:259–272.

PARKE AL & HUGHES GRV (1981) Rheumatoid arthritis and food: a case study. *Br Med J* **282**:2027–2029.

PARKER JL, YUNGINGER JW & SWEDLUND HA (1981) Anaphylaxis after ingestion of millet seeds. *J Allergy Clin Immunol* **67**:78–80.

PASTINSZKY I (1959) The allergic diseases of the male genitourinary tract with special reference to allergic urethritis and cystitis. *Urol Int* **9**:288–305.

PASTORELLO E, ORTOLANI C, LURAGHI MT *et al.* (1985) Evaluation of allergic etiology in perennial rhinitis. *Ann Allergy* **55**:854–856.

PELIKAN Z (1987) Rhinitis and secretory otitis media: a possible role of food allergy. In Brostoff J & Challacombe SJ (eds) *Food Allergy and Intolerance*, pp. 467–485, Baillière Tindall, London.

PELIKAN Z (1988) Nasal response to food ingestion challenge. *Arch Otolaryngol Head Neck Surg* **114**:525–530.

PELIKAN Z & PELIKAN-FILIPEK M (1989) Effects of oral cromolyn on the nasal response due to foods. *Arch Otolaryngol Head Neck Surg* **115**:1238–1243.

POLLOCK I & WARNER JO (1990) Effect of artificial food colours on childhood behaviour. *Arch Dis Child* **65**:74–77.

POWELL NB (1961) Allergies of the genito-urinary tract. *Ann Allergy* **19**:1019–1025.

POWELL NB, BOGGS PB & McGOVERN JP (1970) Allergy of the lower urinary tract. Ann Allergy **28**:252–255.

POWELL NB & POWELL EB (1954) Vesical allergy in females. *South Med J* **47**:841–848.

POWELL NB, POWELL EB, THOMAS OC, QUENG JT & McGOVERN JP (1972) Allergy of the lower urinary tract. *J Urol* **107**:631–634.

PRIER A (1988) Effets des manipulations diététiques sur l'évolution de la polyarthrite rhumatoïde. *Presse Médicale* **17**:1181–1183.

PRYSE-PHILLIPS W (1987) Dietary precipitation of vascular headaches. In Chandra RK (ed) *Food Allergy*, pp. 237–252, Nutrition Research Education Foundation, Newfoundland.

RANDOLPH TG (1947) Allergy as a causative factor of fatigue, irritability, and behaviour problems of children. *J Pediat* **31**:560–572.

RAPHAEL G, RAPHAEL MH & KALINER M (1989) Gustatory rhinitis: a syndrome of food-induced rhinorrhea. *J Allergy Clin Immunol* **83**:110–115.

RAPOPORT JL, BERG CJ, ISMOND DR, ZAHN TP & NEIMS A (1984) Behavioral effects of caffeine in children. Relationship between dietary choice and effects of caffeine challenge. *Arch Gen Psychiat* **41**:1073–1079.

RAPP DJ (1979) *Allergies and the Hyperactive Child*, Simon & Schuster, New York.

RAPP DJ (1987) Management of allergy-related serous otitis. *Am J Otolaryngol* **5**:463–467.

RATNER D, ESHEL E & VIGDER K (1985) Juvenile rheumatoid arthritis and milk allergy. *J Roy Soc Med* **78**:410–413.

RICHET C (1931) Food anaphylaxis. *J Allergy* **2**:76–84.

RUBENSTEIN L (1950) Sensitivity to sesame seed and sesame oil. *NY State J Med* **50**:343–344.

RUBIN JM, SHAPIRO J, MUEHLBAUER P & GROLNICK M (1965) Shock reaction following ingestion of mango. *J Am Med Ass* **193**:147–398.

RUDD P & MANUEL P & WALKER-SMITH J (1981) Anaphylactic shock in an infant after feeding with a wheat rusk. A transient phenomenon. *Postgrad Med J* **57**:794–795.

RUOKONEN J, PAGANUS A & LEHTI H (1982) Elimination diets in the treatment of secretory otitis media. *Int J Pediat Otorhinolaryngol* **4**:39–46.

SABBAH A, DROUET M, MILLET B & BISET T (1990) Rhinite perannuelle par allergie alimentaire. *Allergie Immunol* **22**:51–55.

SALFIELD SAW, WARDLEY BL, HOULSBY WT *et al.* (1987) Controlled study of exclusion of dietary vasoactive amines in migraine. *Arch Dis Child* **62**:458–460.

SANDBERG D (1987) Food sensitivity: the kidney and bladder. In Brostoff J & Challacombe SJ (eds) *Food Allergy and Intolerance*, pp. 755–767, Baillière Tindall, London.

SANDBERG DH, McINTOSH RM, BERNSTEIN CW, CARR R & STRAUSS J (1977) Severe steroid-responsive nephrosis associated with hypersensitivity. *Lancet* **1**:388–390.

SANDLER M, YOUDIM MBH & HANINGTON E (1974) A phenylethylamine oxidising defect in migraine. *Nature* **250**:335–337.

SCHIFFMAN SS, BUCKLEY CE, SAMPSON HA et al. (1987) Aspartame and susceptibility to headache. *New Engl J Med* **317**:1181–1185.

SCHWARTZ RM, BOYES S & AYNSLEY-GREEN A (1989b) Metabolic effects of three ketogenic diets in the treatment of severe epilepsy. *Dev Med Child Neurol* **31**:152–160.

SCHWARTZ RH, EATON J, BOWER BD & AYNSLEY-GREEN A (1989a) Ketogenic diets in the treatment of epilepsy: short-term clinical effects. *Dev Med Child Neurol* **31**:145–151.

SCHWEITZER JW, FRIEDHOFF AJ & SCHWARTZ R (1975) Chocolate, β-phenethylamine and migraine re-examined. *Nature* **257**:256.

SCOTT RB, GALL DG & MARIC M (1990) Mediation of food protein-induced jejunal smooth muscle contraction in sensitised rats. *Am J Physiol* **259**:G6–G14.

SKÖLDSTAM L & MAGNUSSON KE (1991) Fasting, intestinal permeability, and rheumatoid arthritis. *Rheum Dis Clin N Am* **17**:363–371.

SMITH LH (1976) *Improving Your Child's Behavior Chemistry*, Pocket Books, New York.

SMITH T (1990) Allergy to peanuts. Reactions may be severe and patients should be prepared. *Br Med J* **300**:1354.

STEVENS LJ & STONER RB (1979) *How to Improve Your Child's Behavior Through Diet*, Signet, New York.

TAYLOR DC (1992) Outlandish factitious illness. In David TJ (ed) *Recent Advances in Paediatrics*, vol. 10, pp. 63–76, Churchill Livingstone, London.

TAYLOR E (1985) *The Hyperactive Child. A Parents' Guide*, Martin Dunitz, London.

TEAHON K, BJARNASON I & LEVI AJ (1988) Elemental diets in the management of Crohn's disease – a 10 year review (abstract). *Gastroenterology* **94**:A457.

THOMAS JW & WICKSTEN VP (1944) Allergy in relation to the genito-urinary tract. *Ann Allergy* **2**:396–403.

THORLEY G (1984) Pilot study to assess behavioural and cognitive effects of artificial food colours in a group of retarded children. *Dev Med Child Neurol* **26**:56–61.

TOGOOD JH (1988) Risk of anaphylaxis in patients receiving beta-blocker drugs. *J Allergy Clin Immunol* **81**:1–5.

TORSNEY PJ (1964) Hypersensitivity to sesame seed. *J Allergy* **35**:514–519.

UNGER DL, KUBIK F & UNGER L (1959) Urinary tract allergy. *J Am Med Ass* **170**:1308–1309.

UVITSKY IH (1956) Sensitivity to sesame seed. *J Allergy* **22**:377–378.

VAN SOMEREN VV, ROBINSON RO, McARDLE B & STURGEON N (1990) Restricted diets for treatment of migraine. *J Pediat* **117**:509–510.

VARLEY CK (1984) Diet and behavior of children with attention deficit disorder. *J Am Acad Child Psychiat* **23**:182–185.

VAUGHAN WT & HAWKE EK (1931) Angioneurotic edema with some unusual manifestations. *J Allergy* **2**:125–129.

VISCOMI GJ (1975) Allergic secretory otitis media: an approach to management. *Laryngoscope* **85**:751–758.

WARREN JB, DOBLE N, DALTON N & EWAN PW (1986) Systemic absorption of inhaled epinephrine. *Clin Pharmacol Ther* **40**:673–678.

WARREN JB, MCCUSKER M & FULLER RW (1988) Systemic adrenaline attenuates skin response to antigen and histamine. *Clin Allergy* **18**:197–199.

WELSH CJR, HANGLOW AC, CONN P & COOMBS RRA (1986) Comparison of the arthritogenic properties of dietary cow's milk, egg albumin and soya milk in experimental animals. *Int Arch Allergy Appl Immunol* **80**:192–199.

WENDER EH & SOLANTO MV (1991) Effects of sugar on aggressive and inattentive behavior in children with attention deficit disorder and hyperactivity and normal children. *Pediatrics* **88**:960–966.

WILKEN-JENSEN K & MELCHIOR JC (1970) Food allergy, anaphylactic shock and neurological symptoms. *Ann Allergy* **28**:539–542.

WILLIAMS AC & FRANKLIN I (1989) Migraine after bone-marrow transplantation. *Lancet* **2**:1286–1287.

WILLIAMSON JW (1961) Anaphylactoid reaction to oranges. *J Florida Med Ass* **48**:247.

WOJTULEWSKI JA (1987) Joints and connective tissue. In Brostoff J & Challacombe SJ (eds) *Food Allergy and Intolerance*, pp. 723–735, Baillière Tindall, London.

WRAITH DG (1982) Asthma and rhinitis. *Clin Immunol Allergy* **2**:101–112.

YUNGINGER JW, SWEENEY KG, STURNER WQ *et al.* (1988) Fatal food-induced anaphylaxis. *J Am Med Ass* **260**:1450–1452.

ZALESKI A, SHOKEIR MK & GERRARD JW (1972) Enuresis: familial incidence and relationship to allergic disorders. *Can Med Ass J* **106**:30–31.

Part 16   Elimination Diets

70 General principles of elimination diets
Precise definition is important

Purpose
Elimination diets are used either for the diagnosis or the treatment of food intolerance, or for both. It is important to remember that a diet may be associated with an improvement in symptoms for one or more of three main reasons:
1 intolerance to the food avoided;
2 coincidence;
3 placebo effect.

Degree of avoidance
The degree of avoidance that is necessary to prevent symptoms is highly variable. At one extreme, there are patients who are extremely sensitive to even minute traces of a food. An example would be an urticarial reaction following exposure to the odour of food being cooked (Horesh 1943; Derbes & Krafchuk 1957). Clearly complete avoidance will be required if symptoms are to be prevented. At the other extreme, some patients are able to tolerate moderate amounts of a food, and only react adversely to larger quantities. For example, Hill *et al.* (1988) found that some patients with late onset symptoms of cow's milk protein intolerance required 600–700 ml of milk daily for more than 48 hours before symptoms developed. In between these two extremes are, for example, patients with cow's milk protein intolerance in whom 60–70 ml of milk is adequate to provoke a clinical symptoms (Hill *et al.* 1988).

Some patients only need to avoid specific foods when these are taken under certain circumstances. An example would be food-provoked exercise-induced anaphylaxis, where anaphylaxis only occurs if a specific food is taken shortly before exercise (see chapter 58).

Are *symptoms* the important end-point?
This is an important area of uncertainty. Clearly in a patient with severe symptoms (e.g. anaphylactic shock) one would wish to minimize the risks of exposure to even small traces of a food. However, there are a number of unanswered questions. In a child with food intolerance, does it matter if the child occasionally takes small amounts of the food trigger, leading to minor symptoms (e.g. mild transient skin erythema) which are easily tolerated? Could this be harmful, and be associated either with increasing sensitivity to the food, or alternatively could it be associated with occult

symptoms (e.g. iron deficiency or mild malabsorption in a child with cow's milk protein intolerance)? Or could repeated exposure in some circumstances lead to either hyposensitization or help the child to grow out of the food intolerance? In general, these issues have not been objectively addressed.

Coeliac disease – exception or rule?

In coeliac disease it is established that lapses in a gluten-free diet, although not necessarily associated with obvious symptoms such as diarrhoea, may well be associated with less apparent symptoms, such as iron deficiency, growth failure, or in adults, sub-fertility (Branksi & Lebenthal 1989).

what is gluten-free?

Even here, however, there is uncertainty about what really constitutes a gluten-free diet, for it is evident that such diets often do contain small amounts of gluten (see chapter 26).

need for strict diet?

Patients with coeliac disease are advised to pursue a very strict avoidance diet on the theory that ingestion of even small amounts of gluten will lead to intestinal damage and recurrence of symptoms. These diets eliminate all products made from wheat, rye, barley and oats, including many products that may contain no gluten or only traces of this protein such as wheat starch and hydrolysed vegetable protein (Hartsook 1984). These strict diets are a prudent choice in the absence of proof that these products contain absolutely no gluten or that traces of gluten will not aggravate the illness. Research is needed to define the reactions of patients with coeliac disease to traces of gluten, and to identify foods made from wheat, rye, barley and oats that contain no gluten. The results might remove the requirement for patients to be on such strict avoidance diets (Taylor *et al.* 1987).

Rotation diets

In a so-called rotation diet, a food or a food family eaten on day 1 is then avoided for anything from 3–30 days. The aim is to 'give the body a rest from each food family', to 'prevent new or increased sensitivity to foods developing' (Monro 1987). However, there is no objective evidence that the development of food intolerance can be prevented in this way. Considering that cross-reactivity between different foods in a family is unusual (see chapter 71), diets which are based on the avoidance of entire food families are illogical.

Duration of diet

The duration required for a diet varies. The durations required for diagnostic diets are shown in Table 70.1. The duration required depends on how long the child remains intolerant to a food. In some cases, for example food additives, intolerance may only last a few months or years (Pollock & Warner 1987) but in others, most

Table 70.1 Duration required to determine therapeutic response to a diagnostic elimination diet

Clinical problem	Duration of diet required	Comments
Atopic eczema – milk- and egg-free diet	1–2 weeks	This is the minimum period. The natural fluctuation in disease severity means that a longer therapeutic trial (e.g. 6 weeks) is more likely to avoid confusion resulting from chance improvement or placebo response
Severe atopic eczema – few-food diet	6 weeks	Longer period required: (a) because of time taken for severe disease to improve, if it is going to; (b) diet is so disruptive it is important to get a clear idea of possible benefit; and (c) early placebo benefit common
Severe atopic eczema – elemental diet (e.g. Vivonex, 028)	4–6 weeks	Same comments as for few-food diet apply, but shorter time acceptable if a clear positive or negative outcome at 4 weeks (see Devlin *et al.* 1990)
Suspected cow's milk protein intolerance in infancy with prominent gastrointestinal symptoms, e.g. loose stools vomiting, irritability	1–3 days	Response should be very rapid, except in the presence of enteropathy and failure to thrive, where resolution may take a week or two to occur and possibly a few weeks to detect; here a trial period of 2–4 weeks may be more appropriate
Chronic urticaria	6–12 weeks	Depends on frequency of symptoms; if episodes only occur every week or two then it may take a few months to be certain of success or failure
Migraine	6–12 weeks	Depends on frequency of attacks; as with chronic urticaria it may take a few months to be certain of success or failure

notably intolerance to peanuts (Bock & Atkins 1989), it may be life-long.

Need for definition of duration

If one is to avoid leaving patients on unnecessary diets for many years, then it is essential to define for how long any diet is required. A diagnostic diet must always be accompanied by plans to re-assess the patient after a defined period, to see if the diet was helpful, and to determine whether it needs to be continued and if so for how long. A therapeutic diet must be accompanied by recommendations about duration. Apart from patients with life-threatening reactions, periodic food re-introductions are recommended (e.g. every 6 months) to detect the development of tolerance.

Cost

It is often stated that elimination diets are very costly (Nieborg-Eshuis 1991) and that diets are sometimes abandoned because of the 'immense financial burden' (Hathaway & Warner 1983) but there is little evidence to support this. The only systematic study is that

Table 70.2 Estimated (in 1986) weekly cost of elimination diets[1]

Diet	4-year-old boy	8-year-old boy	15–17-year-old boy
Calculated cost of normal diet based on DHSS figures for recommended daily amounts[2]	£5.40	£6.80	£9.46
Cow's milk-free diet[3]	£5.41	£6.22	£8.39
Gluten-free diet	£5.58	£6.81	£9.38
Wheat-free diet	£7.68	£9.33	£12.77
Leeds elimination diet of milk substitute[4], rice, lamb, 7-Up lemonade, carrots, pears, peaches, apricots, milk-free margarine, sugar, salt, 'Polo' mints	£11.29	£13.01	£16.30

[1] Based on data collected in Leeds, England—see Macdonald & Forsythe (1986).
[2] Department of Health and Social Security (1979).
[3] Milk substitute available free on prescription.
[4] Available free on prescription.

of Macdonald & Forsyth (1986) who were able to demonstrate a marginal increase in cost of gluten- or wheat-free diets when compared with the cost of a normal diet. They noted a marked increase in cost of a rather unconventional elimination diet, but it was unclear to what extent certain unusually expensive items, such as peaches and apricots, may have contributed to the overall high cost. On the other hand, a milk-free diet was cheaper than normal diet at certain ages, because of the availability of a cow's milk substitute free on prescription (Table 70.2).

Psychological effects

The potentially handicapping psychological effects of elimination diets are often overlooked, presumably on the grounds that such problems are outweighed by the impact of the intolerance itself. In some situations (e.g. life-threatening reactions or coeliac disease) the need for some sort of food avoidance is absolute. In other situations, however, the benefits of food avoidance may be offset by the disadvantages. An elimination diet may require a child to avoid foods given to siblings or contemporaries at school, but the obvious drawbacks of such situations, although important, have never been quantified. In short, the diet may be worse than the disease, and even where food intolerance is strongly suspected, food avoidance is not necessarily the best solution. The fact that the psychological drawbacks to food avoidance have not been quantified should not be taken as evidence of safety. We have no idea of the possible long-term effects of elimination diets on adult behaviour or eating patterns, and it would be surprising if there were none.

Adherence

If children are to adhere to a dietary regimen, it is important that the parents and child understand the reasons why a diet is being used, and how the relevant foods are to be avoided. Without knowledge and understanding, adherence is impossible. The main reasons for non-adherence to a dietary regimen are listed in Table 70.3.

non-adherence

Diets are easy to prescribe but difficult to follow. Non-adherence (sometimes called non-compliance, a rather judgemental term which implies failure to follow commands) to dietary regimens has received little systematic attention, the main exception being diets for diabetes mellitus (Thomas, 1988). One study which did address this problem examined 40 children with atopic eczema who were treated with a variety of elimination diets (Hathaway & Warner, 1983). Despite some degree of benefit from the diets, three out of 14 children (21%) under 3 years of age and 12 of 26 children (46%) over 3 years of age gave up their diets, with subsequent relapse of their eczema.

Key references 70.1

POLLOCK I & WARNER JO (1987) A follow-up study of childhood food additive intolerance. *J Roy Coll Phys Lond* **21**:248–250. In 76% of 34 children with additive intolerance, the intolerance was transient, and disappeared by the time of repeat challenges 1–5 (mean 2.8) years after the original diagnosis and positive challenge. *Additive intolerance in children is mainly a transient phenomenon.*

70.2

BOCK SA & ATKINS FM (1989) The natural history of peanut allergy. *J Allergy Clin Immunol* **83**:900–904. Of 32 children with intolerance to peanut who were followed up for 2–14 years, none had outgrown their intolerance. Challenge studies showed intolerance to soya in one child and pea in another. Although skin-prick tests were often positive to other nuts, no patient with a positive double-blind peanut challenge had a positive challenge to any other nut. In 14 other children with positive challenges to either walnut (seven), pecan (six), pistachio (two) or filbert (one), one patient reacted to five nuts, one patient

Table 70.3 Reasons for failure to adhere to dietary regimen

Insufficient knowledge or understanding by family

Diet too intrusive to be acceptable to patient or family

Diet fails to reduce or abolish symptoms

Excessive expectations of benefit from diet (e.g. cure rather than improvement in atopic eczema)

Diet no longer needed (child grown out of food intolerance)

reacted to two nuts, and the other 12 reacted to a single nut each. None of the 14 reacted to peanut. *Peanut intolerance is likely to be life-long and not associated with intolerance to other nuts.*

70.3   Macdonald A & Forsythe WI (1986) The cost of nutrition and diet therapy for low-income families. *Hum Nutr Appl Nutr* **40A**:87–96. The authors calculated the cost of a normal diet, a gluten-free diet, a wheat-free diet, an unusual type of elimination diet for food intolerance, a milk-free diet, a reducing diet, a diabetic diet, and two types of cystic fibrosis diet. Figures were given for a 4-year old boy, an 8-year old boy, a 15–17-year old boy, and a 'moderately active man'. *Most diets were more expensive than a normal diet, the main exception being milk-free diets, where the cost was reduced by the availability of a milk substitute free on prescription.*

70.4   Hathaway MJ & Warner JO (1983) Compliance problems in the dietary management of eczema. *Arch Dis Child* **58**:463–464. A number of rather different diets were used in the management of atopic eczema. Out of an unstated total number of cases thus treated, 40 appeared to benefit. However 15 of 40 patients abandoned their diet. *Diet response is either due to food trigger avoidance, placebo effect, or coincidence. Those in the latter groups are likely to abandon their diets, and this is of course quite appropriate. Those with atopic eczema and genuine food intolerance may benefit from a diet but they may also find that the diet is more inconvenient than the disease and chose to abandon the diet.*

Summary 70   Elimination diets are used either for the diagnosis or the treatment of food intolerance, or for both. A diet may be associated with an improvement in symptoms because of intolerance to the food, a placebo effect, or the improvement may have been a coincidence. The degree of avoidance that is necessary to prevent symptoms is highly variable. Some patients are intolerant to minute traces of food, but others may be able to tolerate varying amounts. Strict avoidance and prevention of symptoms are the aims in certain instances, but in many cases it is unknown whether allowing small amounts of a food trigger could lead to either enhanced sensitivity or to the reverse, increasing tolerance. The duration required for dietary avoidance varies; for example, intolerance to food additives may last only a few years, whereas intolerance to peanuts is usually lifelong. If one is to avoid patients being left on unnecessary diets for many years, then it is essential to define for how long any diet is required. The possible adverse psychological effect of elimination diets is an important but neglected subject.

71 Specificity and cross-reaction
Apart from animal milks, cross-reactions are uncommon

Specificity for a food It is sometimes unclear to what extent a certain food should be avoided. Should a patient with soya intolerance be advised to avoid all products made from soya beans (see chapter 21), including soya oil, soya sauce, hydrolysed vegetable protein, and soya lecithin? The child with severe reactions may be advised to avoid all products from the offending food, but does this have a sound basis?

protein component The offending allergen is likely to be part of the protein component of the food, but in food products, such as peanut oil and soya oil, it is unclear whether protein is always present (see chapter 4).

hydrolysed protein In other foods, such as soya sauce or hydrolysed vegetable protein, the protein is partially or completely hydrolysed. In the case of hydrolysed peanut protein, this failed to compete with a crude peanut extract in a RAST inhibition test, suggesting that the hydrolysed protein may not be allergenic (Nordlee *et al.* 1981). The degree of hydrolysis is likely to be important, and studies of cow's milk protein intolerance show that hydrolysis of casein or whey is no guarantee that the resulting items will be tolerated by all patients (see chapter 18).

'hidden' protein Protein may be found to be 'hidden' in various manufactured foods. Examples are lecithin from soya, which contains 1–27 mg/g soya protein, gum arabic, from *Acacia senegal* or related species of *Acacia*, which contains approximately 2% of protein, and guar gum which may contain in excess of 10% protein (Porras *et al.* 1985; Randall *et al.* 1989; Bindels & Verwimp 1990; Lagier *et al.* 1990). One could speculate that this might be particularly important for vegetable gums such as gum arabic, to which sensitization during occupational exposure (inhalation and skin contact) is a well recognized cause of rhinitis, asthma, urticaria and contact dermatitis (Gelfand 1943, 1949). There is a report of an adult in whom asthma and urticaria resulted from the ingestion of gum tragacanth which was an excipient in a tablet (Brown *et al.* 1947).

Empirical advice unavoidable The more complicated a diet, the more room there is for mistakes or non-adherence. Diets are often simplified merely to avoid confusion. For example, those with cow's milk protein intolerance are advised to avoid all forms of cow's milk, including heat-treated forms such as evaporated or condensed milk. In fact, a small number of subjects with milk protein intolerance will tolerate these milks, but the trouble required to identify this minority makes such a tailor-made diet impractical.

Cross-reactivity   If a child is intolerant to one food (e.g. a nut, fish or bean), is it necessary to avoid other foods from the same family (i.e. other nuts, fish or beans)? There is no simple answer, and this is a major area of uncertainty. However, it is clear that although skin-prick tests and *in vitro* tests for IgE antibodies commonly demonstrate cross-reactivity among members of a botanical or animal family (e.g. Vaughan 1930; Barnett *et al.* 1987; Bernhisel-Broadbent *et al.* 1989), with the exception of animal milk, clinical evidence of such cross-reactivity is much less common.

animal milk   It appears that there is a high degree of cross-reactivity between the milk of cows, goats and sheep. In one study, 22 of 28 infants and children with cow's milk protein intolerance were also intolerant to goats' milk (Juntunen & Ali-Yrkkö 1983), but there is little other firm data (see chapter 15).

eggs   As with milk, it appears that there is a high degree of cross-reactivity between the eggs of chickens, ducks, geese and turkeys, but there is scanty firm data (see chapter 23).

seafood   The taxonomic diversity (fish, molluscs, crustaceans) suggests that complete cross-reactivity for all seafood is unlikely to be common. However, there is a lack of useful clinical data on the subject. In one study (de Martino *et al.* 1990), of 20 children with a history of intolerance to cod, there was a history of intolerance to sole in 11 (55%), tuna in seven (35%), and mackerel, anchovy, sardine, red mullet and salmon each in one (5%). The remaining major studies of cross-reactivity are based on skin-prick and IgE antibody test results (e.g. McCants & Lehrer 1985; Waring *et al.* 1985) which are of little relevance to clinical sensitivity (see chapter 43).

legumes   It is not always obvious which plants belong to the same family, and an example would be the Leguminosae (Table 71.1), which includes beans, peas, soya, lentils, peanuts, liquorice, carob and gum arabic. Cross-reactivity has been reported (Gall *et al.* 1990), but it appears to be uncommon (Bernhisel-Broadbent & Sampson 1989), and the degree of genetic relationship may be of little relevance. Thus, for example, patients with soya intolerance often give a history of peanut intolerance (e.g. Bush *et al.* 1985; Herian al 1990), although the two legumes are not closely related.

Table 71.1 Genetic relationships between some members of the Leguminosae family[1]

Common name	Sub-family	Tribe	Sub-tribe	Genus	Species
Peanut	Papilionoideae	Hedysareae	Stylosanthinae	*Arachis*	*hypogea*
Soya bean	Papilionoideae	Phaseoleae	Glycininae	*Glycine*	*max*
Scarlet runner bean	Papilionoideae	Phaseoleae	Phaseolinae	*Phaseolus*	*coccineus* or *multiflorus*
French bean	Papilionoideae	Phaseoleae	Phaseolinae	*Phaseolus*	*vulgaris*
Asparagus or Goa tertragonolobus bean	Papilionoideae	Phaseoleae	Phaseolinae	*Psophocarpus*	
Lima bean (butter bean)	Papilionoideae	Phaseoleae	Phaseolinae	*Phaseolus*	*lunatus*
Mung bean	Papilionoideae	Phaseoleae	Phaseolinae	*Vigna*	*aureus*
Yam	Papilionoideae	Phaseoleae	Phaseolinae	*Pachyrhizus*	*erosus*
Broad bean	Papilionoideae	Vicieae	−	*Vicia*	*faba*
Garden pea	Papilionoideae	Vicieae	−	*Pisum*	*sativum*
Chick pea or garbanzo bean	Papilionoideae	Vicieae	−	*Cicer*	*arietinum*
Grass pea or chickling vetch	Papilionoideae	Vicieae	−	*Lathyrus*	*sativus*
Lentil	Papilionoideae	Vicieae	−	*Lens*	*culinaris*
Tragacanth	Papilionoideae	Galegeae	Astragalinae	*Astragalus*	*gummifer*
Liquorice	Papilionoideae	Galegeae	Astragalinae	*Glycyrrhiza*	*glabra*
Guar	Papilionoideae	Galegeae	Indigoferinae	*Cyamopsis*	*tetragonoloba*
Fenugreek	Papilionoideae	Trifolieae	−	*Trigonella*	*foenum-graecum*
Carob bean	Caesalpiniodeae	Cassieae	−	*Ceratonia*	*siliqua*
Gum arabic	Mimosoideae	Acacieae	−	*Acacia*	*senegal*

[1] Source: Brouk (1975).

food and pollen

Cross-reactions can occur between inhaled pollen and ingested food allergens. Patients with allergy to mugwort pollen can have concomitant intolerance to celery (Pauli *et al.* 1985). A similar association has often been noted between birch tree pollen allergy and intolerance to a variety of foods such as apple, carrot, celery, potato, hazel nut, orange, tomato and peanut (Dreborg 1988). It has been suggested, but not proven, that this association might be explained by a structural similarity between birch pollen allergens and some antigens in these foods (Eriksson 1978).

Key references 71.1   TAYLOR SL, BUSH RK & BUSSE WW (1987) Avoidance diets − how selective should they be? In Chandra RK (ed) *Food Allergy*, pp. 253−266, Nutrition

Research Education Foundation, St. John's, Newfoundland. Review, of the degree of tolerance, specificity and cross-reactivity, which delivers the message that some elimination diets are needlessly strict. *Unfortunately the authors equate the presence of specific IgE antibodies with clinical intolerance, which diminishes the accuracy of some of the review's content.*

71.2   BERNHISEL-BROADBENT J & SAMPSON HA (1989) Cross-allergenicity in the legume botanical family in children with food hypersensitivity. *J Allergy Clin Immunol* **83**:435–440. Sixty-nine patients with positive skin-prick tests to legumes were studied with double-blind placebo-controlled food challenges. Only two patients had symptomatic intolerance to two legumes. *The results of food challenges demonstrate that despite laboratory evidence of extensive immunological cross-reactivity, clinically important cross-sensitivity to legumes in children is rare.*

71.3   DREBORG S (1988) Food allergy in pollen-sensitive patients. *Ann Allergy* **61**:41–46. *Useful review.*

71.4   DE MARTINO M, NOVEMBRE E, GALLI L et al. (1990) Allergy to different fish species in cod-allergic children: in vivo and in vitro studies. *J Allergy Clin Immunol* **86**:909–914. Twenty children with intolerance to cod were studied, and compared with 40 control children with a history of intolerance to foods other than cod. Of the 40 controls, there was a history of intolerance to sole in two and to tuna in one. In the study group, 55% gave a history of reacting to sole, 35% to tuna, and 5% to mackerel, anchovy, sardine, red mullet and salmon. However these percentages partly reflect a history of having consumed a particular fish; thus, all 20 had eaten sole, but only one (5%) had eaten salmon. Although all 20 of the study group and all 40 controls had eaten dogfish, there were no reports of intolerance to this.

71.5   ERIKSSON NE (1984) Clustering of foodstuffs in food hypersensitivity. An inquiry study in pollen allergic patients. *Allergol Immunopathol* **12**:28–32. Six hundred pollen allergic patients were questioned about intolerance to a range of foods, and reports of intolerance to one food were correlated with reports of intolerance to other foods. Thus, for example, for the 209 who reported reactions to apple, there was a correlation coefficient of 0.61 with intolerance to hazelnut. *The drawback to the data is that food intolerance was unconfirmed by challenges.*

71.6   BROUK B (1975) *Plants Consumed By Man*, Academic Press, London. *Invaluable source of information about the geographical origin, taxonomy, and a brief description of the edible portion, for all edible plants.*

Summary 71   It is not always clear to what extent a certain food (e.g. soya) should be avoided. Certain products of a food (e.g. soya oil) may be free from allergenic material, and tolerated, whereas other products (e.g. hydrolysed vegetable protein or soya lecithin) may contain sufficient allergenic material to provoke an adverse reaction in some intolerant individuals. Although tests for specific IgE antibodies commonly demonstrate cross-reactivity among members of a botanical family or animal species, clinical evidence of cross-reactivity is the exception rather than the rule.

72 Nutritional hazards
Malnutrition is a major risk of unsupervised diets

Depends on foods excluded

The nutritional adequacy of a diet depends largely on the food or foods being avoided. Avoidance of a single food such as strawberries or tomatoes is relatively simple, and not likely to cause any nutritional deficiencies. However, the avoidance of other foods such as cow's milk, poses important nutritional problems, especially in young children, where milk is an important source of protein, energy, calcium and vitamins.

What is nutritional adequacy?

It is self evident that a child must eat enough of the right foods to thrive and grow. It is far from clear, however, how to define an adequate intake for an individual child, and this is an important area of uncertainty. The figures for recommended daily amounts (World Health Organisation 1974; Department of Health & Social Security 1979; Committee on Dietary Allowances 1980) are subject to major drawbacks:

1 They were intended to be applied to groups of children, and not individuals. Individual needs are bound to vary from one child to another.

2 The figures were drawn up by a committee, rather than based on objective studies.

3 The figures are designed to err on the side of safety, safety being equated with an intake above an unstated minimum.

Dietary reference values

The old and unsatisfactory term of recommended daily amount has recently been abandoned in the UK. A new report from the Committee on Medical Aspects of Food Policy has introduced two new concepts (Department of Health 1991). One is the reference nutrient intake, which is defined as the amount of the nutrient that is enough, or more than enough, for about 97% of people in a group. The other is the estimated average requirement, which is defined as the requirement of a nutrient for a group of people, about half of whom will usually need more than the estimated average requirement, and half less. The committee set up a number of expert working groups to consider the requirements of children and adults for about 40 different nutrients, and their recommendations are accompanied by a discussion of the function, metabolism and age-related requirements for each nutrient.

Determining intake To establish whether a child's diet is adequate one needs to know the intake of individual nutrients, but this is not easy to discover. A simple diet history may give sufficient information to establish whether or not an intake is reasonable, particularly in a child with a normal or near-normal diet (the possible meaning of the term 'normal diet' is outside the scope of this book). Otherwise some record needs to be made of the child's intake over a few days (Marr 1971; Todd *et al.* 1983). This either involves weighing all food before it is eaten, which is a cumbersome method only suitable for research studies, or the parents making a record of approximate amounts of food consumed, in terms of simple household measures. To even out variations in intake, such studies are usually conducted over 3, 5 or 7 days. The analysis of such records is extremely laborious, though it can be speeded up with the use of a microcomputer on which is stored nutritional data (Holland *et al.* 1992) from a large range of foods (Bassham *et al.* 1984).

Intake only one aspect Nutrient intake is only one aspect of nutrition. An individual child may have, for example, higher energy or protein requirements because of malabsorption or chronic disease. An intake can only be defined as adequate when it equals or exceeds the individual's requirements, which may vary. An example which illustrates the complexity of the problem, is that children with severe atopic eczema may have hypoalbuminaemia (Goodyear & Harper 1989; David *et al.* 1990), and it is possible that in such cases a normal diet may be inadequate to meet the increased needs of the individual. Note, however, that this statement makes the assumption that increasing the food intake in such children will correct the hypoalbuminaemia, but in fact this has never been demonstrated.

Need for a dietitian The dietitian has three roles in this context. One is to ensure that the resulting diet is nutritionally adequate, and prevent potential deficiency states by recommending appropriate amounts of infant milk formula, and supplements of calcium, vitamins and so on. Another role is to advise the parents how to avoid specific foods, particularly in manufactured foods, and if appropriate to provide recipes to help in the preparation and inclusion of unusual or unfamiliar ingredients. The third role of the dietitian is to give suggestions as to how to make the diet practical and palatable, and suggest recipes for the use of a limited range of foods (e.g. how to make biscuits with potato flour).

Calcium Cow's milk is an important source of calcium, and avoidance of cow's milk and its products carries the risk of an inadequate intake of calcium. Unfortunately, it is far from clear what constitutes an adequate intake. The subject is discussed further in chapters 15 and 72.

Protein, energy

Milk, eggs, fish, meat, wheat and their respective manufactured food products, are important sources of protein and energy. Avoidance of these without the provision of alternative sources of protein and energy runs the risk of an inadequate intake, and growth failure and serious malnutrition are well documented sequelae of unsupervised and inappropriate dietary elimination (Editorial 1978; Lloyd-Still 1979; Roberts *et al.* 1979; Tripp *et al.* 1979; Tarnow-Mordi *et al.* 1984; David 1985; Hughes *et al.* 1986; David 1987; Labib *et al.* 1989; Dagnelie *et al.* 1991).

Iodine

Cow's milk and dairy products are an important source of dietary iodine. A child has been reported in whom the unsupervised exclusion of cow's milk products and a number of other items from the diet, coupled with the consumption of large amounts of soya milk, which has been reported to cause hypothyroidism by increasing faecal loss of thyroxine, resulted in hypothyroidism and growth failure due to dietary iodine deficiency (Shepard *et al.* 1960; Labib *et al.* 1989).

Special danger situations

Elimination diets may pose special nutritional problems. Situations where there is a special risk are:

1 *Unsupervised diets*: risk of malnutrition (David 1985).

2 *Parental obsession*: risk of inappropriate escalation of dietary avoidance (David 1985, 1987).

3 *Chronic disease* prior to diagnosis, or concurrent chronic disease such as severe atopic eczema. Child's nutrient requirements may be increased.

4 *Malabsorption or enteropathy*: risk of malabsorption of nutrients.

5 *Child avoiding sunlight*: risk of vitamin D deficiency compounding the effects of a low calcium intake (David 1989).

6 Where a child is *already on a diet* which excludes multiple foods, e.g. vegan or macrobiotic diet (Dagnelie *et al.* 1991).

Key references 72.1

DAVID TJ, WADDINGTON E & STANTON RHJ (1984) Nutritional hazards of elimination diets in children with atopic eczema. *Arch Dis Child* **59**:323–325. The intake of nutrients over 5 days was studied in 23 children with atopic eczema who were on an elimination diet, and 23 healthy controls not on a diet. Significantly low intakes of calcium were discovered in 13 patients but not in controls.

72.2

DEVLIN J, STANTON RHJ & DAVID TJ (1989) Calcium intake and cows' milk free diets. *Arch Dis Child* **64**:1183–1184. In children with atopic eczema on elimination diets, the calcium intake was, as one might have predicted, below the estimated daily requirement in 15 out of 20 who were avoiding cow's milk and received no milk substitute. However, of the 26 who were avoiding cow's milk but had been provided with a soya or casein-hydrolysate infant formula, three had a calcium intake below the estimated requirement. *It is unsafe to assume that calcium requirements will be adequately provided by the prescription of a cow's milk substitute. Such formulae have a lower calcium content than cow's milk formulae, the child may stop drinking the milk because of poor palatibility, and calcium intake may be further compromised by other dietary restrictions.*

72.3   DAVID TJ (1987) Unhelpful recent developments in the diagnosis and treatment of allergy and food intolerance in children. In Dobbing J (ed) *Food Intolerance*, pp. 185–214, Baillière Tindall, London. Review of a range of unorthodox allergy treatments, including report of severe malnutrition in a 13-month old infant, resulting from a severely restricted diet.

72.4   BASSHAM S, FLETCHER LR & STANTON RHJ (1984) Dietary analysis with the aid of a microcomputer. *J Micromcomputer Applic* **7**:279–289. Describes the design, development, implementation and use of a microcomputer software package to assist dietitians with the arithmetical drudgery of computing the nutritional composition of food.

Summary 72   Unsupervised restriction of a child's diet risks an inadequate intake of nutrients, resulting in specific deficiencies, growth failure and malnutrition. Dietetic supervision is designed to help prevent malnutrition by the use of appropriate supplements, and to ensure complete avoidance of individual foods. A major area of uncertainty is the lack of validated data on what constitutes age-related adequate intakes for specific nutrients. Current recommendations are empirical, are intended for groups of subjects and not individuals, and err on the side of safety, equating safety with an intake above an unstated minimum.

73 Cow's milk-free diets
The major trap is manufactured food

Cow's milk protein intolerance   Cow's milk protein intolerance is described in detail in chapters 5 to 15.

Ask the dietitian   The details given here, and in chapter 15, are not exhaustive. The composition of manufactured foods is constantly changing, and varies from country to country. The dietitian should be consulted, as he or she will have access to an up-to-date list of milk-free manufactured foods, and in addition can give parents useful tips and warn of special pitfalls.

Cow's milk   Any form of cow's milk, whether fresh, skimmed, condensed or evaporated, needs to be avoided. The rationale for avoiding heat-treated milk, such as condensed milk, which might be tolerated by a minority of patients, is discussed in chapter 16. Also forbidden are milk products such as casein, whey and non-fat milk solids.

Milk substitutes   The choice lies between formulae based on soya protein, casein hydrolysate or whey hydrolysate (see Table 17.1). Soya formulae are cheaper, but unsuitable for those who are also intolerant to soya.

Butter, margarine, milk products   Butter, margarine, cream, cheese, ice-cream and yoghurt all need to be avoided. Fats which can be used instead include margarines made from pure vegetable fat (e.g. Tomor) and lard.

'Vegetarian' cheese differs from ordinary cheese only by the use of non-animal rennet, and is unsuitable.

Meat, game, poultry   Meat, game and poultry are all allowed, but sausages and pies should be avoided unless it is known that they are milk-free. Intolerance to cow's milk protein is not a reason to avoid beef.

Eggs   Eggs are allowed, but not custard or scrambled egg which may contain milk.

Fish   Fish is allowed, unless it is cooked in batter (which unless otherwise stated should be assumed to contain milk) or milk.

Confectionery   Sugar (except for hydrolysed milk sugar), jam, honey, mincemeat, jelly, boiled sweets, pastilles and gums are allowed. Lemon curd, chocolate spread, chocolate (unless stated to be milk-free), toffee, fudge, caramels and butterscotch are all unsuitable.

Cereals   All ordinary cereals (e.g. oats) are allowed, but caution is required with manufactured breakfast cereals, some of which contain milk powder.

Baby foods   Caution is required, as a large number of manufactured products contain milk protein. For example, rusks may contain milk protein.

Flour products   Items such as bread, cakes, biscuits and puddings are freely allowed, provided they are not made with milk, milk solids, butter or margarine.

Vegetables, fruit   Vegetables and fruit, whether fresh, frozen or tinned, are suitable, but vegetables cooked with butter or milk (e.g. instant potato, creamed potato, cauliflower cheese) must be avoided.

All manufactured foods   It is essential to check the list of ingredients on the label. Beware of unwrapped foods, such as bread, sausages or confectionery, where it is impossible to know the ingredients used in manufacture. In Britain, beware of chocolate products, which are exempt from labelling regulations and may contain a number of unexpected ingredients such as milk or egg.

Contamination   Contamination of manufactured foods with food proteins can occur. Six children with cow's milk protein intolerance who experienced adverse reactions to non-milk products were investigated. In each case, with the use of a sensitive inhibition enzyme-linked immuno-assay, traces of cow's milk protein were found in the 'non-dairy' foods which had been implicated (Gern *et al.* 1991). The products were tofu, hot dogs, a rice desert, a hot dog, bologna and canned tuna fish. In some cases it was unclear how contamination had occurred, while in others the problem was that casein had been omitted from the list of ingredients. In another example, inadequate cleaning of a food processing machine following peanut butter production allowed the contamination by peanut butter of subsequently manufactured jars of sunflower butter (Yunginger *et al.* 1983). The consumption of this sunflower butter caused an adverse reaction in a child known to be intolerant to peanuts.

Key references   73.1   Francis DEM (1987) *Diets for Sick Children*, 4th edn, Blackwell Scientific Publications, Oxford. Useful review of milk-free diets.

73.2   Thomas B (1988) (ed) *Manual of Dietetic Practice*, Blackwell Scientific Publications, Oxford. Useful review of milk-free diets.

73.3   Gern JE, Yang E, Evrard HM & Sampson HA (1991) Allergic reactions to milk-contaminated 'non-dairy' products. *New Engl J Med* **324**:976–979. Detailed report of six children with cow's milk protein intolerance who experienced adverse reactions after consuming food products which were supposedly milk-free but which upon analysis were found to contain cow's milk protein. *The problem partly arose because of previous food-labelling regulations in the US which permitted the inclusion of casein in manufactured foods as 'natural flavouring', but in most cases was due to contamination of foods during manufacture.*

73.4   Yunginger JW, Gauerke MB, Jones RT, Dahlberg MJOE & Ackerman SJ (1983) Use of radioimmunoassay to determine the nature, quantity and source of allergenic contamination of sunflower butter. *J Food Protection* **46**:625–628. A girl known to be intolerant to peanuts experienced an immediate adverse reaction (oral soreness and itching followed by vomiting) after eating sunflower butter. The authors discovered that the manufacturing plant also produced peanut butter, and peanut butter contamination was found (by a solid-phase radioimmunoassay) in six of eight sunflower butter samples. Investigation suggested that inadequate cleaning of manufacturing equipment after peanut butter production led to contamination of sunflower butter manufactured with the same machinery.

Summary 73   All foods which contain cow's milk, such as milk, cream, butter, margarine, yoghurt, cheese, whey and casein, must be completely avoided. For manufactured foods this requires careful scrutiny of the list of ingredients on the label. Special caution is required for foods which are not wrapped and therefore do not have a list of ingredients, and chocolate products which are not required to state their full ingredients. The help of a dietitian, who will have an up-to-date list of milk-free manufactured foods and who can warn parents of special pitfalls, is recommended.

74   Egg-free diets
Minute traces may be sufficient to provoke symptoms

Egg intolerance   Egg intolerance is described in chapters 22 to 25.

Ask the dietitian   The dietitian will have an up-to-date list of egg-free manufactured foods, and in addition can give parents useful tips and warn of special pitfalls. Coping without a dietitian requires some knowledge of cookery and food manufacture. The following are special problems.

Albumen   Products which contain albumen must be avoided.

Cakes   Eggs are widely used to make cakes, such as sponge cakes, angel cakes or fruit cakes.

Bread   Eggs are sometimes used in the manufacture of bread, and this is a special problem because, as with cakes, a list of ingredients is usually not supplied, so that one depends on information provided by shopkeepers, who in turn may not be familiar with the ingredients.

Rolls, buns, baps   Egg wash or glaze is commonly brushed on to the surface of rolls, buns or baps, and also bread, cakes and pastry used in puddings (e.g. apple pie). This is done either to give a shiny glazed appearance, or to serve as an adhesive to attatch other items to the surface of the product. Thus it is not uncommon for parents to report that their child has had an urticarial reaction to sesame seeds after eating a burger bun or bap coated with sesame seeds. In practice the reaction is more likely to come from the egg wash.

Confectionery In the context of food intolerance, sweets are a special trap because they are usually sold without information about ingredients. Egg has been included in several, such as 'dolly mixture' and Opal Fruits (Francis 1987).

Custard, mayonnaise Mayonnaise should contain egg; custard usually does not, with the exception of egg custard and egg custard tarts.

Souffles Eggs are an essential ingredient of souffles.

Sauces Eggs are an essential ingredient of certain sauces, such as Bearnaise or Hollandaise sauce.

Chicken Egg intolerance is not a reason to avoid eating chicken.

Eggs of other birds As well as hen's eggs, eggs of other birds, such as geese, turkeys, quails, must be avoided.

Yolk is not safe Because egg yolk contains small amounts of egg white proteins (see chapters 22 and 23), egg yolk must be avoided.

Key references 74.1 FRANCIS DEM (1987) *Diets for Sick Children*, 4th edn, Blackwell Scientific Publications, Oxford. *Useful review of egg- and milk-free diets.*

74.2 THOMAS B (1988) (ed) *Manual of Dietetic Practice*. Blackwell Scientific Publications, Oxford. *Advice on egg avoidance and egg substitutes.*

Summary 74 All foods which contain the white or yolk of egg must be avoided, regardless of whether the egg was from a hen, goose, turkey or other bird. Common traps are egg wash on buns, baps, cakes and pastry, and confectionery which contains egg.

75 Avoidance of other foods and additives: common pitfalls
Beware chocolate, egg wash, sweets and sausages

Gluten-free   Detailed accounts of gluten-free diets are available elsewhere (Francis 1987; Thomas 1988) and will not be elaborated upon here. Some problems relating to the term 'gluten-free', which does not always mean quite that, are discussed in chapter 27.

Soya-free   Soya intolerance is described in chapter 21. The major pitfalls are mass-produced bread, which in the UK usually contains soya flour as a minor ingredient, manufactured products which contain hydrolysed or textured vegetable protein, and minced beef which unless described as pure beef has been known to include quantities of soya protein.

Food additives   Food additives are most simply avoided by basing a diet on fresh foods. Intolerance to food additives is discussed in chapters 33 to 37. Detailed accounts of additives and their avoidance are given elsewhere (Francis 1987; Hanssen & Marsden 1987; Thomas 1988) and will not be elaborated upon here.

Atopic disease   The dietary management of atopic disease, such as the few-food diet, is discussed in chapter 56. Elemental diets are discussed in chapters 19 and 56.

Common pitfalls   A number of common misunderstandings, pitfalls and traps are listed below.

Vegetarian cheese   Vegetarian cheese is often bought by those on cow's milk protein-free diets, the error being to assume that vegetarian means that no animal product (and therefore no milk) is included. In fact vegetarian cheese differs from ordinary cheese only by the use of non-animal rennet, and contains just as much milk protein as ordinary cheese.

Sausages   Sausages, which may be sold without any packaging (and therefore with a label to indicate the ingredients), often contain cow's milk protein.

Batter   Some recipes for batter comprise flour and water, but others include milk. Since labels usually describe batter without giving the

459

ingredients, it should be assumed to contain milk unless the product is specifically stated to be milk-free.

Ice-cream   Just because an ice-cream is said to contain non-milk fat does not mean it is free from cow's milk protein. The same applies to coffee-whiteners or coffee-creamers, which are often said to contain non-milk fat.

Chocolate products   In Britain, beware of chocolate products, which are exempt from the usual labelling regulations, and may contain a number of unexpected ingredients such as milk or egg. Even plain dark chocolate may contain milk and/or butter.

Baby cereals   Baby cereals, savouries and desserts, particularly the instant powder varieties, frequently contain milk powder, soya and wheat (Francis 1987).

Flour   Iron and vitamin B1 are often added to flour to bring the levels up to those required by statutory standards (Egan *et al.* 1981). Although only caramel may be used for colouring, flour may contain a wide range of bleaching and improving agents (Egan *et al.* 1981). There is no requirement to declare these ingredients on labels. In practice the only problem is for those with soya intolerance.

Potato crisps   The oil used to make crisps is rarely identified, and it may also contain antioxidants. Flavoured crisps may contain milk protein, even the 'salt & vinegar' type (Francis 1987).

Sweets   Hydrolysed whey sugar contains up to 10% milk protein, and is used in the manufacture of certain confectionery.

Wheat starch   Wheat starch is unsuitable for wheat- or cereal-free diets.

Key reference 75.1   THOMAS B (1988) (ed) *Manual of Dietetic Practice*, Blackwell Scientific Publications, Oxford. *Useful review of food and food additive avoidance, with practically based dietetic advice.*

Summary 75   The major traps are associated with foods which are sold without a full list of ingredients, such as flour, bread, confectionery and chocolate products.

References to Chapters 70–75

BARNETT D, BONHAM B & HOWDEN MEH (1987) Allergenic cross-reactions among legume foods – an in vitro study. *J Allergy Clin Immunol* **79**:433–438.

BASSHAM S, FLETCHER LR & STANTON RHJ (1984) Dietary analysis with the aid of a microcomputer. *J Micromcomputer Applic* **7**:279–289.

BERNHISEL-BROADBENT J & SAMPSON HA (1989) Cross-allergenicity in the legume botanical family in children with food hypersensitivity. *J Allergy Clin Immunol* **83**:435–440.

BERNHISEL-BROADBENT J, TAYLOR S & SAMPSON HA (1989) Cross-allergenicity in the legume botanical family in children with food hypersensitivity. II. Laboratory correlates. *J Allergy Clin Immunol* **84**:701–709.

BINDELS JG & VERWIMP J (1990) *Allergenic Aspects of Infant Feeding*, Nutricia Research Communications: 2. Zoetermeer, Holland, N.V. Verenigde Bedrijven Nutricia.

BOCK SA & ATKINS FM (1989) The natural history of peanut allergy. *J Allergy Clin Immunol* **83**:900–904.

BRANSKI D & LEBENTHAL E (1989) Gluten-sensitive enteropathy. In Lebenthal E (ed) *Textbook of Gastroenterology and Nutrition in Infancy*, 2nd edn, pp. 1093–1106, Raven Press, New York.

BROUK B (1975) *Plants Consumed By Man*, Academic Press, London.

BROWN EB & CREPEA SB (1947) Allergy (asthma) to ingested gum tragacanth. A case report. *J Allergy* **18**:214–215.

BUSH RK, TAYLOR SL, NORDLEE JA & BUSSE WW (1985) Soybean oil is not allergenic to soybean-sensitive individuals. *J Allergy Clin Immunol* **76**:242–245.

COMMITTEE ON DIETARY ALLOWANCES (1980) *Recommended Dietary Allowances*, 9th edn, National Academy of Sciences, Washington DC.

DAGNELIE PC, VAN STAVEREN WA & HAUTVAST JGJA (1991) Stunting and nutrient deficiencies in children on alternative diets. *Acta Paediat Scand* **374** (suppl.):111–118.

DAVID TJ (1985) The overworked or fraudulent diagnosis of food allergy and food intolerance in children. *J Roy Soc Med* **78** (suppl. 5):21–31.

DAVID TJ (1987) Unhelpful recent developments in the diagnosis and treatment of allergy and food intolerance in children. In Dobbing J (ed) *Food Intolerance*, pp. 185–214, Baillière Tindall, London.

DAVID TJ (1989) Short stature in children with atopic eczema. *Acta Derm Venereol (Stockh)* (suppl. 144):41–44.

DAVID TJ, WADDINGTON E & STANTON RHJ (1984) Nutritional hazards of elimination diets in children with atopic eczema. *Arch Dis Child* **59**:323–325.

DAVID TJ, WELLS FE, SHARPE TC, GIBBS ACC & DEVLIN J (1990) Serum levels of trace metals in children with atopic eczema. *Br J Dermatol* **122**:485–489.

DE MARTINO M, NOVEMBRE E, GALLI L *et al.* (1990) Allergy to different fish species in cod-allergic children: in vivo and in vitro studies. *J Allergy Clin Immunol* **86**:909–914.

DEPARTMENT OF HEALTH AND SOCIAL SECURITY (1979) Report on Health and Social Subjects 15. *Recommended Daily Amounts of Food Energy and Nutrients for Groups of People in the United Kingdom*, Her Majesty's Stationery Office, London.

DEPARTMENT OF HEALTH (1991) Report on Health and Social Subjects 41. *Dietary Reference Values for Food Enery and Nutrients for the United Kingdom. Report of the Panel on Dietary Reference Values of the Committee on Medical Aspects of Food Policy*, Her Majesty's Stationery Office, London.

DERBES VJ & KRAFCHUK JD (1957) Osmylogenic urticaria. *Arch Dermatol* **76**:103–104.

EDITORIAL (1978) Exotic diets and the infant. *Br Med J* **2**:804–805.

EGAN H, KIRK RS & SAWYER R (1981) *Pearson's Chemical Analysis of Foods*, 8th edn, pp. 227–262, Longman, Harlow.

ERIKSSON NE (1978) Food sensitivity reported by patients with asthma and hay fever. *Allergy* **33**:189–196.

FRANCIS DEM (1987) *Diets for Sick Children*, 4th edn, Blackwell Scientific Publications, Oxford.

GALL H, FORCK G, KALVERAM KJ & VON LERSNER-LENDERS S (1990) Soforttypallergie auf Hülsenfrüchte (Leguminosen). *Allergologie* **13**:352–355.

GELFAND HH (1943) The allergenic properties of the vegetable gums. A case of asthma due to tragacanth. *J Allergy* **14**:203–219.

GELFAND HH (1949) The vegetable gums by ingestion in the etiology of allergic disorders. *J Allergy* **20**:311–321.

GERN JE, YANG E, EVRARD HM & SAMPSON HA (1991) Allergic reactions to milk-contaminated 'nondairy' products. *New Engl J Med* **324**:976–979.

GOODYEAR HM & HARPER JI (1989) Atopic eczema, hyponatraemia, and hypoalbuminaemia. *Arch Dis Child* **64**:231–232.

HANSSEN M & MARSDEN J (1987) *The New E For Additives. The Completely Revised Bestselling E Number Guide*, Thorsons, Wellingborough.

HARTSOOK EL (1984) Celiac sprue: sensitivity to gliadin. *Cereal Foods World* **29**:157–158.

HATHAWAY MJ & WARNER JO (1983) Compliance problems in the dietary management of eczema. *Arch Dis Child* **58**:463–464.

HERIAN AM, TAYLOR SL & BUSH RK (1990) Identification of soybean allergens by immunoblotting with sera from soy-allergic adults. *Int Arch Allergy Appl Immunol* **92**:193–198.

HILL DJ, BALL G & HOSKING CS (1988) Clinical manifestations of cow's milk allergy in childhood. I. Associations with in-vitro cellular immune responses. *Clin Allergy* **18**:469–479.

HORESH AJ (1943) Allergy to food odors. Its relation to the management of infantile eczema. *J Allergy* **14**:335–339.

HUGHES M, CLARK N, FORBES L & COLIN-JONES DG (1986) A case of scurvy. *Br Med J* **293**:366–367.

JUNTUNEN K & ALI-YRKKÖ S (1983) Goat's milk for children allergic to cow's milk. *Kiel Milchwirt Forschungsber* **35**:439–440.

LABIB M, GAMA R, WRIGHT J, MARKS V & ROBINS D (1989) Dietary maladvice as a cause of hypothyroidism and short stature. *Br Med J* **298**:232–233.

LAGIER F, CARTIER A, SOMER J, DOLOVICH J & MALO J-L (1990) Occupational asthma caused by guar gum. *J Allergy Clin Immunol* **85**:785–790.

LLOYD-STILL JD (1979) Chronic diarrhea of childhood and the misuse of elimination diets. *J Pediatr* **95**:10–13.

MACDONALD A & FORSYTHE WI (1986) The cost of nutrition and diet therapy for low-income families. *Hum Nutr Appl Nutr* **40A**:87–96.

MARR JW (1971) Individual dietary surveys: purposes and methods. *World Rev Nutr Diet* **13**:105–164.

MCCANTS ML & LEHRER SB (1985) Detection of IgE antibodies to oyster (abstract). *Ann Allergy* **55**:307.

MONRO J (1987) Food families and rotation diets. In Brostoff J & Challacombe SJ (eds) *Food Allergy and Intolerance*, pp. 303–343, Baillière Tindall, London.

NIEBORG-ESHUIS NH (1991) Practical aspects of food allergy and food intolerance. A consumer's perspective. In Somogyi JC, Müller HR & Ockhuizen T (eds) *Food Allergy and Food Intolerance. Nutritional Aspects and Developments*, pp. 138–148, Karger, Basel.

NORDLEE JA, TAYLOR SL, JONES RT & YUNGINGER JW (1981) Allergenicity of various peanut products as determined by RAST inhibition. *J Allergy Clin Immunol* **68**:376–382.

HOLLAND B, WELCH AA, UNWIN ID, BUSS DH, PAUL AA & SOUTHGATE DAT (1992) *McCance and Widdowson's The Composition of Foods*, 5th edn, Royal Society of Chemistry and Ministry of Agriculture, Fisheries and Food, Cambridge.

PAULI G, BESSOT JC, DIETEMANN-MOLARD A, BRAUN PA & THIERRY R (1985) Celery sensitivity: clinical and immunological correlations with pollen allergy. *Clin Allergy* **15**:273–279.

POLLOCK I & WARNER JO (1987) A follow-up study of childhood food additive intolerance. *J Roy Coll Phys Lond* **21**:248–250.

PORRAS O, CARLSSON B, FÄLLSTRÖM SP & HANSON LÅ (1985) Detection of soy protein in soy lecithin, margarine and, occasionally, soy oil. *Int Arch Allergy Appl Immunol* **78**:30–32.

RANDALL RC, PHILLIPS GO & WILLIAMS PA (1989) Fractionation and characterization of gum from *Acacia senegal*. *Food Hydrocolloids* **3**:65–75.

ROBERTS IF, WEST RJ, OGILVIE D & DILLON MJ (1979) Malnutrition in infants receiving cult diets: a form of child abuse. *Br Med J* **1**:296–298.

SHEPARD TH, PYNE GE, KIRSCHVINK JF & MCLEAN M (1960) Soybean goiter. *New Engl J Med* **262**:1099–1103.

TARNOW-MORDI WO, MOSS C & ROSS K (1984) Failure to thrive owing to inappropriate diet free of gluten and cows' milk. *Br Med J* **289**:1113–1114.

TAYLOR SL, BUSH RK & BÜSSE WW (1987) Avoidance diets – how selective should they be? In Chandra RK (ed) *Food Allergy*, pp. 253–266, Nutrition Research Education Foundation, St. John's, Newfoundland.

THOMAS B (1988) (ed) *Manual of Dietetic Practice*, pp. 108–109, Blackwell Scientific Publications, Oxford.

TODD KS, HUDES M & CALLOWAY DH (1983) Food intake measurement: problems and approaches. *Am J Clin Nutr* **37**:139–146.

TRIPP JH, FRANCIS DEM, KNIGHT JA & HARRIES JT (1979) Infant feeding practices: a cause for concern. *Br Med J* **2**:707–709.

VAUGHAN WT (1930) Food allergens. I. A genetic classification, with results of group testing. *J Allergy* **1**:385–402.

WARING NP, DAUL CB, DE SHAZO RD, MCCANTS ML & LEHRER SB (1985) Hypersensitivity reactions to ingested crustacea: clinical evaluation and diagnostic studies in shrimp-sensitive individuals. *J Allergy Clin Immunol* **76**:440–445.

WORLD HEALTH ORGANISATION (1974) Monograph series no.61. *Handbook of Human Nutritional Requirements*, World Health Organisation, Geneva.

YUNGINGER JW, GAUERKE MB, JONES RT, DAHLBERG MJOE & ACKERMAN SJ (1983) Use of radioimmunoassay to determine the nature, quantity and source of allergenic contamination of sunflower butter. *J Food Protection* **46**:625–628.

Part 17 Drug Treatment

76 Drug treatment
Cromoglycate and antihistamines occasionally helpful

Role for drugs

Where a specific food intolerance has been identified, the simplest approach is usually avoidance of the food. In practice, there are a number of reasons why drug treatment may be necessary (Table 76.1).

Atopic disease and other disorders

Even if food intolerance plays a part in provoking exacerbations of atopic disease, such as atopic eczema, it is rarely the sole cause, and some sort of drug treatment is likely to be required even if it is possible to identify and avoid specific food triggers. The treatment of specific disorders are dealt with elsewhere in this book: (a) asthma, see chapter 53; (b) eczema, see chapter 54; (c) urticaria, see chapter 60; and (d) anaphylaxis, see chapter 63.

Sodium cromoglycate

origin

Khellin, a naturally occurring constituent of the eastern Mediterranean plant *Amni visnaga*, known since Biblical times for its bronchodilating properties. Efforts to enhance its smooth muscle relaxant action and reduce toxicity led to the synthesis in 1965 of the sodium salt of a bis-chromone carboxylic acid, sodium cromoglycate. Although inhibition of mediator release from mast cells is an important effect of sodium cromoglycate, this does not explain all its effects, and the exact mechanism of action is not fully understood (Altounyan 1980).

only for prevention

If sodium cromoglycate has any role at all in the treatment of food intolerance, then it is in the prevention of reactions to food, giving the drug orally, a route by which little drug is absorbed systemically. Once a reaction is established, the drug is no use, and this probably explains the fairly consistent reports of treatment failure in those with chronic symptoms, such as atopic eczema (see below).

Table 76.1 Reasons why drug treatment may be needed

Treatment of symptoms caused by accidental ingestion of food trigger

Treatment of symptoms where causal food trigger has not been identified

Treatment of symptoms of associated atopic disease, such as asthma, eczema, conjunctivitis, rhinitis or urticaria

Decision to use drug therapy rather than food avoidance

467

unhelpful in most

It is established that quick-onset reactions to food triggers can be prevented by the prior administration of oral sodium cromoglycate in a small number of patients (Vaz *et al.* 1978). One wonders whether it would have been simpler to avoid the food rather than swallow sodium cromoglycate before every meal which contained the trigger food. Most reports of efficacy are of greater theoretical interest (in throwing some light on the mechanisms involved) than of practical value. In the author's experience, memorable reports of striking efficacy are overshadowed by the majority of patients in whom the drug appeared to be of no value.

any place for oral therapy?

It is doubtful whether oral sodium cromoglycate has anything other than a very occasional place in the management of food intolerance, although there are some (especially in Italy) who take a more enthusiastic standpoint (Businco & Cantani 1990, 1991). The relative safety, the lack of side effects, and the very occasional success story may be sufficient to encourage one to conduct a short therapeutic trial when simpler approaches have been unsuccessful.

dosage

The doubtful efficacy of oral cromoglycate means that recommendations for dosage are pure guesswork. One approach is simply to give the drug four times a day in the form of capsules which contain 200 mg of sodium cromoglycate powder. Another approach is to give the drug about 20 min before any form of food or drink. A further approach, which is designed to enable the drug to reach the buccal mucosa, is to dissolve the contents of a capsule in water, and swill the solution around the mouth before swallowing. It has been suggested that one should commence with a very low dose (e.g. 20 mg) and slowly increase the dose, but there are no objective data to compare different regimens. The principal adverse effect is marked worsening of pre-existing atopic eczema (Settipane *et al.* 1979; Eveleigh & Edwards 1984; Fairris 1984), and this plus lack of efficacy (Atherton *et al.* 1982) severely restrict its use in this disorder.

topical cromoglycate

Although beyond the scope of this book, the lack of efficacy when given by mouth for food intolerance is in marked contrast to the proven value of sodium cromoglycate when given by inhalation in the prevention of asthma and rhinitis.

Histamine antagonists

Histamine exerts its actions via H1 and H2 receptors. Histamine acts on the sensory nerves (H1), bronchial smooth muscles (H1), airway glands (H2), blood vessels (H1 and H2), gastric glands (H2), and mast cells and lymphocytes (H2).

H1-receptor antagonists

H1-receptor antagonists are sometimes used, without validation from objective studies, in the treatment of symptoms caused by adverse reactions to foods, particularly where the symptoms suggest that histamine has already been released (e.g. urticaria). The rationale is presumably to attenuate or prevent the effects of histamine release. It is unclear, however, whether it is helpful to use histamine-receptor antagonists in this way, *after* symptoms have developed. The principal requirement in this situation is speed of absorption from the gastrointestinal tract and speed of action. These criteria are fulfilled by old fashioned H1-receptor antagonists such as chlorpheniramine or promethazine, but for oral use these agents have been eclipsed by the availability of non-sedating H1-receptor antagonists (Rimmer & Church 1990; Simons 1990), particularly the quick-acting compound terfenadine (Table 76.2).

ketotifen

Suggestions that ketotifen, an H1-receptor antagonist, might be useful in the prevention of symptoms caused by food intolerance (Ciprandi *et al.* 1987; Molkhous & Dupont 1989) have not been confirmed, and in the UK the drug is not licensed for use in the prevention or treatment of food intolerance.

H2-receptor antagonists

There is no evidence that H2-receptor antagonists such as ranitidine or cimetidine are of any value in the management of food intolerance.

Table 76.2 Oral antihistamine dosages

Drug	<1 year	1–5 year	6–12 year	Adult	Comments
Chlorpheniramine	1 mg	1–2 mg	2–4 mg	4 mg	Up to × 3 daily
Promethazine	2.5–5 mg[1]	5–15 mg	10–25 mg	25 mg	Up to × 2 daily; very sedating
Trimeprazine	2.5–5 mg[1]	5–15 mg[1]	10–30 mg	30 mg	Up to × 2 daily; very sedating
As bedtime sedative in atopic eczema	10–30 mg[1]	20–50 mg	up to 60 mg	up to 60 mg	Given as single dose an hour before bedtime; main problem is drowsiness in the morning
Terfenadine	7.5 mg[1]	15 mg[1]	30 mg	60 mg	Given twice daily; non-sedating

[1] Problem in the UK: many drugs, although widely used in infancy and childhood, are not licensed for use below certain ages. This is generally either because of the difficulty in obtaining the necessary data for safety or efficacy in small children, or because it is not commercially worthwhile for companies to go to the expense of collecting the relevant data. The ages below which these antihistamines were not licensed for oral use at the time of writing were: promethazine 1 year, trimeprazine 2 years, and terfenadine 3 years.

Corticosteroids   Corticosteroids are of no proven value in the treatment of adverse reactions to foods, and it takes 4–6 hours before their clinical effects are detectable in disorders such as acute asthma. Some years ago it was noted that when children with asthma were started on inhaled beclomethasone, co-existing atopic eczema improved, and this led to a formal study of oral and inhaled beclomethasone in atopic eczema (Heddle *et al.* 1984). The results, which require confirmation, suggested some clinical benefit, but direct evidence of possible adverse effects such as growth impairment was not sought. Whether these observations have anything to do with food intolerance is unknown.

Aspirin   Uncontrolled anecdotal observations have suggested that on rare occasions aspirin, or other non-steroidal anti-inflammatory agents which inhibit cyclo-oxygenase, may be able to prevent gastrointestinal reactions to foods. In one adult with arthritis, the use of ibuprofen enabled the patient to eat without ill-effects shellfish, which had previously caused severe vomiting and loose stools (Buisseret *et al.* 1978). Elevation of the serum levels of the prostaglandins, PGE_2 and $PGF_{2\alpha}$ coincided with reactions in this patient, suggesting that a prostaglandin-mediated process was responsible for the adverse food reaction in this patient. Youlten (1987) has anecdotally reported that the induction of tolerance to aspirin in patients with urticaria and salicylate intolerance (see chapter 38) may sometimes be associated with the development of tolerance to foods which previously provoked urticaria. These anecdotal observations of possible benefit of aspirin must be set against clear proof of intolerance to salicylates in other patients (see chapter 38) and a report that the use of aspirin was associated with greatly enhanced sensitivity to a food (Cant *et al.* 1984).

Adrenaline   For the use of adrenaline, see chapter 63.

Calcium supplements   For calcium supplements for those who are on cow's milk-free diets, see chapter 15.

Key references   76.1   Youlten LJF (1987) Drug treatment of food allergy and intolerance. In Brostoff J & Challacombe SJ (eds) *Food Intolerance*, pp. 977–984, Ballière Tindall, London. Review of possible uses of oral sodium cromoglycate in food intolerance. Efficacy is most readily demonstrated in subjects who have clear cut symptoms precipitated acutely by the ingestion of single specific foods.

76.2   Rimmer SJ & Church MK (1990) The pharmacology and mechanisms of action of histamine H1-antagonists. *Clin Exper Allergy* **20** (suppl. 2):3–17. *Review.*

76.3   Buisseret PD, Youlten LJF, Heinzelmann DI & Lessof MH (1978) Prostaglandin-synthesis inhibitors in prophylaxis of food intolerance. *Lancet* **1**:

906–908. Prophylactic doses of aspirin, indomethacin, or ibuprofen prevented symptoms of food intolerance in five patients with acute gastrointestinal symptoms after the ingestion of specific foods. Blood and stool prostaglandins PGE_2 and $PGF_{2\alpha}$ concentrations during unprotected challenge were consistent with the hypothesis that these symptoms were mediated through prostaglandin release. *Prostaglandin synthetase inhibitors may benefit some patients with food intolerance. Further studies are needed.*

76.4   BUSINCO L & CANTANI A (1991) Oral sodium cromoglycate in the management of atopic dermatitis in children. *Allergy Proc* **12**:333–338. *Review, somewhat biased in favour of the drug.*

Summary 76   Drug treatment of the effects of food intolerance is unlikely to be as effective as avoidance of specific food triggers. Although oral sodium cromoglycate may sometimes prevent symptoms precipitated acutely by the ingestion of specific foods, the use of this agent is unhelpful in the management of chronic atopic disorders where specific food triggers are suspected of provoking symptoms. Quick acting H1-receptor antagonists, such as chlorpheniramine or the non-sedating agent terfenadine, are sometimes used to treat a symptom (e.g. urticaria) suggestive of histamine release, although it is possible that giving such drugs at this stage is too late. Corticosteroids are of no value in the management of food intolerance.

References to Chapter 76

ALTOUNYAN REC (1980) Review of clinical activity and mode of action of sodium cromoglycate. *Clin Allergy* **10** (suppl.):481–489.

ATHERTON DJ, SOOTHILL JF & ELVIDGE J (1982) A controlled trial of oral sodium cromoglycate in atopic eczema. *Br J Dermatol* **106**:681–685.

BUISSERET PD, YOULTEN LJF, HEINZELMANN DI & LESSOF MH (1978) Prostaglandin-synthesis inhibitors in prophylaxis of food intolerance. *Lancet* **1**:906–908.

BUSINCO L & CANTANI A (1990) Food allergy in children: diagnosis and treatment with sodium cromoglycate. *Allergol Immunopathol* **18**:339–348.

BUSINCO L & CANTANI A (1991) Oral sodium cromoglycate in the management of atopic dermatitis in children. *Allergy Proc* **12**:333–338.

CANT AJ, GIBSON P & DANCY M (1984) Food hypersensitivity made life threatening by ingestion of aspirin. *Br Med J* **288**:755–756.

CIPRANDI G, SCORDAMAGLIA A, BAGNASCO M & CANONICA GW (1987) Pharmacologic treatment of adverse reactions to foods: comparison of different protocols. *Ann Allergy* **58**:341–343.

EVELEIGH HA & EDWARDS AM (1984) Generalised eczema caused by sodium cromoglycate. *Br Med J* **289**:837.

FAIRRIS GM (1984) Generalised eczema caused by sodium cromoglycate. *Br Med J* **289**:470.

HEDDLE RJ, SOOTHILL JF, BULPITT CJ & ATHERTON DJ (1984) Combined oral and nasal beclomethasone diproprionate in children with atopic eczema: a randomised controlled trial. *Br Med J* **289**:651–654.

MOLKHOUS P & DUPONT C (1989) Ketotifen treatment of atopic dermatitis and other food allergy diseases. *Allergy* **44** (suppl. 9):117–123.

RIMMER SJ & CHURCH MK (1990) The pharmacology and mechanisms of action of histamine H1-antagonists. *Clin Exper Allergy* **20** (suppl. 2):3–17.

SETTIPANE GA, KLEIN DE, BOYD GK, STURAM JH, FREYE HB & WELTMAN JK (1979) Adverse reactions to cromolyn. *J Am Med Ass* **241**:811–813.

SIMONS FER (1990) New H1-receptor antagonists: clinical pharmacology. *Clin Exper Allergy* **20** (suppl. 2):19–24.

VAZ GA, TAN LKT & GERRARD JW (1978) Oral cromoglycate in treatment of adverse reactions to foods. *Lancet* **1**:1066–1068.

YOULTEN LJF (1987) Drug treatment of food allergy and intolerance. In Brostoff J & Challacombe SJ (eds) *Food Intolerance*, pp. 977–984, Ballière Tindall, London.

Part 18 Unorthodox Methods

77 Unorthodox investigations
Adventures into the bizarre

Background

The lack of simple and reliable conventional tests for the diagnosis of food intolerance (see chapters 39 to 49) and allergy in general is one factor which has led to the development of unorthodox methods (David 1987). This chapter reviews unorthodox methods of investigation, and the next chapter examines unconventional forms of treatment.

Why go unorthodox?

There are a number of reasons why parents seek unorthodox or alternative approaches to diagnosis and treatment (Table 77.1).

Radionics

Radionics, radiesthesia, psionic medicine and dowsing are closely related practices and all employ extra-sensory perception. Radionics is based on the concept that man is submerged in an energy field which lies beyond the electromagnetic spectrum and is therefore undetectable by scientific instruments. The patient does not need to be present for radionic diagnosis or treatment, for the doctor and patient are said to be connected by a beam of energy, along which information can be transmitted that is relevant to the patient's health (Fulder 1984). The method uses a pendulum (Reyner *et al.* 1982), accompanied by a 'witness' of the patient, usually a sample of hair. Some with special gifts claim they can dispense with the pendulum and the witness, and test using merely the patient's name. It is said that radionics can be used for the detection of all allergies, for the diagnosis of virtually all common diseases, and also for the identification of most individual bacterial pathogens.

Table 77.1 Some reasons why parents seek unorthodox or alternative approaches

Desire to play a more active part in child's treatment (e.g. employing a diet, or giving physiotherapy)

Chronic disease which is poorly responsive to conventional treatment (e.g. atopic disease, arthritis)

Fear of side effects of conventional treatment (e.g. topical steroids for eczema)

Dissatisfaction with present doctor

Dramatic but uncritical media coverage of individual 'success' stories and general media misinformation

Belief that treatment which is paid for is superior to that given 'free' on the National Health Service

Impressive claims made for efficacy of unorthodox or alternative treatment validation Radionics has never been objectively evaluated, and it is claimed that radionic techniques are not amenable to any sort of scientific study. It is said that radionics 'does not have a place within such a restrictive belief system as orthodox science. Radionics is an interface with higher dimensions of reality and consciousness, where the gods of logic and reason do not necessarily hold sway' (Tansley 1982).

Scientific study is reportedly precluded by the notion that disbelief either in the patient's mind or that of a third part destroys the reliability of the testing process (Simmonds 1984): 'it has been known, for example, for a sceptical doctor to refer a case for psionic medical diagnosis as a sort of test; perhaps even to discredit the technique. This scepticism conveys itself to the practitioner, either directly or through the patient, and unless he is able to preserve his integrity of mind, failure is inevitable... The weight of prejudice is immense and it is usually sufficient to render the dowser incapable of attaining the necessary freedom and innocence of mind to be able to function... It therefore behoves every practitioner... to avoid any occasion where there is likely to be a climate of disbelief. Psionic medicine requires of the practitioner a mind undisturbed by the clash of disputation − a state not easy to attain in the presence of those whose coin is dispute' (Reyner *et al.* 1982).

Pulse testing Coca, who with Cooke first introduced the term '*atopy*' (Coca & Cooke 1922), classified allergic disease into four main categories, but in addition he proposed a fifth group, familial non-reaginic food allergy, which he named 'idioblapsis' (Coca 1953). The 11 most frequent symptoms of this supposed disorder are listed in Table 77.2. The features of this proposed condition were that the individual sensitivities were not attributable to circulating antibodies but to the sympathetic nervous system, and that the allergic reaction reliably caused an acceleration of the pulse rate (Coca 1953). Coca claimed that at least 90% of the population suffered from idioblaptic allergy. He said that an increase in the pulse rate was a reliable pointer to food allergy and he recommended identification of idioblaptic allergy by observing a tachycardia 5−90 min after exposure to a food or inhaled allergen.

an art Coca described the interpretation of the pulse as 'an art' because of multiple confounding factors, including a latent period of lost sensitivity, and aluminium sensitivity. Other authorities have suggested that a slowing of the pulse is equally reliable in the diagnosis of food allergy (Radcliffe 1982). Using pulse testing, Coca claimed cures for food intolerance as well as a miscellaneous

Table 77.2 The eleven most common symptoms of idioblaptic allergy[1]

Headaches
Indigestion
Constipation
Hives
Chronic rhinitis
Canker-sores in mouth
Heartburn
Dizziness
Nervousness
Neuralgia
Abnormal tiredness

[1] Source: Coca (1953).

collection of disorders including headaches, urticaria, eczema, indigestion, colitis, haemorrhoids, hypertension, dysmenorrhoea, subfertility, frigidity and glaucoma (Coca 1982).

validation   There have been no published attempts to validate pulse testing for the diagnosis of food intolerance. The Royal College of Physicians and British Nutrition Foundation joint report on food intolerance and food aversion (1984) declared that the pulse test was of no diagnostic value.

Auricular cardiac reflex test   It is claimed that if a substance to which a patient is allergic is brought within half an inch of the skin, then the auricular cardiac reflex (derived from a form of acupuncture – see Nogier 1981) changes the wave form of the pulse at the wrist, enabling detection of the allergy (Lewith & Kenyon 1985). Such testing currently uses dried food samples mounted in specially prepared filters, and it is said that using this technique 50 foods or chemicals can be tested in 15 min (Lewith & Kenyon 1985).

validation   There have been no published attempts to validate objectively the auricular cardiac reflex or its use for the diagnosis of allergy.

Applied kinesiology   Using applied kinesiology, it is alleged that if an allergen to which a subject is allergic – for example an egg – is held near the patient's body, placed in the patient's palm, or administered as drops under the tongue, it will instantly cause pronounced loss of muscle power which is easily detected by an observer (Valentine & Valentine 1986). Where a patient is too young to co-operate, a surrogate is used. The surrogate is tested alone, and then retested holding the child's hand, and the results from the two tests are subtracted to show the patient's allergies.

validation   An objective study of applied kinesiology has shown it to be useless for the diagnosis of allergy (Garrow 1988).

Vega testing   Vega testing is one of the so-called bio-electronic regulatory techniques. It is based on the idea that all biological events are basically electrical changes (Kenyon 1986), and that electrical pathology predates actual structural changes, enabling diagnosis of disease prior to any detectable cellular change (Kenyon 1986). Vega testing employs a Vegatest electrical device. The method relies on changes in the resistance to the flow of electricity over acupuncture points on the ends of fingers and toes, brought about by bringing particular substances, in glass phials, into series in the circuit (Kenyon 1986). When used to test for food intolerance, Vega testing is claimed to be 80% accurate 'in skilled hands' (Lewith & Kenyon 1985).

validation   There have been no published attempts to objectively validate Vega testing, although there is an unsubstantiated report of double-blind testing which showed that consistent results could not be obtained (McEvoy 1991). It has been postulated that Vega testing is partially dependent on the 'psyche' of the practitioner, to the extent that 'changes in readings noted are partially psychokinetic effects (literally "mind-caused" effects), which may in some cases be observed extra sensorily' (Kenyon 1986).

Trace metal hair analysis   It has been claimed that an imbalance or lack of trace metals, detectable by analysis of the trace metal concentration in scalp or pubic hair, may cause food intolerance, and that trace metal supplements may then benefit the patient (Bland 1983; Lewith & Kenyon 1985).

validation   There is no evidence that measuring the level of trace metals in hair samples is of any clinical relevance to food intolerance. Nor is there any evidence that mineral supplements based on such tests confer any clinical benefit. It has been shown that properly performed hair analysis provides results that are of little or no clinical value (Fletcher 1982; Hambidge 1982; Rivlin 1983; Taylor 1986). Increasing distance from the scalp clearly affects concentrations of hair trace elements, as do age, sex, drugs, and various forms of hair washing (Assarian & Oberleas 1977; Deeming & Weber 1978; McKenzie 1978). A recent study of laboratories providing a hair analysis service showed that the reported levels of most minerals varied considerably between identical samples sent to the same laboratory, and also between identical samples sent to different laboratories (Barrett 1985).

The cytotoxic test   This is also known as the leucocyte cytotoxicity test or the leucocyte food allergy test. The test consists of the observation of morphological changes in blood cells, primarily polymorphonuclear leucocytes, incubated simultaneously with the appropriate antigen and the patient's serum (Black 1956; Ulett & Perry 1974). The presence or absence and degree of damage caused to the leucocytes is claimed to 'be an indicator of the presence of food and/or chemical sensitivity' and to give 'some indication as to its degree' (Lewith & Kenyon 1985).

spontaneous cytotoxicity   The cytotoxic test should not be confused with the putative phenomenon, alleged to be enhanced by the presence of food intolerance, of spontaneous allergic cytotoxicity where '*in vivo* autoactivated cells are programmed for a suicidal reaction thus culminating in killing themselves' (Podleski 1985, 1986a, b).

validation   There are several anecdotal claims that the cytotoxic test may be of value in the diagnosis of food intolerance (Black 1956; Bryan & Bryan 1960; Ulett & Perry 1974; Boyles 1977; Ruokonen *et al.* 1981). However, an objective study by Chambers *et al.* (1958) showed that the cytotoxic test revealed genuine intolerance in only one out of 24 known examples, and that in 70% of the test results definite interpretation of the microscopic appearances could not be made. The observers only agreed on two-thirds of the test preparations. Further evaluation of the cytotoxic test demonstrated a high incidence of false positive results, poor ability to identify patients with known food intolerance, poor inter-observer correlation, and marked day-to-day variation in the results of the test (Lieberman *et al.* 1975; Benson & Arkins 1976; Holopainen *et al.* 1980; Lehman 1980a). The Royal College of Physicians and British Nutrition Foundation (1984) joint report on food intolerance and food aversion declared the results of cytotoxic food testing 'of no diagnostic value' and referred to one British laboratory which had failed to obtain reproducible results on duplicate blood samples taken from the same subject.

Key reference 77.1   DAVID TJ (1987) Unhelpful recent developments in the diagnosis and treatment of allergy and food intolerance in children. In Dobbing J (ed) *Food Intolerance*, pp. 185–214, London, Baillière Tindall. *Detailed review of unorthodox methods of diagnosis and treatment.*

Summary 77   Radionics, pulse testing, auricular cardiac reflex testing, applied kinesiology, Vega testing, lymphocyte cytotoxicity testing, and trace metal hair analysis are unorthodox and unproven methods for the diagnosis of food intolerance. Not all methods have been evaluated objectively, but those that have were found to be useless.

78 Unorthodox treatments
Useless or unproven, costly, and sometimes hazardous

Urine therapy   This comprises the child drinking his own urine, having injections of urine, or having urine rubbed on the skin or applied to the skin in compresses (Armstrong 1981; Dunne 1981). The basis for such treatment is obscure. The dose of urine for injection ranges from 2 ml for an infant to 8 ml for an adult. It is claimed that urine therapy can cure numerous diseases including eczema, asthma and bed-wetting. The concept of 'auto-immune urine therapy', which has also been used to treat 'intra-familial sensitivity', a term used to describe the putative disorder of allergy to members of one's family (Wilson 1983), is based on the theory that a therapeutic dose of antigen is excreted in the urine.

validation   There have been no reported attempts to validate urine therapy in the treatment of atopic disease, food intolerance or allergy. The National Center for Health Care Technology in the USA declared in 1981 that urine autoinjection and autogenous urine immuniza-tion is an 'untested and unproven procedure that lacks a reason-able theoretical basis' (1981). The American Academy of Allergy (1981) have declared that the method is not acceptable medical practice, and have warned that such treatment might induce glomerulonephritis.

Intestinal candidiasis   In this supposed condition and the related putative entity 'dysbiosis' (Kenyon 1986) it is alleged that there is an imbalance of the flora of the gastrointestinal tract, which leads to a proliferation of *Candida albicans*. It is claimed that food intolerance and a number of other disorders ranging from schizophrenia to rheumatoid arthritis are 'yeast-related diseases' and that anti-yeast therapy results in recovery (Truss 1982; Crook 1984; Kroker 1986). It is further claimed that where intestinal candidiasis underlies food intolerance, the food intolerance will not respond to a diet or hyposensitization until the candidiasis itself has been diagnosed and treated (Crook 1984). The recommended treatment is either with anti-Candida agents such as nystatin, given orally or rectally, or with sublingual drops (Crook 1984).

validation   There is no published evidence to support the notions that food intolerance can be related to *Candida albicans*, or that anti-candida

480

therapy will have any effect on food intolerance. Under double-blind placebo-controlled conditions, anti-*Candida* therapy failed significantly to reduce symptoms in a study of women with presumed candidiasis (Dismukes *et al.* 1990).

Enzyme potentiated transepidermal desensitization

This technique, exploits a putative potentiating effect of the enzyme betaglucuronidase when this is added to dilute mixtures of 70 or more antigens (McEwen *et al.* 1967, 1973; McEwen & Starr 1972; McEwen 1973; McEwen 1975; Eaton *et al.* 1982). The antigen mixture is placed in a cup which is held in place for 24 hours over an area of skin which has been scarified with a blunt scalpel. In a recent variation, the mixture is injected intradermally (Fell & Brostoff 1990). The large number of antigens which can be employed is claimed to remove the need to identify individual antigens. Treatment is given monthly for 3 months, with booster doses every 4 months. 'The average patient with multiple food sensitivities can develop tolerance to his sensitive foods in 6–12 months from starting treatment' (Lewith & Kenyon 1985). The treatment is said to be safe, and is claimed to bring about varying degrees of improvement in 80% of subjects treated.

validation

There is no objective evidence that this method is of any benefit in the management of food intolerance in childhood, or of disorders such as atopic eczema. The claim that treatment may take 1–2 years to result in benefit should be borne in mind, since a high proportion of children with food intolerance or atopic eczema spontaneously grow out of their problem within this period of time. In one study, enzyme-potentiated desensitization was reported to be associated with sigmoidoscopic improvement and decreased steroid usage 14 and 28 months after treatment had been initiated in adults with ulcerative colitis (McEwen 1987). These results were said to indicate that 'food allergy is a likely cause of ulcerative colitis' (McEwen 1987). This approach is unlikely to be taken up unless supported by further data.

Intradermal skin testing and neutralization therapy

Conventional intradermal testing, which is of no value in the diagnosis of food intolerance, is discussed in chapter 41. A bizarre alternative technique of intradermal testing has been widely adopted by ecologists, and is claimed to be applicable for both diagnosis and treatment.

method

In this form of intradermal testing, antigens are diluted with benzyl alcohol and normal saline to produce nine successively weaker concentrations (Williams 1965; Willoughby 1965; Lee *et al.* 1969a; Williams 1971; Willoughby 1974; Cowen 1981; Podell 1983; Maclennan

1984; Mansfield 1984; King *et al.* 1988a). Usually 0.05 ml of each dilution is injected intradermally, producing a weal measuring 4 mm (Mumby 1986) to 7 mm (Mansfield 1984) in diameter. 'The behaviour of this weal is observed after 10 min and features such as lateral increase in size, blanching, hardness and well-demarcated edges are assessed. After 10 min, a positive weal has retained most of these features and has grown at least 2 mm in diameter. Negative weals lose these characteristics and grow less than 2 mm in diameter' (Mansfield 1984).

provocation & neutralization

Using this method it is reported that though injection of, for example, a food concentrate may produce no reaction, injection of a diluted solution may result in a weal. Further, it is claimed that at the same time as the weal enlarges, symptoms related to the patient's complaint are provoked in 70% of patients. It is further claimed that if increasing dilutions are injected at half-hourly intervals, when a dilution is reached which causes no wealing the injection of this is accompanied by an almost instantaneous cessation of symptoms (Lewith & Kenyon 1985). This dilution is then employed in neutralization therapy (see below).

mechanism

The mechanism for this almost instantaneous 'switch-off' of symptoms is obscure. The ecological view is that it involves 'an electrical mechanism of an ill-understood nature' (Lewith & Kenyon 1985).

neutralization therapy

Having determined the 'neutralizing dose' with the above methods, neutralizing solutions are then administered either by sublingual drops or by subcutaneous injection (Lee *et al.* 1969b; Miller 1972, 1977, 1987; Mansfield 1983, 1984; Rea *et al.* 1984; Finn *et al.* 1986; King *et al.* 1988b). Sublingual drops are said to be beneficial for 5 hours, while injections last at least 2 days (Mansfield 1984). It is suggested that after a few weeks, the injections can be given every 3 days, and it is claimed that symptom control occurs almost immediately, though 'permanent desensitization often requires a few years of therapy' (Mansfield 1984). Drawbacks to the method include patients who constantly develop 'new allergies' (Mumby 1985) and patients in whom the 'end-points' change daily (Lewith & Kenyon 1985).

validation

Controlled double-blind studies have failed to confirm the reproducibility or validity of symptom provocation or neutralization therapy (Caplin 1973; Kailin & Collier 1980; Lehman 1980b; Grieco 1982; Van Metre 1983; Jewett *et al.* 1990).

Rotation diets   There is no rational basis for rotation diets, which have never been objectively validated. These diets are discussed further in chapter 70.

Does it matter?   There are a number of adverse sequelae associated with the use of these unorthodox methods (David 1987).

1 *Treatment failure*: the treatment may simply fail to help the patient (David 1987).

2 *False diagnosis of non-existent disorders*: radionic testing, cytotoxic testing, Vega testing, pulse testing and intradermal testing have been associated with false positive results, and with the creation of fictional entities such as allergy to North Sea gas (David 1987).

3 *Failure to diagnose and treat genuine disease*: the tendency to overdiagnose food intolerance is inevitably associated with a failure to recognize and treat the true cause of a patient's symptoms (David 1987; Robertson *et al.* 1988).

4 *Dietary restriction leading to inadequate diet*: unsupervised and inappropriate diets carry the risk of malnutrition and death (Editorial 1978; Lloyd-Still 1979; Roberts *et al.* 1979; Tripp *et al.* 1979; Tarnow-Mordi *et al.* 1984; David 1987; Robertson *et al.* 1988).

5 *Unnecessary dietary restriction leading to dietary obsession*: a permanent obsession with food intolerance is a risk of unnecessary dietary treatment (David 1987; Taylor 1992).

6 *Financial loss*: many of the above unorthodox approaches are extremely costly (David 1987).

What to advise?   Many parents of children with chronic disease desire to try alternative approaches. Treatments which involve the parents in 'doing something' to help their own child, such as a special diet, or physiotherapy, are particularly appealing. In the past, the medical advice to such parents has often been rather passive – 'why not give it a try?'. This tacit approval is unhelpful, and there is a duty to warn parents of the possible hazards and doubtful efficacy associated with unorthodox approaches.

Key references 78.1   DAVID TJ (1987) Unhelpful recent developments in the diagnosis and treatment of allergy and food intolerance in children. In Dobbing J (ed) *Food Intolerance*, pp. 185–214, London, Baillière Tindall. *Detailed review of unorthodox methods of diagnosis and treatment. The sequelae of these methods include the false diagnosis of non-existent disease, allergy or intolerance, failure to diagnose and treat genuine disease, and unsupervised dietary restriction leading to inadequate diet.*

78.2   ROBERTSON DAF, AYRES RCS, SMITH CL & WRIGHT R (1988) Adverse consequences arising from misdiagnosis of food allergy. *Br Med J* **297**:719–720. A report of three patients in whom serious sequelae were the result of the incorrect diagnosis of food intolerance by unorthodox practitioners. In a 43-year-old man with anaemia, diagnosis of colonic carcinoma was delayed by 6 months of treatment for supposed food intolerance. By the time he presented to the surgeons, multiple hepatic metastases were present and he died. In a 23-year-old woman with abdominal pain, weight loss and bloody diarrhoea, treatment for supposed milk allergy which was diagnosed by Vega testing, delayed the final discovery of Crohn's disease of the rectum. A 13-year-old girl with anorexia nervosa, who was already on a highly restrictive diet and refusing to accept conventional treatment, was diagnosed by an allergist as suffering from multiple food intolerance and placed on an even more restrictive diet and treated with enzyme potentiated desensitization. The patient and her mother declined any food unless it was discussed with the allergist, and the girl collapsed and died of bronchopneumonia due to anorexia nervosa.

Summary 78   Urine therapy, treatment of so-called intestinal candidiasis, trans-epidermal enzyme potentiated desensitization, symptom provocation and neutralization therapy, and rotation diets are unorthodox and unproven methods for the treatment of food intolerance. Not all methods have been evaluated objectively, but those that have been were found to be useless. Adverse sequelae associated with these methods include treatment failure, false diagnosis of non-existent disease entities, inadequate nutritional intake, persistent obsession with the diet, and financial loss.

References to Chapters 77 and 78

AMERICAN ACADEMY OF ALLERGY (1981) Position statements – controversial techniques. *J Allergy Clin Immunol* **67**:333–338.

ARMSTRONG JW (1981) *The Water of Life. A Treatise on Urine Therapy*, 2nd edn, Health Science Press, Saffron Walden.

ASSARIAN GS & OBERLEAS D (1977) Effect of washing procedures on trace-element content of hair. *Clin Chem* **23**:1771–1772.

BARRETT S (1985) Commercial hair analysis. Science or scam? *J Am Med Ass* **254**:1041–1045.

BENSON TE & ARKINS JA (1976) Cytotoxic testing for food allergy: evaluation of reproducibility and correlation. *J Allergy Clin Immunol* **58**:471–476.

BLACK AP (1956) A new diagnostic method in allergic disease. *Pediatrics* **17**: 716–724.

BLAND J (1983) *Hair Tissue Mineral Analysis. An Emergent Diagnostic Technique*, Thorsons, Wellingborough.

BOYLES JH (1977) The validity of using the cytotoxic food test in clinical allergy. *Ear, Nose Throat J* **56**:35–43.

BRYAN WTK & BRYAN MP (1960) The application of in vitro cytotoxic reactions to clinical diagnosis of food allergy. *Laryngoscope* **70**:810–823.

CAPLIN I (1973) Report of the committee on provocative food testing. *Ann Allergy* **31**:375–381.

CHAMBERS VV, HUDSON BH & GLASER J (1958) A study of the reactions of human polymorphonuclear leukocytes to various allergens. *J Allergy* **29**:93–102.

COCA AF (1953) *Familial Nonreaginic Food-Allergy*, 3rd edn, Charles C Thomas, Illinois.

COCA AF (1982) *The Pulse Test. Easy Allergy Detection*, Arco Publishing Inc, New York.

COCA AF & COOKE RA (1922) On the classification of the phenomena of hypersensitiveness. *J Immunol* **8**:163–182.

COWEN DE (1981) Serial-dilution titration: technique and application. In King HC (ed) *Otolaryngologic Allergy*, pp. 179–206, Symposium Specialists, Florida.

CROOK WG (1984) *The Yeast Connection. A Medical Breakthrough*, 2nd edn, Professional Books, Tennessee.

DAVID TJ (1987) Unhelpful recent developments in the diagnosis and treatment of allergy and food intolerance in children. In Dobbing J (ed) *Food Intolerance*, pp. 185–214, Baillière Tindall, London.

DEEMING SB & WEBER CW (1978) Hair analysis of trace minerals in human subjects as influenced by age, sex, and contraceptive drugs. *Am J Clin Nutr* **31**:1175–1180.

DISMUKES WE, WADE JS, LEE JY, DOCKERY BK & HAIN JD (1990) A randomized, double-blind trial of nystatin therapy for the candidiasis hypersensitivity syndrome. *New Engl J Med* **323**:1717–1723.

DUNNE AP (1981) The use of injected and sublingual urine in the treatment of allergies. *Irish Med Times* **19**:24–26.

EATON K, ADAMS A & DUBERLEY J (1982) *Allergy Therapeutics*, Ballière Tindall, London.

EDITORIAL (1978) Exotic diets and the infant. *Br Med J* **2**:804–805.

FELL P & BROSTOFF J (1990) A single dose desensitisation for summer hay fever. Results of a double blind study – 1988. *Eur J Clin Pharmacol* **38**:77–79.

FINN R, BARKER DP & BARLETT AN (1986) A clinical trial of low dose desensitization and environmental control. *Clin Ecology* **4**:75–76.

FLETCHER DJ (1982) Hair analysis. Proven and problematical applications. *Postgrad Med* **72**:79–88.

FULDER S (1984) *The Handbook of Complementary Medicine*, Hodder and Stoughton, London.

GARROW JS (1988) Kinesiology and food allergy. *Br Med J* **296**:1573–1574.

GRIECO MH (1982) Controversial practices in allergy. *J Am Med Ass* **247**:3106–3111.

HAMBIDGE KM (1982) Hair analyses: worthless for vitamins, limited for minerals. *Am J Clin Nutr* **36**:943–949.

HOLOPAINEN E, PALVA T, STENBERG P, BACKMAN A, LEHTI H & RUOKONEN J (1980) Cytotoxic leukocyte reaction. *Acta Otolaryngol* **89**:222–226.

JEWETT DL, FEIN G & GREENBERG MH (1990) A double-blind study of symptom provocation to determine food sensitivity. *New Engl J Med* **323**:429–433.

KAILIN EW & COLLIER R (1971) 'Relieving' therapy for antigen exposure. *J Am Med Ass* **217**:78.

KENYON JN (1986) *21st Century Medicine. A Layman's Guide to the Medicine of the Future*, Thorsons, Wellingborough.

KING WP, RUBIN WA, FADAL RG et al. (1988a) Provocation-neutralization: a two-part study. Part I. The intracutaneous provocative food test: a multi-center comparison study. *Otolaryngol Head Neck Surg* **99**:263–271.

KING WP, FADAL RG, WARD WA *et al.* (1988b) Provocation-neutralization: a two part study. Part II. Subcutaneous neutralization therapy: a multi-center study. *Otolaryngol Head Neck Surg* **99**:272–277.

KROKER GF (1986) Chronic candidiasis and allergy. In Brostoff J & Challacombe SJ (eds) *Food Allergy and Intolerance*, pp. 850–872, Ballière Tindall, London.

LABIB M, GAMA R, WRIGHT J, MARKS V & ROBINS D (1989) Dietary maladvice as a cause of hypothyroidism and short stature. *Br Med J* **298**:232–233.

LEE CH, WILLIAMS RI & BINKLEY EL (1969a) Provocative inhalant testing and treatment. *Arch Otolaryngol* **90**:173–177.

LEE CH, WILLIAMS RI & BINKLEY EL (1969b) Provocative testing and treatment for foods. *Arch Otolaryngol* **90**:113–120.

LEHMAN CW (1980a) The leukocytic food allergy test: a study of its reliability and reproducibility. Effect of diet and sublingual food drops on this test. *Ann Allergy* **45**:150–158.

LEHMAN CW (1980b) A double-blind study of sublingual provocative food testing: a study of its efficacy. *Ann Allergy* **45**:144–149.

LEWITH GT & KENYON JN (1985) *Clinical Ecology. A Therapeutic Approach to Understanding and Treating Food and Chemical Sensitivities*, Thorsons, Wellingborough.

LIEBERMAN P, CRAWFORD L, BJELLAND J, CONNELL B & RICE M (1975) Controlled study of the cytotoxic food test. *J Am Med Ass* **231**:728–730.

LLOYD-STILL JD (1979) Chronic diarrhea of childhood and the misuse of elimination diets. *J Pediatr* **95**:10–13.

MACLENNAN JG (1984) Clinical titration principles and techniques. Part 1. *Clin Ecology* **2**:151–158.

MANSFIELD J (1984) Symptoms and their solutions. *Mims Magazine* **1**:19–22.

MANSFIELD JR (1983) Food allergies: clinical aspects and natural allergens. In Conning DM & Lansdown ABG (eds) *Toxic Hazards in Foods*, pp. 275–291, Croom Helm, London.

MCEVOY RJ (1991) Vega testing in the diagnosis of allergic conditions. *Med J Aust* **155**:350.

MCEWEN LM (1973) Enzyme-potentiated hyposensitisation. Effects of glucose, glucosamine, N-acetylamino-sugars and gelatin on the ability of F β-glucuronidase to block the anamnestic response to antigen in mice. *Ann Allergy* **31**:79–83.

MCEWEN LM (1975) Enzyme potentiated hyposensitization: V. Five case reports of patients with acute food allergy. *Ann Allergy* **35**:98–103.

MCEWEN LM (1986) Hyposensitization. In Brostoff J & Challacombe SJ (eds) *Food Allergy and Intolerance*, pp. 985–994, Ballière Tindall, London.

MCEWEN LM (1987) A double-blind controlled trial of enzyme potentiated hyposensitization for the treatment of ulcerative colitis. *Clin Ecology* **5**:47–51.

MCEWEN LM, GANDERTON MA, WILSON CMW & BLACK JHD (1967) Hyaluronidase in the treatment of allergy. *Br Med J* **2**:507–508.

MCEWEN LM, NICHOLSON M, KITCHEN I & WHITE S (1973) Enzyme-potentiated hyposensitisation. III. Control by sugars and diols of the immunological effect of β glucuronidase in mice and patients with hay fever. *Ann Allergy* **31**: 543–550.

MCEWEN LM & STARR MS (1972) Enzyme-potentiated hyposensitisation. I. The effect of pre-treatment with β-glucuronidase, hyaluronidase, and antigen on anaphylactic sensitivity of guinea-pigs, rats and mice. *Int Arch Allergy* **42**:152–158.

McKenzie JM (1978) Alteration of the zinc and copper concentration of hair. *Am J Clin Nutr* **31**:470–476.

Miller JB (1972) *Food Allergy. Provocative Testing and Injection Therapy*, Charles C Thomas, Springfield.

Miller JB (1977) A double-blind study of food extract injection therapy: a preliminary report. *Ann Allergy* **38**:185–191.

Miller JB (1987) *Relief At Last! Neutralization for Food Allergy and Other Illnesses*, Charles C Thomas, Springfield.

Mumby K (1986) *Allergies . . . What Everyone Should Know*, Unwin, London.

National Center for Health Care Technology (1981) Summary of assessments 1981. *J Am Med Ass* **246**:1499.

Nogier PMF (1981) *Handbook of Auriculotherapy*, Maisonneuve, Moulins-Lès-Metz, France.

Podell RN (1983) Intracutaneous and sublingual provocation and neutralization. *Clin Ecology* **2**:13–20.

Podleski WK (1985) Cytodestructive mechanisms provoked by food antigens. II. Antibody-dependent, allergic autocytotoxicity. *Allergy* **40**:166–172.

Podleski WK (1986a) Broncho-Vaxom and spontaneous allergic autocytotoxicity (spACT) in bronchial asthma associated with food hypersensitivity. *Int J Immunopharmacol* **8**:433–436.

Podleski WK (1986b) Spontaneous allergic autocytotoxicity in bronchial asthma associated with food allergy. *Am J Med* **81**:437–442.

Radcliffe MJ (1982) Clinical methods for diagnosis. *Clin Immunol Allergy* **2**:205–219.

Rea WJ, Podell RN, Williams ML, Fenyves E, Sprague DE & Johnson AR (1984) Elimination of oral food challenge reaction by injection of food extracts. *Arch Otolaryngol* **110**:248–252.

Reyner JH, Laurence G & Upton C (1982) *Psionic Medicine*, 2nd edn, Routledge and Kegan Paul, London.

Rivlin RS (1983) Misuse of hair analysis for nutritional assessment. *Am J Med* **75**:489–493.

Roberts IF, West RJ, Ogilvie D & Dillon MJ (1979) Malnutrition in infants receiving cult diets: a form of child abuse. *Br Med J* **1**:296–298.

Robertson DAF, Ayres RCS, Smith CL & Wright R (1988) Adverse consequences arising from misdiagnosis of food allergy. *Br Med J* **297**:719–720.

Royal College of Physicians and the British Nutrition Foundation (1984) Joint report on food intolerance and food aversion. *J Roy Coll Phys Lond* **18**:83–123.

Ruokonen J, Holopainen E, Palva T & Backman A (1981) Secretory otitis media and allergy. With special reference to the cytotoxic leucocyte test. *Allergy* **36**:59–68.

Simmonds W (1984) Splitting hairs on food allergy. *World Med* **19**:10.

Tansley DV (1982) *Radionics: Science or Magic?* C.W. Daniel, Saffron Walden.

Tarnow-Mordi WO, Moss C & Ross K (1984) Failure to thrive owing to inappropriate diet free of gluten and cows' milk. *Br Med J* **289**:1113–1114.

Taylor A (1986) Usefulness of measurements of trace elements in hair. *Ann Clin Biochem* **23**:364–378.

Taylor D (1992) Outlandish factitious illness. In David TJ (ed) *Recent Advances in Paediatrics*, vol. 10, pp. 63–76, Churchill Livingstone, London.

Tomlinson H (1966) *Medical Divination. Theory and Practice*, Health Science Press, Holsworthy.

Tripp JH, Francis DEM, Knight JA & Harries JT (1979) Infant feeding practices: a cause for concern. *Br Med J* **2**:707–709.

TRUSS CO (1982) *The Missing Diagnosis*, The Missing Diagnosis Inc, Birmingham, Alabama.

ULETT GA & PERRY SG (1974) Cytotoxic testing and leukocyte increase as an index to food sensitivity. *Ann Allergy* **33**:23–32.

VALENTINE T & VALENTINE C (1986) *Applied Kinesiology. Muscle Response in Diagnosis, Therapy and Preventive Medicine*, Thorsons, Wellingborough.

VAN METRE TE (1983) Critique of controversial and unproven procedures for diagnosis and therapy of allergic disorders. *Pediat Clin N Am* **30**:807–817.

WILLIAMS RI (1965) The provocative skin food test. *Laryngoscope* **75**:1428–1437.

WILLIAMS RI (1971) Skin titration: testing and treatment. *Otolaryngol Clin N Am* **4**:507–521.

WILLOUGHBY JW (1965) Provocative food test technique. *Ann Allergy* **23**:543–554.

WILLOUGHBY JW (1974) Serial dilution titration skin tests in inhalant allergy. A clinical quantitative assessment of biologic skin reactivity to allergenic extracts. *Otolaryngol Clin N Am* **7**:579–615.

WILSON CWM (1983) Allergic factors affecting the family. *Nutr Health* **1**:195–207.

Index